# Praise for *The U.S. Healthcare Ecosystem*

## From the Professional Associations

The term "ecosystem" captures the decentralized, multi-component nature of the U.S. healthcare system. By providing clear overviews of each component, Robert Burns informs us as to why this ecosystem often "works" inefficiently. *The U.S. Healthcare Ecosystem* will orient students to the "anatomy and physiology" of U.S. healthcare.

James L. Madara, M.D.
CEO, American Medical Association
Former Dean and CEO, University of Chicago Medical Center
Adjunct Professor, Feinberg School of Medicine, Northwestern University

For decades, Robert Burns has been an exceptional observer and reporter on the complex U.S. healthcare system. As a teacher and mentor of Wharton healthcare students, his expert and wide-ranging understanding of healthcare is now available to all of us. Written with his in-depth mastery of the subject, this textbook covers multiple sectors of the healthcare economy and is a basic primer on the state of the system. It provides a comprehensive overview of the entire healthcare ecosystem, and advances our ability to make informed changes through a more complete understanding of the system's complexity. I recommend it to professionals in the healthcare sector, as well as to analysts as they consider future policy changes.

Rick Pollack
President and CEO
American Hospital Association

## From the Policy Community

If, like me, you have long wished for a single comprehensive, accessible, and accurate textbook that explains the forms, functions, finance, and performance of the maddeningly complex U.S. healthcare system, your wait is over. Professor Burns knows his subject well, and his book is instantly an essential and peerless guide for students, teachers, and practitioners of health management, medicine, policy, economics, and more, and for the interested general public, as well.

Donald M. Berwick, MD, MPP
President Emeritus and Senior Fellow
Institute for Healthcare Improvement

Over the past 50 years of lecturing about how our healthcare system functions, its many problems and possible policy solutions, I could not find in one manuscript the many interrelated issues involved. That is until now. Professor Burns has written the most comprehensive and detailed analysis of what he has labeled the U.S. healthcare "ecosystem." I plan to use it in my courses and public lectures and suggest that many of you that are looking for a useful guide to the U.S. healthcare system do so as well.

Stuart Altman Ph.D.
Chaikin Professor of Health Policy
The Heller School for Social Policy and Management
Brandeis University

In this new text, Professor Burns confronts key topics related to the U.S. healthcare system… The picture that emerges is of a system that is not a coherent system at all, but one in which different components interact in different ways to provide Americans with some of the most advanced care in the world, while at the same time being prohibitively expensive and often out of the reach of many of the people who need it most. Understanding how these components interact is crucial to improving the system's performance and making affordable healthcare more available to everyone who needs it.

Stuart Guterman
Consultant
Former Director of Research, Development, and Information
Centers for Medicare and Medicaid Services (CMS)

Explaining how U.S. healthcare works is a daunting challenge, because it has to explain the often disparate and ever evolving perspectives and interests of the broad range of stakeholders that comprise nearly twenty percent of the country's economy. *The U.S. Healthcare Ecosystem* promises to become the go-to source, not only for students of health administration, business, medicine, and public health, but also for working professionals in the healthcare industry, the media, and policy makers.

Robert Berenson, M.D.
Fellow–The Urban Institute
Former Vice Chairman, Medicare Payment Review Commission

Robert Burns provides a much needed, clear and comprehensive guide to America's seemingly complex, growing and increasingly expensive healthcare system. Based on 40 years of experience teaching healthcare management, he explains in logical and understandable detail how our system operates based on a small number of principles. This book will be an essential guide to the novice entering the field, but should also serve experienced administrators throughout their careers. It's one they should all have on their desk.

Harold M. Koenig, M.D.
Vice Admiral, Medical Corps
United States Navy, Retired
32nd Navy Surgeon General

## From Industry

Driving real impact in healthcare requires having the ecosystem perspective that Robert Burns carefully constructs in his classroom and now in this comprehensive volume. Now more than ever, scientific innovation and care delivery advancement require systemic changes reliant on cross-sector partnership and creativity. *The U.S. Healthcare Ecosystem* provides the deep and integrated perspective into how healthcare works in the U.S.

Maria Whitman, MBA
Managing Principal, ZS Associates
President, Wharton Health Care Management Alumni Association

Robert Burns' textbook is a well-written guide with numerous practical examples and a thoughtfully constructed history of how we have arrived at our current state. More importantly, it provides valuable insight into how to address the problems and challenges of healthcare—including cost, access, and quality—as we move into the future.

I. Steven Udvarhelyi, MD
President and CEO
Blue Cross and Blue Shield of Louisiana

This book will provide a starting point for students learning about this complex industry, but it will also be incredibly valuable to experts working in any one of the many components who wish to understand how the other parts fit in. These other parts can be as different as finance and insurance compared with biochemistry and molecular biology. While experts in these different fields often do not speak the same language, Burns explains in understandable English what these disciplines contribute and how these groups interact to produce important breakthroughs in improved health.

P. Roy Vagelos, MD
Retired Chairman and CEO, Merck & Co., Inc.
Chairman of the Board, Regeneron Pharmaceuticals, Inc.

Robert Burns has been a master analyst of the U.S. healthcare system for decades. For those, who said that "nobody knew that health care could be so complicated," Burns' comprehensive guide provides a detailed map of this complex sector, from hospitals and doctors, to insurance companies and pharma, that helps policy advocates see what they are facing. This book, written to educate college and professional school students, should be "must reading" in the policy community as well.

Ralph W. Muller
CEO, University of Pennsylvania Health System, 2003–19

I had the good fortune of being one of Rob Burns' first Wharton MBA students. I would credit his inspiring, truthful, and real-world overview of the healthcare industry as the primary driver of my decision to spend a career dedicated to transforming U.S. healthcare. As Rob comprehensively and insightfully details in this text, reinvention of healthcare is only possible if we see our industry as an ecosystem, and if we work to align and reform the way that payers, providers, suppliers, and consumers interrelate.

Craig E. Samitt, MD, MBA
President & Chief Executive Officer
BlueCross BlueShield Minnesota

At nearly $4 trillion dollars in 2020, the U.S. healthcare system is of the scale and complexity of a large industrial nation. Hospitals, the largest single institutional component of the health system, represent only a third of health spending; the remaining two thirds are lodged in hundreds of thousands of smaller economic units, which depend on one another for patient flow and revenues. The largest payer in the system, the federal Medicare program, is less than a quarter of total spending. To understand this vast and dynamic sector requires a managerial understanding of the interdependency between financing, technology, and care organization which Burns' volume provides.

Jeff Goldsmith, Ph.D.
President, Health Futures Inc.

For students and others seeking to fix healthcare, Burns' book goes beyond the "anatomy" (structure) of the U.S. delivery system, and brings the "physiology" (processes) to life. His grasp of the players and how they interact allows readers to approach challenges that otherwise might seem overwhelming in their complexity. There are no single, simple solutions for these challenges, but Burns' descriptions of the dynamics that shape the healthcare ecosystem can help define the multi-pronged approaches needed to provide high value healthcare to all.

Thomas Lee, MD, MSc
Chief Medical Officer, Press Ganey
Professor, Harvard Medical School

We do not have a healthcare "system." America has a disassociated clutter of well-meaning health providers whose interactions more closely display chaos theory than systemic order. Professor Burns' book is desperately needed as a presentation and instruction to future healthcare leaders, of today's disorder contrasted with tomorrow's potentially coordinated and powerful diagnostic and therapeutic care. His insightful mind and deep experience create a unique opportunity to learn, and then critique, the least functional but most important area of our economy…

Bryan C. Cressey, JD, MBA
Founder of Four Prominent Healthcare Venture Capital and PE Firms
Pioneer of Healthcare Investment and Growth Strategies
Recipient of Healthcare Lifetime Achievement Award

Robert Burns covers a remarkable range of topics and brings to print what he has uniquely done for so many years in his highly popular introduction to healthcare course. As a physician executive, I would call this a physiological approach rather than the less interesting anatomy and structure of healthcare. I highly recommend this book for students, healthcare executives, physicians, and non-physicians.

Allen L. Smith, MD, MS
Former President, Brigham and Women's Physicians Organization
Former Asst. Vice President for Strategy and Business Planning, Tufts Health Plan

This book is a "must read" for anyone seeking to understand healthcare's value chain, and why the process holds much more importance than its overall structure in its ability to provide high-quality, cost-effective care.

Mark A. Turco, M.D.
Cardiologist and Medical Device Executive
Former Vice-President and Chief Medical Officer – Medtronic's Aortic/Vascular/EndoVenous Division

*The U.S. Healthcare Ecosystem* offers a comprehensive, up to date, and distinctively holistic view of healthcare. Robert Burns draws from the real-world experiences of those in the field to provide an exceedingly practical guide to how healthcare products are created, services are provided, and bills are paid. The text distills complex subject material, such as the emergence and evolution of the biotechnology industry, down to a few key concepts that matter.

Eric Schmidt, Ph.D.
Chief Financial Officer
Allogene Therapeutics

Finally, the definitive book on the U.S. healthcare industry that academics and professionals alike have been waiting for. Robert Burns, through his detailed research and insightful analysis, illuminates and explains one of the world's most complex and interconnected ecosystems and renders it understandable to the reader. This is an essential text for those looking to profit from or fix healthcare.

David Blumberg
Pharmaceutical Sector Lead Partner at KPMG and Accenture (retired)

Professor Burns has performed a Herculean task, providing a detailed understanding of the inner workings of an ecosystem that represents almost 20% of the GDP of the world's largest economy.

Hal Andrews
President and CEO, Trilliant Health

Burns weaves academic and commercial insights in a well-written, approachable and common-sense way. Having co-taught with Rob on the insurance industry for more than a decade, the book is a "mirror" of how he has taught MBA students – real world learning often through case studies. Well done!

Jonathan Lord, M.D.
Chair, Biolase
Former Chief Innovation Officer and Medical Officer for Humana, Inc
Former Chief Operating Officer, American Hospital Association
Former Chief Operating Officer, University of Miami Healthcare System (UHealth)

Insightfully identifying healthcare in America not as an organized system, but as a more organic and dynamic ecosystem, Robert Burns reveals how the healthcare industry really works, from the inside. By focusing more on processes than on structure, he examines the ways in which a remarkable range of players, from specialty clinicians, public and private payers, contractors and medical technology professionals to pharmacy benefits managers and coding and reimbursement specialists, interact, compete, collaborate and sometimes conflict with one another.

C. Martin Harris, M.D., MBA
Associate Vice President and Chief Business Officer of the Health Enterprise
Professor of Medicine
Dell Medical School
The University of Texas at Austin

Robert Burns is one of the most thoughtful and insightful observers of healthcare. It is demonstrated again in his newest book *The U.S. Healthcare Ecosystem*. The book provides an exceptional analysis of the roles, motives, capabilities, and interactions of payers, providers, and suppliers who collectively make up the "ecosystem" of healthcare.

John Glaser, Ph.D.
Executive in Residence
Harvard Medical School Executive Education
Senior Vice President, Population Health, Cerner Corp
CEO, Siemens Health Services
Chief Information Officer, Partners HealthCare

Professor Burns is one of the most astute observers of the entire healthcare system, as witnessed by the depth and breadth of knowledge detailed in this book. I've been in the industry for nearly 40 years (and have taught MBAs for over 20) and have not found a text that covers all of this in such depth.

Bradley Fluegel
Chief Commercial Officer, Walgreens
Chief Strategy Officer, Walgreens
Chief Strategy and External Affairs Officer, Anthem
Head of National Accounts, Aetna
Head of Enterprise Strategy, Aetna

Healthcare professionals and employers, equally, will find the process-driven discussion invaluable in better understanding how to operate and navigate within the ecosystem. A timely work for a rapidly changing, post-Covid world of healthcare.

Mike Taylor
Principal, MT Healthcare Consulting
Former Senior Vice President, Delivery System Transformation, Aon plc
BSc King's College London, MA SUNY Stony Brook, MS SUNY Stony Brook
Advisory Board Member, Boston University School of Public Health
and King's College London Business School
Expert Panel Member, Leavitt Health Partners

## From the Academic Community

In our attempt to simplify our complicated healthcare system, we have tended to look at its individual components and not at the processes and interactions of the whole. The result is that we have duplicated our efforts, driven up costs, and compromised quality of care. In *The U.S. Healthcare Ecosystem*, Robert Burns looks (for the first time that I can tell) at the function of the system as a whole.

Rulon F. Stacey, Ph.D. FACHE
Malcolm Baldrige National Quality Award Recipient
Director of Graduate Programs in Health Administration
University of Colorado Denver

Rather than do his work from the "ivory tower" of academia, Professor Burns has spent considerable time over his illustrious career interviewing healthcare executives for field research projects and delving into conflicts between healthcare organizations through his work as an expert witness. His understanding of healthcare organizations and how they interact with patients, payers, and each other has prepared him to write a text that students will find to be highly relevant.

Paul B. Ginsburg, Ph.D.
Director, USC-Brookings Schaeffer Initiative for Health Policy
Leonard D. Schaeffer Chair in Health Policy Studies, The Brookings Institution
Professor of Health Policy and Director of Public Policy, Schaeffer Center for
Health Policy and Economics, University of Southern California

There is no shortage of books on the U.S. healthcare "system." While all these books provide value, they often employ a framing that does not lend itself to a more holistic "on the ground" understanding of how the healthcare system works (or doesn't) and the important interrelationships among its various components. In this text, Burns takes advantage of his decades of business school teaching by employing a no-nonsense, business perspective on how the system operates as an ecological system. The need for such a text is great as students of health administration or business management rightfully expect material that equips them to operate in a challenging and changing industry.

Jeffrey Alexander, Ph.D.
Professor of Health Management and Policy, emeritus
School of Public Health
University of Michigan

*The U.S. Healthcare Ecosystem* fills a void in introductory textbooks by providing insightful analysis on how the entire healthcare industry operates. Its unique focus on processes rather than structure is revealing and instructive. The volume is comprehensive in its coverage of the many moving parts that constitute healthcare delivery, including the workforce, which makes the text valuable in courses for nurses, physicians, management, and health policy.

Linda H Aiken, Ph.D., RN, FAAN
The Claire M Fagin Professor of Nursing
Professor of Sociology
Director, Center for Health Outcomes and Policy Research
University of Pennsylvania

This is an outstanding textbook, and one that we have needed for a long time. The book's most distinctive and valuable contribution is the perspective it takes: to improve the U.S. healthcare system, we need to understand how it operates from an ecological perspective that emphasizes how a variety of key actors and systems interact with each other. In short, this book focuses on the physiology of our healthcare system, not simply its anatomy.

Thomas D'Aunno, Ph.D.
Professor of Management
Wagner Graduate School of Public Service
New York University

What sets this text apart from others in the field is its focus on process—how things get done—within the current and emerging structures of the healthcare ecosystem.

Jacqueline Zinn, Ph.D., M.B.A.
Professor Emeritus
Fox School of Business, Temple University

Over the past 20 years, I have taught an introductory course on the U.S. healthcare system at the undergraduate and graduate level in various settings aimed at students interested in business, medicine, nursing, public health, and public policy. This is the first textbook that covers the key actors in the healthcare system with the right balance of breadth and depth.

Daniel Polsky, PhD
Bloomberg Distinguished Professor of Health Policy and Economics
Carey Business School
Department of Health Policy and Management, Bloomberg School of Public Health
Johns Hopkins University

A *la* Clayton Christensen, Burns differentiates the appearance from the reality of innovation. He provides us with a clear, consistent, and comprehensive account of healthcare flows of money, information, products, and influence. This is "must reading" for management and business students and working professionals in all health disciplines and schools.

Anthony R Kovner, Ph.D.
Professor Emeritus of Public and Health Management
Robert F. Wagner Graduate School of Public Service

The *U. S. Healthcare Ecosystem* is a novel text and refreshing departure from other introductory books on our healthcare industry. Students will benefit from the emphasis on the strategic decisions and processes involved as opposed to the traditional emphasis on the structure of the system.

Stephen M. Shortell, PhD, MBA, MPH
Professor of the Graduate School
Blue Cross of California Distinguished Professor of Health Policy and
Management Emeritus
Co-Director, Center for Healthcare Organizational and Innovation Research (CHOIR)
Co-Director, Center for Lean Engagement and Research (CLEAR)
Dean Emeritus, School of Public Health
Professor of Organization Behavior, Emeritus, Haas School of Business
UC-Berkeley

In a field that is changing at a breathtaking pace with no signs of letting up, how much more productive it is to help students understand the actions and interactions of healthcare players than having them focus on statistics and descriptions of them that are destined to be out of date before the end of the term. Another advantage of the text is the inclusion of many areas that are not covered by other texts, since a segment of the delivery system that seems insignificant today may be driving important changes tomorrow. This was a book worth waiting for.

Cindy (Carolyn) A. Watts, Ph.D.
Professor
Department of Health Administration
College of Health Professions
Virginia Commonwealth University

I fully expect this text to become the standard in U. S. healthcare administration programs, benefiting faculty as well as students. It will be exciting to see its impact in the classroom and beyond.

Jon B. Christianson, PhD
James A. Hamilton Chair in Health Policy and Management
Professor, Division of Policy and Management
School of Public Health, University of Minnesota

This outstanding text describes how the U.S. healthcare industry functions as an ecosystem of complementary organizations, rather than a set of stand-alone actors. This has become all too evident during the COVID pandemic, where lack of coordination between different organizations in local and national ecosystems has damaged our ability to respond. The book describes the elements of the healthcare ecosystem, identifies the points of contact among actors, and highlights areas where we need drastic improvement.

Will Mitchell, Ph.D.
Anthony S. Fell Chair in New Technologies and Commercialization
Academic Co-director Global Executive MBA in Healthcare and Life Sciences
Rotman School of Management, University of Toronto

Professor Burns, a seasoned observer of the U.S. healthcare industry, has written a volume of unusual breadth and depth. He includes topics that are rarely covered well in introductory courses – for example health information technology, biotechnology, and medical technology – and brings a thoughtful, critical eye to controversies of each topic.

Lawrence P. Casalino, M.D., Ph.D.
Livingston Farrand Professor of Public Health
Chief, Division of Health Policy and Economics
Department of Population Health Sciences
Weill Cornell Medical College

Robert Burns, an internationally renowned healthcare expert, has prepared an outstanding text book on the U.S. system. The book is both comprehensive and insightful as a resource for understanding why and how healthcare is currently delivered. Most impressive is the book's elucidation of the organizational, financial, and public policy considerations that shape the way healthcare is delivered at every level of the industry. The book thoroughly covers topics that other textbooks on U.S. healthcare tend to overlook, particularly the sectors responsible for medical technology and drugs. It is really a "must read" for students pursuing careers in healthcare management and for healthcare professionals who seek a deep understanding of the world in which they work.

Gary J. Young, J.D., Ph.D.
Director, Northeastern University Center for Health Policy and Healthcare Research
Professor, D'Amore-McMim School of Business and Bouve College of Health Sciences Northeastern University

As the 45th President learned, "Nobody Knew Health Care Could Be So Complicated!" For anyone interested in a career in healthcare, it's critical to understand all of the pieces and how they fit together—sometimes in competition, sometimes in collaboration, and seemingly always with critical relationships in flux. I know of no other volume that addresses this entire system in such a comprehensive, accessible, and informative manner.

Kevin Schulman, M.D.
Professor of Medicine, Stanford University School of Medicine
Professor of Economics (by courtesy), Stanford Graduate School of Business
President, Business School Alliance for Health Management

Robert Burns applies his formidable repertoire of deep and broad insights to create a highly useful guidebook for readers seeking to better understand and navigate the complexities of the largest and fastest growing industry in the U.S. With his holistic emphasis on the interactions between and among key actors, Prof. Burns provides a welcome cohesion and coherence as he expertly addresses the functioning (as well as the dysfunctioning) of our healthcare ecosystem. Bravo!

Edward J. Zajac
James F. Beré Professor of Management and Organizations
Kellogg School of Management
Northwestern University

Any book that describes U.S. healthcare as a "system" must confront the evidence of variability, fragmentation, and disparities, among other challenges. Robert Burns offers a wholly different approach to understanding healthcare in America – as an ecosystem in which different actors and entities transact, innovate, provide, and produce healthcare services and products. His process analysis of how the business of healthcare actually works (or doesn't) is a welcome addition to understanding the healthcare industry.

Denise Anthony, PhD
Professor, Health Management & Policy
School of Public Health
Professor, Sociology
University of Michigan

Few have immersed themselves in the complex inner workings of the U.S. healthcare system like Rob Burns. This expansive yet in-depth survey of the healthcare landscape offers insights not found in typical texts. Recognizing that the U.S. system lacks structural design in its origin, Burns focuses on its evolution—how the diversity of actors have adapted under a mix of market and regulatory pressures, and how their interactions determine the care we get. The book at once applies scholarly rigor to an industry rife with slogans and grounds academic instincts in the reality of how the business works. The result is a must read for thinkers and doers alike.

J. Michael McWilliams M.D., Ph.D.
Warren Alpert Foundation Professor of Health Care Policy
Professor of Medicine
Dept. of Health Care Policy
Harvard Medical School

## ABOUT THE AUTHOR

Lawton Robert Burns, PhD, MBA, is the James Joo-Jin Kim Professor, Professor of Healthcare Management, and Professor of Management at the Wharton School, University of Pennsylvania. He is also Co-Director of the Roy and Diana Vagelos Program in Life Sciences and Management. He received his doctorate in sociology and his MBA in health administration from the University of Chicago. Dr. Burns taught previously in the Graduate School of Business at the University of Chicago and the College of Business Administration at the University of Arizona. Dr. Burns teaches courses on healthcare strategy, strategic change, strategic implementation, organization and management, managed care, and integrated delivery networks. He has analyzed many different sectors of the healthcare industry. He completed a book on supply chain management in the healthcare industry, *The Health Care Value Chain* (Jossey-Bass, 2002), and is also the lead editor of the major texts *Healthcare Management: Organization Design and Behavior* (Delmar, 2019) *and The Business of Healthcare Innovation* (Cambridge University Press, 2020). He has written two books on the healthcare systems in other countries: *India's Healthcare Industry* (Cambridge University Press, 2014) and *China's Healthcare System and Reform* (Cambridge University Press, 2017). More recently, along with two colleagues, he published *Managing Discovery: Harnessing Creativity to Drive Biomedical Innovation* (Cambridge University Press, 2018). He has two new books forthcoming in early 2021: *Big Med: Megaproviders and the High Cost of Health Care in America* (University of Chicago Press) and *The U.S. Healthcare Ecosystem* (McGraw Hill).

# The U.S. Healthcare Ecosystem

*Payers, Providers, Producers*

## Notice

Medicine is an ever-changing science. As new research and clinical experience broaden our knowledge, changes in treatment and drug therapy are required. The author and the publisher of this work have checked with sources believed to be reliable in their efforts to provide information that is complete and generally in accord with the standards accepted at the time of publication. However, in view of the possibility of human error or changes in medical sciences, neither the author nor the publisher nor any other party who has been involved in the preparation or publication of this work warrants that the information contained herein is in every respect accurate or complete, and they disclaim all responsibility for any errors or omissions or for the results obtained from use of the information contained in this work. Readers are encouraged to confirm the information contained herein with other sources. For example and in particular, readers are advised to check the product information sheet included in the package of each drug they plan to administer to be certain that the information contained in this work is accurate and that changes have not been made in the recommended dose or in the contraindications for administration. This recommendation is of particular importance in connection with new or infrequently used drugs.

# The U.S. Healthcare Ecosystem

## Payers, Providers, Producers

**Lawton Robert Burns, PhD, MBA**
The James Joo-Jin Kim Professor
The Wharton School
University of Pennsylvania
Philadelphia, Pennsylvania

New York   Chicago   San Francisco   Athens   London   Madrid   Mexico City
Milan   New Delhi   Singapore   Sydney   Toronto

**The U.S. Healthcare Ecosystem**

2 3 4 5 6 7 8 9  LWI   26 25 24 23 22 21

ISBN 978-1-264-26447-6
MHID 1-264-26447-X

This book was set in Minion Pro by KnowledgeWorks Global Ltd.
The editor was Kay Conerly. The production supervisor was Catherine Saggese.
Project management was provided by Revathi Viswanathan, KnowledgeWorks Global Ltd.
The cover designer was W2 Design.
Cover diagram adapted with permission from Zhongyuan (Annie) Yu, PhD, Research Assistant Professor, School of Systems and Enterprises, Stevens Institute of Technology, Hoboken, NJ.

This book is printed on acid-free paper.

**Library of Congress Cataloging-in-Publication Data**
Names: Burns, Lawton R., author.
Title: The U.S. healthcare ecosystem : payers, providers, producers /
    Lawton Robert Burns.
Description: New York : McGraw Hill, [2021] | Includes bibliographical
  references and index. | Summary: "This text is differentiated from the
  many other healthcare delivery texts available in that it gives equal
  attention to the parties that pay for health care, the parties that
  provide healthcare, and the parties that produce the products used in
  healthcare. To this end, the author weaves a common thread throughout
  every chapter in the book that the goals of healthcare relate to the the
  iron triangle(cost, quality, and access) and the triple aim (per capita
  cost, population, health, and patient experience)"—Provided by
  publisher.
Identifiers: LCCN 2021005675 (print) | LCCN 2021005676 (ebook) | ISBN
  9781264264476 (paperback) | ISBN 9781264264483 (ebook)
Subjects: MESH: Health Services Administration | Delivery of Health Care |
  Health Care Sector | Economics, Medical | United States
Classification: LCC RA418.3.U6  (print) | LCC RA418.3.U6  (ebook) | NLM W
  84 AA1  | DDC 362.10973—dc23
LC record available at https://lccn.loc.gov/2021005675
LC ebook record available at https://lccn.loc.gov/2021005676

McGraw Hill books are available at special quantity discounts to use as premiums and sales promotions or for use in corporate training programs. To contact a representative, please visit the Contact Us pages at www.mhprofessional.com.

*To the Coming Kingdom*

# Contents

# Preface

## PURPOSE OF THIS VOLUME

I have taught a course on the US healthcare system for a long time to an MBA audience at 3 different institutions: the Universities of Chicago, Arizona, and Pennsylvania. The MBAs are a demanding set of students—not necessarily interested in academic theory or research, but very much interested in how the system actually works and, more importantly, where the growth and investment opportunities lie. This is not really the academician's strength; we are not trained to focus on these issues in our research. By contrast, the MBA students frequently have industry experience and often know more about certain topics than we professors do. This makes for a very uncomfortable "information asymmetry" in class.

I had a tough choice to make when I started teaching at Chicago: either continue with a strictly academic focus as I taught the introductory course, or learn how the system operates, master it at least as well as my MBA students, and then try to teach it in an entertaining manner. The task was made even more complex by the continual changes in the healthcare industry, which meant you had to continually update your presentation. MBAs frown upon any professor whose slides and statistics are "out of date." This meant continual learning about issues that we academics studying healthcare management often avoid:

- Business models
- Revenue models
- Growth models
- Capital acquisition
- Market shares
- Service line management
- Coding and reimbursement
- Contracts and contracting
- Profit margins and expense management
- Scale and scope economies
- Outsourcing

My perusal of the current introductory texts on the US healthcare system confirms that our field often ignores these topics. That is why I no longer use them. I used to be partial to the volume edited by Stephen Williams and Paul Torrens (an old friend), but it too avoided these topics.

I choose to confront these and other topics here in this book. My research on integrated delivery networks and quality of care has long convinced me that "process" is more important than "structure" and, thus, that an analysis of how the business of healthcare *works* is more important, interesting, and valuable to students than statistics on the number of professionals, organizations, and beneficiaries. To put this into practice, I focus on how the different players in the healthcare industry interact with one another, contract with one another, and collaborate and conflict with one another. That is why the title of this healthcare book contains the term *ecosystem* (ie, the series of interactions among organisms that all inhabit the same community). I have endeavored to apply this process approach elsewhere to the study of how innovation works in the healthcare industry through a comparative analysis of the business and revenue models of pharmaceutical, biotechnology, medical device, and information technology companies.[1] This volume is meant as a compendium to that volume.

---

[1] Lawton Robert Burns. *The Business of Healthcare Innovation*–Third Edition (Cambridge, UK: Cambridge University Press, 2020).

## THE LONG AND WINDING ROAD

How did I arrive at this approach? In 1976, while I was a doctoral student in sociology at the University of Chicago, my father advised me to study healthcare. When I asked him why, he said, "People are not taking good care of themselves." Given the epidemic of chronic illness that we see today (much of it self-inflicted wounds), he was way ahead of his time. Thankfully, I listened to him (at least this once) and applied my interest in sociology and organization theory to healthcare.

Chicago was a great place to study healthcare, given that it hosted the first graduate program in health administration, founded in 1937 in the Graduate School of Business (GSB), as well as a dedicated research center, the Center for Health Administration Studies (CHAS). GSB was also directly linked by a corridor to the Sociology Department in the Social Sciences Building, which made it easy to traverse the 2 departments. I literally followed in the footsteps of many famous scholars coming out of Chicago who likely did the same thing: Richard Scott, Eliot Freidson, Steve Shortell, Duncan Neuhauser, William Richardson, Doug Conrad, Chuck Phelps, Jeff Goldsmith, Charles Bosk, Wolf Heydebrand, Montague Brown, and Andy Abbott. I traversed that corridor many times and enrolled in several MBA healthcare and management classes taught at GSB while I completed my doctoral work. I also took advantage of the close ties between Sociology and the National Opinion Research Center (NORC, also on campus), where I took many courses on survey design and analysis.

I wrote my dissertation on the role of networks in the diffusion of new forms of hospital organization, partly under the mentorship of James Coleman, who had studied the diffusion of tetracycline among physicians in Indianapolis, and Edward Laumann, who studied social networks in healthcare and other sectors. The dissertation marked my first foray into the business of healthcare management. To conduct the research, I obtained the support of the American Hospital Association (conveniently located in downtown Chicago) and received access to their annual survey data going back to 1955. To support the research, I received a doctoral dissertation grant from Joanne Levy at the Wharton School and its Department of Health Care Management, where I now teach. Odin Anderson at CHAS then wrote a cover letter to hospital CEOs around the country asking them to participate in a survey I had developed; because they all knew and respected Odin, I was able to get a 90% response rate. This was "beginners' luck"; I have come close to this response rate only one time since in 35+ years of survey research.

After completion of my dissertation, Ron Andersen at CHAS helped me to obtain a postdoctoral fellowship at GSB and CHAS. I now was situated full time in a business school. During that year, I worked with Odin Anderson, Ron Andersen, and LuAnn Aday on (1) a study of the comparative development of health maintenance organizations (HMOs) in Minneapolis and Chicago, and (2) the advent of hospital-sponsored primary care physician groups—again, a topic way ahead of its time. That year, Ron also suggested I develop a new course on the organization and management of the healthcare sector, focusing mainly on the providers, to be taught in the MBA program. I had zero experience teaching, but fortunately was paired with Paul Hirsch (an organizational sociologist at GSB, now at Kellogg) who taught me the ropes as we perfected that course over a 4-year run.

My business school exposure continued after my post-doc for an additional 2 years when Ron Andersen suggested I get an MBA in hospital administration (starting in the nighttime program downtown) to supplement my PhD in sociology. Ron believed (rightly, as it turned out) that one might do better research if one understood how the business worked. It was a great idea in some respects. I learned the business school disciplines of finance, accounting, operations research, and marketing (my minor), which I endeavored to utilize in my early research and have drawn on ever since in teaching my students. I also completed an internship at Hospital Corporation of America (HCA) in their Dallas-Fort Worth region and then a residency at Jackson Park Hospital on the South Side of Chicago. The 2 hospitals were "day and night"—for-profit versus nonprofit, suburban versus inner-city, etc. Given the debate taking place in the academic community on investor-owned hospitals, these experiences gave me valuable, on-the-ground insight into what was (and wasn't) true. That was Ron's intent.

The MBA program was also a horrible 2 years in some respects. Think of it: My faculty colleagues during the daytime were my MBA course instructors at night, and my MBA students during the daytime were my teammates in courses at night. Nobody was happy, especially my wife, who now saw me go back to school and need someone to support me.

When I finally finished, I tested the waters to see if I was employable in industry. I was offered a position at Evangelical Health Systems on the South Side of Chicago (now part of Advocate Health) but turned it down because the pay was even lower than in academia. Given my recent trajectory, I instead looked for a faculty position at a business school rather than a school of public health. I took my first faculty position in the College of Business and Public Administration (BPA) at the University of Arizona, where I spent 10 years. I was surrounded by colleagues who played a major role in my academic career, including Jon Christianson (who hired me and provided comments on *all* of my early papers), Doug Wholey (with whom I wrote 27 papers over the next 30 years), and Dean Ken Smith, who financially supported my first survey of physicians—a research endeavor I would continue for decades.

I ended up being dually appointed in Management and Policy and BPA's new School of Public Administration and Policy (MAP and SPAP, for short—an endless source of faculty jokes and parallels to "fric and frac"). In MAP, I taught the core MBA and undergrad course on organization design and management. In SPAP, I taught many of the MBA/MPA courses on healthcare, including (1) Introduction to the Healthcare System, (2) Health Policy, and (3) Comparative Healthcare Management. For the third course, I teamed up with Darrell Thorpe, Chief Medical Officer (and later CEO) of Tucson Medical Center, the largest tertiary hospital in town. Darrell helped me to learn how to teach applied topics on managed care, managing physicians, and integrated delivery networks—topics his own hospital was going through in real time. Darrell and I published several papers together, a practice I continued here at Penn with the CEO of the University of Pennsylvania Health System, Ralph Muller.

In 1994, I moved to my current position in the Department of Health Care Management at the Wharton School, with a dual appointment in the Department of Management. As in Arizona, I taught the core MBA course on organization design for the Management Department (with some top-notch colleagues like Jitendra Singh, Marshall Meyer, Hans Pennings, and Mike Useem), as well as an elective on Strategic Implementation. For the Health Care Management Department, I taught a seminar on Integrated Delivery Networks and then the core, required MBA course on Introduction to the Healthcare System. I have taught that introductory course now at Wharton for over 2 decades in both the daytime program and the weekend MBA executive program.

This volume is intended to capture the insights and lessons from teaching the introductory course on the US healthcare industry. Hopefully, after teaching it for so long, I have been faithful to reproduce it for the reader in its complexity but also in an entertaining and comprehensible way.

Lawton Robert Burns, PhD, MBA
Email: hcecosystem@wharton.upenn.edu

# Acknowledgments

Like everyone else, I stand on the shoulders of giants in my field who have gone before me (and some who have gone with me). I always like to acknowledge them for their assistance and friendship over the years. It is important to be thankful; it is also humbling to work with a lot of people smarter than myself. Some of them are already mentioned in the Preface. They include (in historical order):

- James Coleman, Ed Laumann, Charles Bidwell, Odin Anderson, and Ron Andersen at the University of Chicago
- Steve Shortell, who mentored me for years and agreed to work with me and Ron Andersen on some of my early publications on physician-hospital relationships
- Helen Ingram at the University of Arizona, who awarded me a full-year grant to study the Arizona Health Care Cost Containment System (AHCCCS)—Arizona's Medicaid program—making me 1 of 4 professors who constituted the initial class of "Udall Fellows"
- Howard Zuckerman at Arizona State University (and later the University of Washington), who, along with Ron Andersen, invited me to join their research team studying the early integrated delivery networks (IDNs) that were members of the Center for Health Management Research (CHMR)
- Jeff Alexander and Mike Morrisey, who invited me to join their research team studying IDNs with the Prospective Payment Assessment Commission (ProPAC)
- Gloria Bazzoli at the Hospital Research and Educational Trust (HRET), who asked me to join her in studying IDNs using data from the American Hospital Association

- My Wharton colleague Mark Pauly, who agreed to work with me every few years studying IDNs, price transparency, accountable care organizations (ACOs), and (most recently) B.S. in healthcare
- Other healthcare economists, such as David Dranove, Frank Sloan, Jamie Robinson, Marty Gaynor, Roger Feldman, Bob Town, Lorens Helmchen, and Guy David, who (for some unknown reason) like to work with a sociologist like me
- My Wharton colleagues Harbir Singh, Anjani Jain, Jagmohan Raju, and Ziv Katalan, who facilitated my global immersion and study of the healthcare systems in India and China
- Industry executives and consultants, such as Ralph Muller, Jack Lord, Jeff Goldsmith, Adam Fein, and Brad Fluegel, who have taught me a lot about hospital systems, integrated healthcare, managed care, and the pharmaceutical supply chain

I also owe a great deal of thanks to (1) Joanne Levy, at the Leonard Davis Institute (LDI) at Penn; (2) Richard Bogue at HRET, who awarded me a full-year fellowship to study IDNs; (3) Tom D'Aunno and Jon Chilingerian, who entered the field of healthcare management at the same time I did, joined me in the junior faculty consortium at the Academy of Management (where we all met), and have worked with me occasionally; (4) Tim Hoff, who nominated me to receive the Keith Provan Distinguished Research Award from the Academy of Management; and (5) a host of Wharton doctoral students (Larry van Horn, Steve Walston, Bob DeGraaff, Gilbert Gimm, Andrew Lee, Mike Housman, Adam Powell, Aditi Sen, Ambar

LaForgia, and Steve Schwab) who ably served as my research and teaching assistants and have since gone into academia.

I need to acknowledge the incredible help and support from Kay Conerly, Senior Editor - Medical at McGraw-Hill. Kay was an enthusiastic backer of this book from the beginning, and offered so many good ideas on how to improve it. I have thoroughly enjoyed my collaboration with her in getting this volume to press. I also need to acknowledge the great assistance provided by her colleagues, Revathi Viswanathan, Client Services Manager, and Karunakaran Gunasekaran, Senior Permissions Manager—both at KnowledgeWorks Global Ltd.—who helped with the copy-editing, galley proofs, and the copyright permissions. I also thank Annie Yu for allowing me to use her original artwork as the cover image of this book, as well as Jennifer Pryll who helped to get this image formatted.

I also want to thank several industry executives and colleagues who took the time to read various chapters in this book and offer some judicious edits. These include: Mike Taylor (Chapter 15); Steve Wood and Kirk Twiss at Clear View Solutions, attorney Mark Joffe, and Professor Mark Pauly (Chapter 19); David Blumberg (Chapter 21); and Eric Schmidt (Chapter 22). I have learned a lot from these gentlemen over time; apparently, I am not yet done learning. Any remaining errors in these chapters are mine, not theirs.

I owe special thanks to Tina Horowitz, my administrative assistant, who is a marvel and a professor's dream. An attorney by training, she has carefully edited several of my prior books, dug up the obscure studies I needed to reference, created many of my PowerPoint slides, kept me organized for class, and proofread this entire textbook. Don't even think of hiring her away.

Finally, my family has played a huge role in the foregoing. My wife Alexandra has patiently put up with me over 40 years of marriage and been a constant source of love, support, and encouragement. She also taught me by example what it means to be Christian. At the same time, she and her family (all from Greece) comprise my "big fat Greek in-laws," a continual source of culture clash with my Canadian and Scottish roots. I have just completed 4 decades of postmerger integration with her. I also want to give a "shout out" to my son Brendan, who (like my wife) is a lot smarter than me. He will be the first to tell you. He was the one who encouraged me to write this book. Like my dad, I am glad I listened to him.

# SECTION I

## Foundations of the Ecosystem

# Introduction

## THE INTRO AND THE OUTRO

In 1967, the Bonzo Dog Band from England released their debut album with an opening track (which you have likely never heard but should listen to) called "The Intro and the Outro." The song introduces an endless cast of characters that each play their respective instruments or contribute their voices and whose sounds are layered upon one another in a cyclical, repetitive fashion.[1] Eric Clapton even plays ukulele! The result is entertaining, confusing, and somewhat mind-numbing—and yet, you want to stick around to hear what comes next.

It is an apt metaphor for the US healthcare system. Our system has a seemingly endless cast of characters that have taken the stage over time. We started with some apothecaries, physicians and quasi-physicians (bone setters, herbalists), and quasi-hospitals (almshouses) in the 18th century. In the mid to late 19th century, we added more professionally trained physicians and nurses, hospitals, pharmacies, and pharmaceutical companies. In the 20th century, we then added a succession of other players (in roughly chronological order): private insurers, nursing homes, employers offering health insurance benefits, group purchasing organizations, hospital outpatient departments, public insurers (Medicare and Medicaid), long-term care hospitals, emergency rooms, drug wholesalers, pharmacy benefit managers, hospices, medical device firms, ambulatory surgery centers, biotechnology firms, managed care organizations, home healthcare agencies, information technology firms, and retail clinics.

This proliferation in healthcare occupations and organizations has been going on for over 70 years and perhaps for a century.[2] Decades ago, Milton Roemer documented that the ratio of nonphysician healthcare professionals (eg, nurses, dentists, technologists) to physicians rose from 0.58:1 (in 1900) to 3.35:1 (in 1950) and then to 12:1 (in 1973).[3] More recently, David Lawrence, former chief executive officer of Kaiser Foundation Health Plan and Hospitals, noted that the number of categories of healthcare professionals mushroomed from 10 to 12 in the 1950s to more than 220 by the early 2000s. Similarly, the number of specialties in medicine grew from six to eight following World War II to more than 100.[4] Such proliferation has been interpreted in a variety of ways.[5] First, some view the growing sprawl as evidence of "Taylorism" in healthcare: an increasing specialization and division of labor that leaves professionals in ever narrow, bureaucratically confined roles. Some extrapolate further and suggest that these professionals have been "proletarianized." Second, some view this as a major contributor to the growing "fragmentation" of healthcare, where no one professional or organization takes account of the "whole person" in the delivery of healthcare. Third, some view this as contests among competing professional groups—"turf battles"—for control over healthcare work that used to be dominated by physicians. None of these interpretations sounds good. However, they may all be accurate (see Chapters 9 and 10).

Each year I teach and conduct research, I discover yet another "nook and cranny" in the US healthcare system's "cast of characters" that I had not really embraced, let alone understood. All of these industry characters pile up, one on top of the other, to become an ever-growing jumble. I now teach my students that what we call "the healthcare system" is really a mélange of 20-plus different industries that interact with one another but do not really act together in any systemic way. It is both time-intensive and mind-numbing to keep up with (let alone analyze) all of them. And yet, not that much in healthcare really changes; despite the introduction of new stuff (eg, magnetic resonance imaging [MRI] machines), the old stuff (eg, x-ray machines) keeps on hanging around. I have been at this task now for nearly 4 decades and am *just* beginning to understand it (maybe I'm a slow learner). The lesson is to embrace the complexity, strive to learn as much as you can, and take another bite each day.

Why tell you all this? Because many people mindlessly make the following proclamations:

- "The US healthcare system is broken."
- "We need to fix healthcare."

Such statements presume that our healthcare industry was once whole, unbroken, and functional in the first place. The historical progression described earlier suggests that it never was; it just evolved into a more and more complex *ecosystem* (ie, a community of living organisms that live and interact with each other in a specific environment). These "organisms" include all of the healthcare professions and firms that now occupy the industry. The problems we face today, which lead commentators to claim our healthcare system is broken, are the same problems we faced at least a century ago. Costs of care have been rising since the advent of the modern hospital and new technology (eg, the x-ray machine) in the late 19th and early 20th centuries. The problem of rising costs was evident by the late 1920s, as reported by the Committee on the Costs of Medical Care, which studied the issue from 1927 to 1932.[6]

Fragmentation of care began with the rise of medical and surgical specialties, each with their own professional turf, in the first half of the 20th century. Piecemeal health insurance coverage began with workers' compensation laws in cities between 1910 and 1920, expanded to the early Blue Cross-Blue Shield plans in the 1930s, to the commercial insurance companies in the 1940s, and then to public insurers in the 1960s. We have never covered the entire population for a comprehensive set of services, and even among the highest-income population, insufficient care was the rule.

Not only are some healthcare issues at least a century old, but also some industry trends seem to repeat developments I noticed earlier in my career. This suggests a cyclical pattern may underlie at least part of the unplanned evolution of our healthcare system. For example, when I was a doctoral student just getting into the healthcare field, the second book I read was Edward Lehman's *Coordinating Health Care*, published in 1975.[7] This topic consumes much of our attention today—some of it embodied in research on accountable care organizations—but is clearly not new. This observation raises 2 uncomfortable questions: Just what have we learned? And how much progress are we really making?

This is not meant to be cynical or pessimistic. Indeed, as you will read later in this chapter, you could not have picked a better topic to study—for both mental and career development. My intent is to try to (1) depict the seemingly endless cast of characters that have entered the healthcare system stage, (2) describe the mosaic of their roles and interactions, and (3) make sense of it all. In contrast to other introductory texts, my intent is also to frame the business interests, relationships, and exchanges that increasingly underlie this industry.

## HEALTHCARE: NOT YOUR TYPICAL INDUSTRY

Many of my students are surprised to find out that what they learn about business in their nonhealthcare courses does not seem to transfer over to the healthcare industry. There are several reasons why (Figure 1-1).

First, buyer-seller interactions are more mediated than direct. This is due to the presence of "third-party" payers (ie, insurance companies) that separate consumers from providers (the first 2 parties). Only 11% of healthcare spending is made "out of pocket" by the consumer, and only 7% of healthcare is "shoppable."[8] As a result, consumerism—defined recently as "people proactively using trustworthy, relevant information and appropriate technology to make better-informed decisions about their health care options in the broadest sense, both within and outside the clinical setting"—is more an aspiration than a reality in healthcare

- Low degree of consumerism
- Third parties usually separate buyer and seller
- Third parties are often the initial "payer"
- Government regulation
- Power of professionals
- Nonprofits dominate the provider landscape
- Lack of price transparency
- Lack of information technology and data flows
- Asymmetric information
- Local markets: "all healthcare is local"
- Totally different language

**Figure 1-1** • Healthcare Differs from Other Industries in the United States.

(covered more in Chapter 2).[9] It also means that consumers armed with health insurance may be price insensitive.

Second, healthcare is dominated by professionals (eg, physicians, research scientists) who have extensive postgraduate training. This creates an asymmetry of information between (1) doctors and patients and (2) professionals and the managers of the organizations within which they work. It also confers considerable power over decision making to the knowledge workers.

Third, much of the provider sector in healthcare (eg, hospitals, nursing homes) is dominated by nonprofit firms whose goals are not purely market oriented.

Fourth, the goals pursued in healthcare, such as quality and cost, are difficult to measure, not only by consumers but even by the industry. This leads to problems with transparency of results.

Fifth, of the 3 "flows" that characterize most economic sectors—money, products, and information—healthcare is a laggard on the third. Healthcare information is still largely paper based, and even when it is digitized, the data lack interoperability across information systems.

Sixth, healthcare is one of the most regulated industries in the United States, ranking anywhere from first to ninth, depending on the analysis.[10]

Seventh, as covered in the next chapter, healthcare is primarily a locally organized economic activity that differs from one city to the next.

Eighth, and finally, healthcare (like any scientific field) has a lot of jargon that is impenetrable to the lay public. Much of healthcare is encapsulated in a bewildering array of 3-letter acronyms (TLAs) that require a good memory or a handy glossary.

Many of these features create what economists call "market failure." That means there are noncompetitive market conditions in the healthcare system that inhibit the efficient operation of supply and demand. These features include lack of price information and pricing transparency; lack of data on product quality; the resulting inability to assess the comparative value (defined as quality divided by cost) of products and services; asymmetric information between providers and consumers; imperfect agency relationships between physicians and their patients; the heavy role of government as both a buyer and regulator; and "moral hazard" flowing from insurance coverage (ie, the tendency to overuse healthcare when insurance lowers the marginal, or out-of-pocket, cost). Such features lead to distortions in market efficiency. The presence of such market failures suggests that (1) the invisible hand of the market will not always work the way we want it to and (2) there may be a need for the visible hand of government to correct the distortions, including all of the efforts to gather quality measures (covered in Chapters 5 and 7). It also means that (3) competition may not always ensure lower-cost and higher-quality healthcare.

## THERE'S GOOD NEWS AND BAD NEWS

For anyone electing to study the healthcare system and perhaps make it their chosen field of study and/or employment, consider the words Charles Dickens used to open *A Tale of Two Cities*: "It was the best of times. It was the worst of times."

### The Good News

Adopting the lens of a business school professor, which I have been since 1981, it is easy to deliver the good news. Simply stated, healthcare is the number one, global growth industry. There is something in this statement for everyone. First, healthcare is one of the largest sectors of our economy, accounting for roughly 18% to 19% of the US gross domestic product (GDP). That clearly makes it an important topic of inquiry. Second, it is a growth sector, outstripping the rate of overall growth in the economy by 1% to 2% annually for decades. That explains why healthcare accounts for an increasing percentage of our GDP (see Chapter 6). Third, the size and growth of healthcare is not just a US phenomenon but rather a global reality. Other countries are experiencing the same issues as ours, as you will learn later. Fourth, the healthcare systems of the world are more similar than dissimilar, as I have discovered teaching introductory courses (and writing introductory texts) on healthcare in India and China. That suggests that what you learn studying one country's system may be transferable to understanding and working in another's system. You just have to start somewhere. All of this means that your employment prospects are solid, enduring, and global. You have a job for life, perhaps anywhere in the world. In other words, entering the healthcare space is akin to the full employment act.

But wait … there is more! This growth is not only relentless and global, it is also multisectoral. So many areas of healthcare are growing and, increasingly, integrating with other sectors. You have a wide variety of study and employment options to choose from and can shift (somewhat effortlessly) between them. You will never be bored and will always have quite a buffet menu to choose from. If that were not enough, healthcare is a complex system that requires both clinical and business insight—both of which are hard to gather without formal training. This means there are some natural barriers to entry that improve your competitive advantage as you continue your healthcare studies. Healthcare is opaque to just about everyone; comprehension is not widespread. As President Trump famously noted after his election, "Nobody knew healthcare could be so complicated."[11]

## The Bad News

The bad news about healthcare is that its most important problems are seemingly intractable. Consider the fact that we have worried about the rising cost of care for nearly a century with little success in tackling it. Add to this the following tough issues: an aging population, the attendant rise in chronic illness, the recent opioid epidemic, the growing prevalence of obesity and perhaps mental illness in the population, continuing difficulties with measuring and managing quality, and the continued lack of insurance coverage for all people and important conditions (eg, post-acute care).

Like the good news, the bad news spans multiple sectors of healthcare and is growing and global in nature. The United States has lots of company: every country faces nearly the exact same set of problems that we do. The problems are also buried inside a byzantine system that is virtually unknown to the layman, that is often not fully understood by experts inside the system, and that is usually resistant to externally imposed solutions. As President Trump declared in 2017, healthcare is the only thing more difficult than peace in the Middle East.[12]

## SUMMARY

This chapter argues that the healthcare system in the United States is not so much broken as it is unplanned and evolving without any central direction. It has become a sprawl of occupations and organizations that interact and transact with one another. Healthcare does not operate according to the principles observed in other sectors of the economy. Some call this "market failure." You might alternatively argue that healthcare "walks to the beat of a different drum."

Healthcare offers both boundless opportunities and stubborn problems. But it takes a while to get familiar with the system. This brings to mind the entrance of Leonardo DiCaprio, glass of champagne in hand, in the 2013 remake of The Great Gatsby: "Welcome to the party."

## OVERVIEW OF THE VOLUME

### Chapters 2 to 7: Foundations

Chapter 2 provides an initial "big picture" of the healthcare system and lays out some of the principles by which it operates. It serves as a field guide to "things to watch out for." As you read the daily newsfeeds on the healthcare system, it is helpful to be able to sort through everything you are reading and put it in its proper place. It is also helpful to know the underlying dynamics and principles behind all that you read, so that you can get to the essence of the issue. Finally, it is helpful to develop what I have called a "B.S. detector" to recognize when you are reading nonsense. This will save you time (now) and money (later).

Chapter 3 continues the "big picture" presentation by examining the major frameworks used by economists, management researchers, and policymakers to analyze any country's healthcare system. You will quickly see that 2 "dueling triangles"—the iron triangle and the triple aim—constitute the endpoints in these frameworks. The endpoints are the "dependent variables" of cost, quality, access, and population health. These are the goals we are trying to impact. Everything else in the healthcare system serves as "drivers" or determinants (ie, independent variables) of these endpoints.

Chapter 4 continues the big picture presentation by delving further into a major framework introduced in Chapter 3 that has received increasing attention—population health. Population health considers the societal factors that drive health status, the disease burden in the population, and life expectancy. It also considers the distribution of these health outcomes and why "outcome disparities" occur among population segments.

Chapter 5 introduces the 2 major sets of goals that policymakers and providers seek to achieve. The first is the "iron triangle" of access, quality, and cost; the second is the "triple aim" of care, health, and cost. These 2 sets of goals are not the same but are not necessarily incompatible. You may not be shocked to hear that most people confuse the two and have difficulty in distinguishing them. For many reasons spelled out in the chapter, I feel that you need clarity on both.

Chapter 6 examines the problem of rising healthcare costs. The cost angle is found in both the iron triangle and the triple aim. It is also a major preoccupation for many countries, as they experience rates of increase in healthcare spending that match or exceed the rates in the United States. The chapter reviews the drivers of rising costs in 2 ways: (1) supply and demand drivers and (2) cost and volume drivers. You will see that the problem of rising healthcare costs is often considered "the 800-pound gorilla."

Chapter 7 examines the issue of managing quality of care. This problem is no less thorny than managing cost. Part of the problem is that we don't really know what quality is and, thus, how to measure it. Another problem is that nearly all of the effort we have directed at improving quality (whatever it is) does not seem to have worked that well.

## Chapters 8 to 14: Provider Sectors

Chapters 8 to 14 cover the provider sectors of healthcare. This is where most of the people in the healthcare system work and where most of the money in the healthcare system is spent. In other words, these sectors are important. Chapter 8 provides an introductory view of the number and diversity of providers—the "proliferation" discussed earlier in this chapter. It also provides a glimpse into how they are each paid, suggesting at least one reason why it is hard to align their financial incentives and get them to all work together.

Chapter 9 covers the medical profession. You will see that physicians occupy a unique space in the healthcare system by virtue of their near-monopoly over most of the major decisions (eg, hospital admission, diagnostic test, drug prescription). Physicians account for the second largest destination of healthcare spending, about 20%. And yet, physicians increasingly feel powerless and burned out—much like the "proletarianization" argument raised earlier in this chapter. Chapter 9 unpacks this conundrum.

Chapter 10 analyzes 2 other professional occupations—nurses and pharmacists—and their roles in the delivery of care. The chapter identifies many of the same tensions in these occupations as are found among physicians. This does not bode well for healthcare. It also examines the case for primary care as a way out of the wilderness to reduce cost and improve quality.

Chapter 11 analyzes the hospital sector. This sector is important for so many reasons. It is the single most expensive destination of healthcare spending, composing about 33% of national healthcare expenditures. It is also the site in which many doctors deliver care, with lots of different arrangements between them. This makes the interaction of hospitals with doctors of great strategic importance because they collectively account for over half (53%) of every dollar spent on healthcare.

Chapter 12 analyzes some of the organizational changes pursued by hospitals over the past several decades to respond to the rise of private insurance, public insurance, and government regulation. These changes include outpatient departments, emergency departments, ambulatory care divisions, post-acute care operations, the formation of hospital chains, the formation of vertically integrated delivery networks (IDNs) that encompass physicians, the formation of accountable care organizations (ACOs), and the diversification of hospitals into health insurance. Managing all of this has become a major challenge for hospital executives.

Chapter 13 dives further into "organized" ambulatory care (ie, primary care that is delivered by organizations rather than by physicians or nurses). A host of organizational vehicles to deliver primary care has evolved over time. They include community health centers (CHCs) and federally qualified health centers (FQHCs), rural health clinics (RHCs), community mental health centers (CMHCs), urgent care centers (UCCs), ambulatory surgery centers (ASCs), retail clinics (RCs), and retail pharmacies. You can see the acronyms are multiplying.

Chapter 14 concludes the provider section of the book by examining an increasingly important sector—post-acute care (PAC). PAC providers come in many shapes and sizes, including skilled nursing facilities (SNFs), home healthcare agencies (HHAs), intermediate rehabilitation facilities (IRFs), long-term care hospitals (LTCHs), and hospices. Like ambulatory care, the PAC sector offers the promise of stemming high hospital costs by treating patients in noninstitutional and lower-cost sites of care.

## Chapters 15 to 19: Payer Sectors

Chapters 15 through 19 shift from the provider sectors to the payer sectors. The "payers" are the entities that pay for and/or finance the delivery of healthcare by the providers. Chapter 15 begins with private employers and employer-based health insurance (EBHI). This is the major source of private insurance in the United States, and one that sets the United States apart from most other countries (where the government pays for insurance). The chapter outlines how employers approach the provision of health insurance, how they design the benefits offered to employees, the variation in the plans offered, and the trade-offs they make between access and cost. It also examines the strategies employers use to control their rising outlays on the insurance benefits offered.

Chapter 16 delves into the management of one particular type of benefit offered to employees—coverage for prescription drugs. This benefit is more recent in origin (1980s and 1990s) compared to hospital and medical coverage (starting in the 1930s and 1940s). It receives separate treatment in this book for 2 reasons. First, rising out-of-pocket costs for prescription drugs have occasioned calls for legislative relief by the federal government. Second, the rising spending on pharmaceuticals that followed from offering a drug benefit occasioned the rise of one of the most controversial players in the US healthcare system— the pharmacy benefit managers (PBMs). This chapter unpacks the PBM's role and the controversy surrounding PBMs.

Chapter 17 provides an introduction to private health insurance. It summarizes the role of insurers in the healthcare system, the shift to "managed care" in the 1980s and 1990s, and the types of managed care plans (eg, health maintenance organization [HMO], preferred provider organization [PPO], point of service [POS], high-deductible health plan [HDHP]). It also analyzes the internal value chain of an insurer, the different lines of business that insurers get into, the business model of an insurer (ie, how they make or lose money), and finally some new horizons in the private insurance market.

Chapter 18 analyzes the first of 2 major public insurance programs: Medicare. Medicare covers the elderly (age ≥65 years) and the disabled in the US population. Medicare is basically our country's version of national health insurance: it is a federal program that covers much of the care required by these 2 population segments. It is a complex program that contains 4 parts (creatively labeled Parts A, B, C, and D) and an optional supplement (to cover what the 4 parts do not). The Medicare program is extremely important to know for (at least) 2 reasons. First, the program often serves as a springboard for innovation in how providers are paid by insurers and how providers are organized to render care. Second, it is a major payer for most providers. As a result, changes in Medicare policy occasion changes in provider reimbursement, cash flow, profitability, and incomes.

Chapter 19 analyzes the second of 2 major public insurance programs: Medicaid. Medicaid has traditionally covered the poor, both young and old. Unlike Medicare, Medicaid is a joint federal-state program in which the federal government picks up 50% to 77% of the tab, leaving the remainder to the states. What this means in practice is that we have 51 different Medicaid programs (Puerto Rico has its own) with lots of variation in how they fund care and what services they offer. In contrast to Medicare, Medicaid has evolved in a series of directions over time to cover more and more of the population. In 2010, the Patient Protection and Affordable Care Act (PPACA, also known as Obamacare) expanded the Medicaid-eligible population considerably. Chapter 19 reviews the performance of PPACA in meeting the goals of the iron triangle and triple aim.

## Chapters 20 to 24: Producer (Technology) Sectors

Chapters 20 through 24 cover the "producer" sectors of the healthcare system. These are the sectors that make the technologies and products that providers rely on to treat their patients. Chapter 20 offers an overview of the technology sectors and explains why coverage of the technology sectors in a text like this is so important for students to learn. These sectors have yielded an impressive armamentarium of new therapies and devices that improve our health status but also come with big price tags. They share many similar features but also differ in important ways (eg, their customers, their margins, product cycles, and industry competitiveness).

Chapter 21 analyzes the pharmaceutical sector, defined here as companies that make small-molecule drugs (ie, pills you can take orally). This sector is "fascinating" in some not-so-desirable ways, such as federal investigations and fines for various practices. It is also important given that retail drugs constitute the third highest destination of spending (11%-12%) in the United States, following hospitals and physicians. For the uninitiated, the chapter provides an overview of the research and development (R&D) process (preclinical development, phases I, II, and III) and the issue of "pipeline productivity"—how many new drugs the pharmaceutical sector manages to produce every year.

Chapter 22 analyzes the biotechnology sector, which includes large-molecule products (biologics) that cannot be taken orally as a pill but usually require an injection. Biotechnology differs in many important ways from

pharmaceuticals in terms of its scientific foundation (biology vs chemistry), historical origin (late 20th century vs 19th century), financing (external vs internal capital), and profitability (low vs high). However, biotechnology has advanced considerably in recent decades to become the "farm system" for pharmaceutical firms by virtue of developing a growing share of the new drugs brought to market, many of which have hefty price tags. Many cities and countries are now seeking to ramp up their biotechnology sectors to boost their economies. Biotechnology also poses some interesting challenges in R&D that rely heavily on innovative management techniques.

Chapter 23 changes focus from the life sciences covered in Chapters 21 and 22 to the medical technology sector. This sector includes lots of diverse segments such as coronary stents, pacemakers, implantable defibrillators, heart valves, hip and knee implants, surgical instruments, imaging equipment, and robotics. It differs considerably from the life sciences in that it focuses on a small number of physician specialties as its customers and serves them with a different value proposition. Chapter 23 illustrates this using one set of products: vascular interventions (including stents).

Chapter 24 concludes this section of the book by analyzing healthcare information technology (HCIT). This sector has been "hot" over time, but for different reasons. In the early part of the new millennium, HCIT was hot due to the development of electronic medical records (EMRs). More recently, it has become hot due to the emergence of new players—"big tech" firms like Amazon and Google—who have entered the healthcare space with various solutions to collecting and analyzing the data that pervade the healthcare system. This includes the development of "analytics," "wearables," "machine learning," and "artificial intelligence." Chapter 24 covers this diverse and expanding landscape, which has attracted a lot of investment from venture capitalists.

## Chapters 25 and 26: The Public Sector

Finally, Chapters 25 and 26 examine the public sector of healthcare. Chapter 25 outlines the structure and function of the US healthcare bureaucracy in Washington, DC. This includes the health agencies in the executive branch, as well as the various committees in the legislative branch (House of Representatives and the Senate) that exercise oversight for different aspects of the healthcare system. It also includes an overview of the regulatory functions of the federal government and some of the major areas of investigation and enforcement over time. Chapter 26 outlines the role of government in the provision of public health. Although there is some limited federal role, public health is primarily a function of state and local government. This chapter outlines the structure and function of public health activities at these latter 2 governmental levels.

---

### QUESTIONS TO PONDER

1. What might be ways to combat the fragmentation in healthcare brought about by the proliferation of healthcare occupations and organizations?
2. This chapter argues that healthcare is unlike other industries in several respects. What are the important commonalities that healthcare shares with other industries that help to understand its behavior?
3. Why is healthcare such a "growth" sector?
4. According to the chapter, the occupations and organizations that populate the US healthcare system made a serial entrance for more than a century, without any formal oversight or coordination. What explains this rather chaotic development?

---

### REFERENCES

1. Song available online at: https://www.youtube.com/watch?v=hcrUuCDFLOQ. Accessed on February 24, 2020.
2. See R.A. Davis. "Fresh Thoughts on a Growing Problem: How We Could Arrest Proliferation of Allied Health Professions," *Can Med Assoc J.* 105 (July 24, 1971): 193-194, 213.
3. Milton Roemer. *Ambulatory Health Services in America* (Rockville, MD: Aspen Systems, 1981).
4. David Lawrence. "Bridging the Quality Chasm," in Proctor P. Reid, W. Dale Compton, Jerome H. Grossman, and Gary Fanjiang (Eds.), *Building a Better Delivery System: A New Engineering/Health Care Partnership* (Washington, DC: National Academies Press, 2005): 99-101.
5. See, for example, Darius Rastegar. "Health Care Becomes an Industry," *Ann Fam Med.* 2(1) (2004): 79-83; and Linda Aiken and Karen Lasater. "Commentary on 'The Changing Medical Division of Labor,'" *J Ambul Care Manage.* 40(3) (2017): 176-178.
6. For a summary, see Joseph S. Ross. "The Committee on the Costs of Medical Care and the History of Health Insurance in the United States," *Einstein Quart J Biol Med.* 19 (2002): 129-134.
7. Edward Lehman. *Coordinating Health Care: Exploration of Interorganizational Relations* (Beverly Hills, CA: Sage Publications, 1975).
8. Mark V. Pauly and Lawton R. Burns. "When Is Medical Care Price Transparency a Good Thing (and When Isn't It)?" in Timothy Huerta (Ed.), *Advances in Health Care Management—Price Transparency: Stakeholder and Policy Perspectives on Health Systems* (Bingley, United Kingdom: Emerald Press, 2020).
9. Kristin Carman, William Lawrence, and Joanna Siegel. "The 'New' Health Care Consumerism," *Health Affairs.* March 5, 2019, 10.1377/HBLOG20190304.69786. Available online: https://www.healthaffairs.org/do/10.1377/hblog20190304.69786/full/. Accessed on August 4, 2020.
10. See, for example, "The McLaughlin-Sherouse List: The 10 Most-Regulated Industries of 2014," https://www.mercatus.org/publications/regulation/mclaughlin-sherouse-list-10-most-regulated-industries-2014. Also see "Regulation Nation: What Industries Are Most Carefully Overseen?" https://blogs.findlaw.com/free_enterprise/2016/02/regulation-nation-what-industries-are-most-carefully-overseen.html. Both accessed on August 4, 2020.
11. Kevin Liptak. "Trump: 'Nobody Knew Health Care Could Be So Complicated,'" *CNN Politics,* February 28, 2017. https://www.cnn.com/2017/02/27/politics/trump-health-care-complicated/index.html. Accessed on October 19, 2020.
12. Jake Lahut. "Trump: Health Care Is 'Only Thing More Difficult' Than Middle East Peace," *Politico,* July 13, 2017. https://www.politico.com/story/2017/07/13/trump-health-care-middle-east-peace-comparison-240521. Accessed on October 19, 2020.

# A Guide Through the Wilderness

## THE NEED FOR A GUIDE

As outlined in Chapter 1, the US healthcare system plays host to a dizzying array of occupations and organizations that have taken the stage over the past century. The result is an unplanned, chaotic hodgepodge of players, aptly portrayed in Figure 2-1. This same view has been voiced by the Centers for Disease Control and Prevention (CDC), which developed a slimmed-down version called "Health Run" that (like its title) is still confusing (Figure 2-2).

Nearly 40 years of teaching this material have made me realize there are some invariant principles that help to dispel the darkness and bring order out of chaos. Such principles also serve as a standard by which to evaluate the likely veracity of some new claim and judge the likely durability of some new trend in the industry. These principles are also portable—you can use them to understand any country's healthcare system.

## THE HEALTHCARE QUADRILEMMA

One principle is the interplay between the goals of access, quality, and cost (covered more fully in Chapter 5). Developed by economist Burton Weisbrod, "the healthcare quadrilemma" model suggests that efforts to address problems in access to healthcare by extending insurance coverage to previously uncovered segments of the population have multiple downstream effects (Figure 2-3).[1] These include financial incentives to manufacturers and producers to invest more

in technological research and development (R&D), since the costs of innovation are more likely to be covered. The resultant innovation, with its potential for higher quality, appeals to both providers and patients and thus leads to widespread adoption. The innovation carries a higher price tag as well, leading to simultaneously higher costs and higher quality. As costs rise and care improves, there is subsequent demand for greater insurance coverage. This cycle offers one plausible explanation for the observed trade-offs among these goals that make it hard to achieve all 3 simultaneously.

There is more to the healthcare quadrilemma. It can be likened to a "flywheel" (ie, a mechanical device that efficiently stores kinetic energy). Consider the description offered by Jim Collins[2]:

Picture a huge, heavy flywheel—a massive metal disk mounted horizontally on an axle, about 30 feet in diameter, 2 feet thick, and weighing about 5,000 pounds. Now imagine that your task is to get the flywheel rotating on the axle as fast and long as possible. Pushing with great effort, you get the flywheel to inch forward, moving almost imperceptibly at first. You keep pushing and, after two or three hours of persistent effort, you get the flywheel to complete one entire turn. You keep pushing, and the flywheel begins to move a bit faster, and with continued great effort, you move it around a second rotation. You keep pushing in a consistent direction. Three turns ... four ... five ... six ... the flywheel builds up speed ...

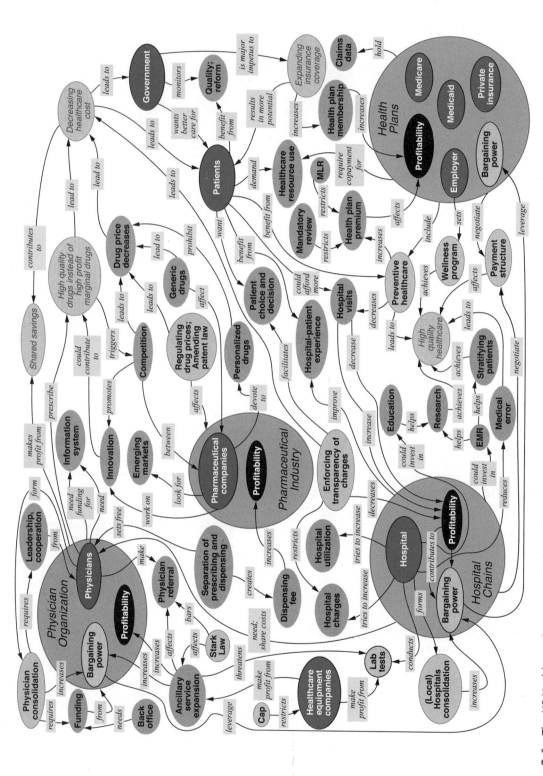

**Figure 2-1 •** The US Healthcare System as a Hodgepodge. EMR, Electronic Medical Record; MLR, Medical Loss Ratio. (Source: Diagram Adapted with Permission from Zhongyuan (Annie) Yu, PhD, Research Assistant Professor, School of Systems and Enterprises, Stevens Institute of Technology, Hoboken, NJ.)

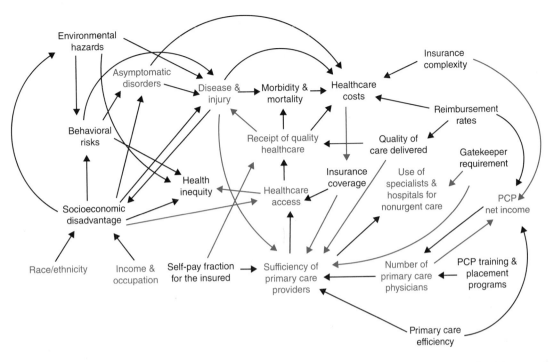

**Figure 2-2** • "Health Run" of the Centers for Disease Control and Prevention. PCP, Primary Care Physician.

seven … eight … you keep pushing … nine … ten … it builds momentum … eleven … twelve … moving faster with each turn … twenty … thirty … fifty … a hundred.

Then, at some point—breakthrough! The momentum of the thing kicks in in your favor, hurling the flywheel forward, turn after turn … whoosh! … its own heavy weight working for you. You're pushing no harder than during the first rotation, but the flywheel goes faster and faster. Each turn of the flywheel builds upon work done earlier, compounding your investment of effort. A thousand times faster, then ten thousand, then a hundred thousand. The huge heavy disk flies forward, with almost unstoppable momentum.

Now suppose someone came along and asked, "What was the one big push that caused this thing to go so fast?" You wouldn't be able to answer; it's just a nonsensical question. Was it the first push? The second? The fifth? The hundredth? No! It was *all* of them added together in an overall accumulation of effort applied in a consistent direction. Some pushes may have been bigger than others, but any single heave—no matter how large—reflects a small fraction of the entire cumulative effect upon the flywheel.

As incremental expansions in insurance coverage accumulate over time, they provide additional momentum to the flywheel, which speeds up and increasingly resists any effort to

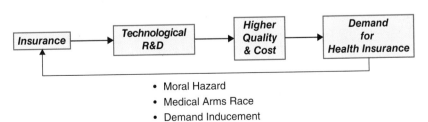

- Moral Hazard
- Medical Arms Race
- Demand Inducement

**Figure 2-3** • The Healthcare Quadrilemma. R&D, Research and Development.

slow it down. This is what is happening in the healthcare quadrilemma: driving greater utilization, higher quality of care, and higher and higher costs. And it is virtually unstoppable!

## MURKY RELATIONSHIPS AMONG GOALS

The world is messy, and simple linear models and/or straightforward relationships are not always observed. Sadly, this is the case with the goals we pursue in healthcare. Take for example the relationship between the quality of care and the cost of care: Is it positive (better healthcare costs less) or negative (better healthcare costs more)? Your gut answer to this question probably says something about your ideology and cherished beliefs. Optimists would say it should be positive, especially if we successfully deal with issues of "waste" and "inefficiency," foster some disruptive innovation that allows cheaper alternatives to enter the market and outcompete more expensive models, and have some wise integrators orchestrating events from above. Pessimists (perhaps realists?) would say the quality-cost relationship is negative due to limited resources, the difficulty in rooting out waste and inefficiency, and necessary trade-offs due to budgetary constraints.

What does the research say?[3] At the population level, there are conflicting findings. Dartmouth Atlas researchers reported a negative quality-cost relationship in the Medicare population; others reported a positive relationship across both Medicare and commercial populations; still others found no relationship. A meta-analysis suggests the overall correlation between quality and cost is nearly zero.

Why might this be the case? One possibility is that the 2 goals are orthogonal. A second possibility is that the data are generated by firms that differ in managerial efficiency so that, although cost and quality trade off in every firm, those firms that choose to produce at high quality are the more efficient, lower-cost firms. A third likely explanation is that cost and quality have a more complex relationship that sums to zero, perhaps as pictured in Figure 2-4. This curve reflects 3 types of "process" measures of quality (see Chapter 5). The upward-sloping part on the left side of the curve suggests that cost and quality are positively correlated for a range of services that are underused. These would include vaccinations, taking prescribed

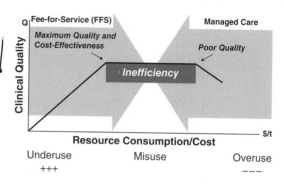

**Figure 2-4** • Quality-Cost Relationship. (Source: Brad Fluegel.)

medications (eg, statins or β-blockers for heart disease), guideline-based care, and both preventive and primary care. The downward-sloping part on the right side of the curve suggests cost and quality are negatively correlated for a different range of services. These include antibiotics for simple infections. Along the flat part of the cost-quality production curve, cost and quality are not related (eg, care involving inappropriate medications for the elderly, prostate-specific antigen testing for colon cancer, imaging for low back pain). This explanation is consistent with that offered by various researchers who suggest that cost and quality can be both positively and negatively correlated.

The lack of a consistent relationship between cost and quality further suggests that their joint pursuit will involve multitasking (and "multiknowledge") by providers to be successful—if someone can discover how to implement such a model and maintain productivity. The efforts and strategies needed to reduce cost may differ from those needed to improve quality and are likely to engender animosity between the quality improvement team and the cost containment team. Providers interested in quality would need to be aware of and reactive to the costs of what they recommend as well as the clinical benefits and how the two compare.

The task may be even more complex than this. As economist Uwe Reinhardt noted, "quality" is a vector of lots of specific quality measures (see Chapter 5)—measures that may not be correlated with one another.[4] Research has discovered that Avedis Donabedian's tripartite quality measures of "structure, process, and outcome" are weakly linked. For example, there is little evidence that nonprofit hospitals (a structural measure) have better patient outcomes than for-profit hospitals and some recent evidence that merging (larger) hospitals have worse outcomes. With regard to the latter finding, research shows that volume in a given procedure may be more important than a hospital's overall volume (size).[5] However, there is evidence that quality is higher in teaching compared to nonteaching hospitals.[6] Similarly, data on pay-for-performance programs show that hospitals that score better on process measures of quality do not achieve sustainably higher levels of outcomes.[7]

This pattern is further illustrated by data released by The Commonwealth Fund on the health system performance of Western countries.[8] They measure performance on 5 dimensions: access, administrative efficiency, care process, equity, and healthcare outcomes. The correlations between these 5 dimensions are depicted in Figure 2-5. The strongest association is between access and equity ($r = 0.74$); most of the associations are modest, ranging from 0.20 to 0.40; one important association (between care process and healthcare outcomes) is negative ($r = -0.37$)!

Thus, efforts to score well on one performance dimension may not work to score well on others. There is now growing recognition of

(1) the "measure mania" on the part of payers who are bombarding providers with too many performance metrics, and thus (2) the need to develop a smaller (but more powerful or more feasible) list that is consistent across multiple payers. But a smaller list of metrics that fails to capture all goals may lead providers to focus on what is measured (eg, surgical outcomes) at the expense of what is not (eg, more equal access to care).

## TRADE-OFFS ARE EVERYWHERE

Another principle is the omnipresence of trade-offs. Trade-offs are a reality in many sectors of healthcare as well as life. When one examines the different health plans that employers offer workers (see Chapters 15 and 17), one finds that those plans that offer a wider choice of provider (more open-network models), such as preferred provider organizations (PPOs), come with higher premiums. That is, PPOs trade off wider access for higher cost. The opposite is the case for

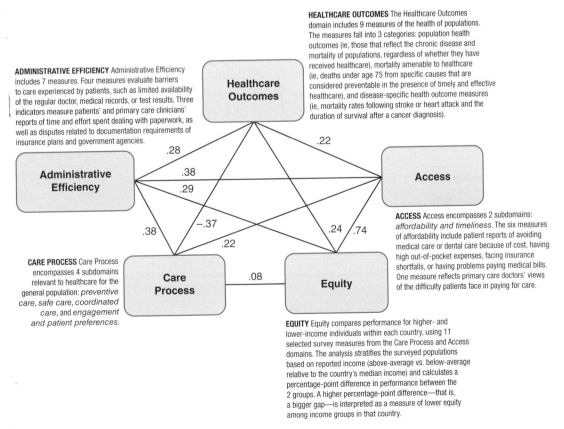

**Figure 2-5** • The Commonwealth Fund Performance Dimensions. (Source: Eric C. Schneider, Dana O. Sarnak, David Squires, et al., Mirror, Mirror 2017. The Common Wealth Fund, 2017. https://interactives.commonwealthfund .org/2017/july/mirror-mirror/#methodology. Reproduced with permission from The Commonwealth Fund.)

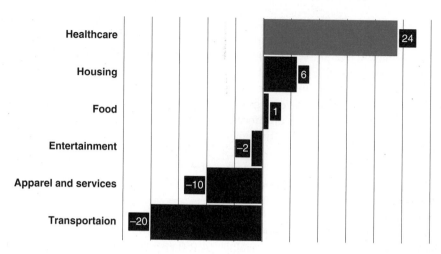

**Figure 2-6** • Percent Change in Middle-Income Basic Household Expenses, 2007-2019. (Source: Statista, US Bureau of Labor Statistics.)

health maintenance organizations (HMOs): You pay a lower premium, but you give up choice of provider in the form of a closed network.

Another illustration of trade-offs can be found in the increasingly popular high-deductible health plans (HDHPs). Roughly one-third of US workers have opted into such health plans. Why? Because they offer coverage at the lowest premium. There is a downside, however: They face high deductibles (up to several thousand dollars) that must be paid out of pocket before their insurance coverage kicks in. So, the trade-off here is lower premium cost for higher out-of-pocket expense. The same trade-off is baked into the "metal plans" on the state insurance exchanges (Obamacare): Bronze and silver plans have lower premiums but more cost sharing compared to the gold and platinum plans.

Another illustration of trade-offs is the focus on healthcare versus other goods and services. At the household level, data suggest that spending on healthcare increased 24% between 2007 and 2019, whereas spending on other basic needs decreased (Figure 2-6). At the state level, increased spending on healthcare between 2001 and 2011 in the Commonwealth of Massachusetts following their healthcare reform crowded out other public spending (Figure 2-7).

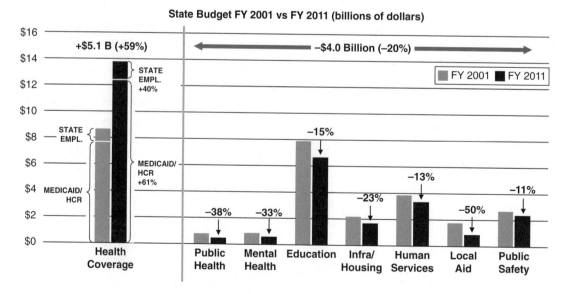

**Figure 2-7** • Massachusetts Health Costs Crowd Out Other State Priorities. FY, Fiscal Year; EMPL., Employee; HCR, Health Care Reform. (Source: Massachusetts Budget and Policy Center, Budget Browser.)

The necessity of making such trade-offs has been exacerbated by the COVID-19 crisis as people have lost their jobs, taken pay cuts, or absorbed family members back into their homes.[9]

A final illustration of trade-offs is found in the choice of practitioners to see. One example is the choice of seeing a generalist physician (eg, family practitioner, general internist) versus a specialist. According to the old adage, the generalist knows less and less about more and more, whereas the specialist knows more and more about less and less. That is, generalists offer more integration and continuity of care, whereas specialists offer more in-depth expertise that comes with a division of labor.[10] Research suggests that specialists provide higher quality of care but at a higher price. Another example is the use of "retail clinics" located in neighborhood pharmacies. The clinics offer very convenient access to primary care, evidenced by ample parking, short walking distances, and little or no waiting to be seen. They are also very inexpensive, with a stipulated low cost per visit. However, the patient sees a nurse practitioner rather than a physician, suggesting a possible trade-off in quality of care (according to the medical profession).

Trade-offs also come in the form of "rationing"—a term that has become politically incorrect in the United States (but not in other countries).[11] Although rationing connotes a central governmental authority allocating care (what the United Kingdom does), it can also occur more informally. The lack of price controls in the United States allows providers and manufacturers to charge what they want, thereby limiting access to those without means. Regardless of the mechanism, rationing is a reality. My former colleague, William Kissick, stated that "No society in the world has ever been—or will ever be—able to afford providing all the health services its population is capable of utilizing."[12] Health economists, such as William Hsiao, make the same observation:

No nation, rich or poor, is able to fund every health service wanted by its population. At the minimum, a portion of health care has to be rationed. Health services can be rationed by price, waiting time, competency of providers, right of patients to choose physicians, availability of complementary goods such as

drugs and surgical supplies, and friendliness of providers. Rationing is primarily accomplished through the financing control knob by deciding what services are funded, and how much to pay.[13]

## HEALTH AND WEALTH

Another principle summarizes the association between wealth (as measured by gross domestic product [GDP] per capita) and health (as measured by life expectancy). This association is depicted in the Millennium Preston curve (Figure 2-8). The logic behind the association depicted in the curve is straightforward. Increased societal wealth can be channeled to greater investments in education, housing, nutrition, and public health, as well as purchases of health insurance and healthcare services that improve health status and longevity. Some summarize this as "health is a luxury good."[14]

The Millennium Preston curve suggests that further improvements in health status (ie, reduced mortality) may be achieved in developing countries by greater societal spending on healthcare as a percentage of GDP. Not all economists agree, however, that the relationship in the curve is causal (ie, that increasing income leads to longer life expectancy).[15] Indeed, improvements in health can come without any increase in societal wealth, and vice versa. In some developing countries like India and China, the dramatic improvements in health occurred prior to periods of great economic growth or during only small intervals of those growth periods. To the degree there is any causality, it may be more that increasing health leads to increased societal wealth. For example, improvements in health status allow investments in education and literacy, which improve productivity, as well as promote a more favorable sociodemographic profile (eg, younger workforce), all of which contribute to economic growth. The mechanisms explaining the mutual causation between wealth and health are depicted in Figure 2-9.

Not all spending is productive toward the end of greater longevity—as suggested by the flattening of the curve in Figure 2-8. Recent research suggests that greater spending on "homerun" technologies and treatments (ie, those that are cost-effective and useful for nearly all patients in the population, such as antibiotics for bacterial infections, aspirin and β-blockers for heart attack

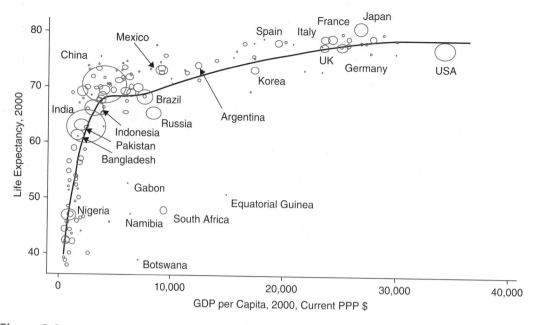

**Figure 2-8 •** The Millennium Preston Curve. GDP, Gross Domestic Product; PPP, Purchasing Power Parity. (Source: Deaton A. Health in an Age of Globalization. Brookings Trade Forum 2004; 2004: 83-130.)

patients, antiretroviral drugs for patients with HIV/AIDS, and improved health behaviors) contributes the most to improved health outcomes and survival. Greater spending on potentially cost-effective technologies with heterogeneous benefits across patients (eg, angioplasties with stents, imaging tests, antidepressants, cesarean sections) can also improve productivity and health but with rapidly diminishing returns as more of the population receives these treatments. Finally, greater spending on technologies with modest or uncertain effectiveness (eg, arthroscopic surgery for knee osteoarthritis, referrals to specialist physicians, vertebroplasty, intensity-modulated radiation therapy for prostate cancer) is likely to result in only marginal health improvements while substantially increasing costs.[16]

A related explanation for the flattening portion of the curve in Figure 2-8 is that much

of the increased spending is devoted to treating the chronically ill population.[17] Such spending does not cure chronic illness but only helps to manage chronic conditions. Research from the United States documents that 46% of the population with one or more chronic conditions account for 84% of all healthcare spending.[18]

A third perspective on the flattening curve is historical. Research suggests that declines in mortality (and thus increases in life expectancy) have traversed 3 phases: improved nutrition and economic growth (mid-1700s to mid-1800s), investments in public health (mid-1800s to early 1900s), and investments in medical interventions such as antibiotics and vaccines and medical technology (1930s to the present).[19] In the poorer countries of the world, recent improvements in life expectancy have occurred as a result of the rapid introduction of public health measures and

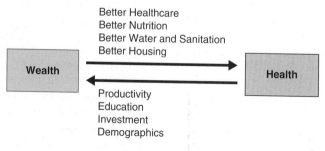

**Figure 2-9 •** Mutual Causation of Wealth and Health.

basic medical interventions, as well as broader social factors such as rising incomes, literacy, and nutrition. Once these rapid gains have been achieved, further progress proves more difficult. A final explanation for the flattening curve is that increased spending on healthcare is not always associated with increased quality or other health outcomes, as noted earlier.

## ALL HEALTHCARE IS LOCAL

The next principle is also a paradox: although all countries face the same healthcare problems, all healthcare is local. This is a paraphrase of US House of Representatives Speaker Tip O'Neill's famous remark that all politics are local. What O'Neill meant is up for some debate. Some say it reflects the politician's needs to understand their local constituents and "bring home the bacon" to their district; others state that politicians need local skills to win the primary election and back-room political skills to keep their legislative seats.

"All healthcare is local" means lots of things too. At the patient level, people's health and healthcare utilization vary by local geography. During the 1970s, economist Victor Fuchs drew an interesting contrast in the health status and healthy (or unhealthy) behaviors between the populations in the contiguous states of Utah and Nevada.[20] At the same time, John Wennberg, MD, began to document the variations across local areas in their utilization of health services. He found that surgical rates for the same condition varied significantly between nearby states (Rhode Island, Maine, and Vermont) and cities (Boston and New Haven), suggesting the imprint of different physician practice styles ("medical signatures") in different markets.[21] These "small-area" variations were later embodied in the statistics compiled in the Dartmouth Atlas.[22]

Over time, we have come to appreciate the importance of locale in healthcare. For example, the recent adage that "geography is destiny" builds upon the work of the Dartmouth Atlas.[23] One's zip code is associated with one's health status, one's sociodemographic status, and other factors that determine one's health, including having health insurance coverage, stress levels, healthcare prices, aggregate healthcare spending, the supply of physicians and hospitals, mortality rates, life expectancy, and the health of the local economy. These variations are now labeled "disparities."

During the 1990s, researchers taught us that the adage "all healthcare is local" also characterized the structure of employers, insurers, and providers in local markets, as well as the balance of power between them. Researchers at the Center for Studying Health System Change explored the dynamics of healthcare in 12 randomly selected local communities from 1995 to 2013, including site visits and interviews, surveys of physicians and consumers, and case studies.[24] They found that the communities varied in the "market concentration" (ie, degree to which a small number of players control a large share of the market) of insurers, hospitals, physicians, and employers—all of which meant that their power structures differed. In some communities, the hospitals were the dominant players; in other communities, the insurers were dominant; employers were seldomly the most powerful player. They likewise found that the bargaining and contracting relationships among these parties varied considerably.

Finally, we need to recognize that much of the action in healthcare is regulated at the state level. This includes (1) licensing of physicians, nurses, hospitals, and other providers; (2) regulation and licensure of health insurers; and (3) management of the Medicaid program. Such state-level regulation limits the ability of medical professionals and insurers to offer their services across state lines.

## *TERROIR*

These small area variations are important for several reasons. First, if you are a product manufacturer (eg, pharmaceutical firm, medical device firm, hospital supply firm), you now have 350+ markets to serve (defined by the Census Bureau as Metropolitan Statistical Areas [MSAs]) that differ in the characteristics of their 2 major customers: patients and providers. Second, if you are an insurer, you have to develop contracts with the providers in your network on an MSA-by-MSA basis; moreover, the rates you will pay these providers will vary depending on each side's bargaining power (which varies by the degree of market concentration). Third, if you are a patient, your insurance coverage and provider network to use are determined locally and may not be transportable to other areas of the country.

Even more important is the notion of *terroir*, which explains why the finest champagne grapes grow only in a small district in northeastern France, characterized by rolling hills and a chalky limestone subsoil that provides a steady level of moisture and imparts a mineral note to the wine's flavor.[25] The concept of *terroir* also applies in healthcare. Health policy advocates have sought for generations to propagate promising forms of healthcare organization across the country, such as the model of Kaiser Permanente. Yet one finds repeatedly that some forms of organization that prosper in one part of the country fail to thrive in others.[26] This means that solutions to healthcare problems may need to be developed and grown locally rather than imported from other cities, states, and countries. There seems to be almost nothing except Medicare that is truly national about our health system. Fort Lauderdale (Florida), Hastings (Nebraska), and Seattle (Washington) are actually in different countries culturally and politically. Those significant cultural and political differences have economic and historical roots and uniquely color the traditions of medical practice and healthcare organization that prevail in those communities.

---

### Critical Thinking Exercise: Case Study

My friend and colleague, Zeke Emanuel, recently published a book on 12 "transformational practices" to make medical provider organizations more effective.[27] Such practices, drawn from 19 organizations he examined, constitute "action items" that providers can and should follow in any market place. These principles include:

- Scheduling
- Performance measurement
- Chronic care coordination
- Site of service
- Registration and rooming
- Standardization of care

- De-institutionalization
- Behavioral health
- Shared decision making
- Palliative care
- Community interventions
- Lifestyle interventions

If the concept of *terroir* is true, then is it possible to document best practices in healthcare that all providers should follow? How would you evaluate the practices Zeke Emanuel has enunciated that you are familiar with? Alternatively, if Zeke is correct, then what does that say about *terroir*?

---

## WATCH OUT FOR THE B.S.

The healthcare industry, like the general business landscape, is full of B.S. (pardon my French). B.S. is found in simplistic claims or principles that usually lack any evidence base but sound pretty cool. They tend to have rapid uptake among providers and consultants and take the form of faddish movements. It took me and my colleague, Mark Pauly, 2 lengthy blogs to lay out 19 different manifestations of B.S. in healthcare.[28]

- Top-down solutions
- One-size-fits-all (off-the-shelf) solutions
- Silver bullet prescriptions
- Follow the guru
- Disruption
- Stage models
- Excel sheet planning
- Bandwagons
- Be like Mike (eg, best practices)

- Buzz/buzzwords (eg, paradigm, ramp up, secret sauce, leapfrog)
- Scale economies
- Roll-ups
- Synergy
- One-stop-shop (cross-selling)
- Physician alignment
- Patient engagement
- Killer app/breakthrough technology
- Platform
- Big data

Little "critical thinking" is applied to these claims and principles. They get repeated mindlessly and so often that everyone believes they are true. Critical thinking, by contrast, involves "reflective skepticism" and requires asking yourself, "Is what I just heard really true?" Unfortunately, these claims and principles tend to yield little success and can be very hazardous to your health and wealth. I examine 3 of these below.

## Scale

As an example, most healthcare mergers and acquisitions (M&As) are touted for (and sold to the public based on) their purported ability to realize economies of scale (ie, bigger is more efficient). There is virtually no evidence for this claim across most sectors of the healthcare ecosystem. Healthcare players mistakenly think that they can "scale themselves" out of their problems. Often, however, larger scale just turns them into more inefficient, bigger bureaucracies that cannot adapt very quickly. They can also require huge outlays of capital and time that divert providers from other, worthwhile endeavors, such as trying to improve quality of care at the patient level. Sometimes M&As and scale strategies are pursued to improve one's market power over other players, thereby diminishing the competitiveness of the healthcare industry.

## Disruption

As another example, many policy analysts express the hope that disruptive innovation will provide an avenue to solve the issue of trade-offs (eg, deliver products and services of higher quality at lower cost). A little critical thinking is required here to evaluate the promise. Let's start at the beginning with Joseph Schumpeter, an Austrian economist who devoted just 6 pages in his 400+ page book, *Capitalism, Socialism, and Democracy*, to the idea of "creative destruction."[29] According to Schumpeter, there is a perennial gale of creative destruction inherent in capitalism that revolutionizes the economic order from within and replaces one industry (eg, horse-drawn carriages) with another (eg, automobiles). In the short term (sometimes forever), jobs are lost, companies are ruined, and industries vanish; in the long term, societies become more productive and wealthier.

Five decades later, Harvard Business School professor Clay Christensen introduced the related idea of "disruptive innovation."[30] Simply stated, Christensen's model suggests that disruptors (new industry entrants) start by making low-quality, low-cost products to address the unmet needs of consumers who are underserved, are not served at all by industry incumbents, or are less demanding. Industry incumbents (market leaders) are not concerned with any competitive threat by the disruptors, since the leaders already offer something better that earns them higher

margins. Over time, the disruptors improve their products' quality and, with the advantages of lower cost and perhaps greater convenience, move upstream to nibble away at the incumbents' customer base. By the time the incumbents recognize what is happening to them, it is too late and the disruptors outcompete them.

Christensen and his colleagues soon applied this model to the healthcare industry over several publications starting in 2000.[31] They cited single-specialty hospitals, ambulatory surgery centers, and retail clinics as illustrations of disruption (the latter 2 are covered in Chapter 13). None of them turned out to be disruptive.[32] The lack of success achieved in applying his theory to healthcare is evident from the title of one of his last reports: "How Disruption Can *Finally* Revolutionize Healthcare" (emphasis added).[33] In this latter work, he cast about for other possible candidates of disruption, hitting upon health coaches, coordinated care teams, community health workers, and Medicare Advantage plans. There is nothing wrong with investing in these efforts, but they are not disruptive according to his own definition. As my colleague Mark Pauly once wrote about the prospects for disruptive innovation in provider and insurer markets, there is no clear sales appeal or value proposition to the idea that "We Aren't Quite as Good, but We Sure Are Cheap."[34]

## Patient Engagement and Consumerism

An increasingly popular vehicle to engage patients are HDHPs. HDHPs entail 3 types of cost sharing to give consumers "skin in the game": the annual deductible to be paid before coverage begins, the percentage of cost sharing (coinsurance) once the insurance coverage kicks in, and the annual out-of-pocket maximum. HDHPs are designed to make the healthcare system more responsive to consumers and make consumers more responsible for the cost of healthcare by exposing them to larger, up-front out-of-pocket expenses.

The evidence on the impact of HDHPs is mixed. There is some evidence that healthcare spending is less for those enrolled in HDHPs and that patients switch to lower-cost providers. The prospect that HDHPs will increase consumerism and engagement, however, has been less rosy. A recent study of consumer behaviors found that most Americans who are enrolled in HDHPs do not use information about price or quality of services, talk to providers about costs, or negotiate prices. When prices are compared or discussions with providers occur, however, it is predominantly for prescription drugs.

More generally, workers may not be fully informed when making their choice among health plans and the types of cost sharing they entail. In one study, when presented with descriptions of possible provider network features, 50% or fewer of consumers could correctly describe HMO and PPO network characteristics.[35] In another study, only 14% of individuals could correctly identify 4 basic components of traditional insurance design: deductible, copay, coinsurance, and out-of-pocket maximum.[36] Employers have voiced similar concerns. In a 2018 survey, employers were asked what they considered the biggest challenges with HDHPs.[37] One-quarter of employers mentioned lack of member understanding of how deductibles work, and nearly one-fifth (19%) mentioned lack of member engagement.

## WHY HEALTHCARE IS SO HARD TO CHANGE

The previous discussion about disruption is sobering and, to some, may be a bitter pill to swallow. It suggests that we may not be able to "disrupt ourselves" out of our problems. We may need to confront the reality that the healthcare system is not only hard to change due to its complexity, but also may actively resist efforts to change it. Economist Henry Aaron said, "The U.S. healthcare system has been designed as if, with enormous intelligence and intent, it was to be as resistant to cost control as possible."[38]

There are many observations to support this contention. First, as noted earlier, the industry is susceptible to (1) bandwagons that do not pan out and (2) B.S. that is untrue—both of which lead to lots of misplaced and wasted efforts. Second, as noted in Chapter 1, the healthcare industry is populated by a horde of stakeholders, each with their own interests and incentives. Any effort to change (let alone reform) the system must contend with many parties likely opposed to what you are trying to alter. Third, these parties are arrayed in a set of nested ecosystems that interpenetrate one another (see

Chapter 3), requiring a multilevel change effort. To paraphrase Dr. Spencer Johnson, this is a lot of "cheese to move."[39] Fourth, the healthcare provider sector is populated with many different professions, each of which has a distinctive knowledge base and each of which believes it should control the content of their work.[40] There is widespread recognition that physicians tend to stick with habits of practice that not only lack an evidence base but may be contradicted by new evidence. Fifth, due to market failure, the healthcare industry is heavily regulated, reducing the effectiveness of market-based-only change efforts. Sixth, the thrust of prior change efforts may have been misdirected by focusing on changing (1) the structure of the system rather than the processes by which it operates and (2) the processes of healthcare delivery rather than the outcomes that patients desire. We have already noted earlier how weakly coupled are structure, process, and outcomes. Seventh, change efforts have been limited by a strong degree of risk aversion, evidenced by an emphasis on slowdowns in new drug approvals by the US Food and Drug Administration, physicians' perceptions of the malpractice environment, and the new focus on patient safety. Eighth, and finally, healthcare providers often play "aggressive defense" to fend off efforts to change them. Hospitals responded to so-called disruptive innovations such as single-specialty hospitals, ambulatory surgery centers, and retail clinics by starting their own competitive versions or partnering with existing ones to blunt the impact of newcomers.[41]

## "SOLUTIONS" THAT ONLY SQUEEZE THE BALLOON

Many of the innovations introduced into healthcare to solve the problem of rising costs have not panned out as well as we had hoped. Diagnosis-related groups (DRGs) became the standard payment methodology used by Medicare to reimburse hospitals in 1983. DRGs were a radical departure from fee-for-service medicine, in that they gave hospitals a lump-sum payment (budget) for each patient they admitted based on the patient's diagnosis. The intent was to give hospitals an incentive to be efficient and provide care at a cost lower than the budgeted amount; any surplus thus earned accrued to the hospital as profit. Another goal of DRGs was to foster greater use of ambulatory care, which was considerably cheaper than inpatient care.

What could possibly go wrong? The DRG-budgeted amount meant that hospitals received less revenue than they had under the prior fee-for-service system (where the more they did and spent, the more they made). Conversely, shifting patients to the less expensive outpatient setting meant lower revenue as well. So, how did hospitals respond? They indeed reduced admissions and lengths of stay to stay within the budget limits set by the DRG, reduced the rate of growth in hospital spending, and shifted patients to outpatient settings.[42] However, hospitals also increased utilization of outpatient care—surgical and other procedures, visits associated with inpatient episodes—to make up for the revenues lost on the inpatient side. Moreover, physician billing under Medicare shifted from inpatient to outpatient care. Thus, the reduced growth in inpatient hospital payments was partially offset by higher growth in outpatient (and other types of) care, with little success in controlling the overall growth of US national health expenditures.[43] Another reason may be that hospitals began to charge higher inpatient rates to commercial insurers to make up for the decreased inpatient payments from Medicare.[44]

The principle here is "squeezing the balloon": When you squeeze on the inpatient side, it enlarges on the outpatient side. The same principle has been observed more recently in hospitals' utilization of post-acute care (PAC) to manage under bundled payments. As noted earlier, PAC includes home healthcare agencies (HHAs), skilled nursing facilities, long-term care hospitals, and inpatient rehabilitation facilities. The latter sites of care are much more expensive than HHAs. Physicians and hospitals participating in bundled payment programs are incentivized to reduce the total cost of care. Several recent studies of these programs illustrate that providers are substituting lower-cost PAC sites like HHAs for higher-cost PAC sites, with sometimes higher utilization. The result is that bundled payment programs have achieved limited savings, partially due to squeezing of the healthcare balloon. To be sure, there is nothing wrong with such substitution to lower-cost sites. But do not expect major payment initiatives like DRGs and bundled payments to exert whopping effects; they can be part of the solution, but they are not the silver bullet.

## IMPORTANCE OF HISTORY AND HISTORY REPEATING

For years, I have been teaching my students about the history of the US healthcare system. In the past, I started with 6 hours of lecture on the history of the hospital sector, the medical profession, and the pharmaceutical sector. Sometimes I included the history of the insurance sector. I no longer need to do this, since one of my colleagues, Robert Field, has recently published a fine volume on the history of all 4 sectors.[45] Instead of lecturing on history, I now assign Field's book as recommended reading. I am not alone in my belief that students of healthcare need to know the history of this system. Two other senior colleagues—Zeke Emanuel and Joel Shalowitz—share the same conviction. Joel incorporated a lot of the historical background into his recent introductory text; I have chosen to "outsource" this material to Robert Field.

Why make students study history? There is a *lot* to be learned from history, considering the repeated lesson handed down to us over time:

| | |
|---|---|
| *There is nothing new under the sun.* | Ecclesiastes 1:9 |
| *What's past is prologue.* | Shakespeare, *The Tempest* |
| *Plus ça change, plus c'est la même chose.* | Jean Baptiste Alphonse Karr |
| *Those who cannot remember the past are condemned to repeat it.* | George Santayana |
| *The only thing new in the world is the history you don't know.* | President Harry Truman |
| *It's déjà vu all over again.* | Yogi Berra |

Starting with history lessons helps to give all students in an introductory course a common foundation and a level playing field. This is important at Wharton, where nearly half of the students are international and many students come into the healthcare program from outside the healthcare industry. History is also important because of what management researchers call "path dependence": Where we are today depends on paths taken in the past. Thus, history helps to explain not only why the US healthcare ecosystem looks the way it does,

| 1990s | 2010s |
|---|---|
| Integrated Delivery Network (IDN) | Accountable Care Organization (ACO) |
| Physician-Hospital Organization (PHO) | Clinically Integrated Network (CIN) |
| Hospital Alliance | Hospital Network |
| Seamless Continuum of Care | Care Continuum |
| Health Maintenance Organization (HMO) | Narrow Network |
| Cost-Effectiveness | Value |
| Control Healthcare Cost Inflation | Bend the Trend |
| Iron Triangle | Triple Aim |
| Health Status of Population | Population Health |

**Figure 2-10** • Just a Little Bit of History Repeating?

but also why the United States may *not* adopt solutions developed in other countries. History also reveals the strong roots for the players in the industry and their interests, stretching back a century or more. This serves to highlight the likely resistance to any proposed changes and reforms.

Finally, the healthcare issues and solutions of today eerily resemble the issues and solutions of yesterday. Consider the fact that many of the payment and organizational changes proposed today to reform the healthcare ecosystem originated in the 1990s (Figure 2-10). During the 1990s, singer Shirley Bassey and the Propellerheads released their hit song, "Just a Little Bit of History Repeating." The words in the song were prophetic.

Past history lessons serve as hypotheses to be tested for current events. These lessons also give you some idea of what you might expect to happen going forward, as well as help to anticipate stakeholders and forces likely to oppose what you are advocating. History can also help you to avoid the same mistakes made in the past. Finally, a knowledge of history can help you to avoid "irrational exuberance" about the latest thing, and thereby avoid the time and money trap of investing in the latest bandwagon movement (ie, the B.S.).

Lastly, according to the University of Chicago (my alma mater), history helps the student to develop the following critical skills: understand complexity, understand change over time and the causal relationship between historical events, ask and answer big questions, balance analysis of finely grained evidence with a deep understanding of narrative, learn a method

of encounter with the world that demands critical inquiry, and "live the life of the mind." Isn't this what higher education should be about?

Given all of this, I would be remiss if I did not include at least a little on the history of the US healthcare system.[46] The US system has undergone several important transformations extending back (at least) to the early 20th century. The most widely read text on healthcare transformation by Paul Starr depicts the rise of physician autonomy in the early 20th century and then its gradual erosion by corporatization in the later 20th century—a transformation lasting 80 to 100 years. Another widely known text by Rosemary Stevens describes the transformation of the American hospital from its initial focus as a community institution focusing on health to a corporation increasingly focused on wealth—another transformation lasting roughly a century.[47] Two other important, gradual transformations lasting nearly 80 and 50 years, respectively, have been the ascendance of third-party payment (over out-of-pocket payment) and the growing share of public payment relative to private payment among third-party payers.

The advent of both public and private insurance ushered in fee-for-service (FFS) payment by third parties—1 of the 2 issues addressed in transformation efforts (along with changing how providers are organized). Moral hazard and escalating healthcare expenditures that followed upon insurance coverage and above-cost FFS payment have bedeviled the industry ever since. The HMO Act of 1973 and the rise of managed care—both designed to address the issue of rising costs—have also exerted lasting influences on the industry, as payers of healthcare have sought to assume greater oversight of the quality rendered by providers. The confluence of their roles as both payers and overseers (of quality and quantity) may have set the stage for discussions of "value" in the 21st century and provided a vehicle for managing it. The 1993 Health Security Act (also known as the Clinton Health Plan), even though it died on arrival in Congress in the spring of 1994, exerted an enormous impact by prompting a wave of horizontal and vertical integration strategies by hospitals in subsequent years in anticipation of the strong managed care that was the core of the plan (covered in Chapter 12).

Beyond these momentous long-term shifts, Figure 2-11 depicts many decade-by-decade transformations. The figure is not meant to be comprehensive but illustrative. In the 20th and 21st centuries, these shifts include (by decade):

1910-1920s: The Flexner reforms in medical education, the closure of many medical schools, and the rise of organized medicine and medical specialties

1930-1940s: The advent of private insurance

1940-1950s: The advent of biomedical innovation and the National Institutes of Health

1960s: The enactment of Medicare and Medicaid

1970s: The various federal and state regulatory efforts to try to contain rising healthcare costs (eg, certificate of need)

1980s: The Prospective Payment System and DRGs, the rise of outpatient care and ambulatory surgery centers, and competitive market solutions to healthcare costs (eg, antitrust enforcement)

1990s: The rise of HMOs, managed care, hospital system formations, and disruptive federal legislation (eg, Health Security Act, Balanced Budget Act)

2000s: Advent of consumerism, HDHPs, Medicare Advantage, and retail clinics

2010s: Big data and analytics and additional federal legislation (eg, the Patient Protection and Affordable Care Act of 2010 and Medicare Access and CHIP Reauthorization Act of 2015)

Most of these shifts were not anticipated or accurately forecast. Moreover, many of the shifts depicted in Figure 2-11 did not positively transform the healthcare industry but rather added to its complexity and fragmentation. For example,

the shift to outpatient care and ambulatory surgery centers did not reduce the rate of increase in healthcare spending or improve quality of care; it represented an effort to squeeze the balloon of inpatient costs, which, by increasing access and convenience, led to an increase in outpatient volume and spending. Similarly, biomedical advances in the 1990s such as blockbuster drugs and less invasive procedures (eg, stents) supplanted surgical procedures and hospitalizations; quality of care may have improved but so did utilization and the costs of care, due to the widespread uptake of these new therapies. In sum, transformation, even with the best of intentions and/or the strongest sales pitch, did not usually result in higher quality at reduced cost. Over much of the past century and through today, healthcare costs have continued to rise at a rate well above GDP growth.

## TWO HISTORICAL LESSONS WORTH REMEMBERING

There have been 2 inexorable trends in the US healthcare ecosystem since the late 19th century that continue to shape the industry's present configuration. The first is technological advance. As the healthcare quadrilemma suggests, new technology is a source of quality enhancements that both patients and physicians desire. You should always be on the lookout for new technology entering the healthcare ecosystem and some of the drivers of this entry. Paradoxically, the 2 world wars of the 20th century served as major spurs to new advances in medical equipment, products, and services to treat the wartime injuries that confronted providers. You should also be cognizant of the consequences of new technology entering the system. As this book argues, new technology exerts an impact on the goals of access, quality, and cost.

But technology has other effects as well that are just as important. That leads us to the second trend: specialization. The history of US healthcare teaches us that new technology fosters increased specialization in the training and the practice of healthcare professionals. For example, new inventions such as the ophthalmoscope (1851) led to the emergence of ophthalmologists, whereas the x-ray machine (1895) led to the emergence of radiologists; more recently, the invention of the implantable pacemaker

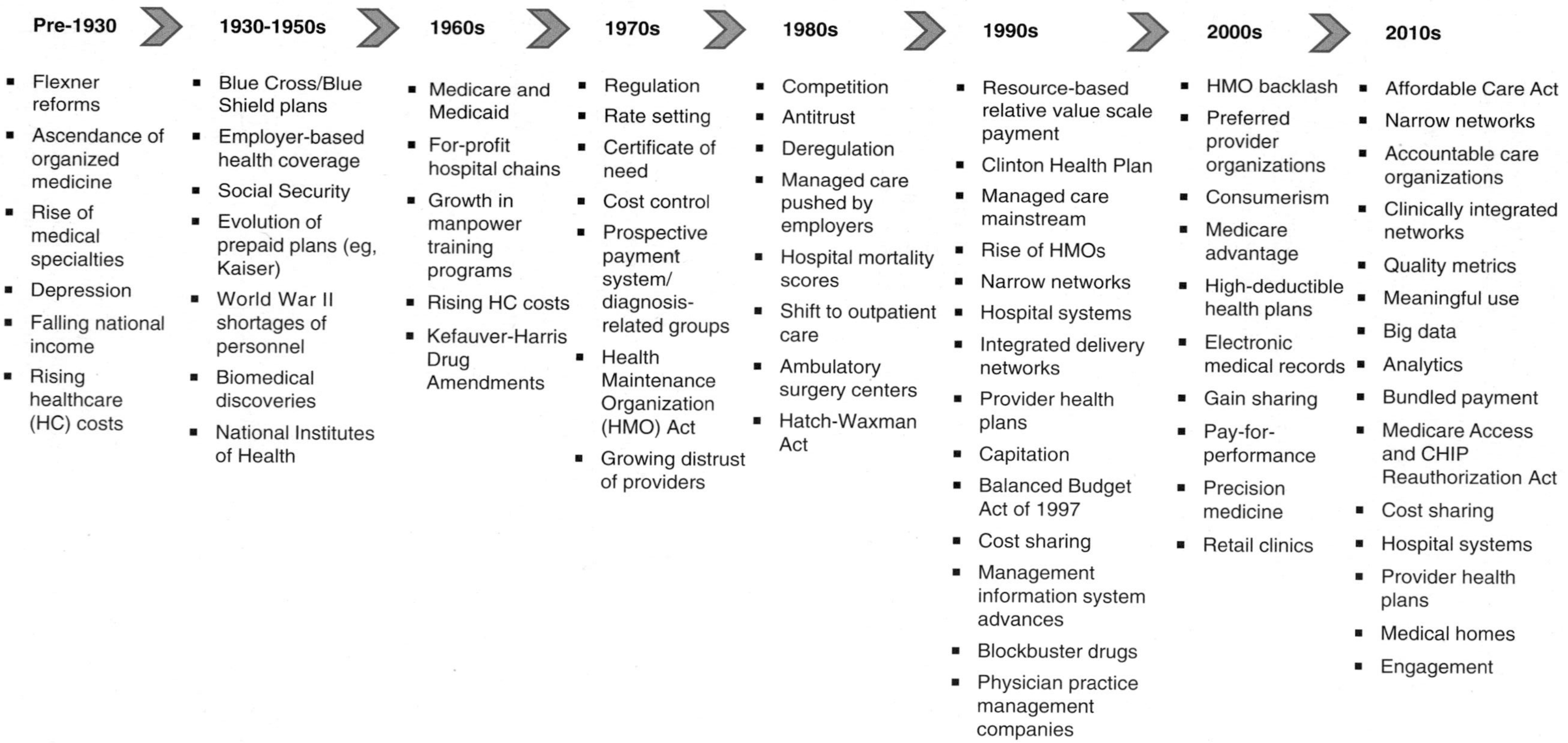

26

| Pre-1930 | 1930-1950s | 1960s | 1970s | 1980s | 1990s | 2000s | 2010s |
|---|---|---|---|---|---|---|---|
| Flexner reforms | Blue Cross/Blue Shield plans | Medicare and Medicaid | Regulation | Competition | Resource-based relative value scale payment | HMO backlash | Affordable Care Act |
| Ascendance of organized medicine | Employer-based health coverage | For-profit hospital chains | Rate setting | Antitrust | Clinton Health Plan | Preferred provider organizations | Narrow networks |
| Rise of medical specialties | Social Security | Growth in manpower training programs | Certificate of need | Deregulation | Managed care mainstream | Consumerism | Accountable care organizations |
| Depression | Evolution of prepaid plans (eg, Kaiser) | Rising HC costs | Cost control | Managed care pushed by employers | Rise of HMOs | Medicare advantage | Clinically integrated networks |
| Falling national income | World War II shortages of personnel | Kefauver-Harris Drug Amendments | Prospective payment system/diagnosis-related groups | Hospital mortality scores | Narrow networks | High-deductible health plans | Quality metrics |
| Rising healthcare (HC) costs | Biomedical discoveries | | Health Maintenance Organization (HMO) Act | Shift to outpatient care | Hospital systems | Electronic medical records | Meaningful use |
| | National Institutes of Health | | Growing distrust of providers | Ambulatory surgery centers | Integrated delivery networks | Gain sharing | Big data |
| | | | | Hatch-Waxman Act | Provider health plans | Pay-for-performance | Analytics |
| | | | | | Capitation | Precision medicine | Bundled payment |
| | | | | | Balanced Budget Act of 1997 | Retail clinics | Medicare Access and CHIP Reauthorization Act |
| | | | | | Cost sharing | | Cost sharing |
| | | | | | Management information system advances | | Hospital systems |
| | | | | | Blockbuster drugs | | Provider health plans |
| | | | | | Physician practice management companies | | Medical homes |
| | | | | | | | Engagement |

**Figure 2-11** • Historical Transformations in US Healthcare. (Adapted from Bradley Fluegel, Presentation to The Wharton School, January, 2017.)

26

(1960) and cardio-defibrillator (1980) occasioned the rise of electrophysiologists. The general principle is that groups of specialized physicians form around new equipment and learn how to harness it. Physician specialization exerts downstream ripple effects on other personnel, leading to specialization among nurses and technicians as well. Why is this important? Because it contributes to the continued entry of new players into the healthcare system discussed at the beginning of Chapter 1 and, thus, the problem of fragmentation.

## SUMMARY

The US healthcare system seems incredibly complex, as depicted in Figures 2-1 and 2-2. Don't let these figures fool you—it really *is* that complex (and more). And yet, the system operates according to a handful of principles that are quite steady and quite sturdy in their explanatory power. They can be usefully employed to illuminate one's path when confronted by a seemingly new development, trend, or potentially disruptive market entrant. Such light often dispels the darkness, the confusion, and the B.S.

---

### QUESTIONS TO PONDER

1. Are the principles enunciated in this chapter unique to the healthcare ecosystem, or do they characterize other US industries as well?
2. Is there any way to stop the "flywheel" of health insurance coverage in the United States?
3. Are trade-offs a fact of life? Are they particularly acute in the US healthcare ecosystem?
4. There is a well-known phrase that "more is better." Is this ever true in healthcare spending?
5. Why is larger scale such a popular strategy in healthcare and corporate America if it doesn't make the company more efficient?
6. What should "engaged patients" look like? How should they behave?
7. If it is true that history repeats itself, why does this happen?

## REFERENCES

1. Burton Weisbrod. "The Healthcare Quadrilemma: An Essay on Technological Change, Insurance, Quality of Care, and Cost Containment," *J Econ Lit.* 29 (2) (1991): 523-552.
2. Jim Collins. *Good to Great* (New York, NY: HarperCollins, 2001).
3. All of the research results cited in these paragraphs are cited in: Lawton R. Burns and Mark V. Pauly. "Transformation of the Health Care Industry: Curb Your Enthusiasm?" *Milbank Quarterly.* 96 (1) (2018): 57-109. Available online: https://onlinelibrary.wiley.com/doi/full/10.1111/1468-0009.12312. Accessed on July 22, 2020.
4. Uwe Reinhardt. "Sense and Nonsense in Defining 'Value' in Health Care," National Institute of Health Care Management. Capitol Hill Briefing on the Future of Health Care in America (October 5, 2016).
5. Frank Sloan, Gabriel Picone, Donald Taylor, et al. "Hospital Ownership and Cost and Quality of Care: Is There a Dime's Worth of Difference?" *J Health Econ.* 20 (1) (2001): 1-21. Nancy Beaulieu, Leemore Dafny, Bruce Landon, et al. "Changes in Hospital Quality After Mergers and Acquisitions," *N Engl J Med.* 382 (1) (2020): 51-59. Anahita Dua, Courtney Furlough, Hunter Ray, et al. "The Effect of Hospital Factors on Mortality Rates After Abdominal Aortic Aneurysm Repair," *Society for Vascular Surgery.* (2014): 1446-1451.
6. Laura Burke, Austin Frakt, Dhruv Kullar, et al. "Association Between Teaching Status and Mortality in US Hospitals," *JAMA.* 317 (20) (2017): 2105-2113.
7. Ashish Jha, Karen Joynt, John Orav, et al. "The Long-Term Effect of Premier Pay for Performance on Patient Outcomes," *N Engl J Med.* 366 (2012): 1606-1615.
8. Eric C. Schneider, Dana O. Sarnak, David Squires, Arnav Shah, and Michelle M. Doty. "Mirror Mirror. 2017: International Comparison Reflects Flaws and Opportunities for Better U.S. Health Care." The Commonwealth Fund. Available online: https://www.commonwealthfund.org/publications/fund-reports/2017/jul/mirror-mirror-2017-international-comparison-reflects-flaws-and. Accessed on July 22, 2020.
9. Tiffany Hsu. "Food, Rent, Health Insurance? Tough Choices in Pandemic Economy," *New York Times* (April 22, 2020).
10. Kenton Johnston and Jason Hockenberry. "Are Two Heads Better Than One or Do Too Many Cooks Spoil the Broth? The Tradeoff Between Physician Division of Labor and Patient Continuity of Care for Older Adults with Complex

Chronic Conditions," *Health Services Res.* 51 (6) (2016): 2176-2205.

11. Ezra Klein. "In the UK's Health System, Rationing Is Not a Dirty Word," *Vox* (January 28, 2020). Available online: https://www.vox.com/2020/1/28/21074386/health-care-rationing-britain-nhs-nice-medicare-for-all. Accessed on July 21, 2020.

12. William Kissick. *Medicine's Dilemmas: Infinite Needs Versus Finite Resources* (New Haven, CT: Yale University Press, 1994).

13. William Hsiao. *What Is a Health System? Why Should We Care?* (August 2003). Available online: https://www.mediastudies.fpzg.hr/_download/repository/Hsiao2003.pdf. Accessed on February 22, 2020.

14. Thomas Getzen. "Health Care Is an Individual Necessity and a National Luxury: Applying Multilevel Decision Models to the Analysis of Health Care Expenditures," *J Health Econ.* 19 (2000): 259-270.

15. David Cutler, Angus Deaton, and Adriana Lleras-Muney. "The Determinants of Mortality," *J Econ Perspect.* 20 (3)(2006): 97-120.

16. Amitabh Chandra and Jonathan Skinner. "Technology Growth and Expenditure Growth in Health Care," *NBER Working Paper 16953* (Cambridge, MA: National Bureau of Economic Research, 2011).

17. Gordon Liu, Yao Yao, Nianyu Du, et al. *Health and Economic Prosperity* (Beijing, China: Peking University National School of Development, 2015).

18. Hamilton Moses, David Matheson, Ray Dorsey, et al. "The Anatomy of Health Care in the United States," *JAMA.* 310 (18) (2013): 1947-1964.

19. David Cutler, Angus Deaton, and Adriana Lleras-Muney. "The Determinants of Mortality," *J Econ Perspect.* 20 (3) (2006): 97-120.

20. Victor R. Fuchs. *Who Shall Live?* (New York, NY: Basic Books, 1974).

21. John Wennberg, Alan Gittelsohn, and Nancy Shapiro. "Health Care Delivery in Maine III: Evaluating the Level of Hospital Performance," *J Maine Med Assoc.* 66 (11) (1975): 298-306. John Wennberg. "Dealing With Medical Practice Variations: A Proposal for Action," *Health Aff.* 3 (2) (Summer 1984).

22. For more information, go to: https://www.dartmouthatlas.org. Accessed on August 4, 2020.

23. Elliott Fisher, David Goodman, and Amitabh Chandra. *Geography Is Destiny: Differences in Health Care Among Medicare Beneficiaries in the United States and California* (Oakland, CA: California Healthcare Foundation, 2008). Available online: https://www.chcf.org/wp-content/uploads/2017/12/PDF-GeographyIsDestiny08.pdf. Accessed on February 11, 2020.

24. Description available online at: Center for Studying Health System Change. http://www.hschange.org/indexb74e.html?file=about. Accessed on February 11, 2020.

25. Jeff Goldsmith and Lawton R. Burns. "Fail to Scale: Why Great Ideas in Health Care Don't Thrive Everywhere," *Health Affairs Blog* (September 29, 2016). Available online at: https://www.healthaffairs.org/do/10.1377/hblog20160929.056856/full/. Accessed on February 11, 2020.

26. Daniel Gitterman, Bryan Weiner, Marisa Domino, et al. "The Rise and Fall of a Kaiser Permanente Expansion Region," *Milbank Memorial Fund Quarterly.* 81 (4) (2003): 567-601.

27. Ezekiel Emanuel. *Prescription for the Future: The Twelve Transformational Practices of Highly Effective Medical Organizations* (New York, NY: Public Affairs, 2017).

28. Lawton R. Burns and Mark V. Pauly. "Detecting BS in Health Care." Available online: https://ldi.upenn.edu/brief/detecting-bs-health-care. Lawton R. Burns and Mark V. Pauly. "Detecting BS in Health Care 2.0." Available online: https://ldi.upenn.edu/brief/detecting-bs-health-care-20.

29. Joseph Schumpeter. *Capitalism, Socialism, and Democracy* (New York, NY: Harper & Row, 1942).

30. Clayton Christensen. *The Innovator's Dilemma: The Revolutionary Book That Will Change the Way You Do Business* (New York, NY: Harper Business, 1997).

31. Clayton Christensen, Richard Bohmer, and John Kenagy. "Will Disruptive Innovations Cure Health Care?" *Harvard Business Review* 78 (2000): 102-112. Clayton Christensen, Jerome Grossman, and Jason Hwang. *The Innovator's Prescription: A Disruptive Solution for Health Care* (New York, NY: McGraw-Hill, 2009).

32. Lawton R. Burns, Guy David, and Lorens Helmchen. "Strategic Response by Providers to Specialty Hospitals, Ambulatory Surgery Centers, and Retail Clinics," *Population Health Management* 14 (2) (2011): 69-77.

33. Clayton Christensen, Andrew Waldeck, and Rebecca Fogg. "How Disruption Can Finally Revolutionize Healthcare," *Industry Horizons* (Spring 2017). Available online: https://www.christenseninstitute.org/wp-content/uploads/2017/05/How-Disruption-Can-Finally-Revolutionize-Healthcare-final.pdf. Accessed on February 11, 2020.

34. Mark Pauly. "'We Aren't Quite as Good, but We Sure Are Cheap.' Prospects for Disruptive Innovation in Medical Care and Insurance Markets," *Health Aff.* 27 (5) (2008): 1349-1352.

35. Source: data extract from AIR's new health insurance literacy measurement tool. See: https://www.air.org/resource/air-index-health-insurance-literacy-america. Accessed on August 4, 2020.

36. George Loewenstein, Joelle Y. Friedman, Barbara McGill, et al. "Consumers' Misunderstanding of Health Insurance," *J Health Econ.* 32 (2013): 850-862.
37. Pharmacy Benefit Management Institute. *Trends in Drug Benefit Design 2018.* Available online: https://www.pbmi.com/ItemDetail?iProduct Code=BDR_2018&Category=BDR. Accessed on January 19, 2020.
38. Ezra Klein. "In the UK's Health System, Rationing Is Not a Dirty Word," *Vox* (January 28, 2020). Available online: https://www.vox.com/2020/1/28/21074386/health-care-rationing-britain-nhs-nice-medicare-for-all. Accessed on July 21, 2020.
39. Spencer Johnson. *Who Moved My Cheese?* (New York, NY: G.P. Putnam's Sons, 1998).
40. Eliot Freidson. *Professional Dominance: The Social Structure of Medical Care* (New York, NY: Aldine-Atherton Press, 1970).
41. Lawton R. Burns, Guy David, and Lorens Helmchen. "Strategic Responses by Providers to Specialty Hospitals, Ambulatory Surgery Centers, and Retail Clinics," *Population Health Manage.* 14 (2) (2011): 69-77.
42. Caroline Davis and Deborah Rhodes. "The Impact of DRGs on the Cost and Quality of Health Care in the United States," *Health Policy.* 9 (2) (1988): 117-131.
43. Robert Coulam and Gary Gaumer. "Medicare's Prospective Payment System: A Critical Appraisal," *Health Care Financing Review.* Annual Supplement (1991): 45-77.
44. Stuart Altman. "The Lessons of Medicare's Prospective Payment System Show That the Bundled Payment Program Faces Challenges," *Health Aff.* 31 (9) (September 2012): 1923-1930.
45. Robert I. Field. *Mother of Invention: How the Government Created "Free Market" Health Care* (New York, NY: Oxford University Press, 2014).
46. The next 2 paragraphs condense material published earlier. See: Lawton R. Burns and Mark V. Pauly. "Transformation of the Health Care Industry: Curb Your Enthusiasm?" *Milbank Quarterly.* 96 (1) (2018): 57-109. Available online at: https://onlinelibrary.wiley.com/doi/full/10.1111/1468-0009.12312. Accessed on July 22, 2020.
47. Paul Starr. *The Social Transformation of American Medicine* (New York, NY: Basic Books, 1982). Rosemary Stevens. *In Sickness and in Wealth* (New York, NY: Basic Books, 1989).

# What Is a Healthcare System?

## WHAT IS A HEALTHCARE SYSTEM?

The phrase "healthcare system" is widely used in discourse on global health but enjoys no agreed-upon definition.[1] "Healthcare system" actually combines 3 nebulous terms: health, care, and system. They should not be confused with one another but often are. The 3 subsections that follow attempt to unpack this phrase.

## Health

According to the World Health Organization (WHO), *health* is "a state of complete physical, mental, and social well-being, and not merely the absence of disease and infirmity."[2] Health has also been defined as an important capability "that enables individuals to pursue things they might value."[3] There are as many indicators of health as there are definitions. These include life expectancy at birth, infant mortality rates, the percentage of children underweight, the percentage of women with body mass index below 18.5, quality-adjusted life-years, disability-adjusted life-years, and disease prevalence (morbidity). These represent measures of *health status*, which constitutes one part of Don Berwick's triple aim (see Chapter 5).

Getting a comprehensive picture of a country across lots of indicators is impossible and probably futile. The United States, for example, is commonly lambasted for ranking relatively poorly among developed countries on infant mortality; on other indicators, however, such as cancer survival, the United States ranks quite highly.

## Care

Care consists of efforts made to maintain or restore physical, mental, or emotional well-being, especially by trained and licensed professionals. This can include taking preventative measures (eg, alterations in a person's lifestyle) or necessary medical interventions (eg, surgical procedure, prescription drugs) to improve a person's well-being. These services are typically offered through organizations in which the licensed professionals work, including ambulatory care offices, retail clinics, ambulatory surgery centers, hospital outpatient departments, and inpatient hospital units. Researchers typically distinguish 3 levels of care:

*Primary care* is medical care provided by the clinician of first contact for the patient. Typically, the primary care physician is a general practitioner, family practitioner, primary care internist, or primary care pediatrician. Primary care may also be administered by health professionals other than physicians, notably, specially trained nurses (nurse practitioners) and physician assistants. Usually, a general practitioner, family practitioner, nurse practitioner, or physician assistant provides only primary care services, but a person with specialty qualifications may provide primary care, alone or in combination with referral services. Thus, it is the nature of the contact (first compared with referred) that determines the care designation rather than the qualifications of the practitioner.

*Secondary care* is medical care provided to a patient when referred by one health professional to another with more specialized qualifications or interests. Secondary care is usually provided by a broadly skilled specialist such as a general surgeon, general internist, or obstetrician.

*Tertiary care* is provided on referral of a patient to a subspecialist, such as an orthopedic surgeon, neurologist, or neonatologist. A tertiary care center is a medical facility that receives referrals from both primary and secondary care levels and usually offers tests, treatments, and procedures that are not available elsewhere. Most tertiary care centers offer a mixture of primary, secondary, and tertiary care services so that it is the specific level of service rendered rather than the facility that determines the designation of care in a given study.

## System

The concept of a *system* is rather elusive. Piecing together definitions from several dictionaries, we might define a system as a whole composed of several interdependent parts that have differentiated roles, are interconnected by 3 processes (input, throughput, and output), and thus are integrated in a holistic fashion. Such a comprehensive definition begs the question: Does any country have a "system" of healthcare? The payer, provider, and producer components found in any country's healthcare industry are surely interdependent and interconnected (in the sense of serving one another as buyers and suppliers). But are they really integrated? And do they commonly focus on the provision of "health" as defined earlier?

The answer to both questions is likely no. There are few collaborative partnerships among these sectors in the United States.[4] As noted earlier, there are huge disconnects between them in terms of their goals and incentives. Moreover, these sectors are commonly oriented to funding and delivering acute *care*, rather than promoting the *health* of the population. The latter would require greater emphasis and funding of prevention, healthcare promotion, and public health activities. Health, as defined in this section, is typically left to the public health system in most countries. The result is the chaotic, hodgepodge network of players depicted in Chapter 2.

What, then, does the United States have if not a system that delivers health? The reality more closely resembles a collection of public and private sector entities (eg, individual professionals, firms, governmental bodies, professional associations) that have taken the stage at different periods in time, pursue their individual interests, pursue one or more desired goals (the efficiency and effectiveness goals discussed later and in Chapter 5), cohabit and interact with one another in the same environment (ie, an "ecosystem"), and may or may not interact with the patient. Harvard University researchers describe a healthcare system in a similar fashion as the collection of:

- Institutions and actors who provide healthcare (eg, doctors, nurses, hospitals, pharmacies, traditional healers)
- The organizations that supply specialized inputs to the providers (eg, training schools, manufacturers of products)
- The financial intermediaries, planners, and regulators who control, fund, and influence the providers (eg, insurers, government agencies, regulatory bodies)
- The organizations that offer preventive services
- The financial flows that finance the provision of healthcare[5]

The WHO defines a healthcare system more simply but more broadly as "all of the activities whose primary purpose is to promote, restore or maintain health."[6] In addition to the list of actors and institutions mentioned in Chapter 1, this definition of a healthcare system also includes health-enhancing interventions such as road improvements and environmental safety efforts. It also includes the efforts of informal healthcare givers in the home, behavioral change interventions conducted by employers or governments, and efforts to promote female education. The WHO explicitly acknowledges that their system definition does not imply any degree of integration among the activities and services performed.

## FRAMEWORKS FOR ANALYZING HEALTHCARE SYSTEMS

There have been several efforts to more formally define a healthcare system. These efforts develop frameworks one can use to analyze a country's healthcare system.[7] An early framework is the Actors framework, which classifies 4 major actors in a health system: providers, payers, regulators, and the population served. Another is the Funds Flow and Payment framework, which identifies 7 major subsystems of financing (eg, out-of-pocket, private reimbursement, public reimbursement).[8] A literature review identified at least 41 different frameworks, which are quite diverse.[9] Some focus on particular segments of the healthcare system ("sub-framework"); some focus on the entire healthcare system ("system framework"); and some focus on how other societal systems interact with the healthcare system ("supra-framework"). This chapter does not review all of these frameworks. However, the chapter concludes with its own integrated framework that resembles the sub-framework, system framework, and supra-framework perspective.

## Health System Typologies

Courses on international health often use typologies that classify the approaches taken by different countries to organize their healthcare systems. One popular typology cross-classifies countries by (1) whether their "financing" of healthcare is private sector versus public sector, and (2) whether their "provision of services" is private sector versus public sector. Another typology focuses on 4 models for paying for healthcare services: national health insurance (eg, the United Kingdom, Scandinavian countries), social health insurance (eg, Germany, Japan), provincial/regional government single payer (eg, Canada, Spain), and voluntary private health insurance (United States). Of course, no country fits purely into one system. In the United States, for example, we have voluntary private insurance for the nonelderly and national health insurance for the elderly (Medicare).

While helpful for classification purposes, these typologies do not really explain how the healthcare systems in different countries actually work. The more you study, the more you will find that each country has a unique history, culture, financing mechanisms, spending patterns, taste for adopting new technologies, and values that make comparisons difficult. Between any 2 countries you compare, there are many similarities and many differences. This is portrayed in Figures 3-1 and 3-2, which contrast the United States and China.[10]

## National Health Accounts

One widely used framework is the analysis of a country's national health accounts (NHA). These accounts rigorously classify the types and purposes of all expenditures made by or to all the actors in a healthcare system. Stated more simply, the accounts depict the sources and destinations of all healthcare spending in that country. The Centers for Medicare and

- Concern with iron triangle
- Affordability of healthcare
- Seeking universal coverage via healthcare reform
- Concern with hospital costs as cause of impoverishment/bankruptcy
- Concern with high costs of technology as percentage of healthcare costs
- Hospital competition via technology wars
- Concern with chronic illness
- Concern with geographic variations in spending and health status
- Concern with conflicts of interest and supplier-induced demand
- Concern with lifestyle issues and behaviors
- Need to develop primary care delivery system

- Hospital waste and inefficiency
- Fee-for-service payment system
- Falling out-of-pocket spending as percentage of healthcare costs
- Mixture of financing mechanism: government, employer, individual
- Fragmentation between federal and state government funding
- Effort to balance market approach with regulatory approach
- Low consumer literacy and information
- Local government competing priorities: education, services, health
- Experimentation with new payment models
- Integrate allopathic with complementary and alternative medicine

**Figure 3-1** • Convergence Between China and the United States.

| System Dimension | China | United States |
|---|---|---|
| • Spend per capita on healthcare | Low | High |
| • Government spend as percentage of NHE | Low | High |
| • Private health insurance | Low | High |
| • Depth and breadth of insurance coverage | Low | High |
| • Role of public sector hospitals | High | Low |
| • Preference for private providers | Low | High |
| • Centralized purchasers | Low | High |
| • Role of central government in healthcare | Low | High |
| • Governance mechanisms to monitor providers | Low | High |
| • Measures of utilization, appropriatensse | Low | High |
| • System of outpatient care/primary care | Low | High |
| • Amount of money spent on pharmaceuticals | High | Low |
| • Integration of hospitals and pharmacies | High | Low |
| • Integration of physicians and hospitals | High | Low |
| • Role of hospitals in public health | High | Low |
| • Locus of conflict | Doctor-patient | Doctor-hospital |
| • Physician payment | Salary | FFS |
| • Standardized doctor training | Low | High |
| • Role of medical profession | Low | High |
| • Hospital length of stays | Long | Short |
| • Smoking viewed as major problem | No | Yes |

**Figure 3-2** • Divergences Between China and the United States. FFS, Fee for Service; NHE, National Health Expenditure.

Medicaid Services (CMS) maintains these data for the United States over time. The Organisation for Economic Co-operation and Development has developed an International Classification for Health Accounts to facilitate international comparisons.[11]

Sources of spending include government (both federal and provincial/state and by public program) and nongovernment entities (employers, community insurance schemes, individual payments out of pocket). Destinations of spending include hospitals, physicians, dentists, retail pharmaceuticals and other products, public health, construction, and so on. Figures 3-3 and 3-4 reproduce these accounts for the United States, based on CMS data. An NHA scheme allows for ongoing analysis of time trends in these money flows, which can serve as the basis for performance appraisal and stewardship. It also follows the old adage, "follow the money."

## Health Systems Strengthening

The NHA scheme itemizes investments at the country level and typically focuses on the investments undertaken by that country. In contrast, developing countries often are also the recipient of investments and income transfers from outside organizations and donors to tackle specific problems. The "health systems strengthening" framework tracks the activities and investments undertaken by different donors and funders to strengthen specific system components.[12] These investments are typically designed to make changes in the healthcare system and accomplish certain system goals. The components targeted include health services (staffing infrastructure, operational support systems), the financing system (eg, health financing policies and legislation, resource generation, fund pooling, provider reimbursement system), monitoring/evaluation and information system (data analysis and reporting, disease surveillance), and stewardship and governance (eg, planning, priority setting, management).

## Functions, Objectives, and Priorities

Another method to analyze healthcare systems is to examine what they do (ie, what functions they perform and what objectives they pursue). Functions include the creation of resources and inputs (investments, training), stewardship (oversight) of these resources, financing (pooling and purchasing), and the provision (delivery) of services. Objectives served include the production of health, fairness, and responsiveness to societal expectations.[13] Thus, for example,

| Source of funds | 2012 | 2013 | 2014 | 2015 | 2016 | 2017 | 2018 |
|---|---|---|---|---|---|---|---|
| **Expenditure amount** | | | | | | | |
| NHE, billions | $2,791.10 | $2,875.00 | $3,025.40 | $3,199.60 | $3,347.40 | $3,487.30 | $3,649.40 |
| Health consumption expenditures | 2,637.70 | 2,720.90 | 2,875.60 | 3,045.50 | 3,190.70 | 3,319.00 | 3,475.00 |
| Out of pocket | 319.2 | 326.9 | 331.8 | 341.7 | 357.2 | 365.2 | 375.6 |
| Health insurance | 2,015.80 | 2,079.20 | 2,223.00 | 2,373.40 | 2,487.50 | 2,592.30 | 2,729.00 |
| Private health insurance | 922 | 939.1 | 994.1 | 1,060.90 | 1,119.90 | 1,175.00 | 1,243.00 |
| Medicare | 568.5 | 588.9 | 618.5 | 648.8 | 676.8 | 705.1 | 750.2 |
| Medicaid | 422.9 | 445.2 | 497.8 | 542.6 | 565.4 | 580.1 | 597.4 |
| Federal | 243.4 | 256.9 | 305.7 | 342.6 | 358.1 | 359.3 | 370.9 |
| State and local | 179.5 | 188.4 | 192.1 | 200.1 | 207.2 | 220.8 | 226.5 |
| Other health insurance programs | 102.4 | 105.9 | 112.6 | 121.1 | 125.4 | 132.1 | 138.3 |
| Other third-party payers and programs and public health activity | 302.7 | 314.9 | 320.8 | 330.4 | 346 | 361.5 | 370.5 |
| Investment | 153.3 | 154.1 | 149.8 | 154.1 | 156.7 | 168.3 | 174.4 |
| Population (millions) | 313.3 | 315.5 | 317.9 | 320.1 | 322.5 | 324.6 | 326.6 |
| GDP, billions of dollars | $16,197.00 | $16,784.90 | $17,527.30 | $18,224.80 | $18,715.00 | $19,519.40 | $20,580.20 |
| NHE per capita | $8,908 | $9,113 | $9,518 | $9,995 | $10,379 | $10,742 | $11,172 |
| GDP per capita | $51,695 | $53,200 | $55,143 | $56,932 | $58,025 | $60,128 | $63,004 |
| NHE as percentage of GDP | 17.2 | 17.1 | 17.3 | 17.6 | 17.9 | 17.9 | 17.7 |

**Figure 3-3 •** Sources of Funds (Centers for Medicare and Medicaid Services). GDP, Gross Domestic Product; NHE, National Health Expenditure.

| Spending category | 2012 | 2013 | 2014 | 2015 | 2016 | 2017 | 2018 |
|---|---|---|---|---|---|---|---|
| Expenditure amount | | | | | | | |
| NHE, billions | $2,791.10 | $2,875.00 | $3,025.40 | $3,199.60 | $3,347.40 | $3,487.30 | $3,649.40 |
| Health consumption expenditures | 2,637.70 | 2,720.90 | 2,875.60 | 3,045.50 | 3,190.70 | 3,319.00 | 3,475.00 |
| Personal healthcare | 2,361.10 | 2,431.20 | 2,556.00 | 2,710.20 | 2,838.30 | 2,954.50 | 3,075.50 |
| Hospital care | 902.5 | 937.6 | 978.2 | 1,034.60 | 1,089.50 | 1,140.60 | 1,191.80 |
| Professional services | 743.2 | 759.6 | 792.5 | 837.9 | 883.2 | 924 | 965.1 |
| Physician and clinical services | 557.1 | 569.6 | 595.7 | 631.2 | 665.6 | 696.9 | 725.6 |
| Other professional services | 76.4 | 78.7 | 83 | 87.8 | 92.7 | 97.5 | 103.9 |
| Dental services | 109.7 | 111.2 | 113.8 | 118.8 | 124.9 | 129.6 | 135.6 |
| Other health, residential, and personal care | 139.1 | 144.3 | 151.5 | 164.5 | 173.6 | 183.2 | 191.6 |
| Home healthcare | 78.3 | 81.4 | 84.8 | 89.2 | 93 | 97.1 | 102.2 |
| Nursing care facilities and continuing care retirement communities | 147.4 | 149 | 152.4 | 158.1 | 163 | 166.2 | 168.5 |
| Retail outlet sales of medical products | 350.6 | 359.3 | 396.6 | 425.9 | 436 | 443.2 | 456.3 |
| Prescription drugs | 253 | 258.2 | 292.4 | 317.1 | 322.3 | 326.8 | 335 |
| Durable medical equipment | 43.7 | 45.1 | 46.7 | 48.6 | 51 | 52.4 | 54.9 |
| Other nondurable medical products | 53.9 | 56 | 57.5 | 60.2 | 62.7 | 64.1 | 66.4 |
| Government administration | 34.2 | 37.5 | 42.3 | 42.8 | 44.9 | 44.8 | 47.5 |
| Net cost of health insurance | 165.2 | 173.3 | 195.3 | 206.7 | 218.8 | 228.3 | 258.5 |
| Government public health activities | 77.2 | 79 | 82 | 85.8 | 88.7 | 91.4 | 93.5 |
| Investment | 153.3 | 154.1 | 149.8 | 154.1 | 156.7 | 168.3 | 174.4 |
| Noncommercial research | 48.4 | 46.7 | 46 | 46.4 | 47.4 | 50.1 | 52.6 |
| Structures and equipment | 105 | 107.5 | 103.7 | 107.7 | 109.3 | 118.2 | 121.8 |

**Figure 3-4 •** Destinations of Funds (Centers for Medicare and Medicaid Services). NHE, National Health Expenditure.

one framework analyzes the interplay between 4 functions (regulation, financing, resource allocation, and service provision) and 4 key actors (government, providers, payers, and patients).[14]

A complementary approach is to categorize the country's healthcare priorities (eg, the various initiatives and interventions to reduce the disease burden in the population), the types of provider organizations and incentives given to them to deliver the interventions, the other resource inputs required to achieve these initiatives (budgets, manpower, technology), and the specific financing mechanisms (eg, revenue collection, pooling, purchasing).[15]

## Building Blocks

The WHO has described the framework of a healthcare system in terms of its basic building blocks. These include service delivery of effective, safe, quality personal and nonpersonal interventions; a health workforce that is adequate in numbers, competently trained, and fairly distributed; a health information system that produces, analyzes, and disseminates reliable and timely information; medical products and technologies that are safe, efficacious, cost-effective, and accessible; a financing system that raises adequate funds to ensure the population can use

needed services and is protected from financial catastrophe; and governance and oversight of the above.[16] All 6 building blocks are viewed as essential for improving health outcomes.

## Control Knobs

Economist William Hsiao at Harvard University developed another framework—known as control knobs—that analyzes the policy levers that can be used to impact societal goals for health. This framework, adopted by the World Bank, conceptualizes a healthcare system as a set of relationships between background factors, policy levers, and system goals.[17] The policy levers—the financing, payment, organizational, regulatory, and behavioral initiatives—are at the center of Figure 3-5. They serve as the mechanisms to try to change healthcare systems (hence, "control knobs"). The levers are themselves conditioned by the country's economic, social, and cultural context—found in the left column of Figure 3-5. Such a framework is helpful for understanding the broader societal and regulatory constraints within which a healthcare system operates. It also serves as a causal model whereby system components serve as a means to an end of achieving system goals.

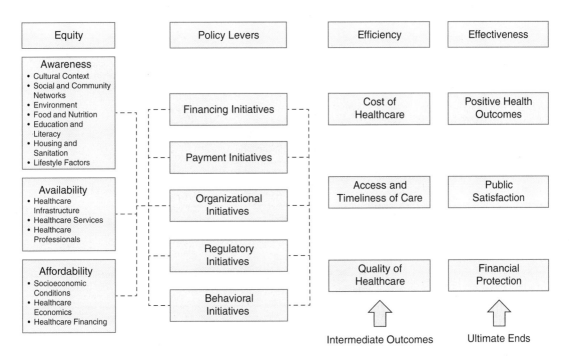

**Figure 3-5** • Control Knobs Framework. (Adapted from Roberts MJ, Hsiao WC, Berman P, Reich MR. 2003. *Getting Health Reform Right.* New York: Oxford University Press.)

The background factors in the left column are particularly worthy of discussion. A country's cultural context exerts a strong influence on what policy levers will be used. Compared to other countries, the US healthcare system balances market-based and regulatory approaches to try to contain healthcare spending. The former is what makes our country distinctive (or an outlier). The market-based approach emanates from the belief that liberty and public good flow from the private sector and individual initiatives, with decentralized decision making and a limited role for government.[18] This has influenced the types of policy levers (eg, financing and payment initiatives) used. For example, the United States has traditionally been financed through individual out-of-pocket payments and private insurance. Regulatory initiatives entered the stage later than in other countries in the 1960s (eg, Medicare and Medicaid) and 1970s (eg, Certificate of Need) to deal with issues the market-based approach could not solve.

As another example of the role of background factors, the United States is now experiencing a litany of problems dealing with lifestyle factors (eg, obesity, drug use), nutrition,

environmental pollution, social isolation, and lack of housing (homelessness), among others. These factors are now labeled *social determinants of health* (SDOHs), a topic developed further in the next chapter. A detailed view of these determinants is presented in Figure 3-6. The growing attention paid to SDOHs is illustrated by newspaper and research article headlines in Figure 3-7. The healthcare system is now being forced to confront these problems to see what it can do to ameliorate them. What is important here is that the health problems that need to be fixed are dumped at the door of the healthcare system from outside the system. There is some consensus that the majority of factors that contribute to one's health status are behavioral, social-environmental, and genetic in nature; the healthcare system exerts a much smaller influence (Figure 3-8).

The policy levers in the center of Figure 3-5 are designed to influence the efficiency and effectiveness of the healthcare system (2 right-hand columns in Figure 3-5). Efficiency encompasses 3 intermediate ends: ensuring access to healthcare, promoting the quality of healthcare, and controlling the cost of healthcare. Effectiveness

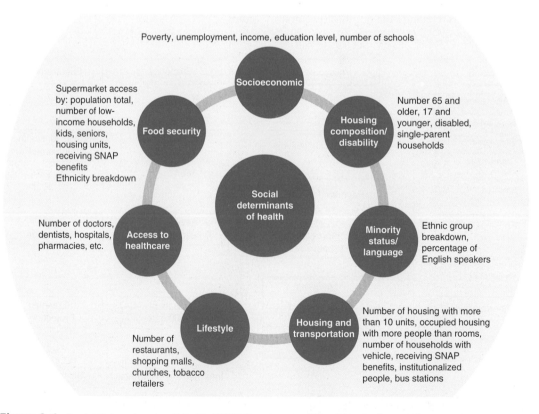

**Figure 3-6** • Social Determinants of Health. SNAP, Supplemental Nutrition Assistance Program.

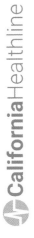
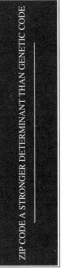
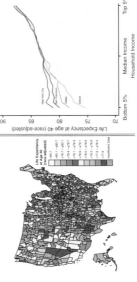
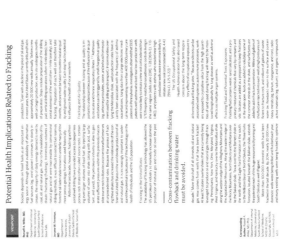
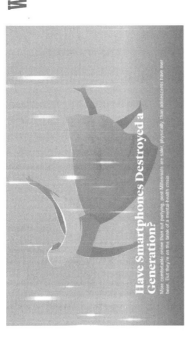

**Figure 3-7 •** Attention Paid to Social Determinants.

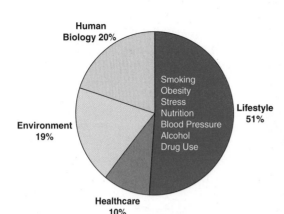

**Figure 3-8 •** Factors Influencing Health Status. (Adapted from McGinnis JM, Foege WH. "Actual Causes of Deaths in the US." *JAMA* 270, no. 18 [1993]: 2207-2212.)

encompasses 3 corresponding ultimate ends: public satisfaction, positive health outcomes, and financial protection. Efficiency and effectiveness represent the "intermediate outcomes" and "ultimate ends" in Figure 3-5. These 2 sets of goals parallel the iron triangle and the triple aim discussed in Chapter 5.

The authors of frameworks like that in Figure 3-5 seldomly discuss how addressing the intermediate outcomes helps to achieve the ultimate ends, however. As stated earlier, things may not be that simple.

Moreover, the model depicted in Figure 3-5 suggests a 1-way causation that is likely inaccurate. Not only are the intermediate and

ultimate ends of a healthcare system impacted by macroeconomic conditions, but they can also determine them. There is growing evidence that societal health shapes societal wealth, as well as vice versa. For example, poor health is positively associated with absence from work, job loss, higher out-of-pocket spending, debt levels, and loan defaults—all of which contribute to lower income. In addition, poor health among pregnant mothers and children is negatively associated with education and long-term cognitive development. There is also evidence that societal health shapes nation-state security, which, in turn, fosters economic growth.[19] Economists argue that a country's health status, incidence of illness, and likelihood of catastrophic illness heavily influence the country's labor force participation rates, labor productivity, savings and poverty rates, and healthcare demand and consumption. These latter forces influence, in turn, inflation rates, wage rates, exchange rates, and the country's fiscal health.[20]

## Value Chain

Every country's healthcare system resembles a value chain, as depicted in Figure 3-9.[21] According to this framework, a healthcare system can be studied in terms of the buyers and suppliers of products and services that make up this chain, who engage in the important market exchanges that compose this system, and whose activities add value to system outputs as they

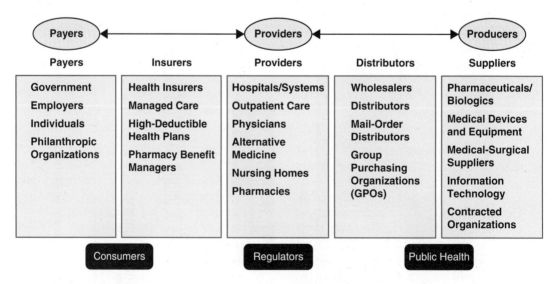

**Figure 3-9 •** The Healthcare Value Chain. (Source: Burns LR. 2002. *The Health Care Value Chain.* San Francisco: Jossey-Bass.)

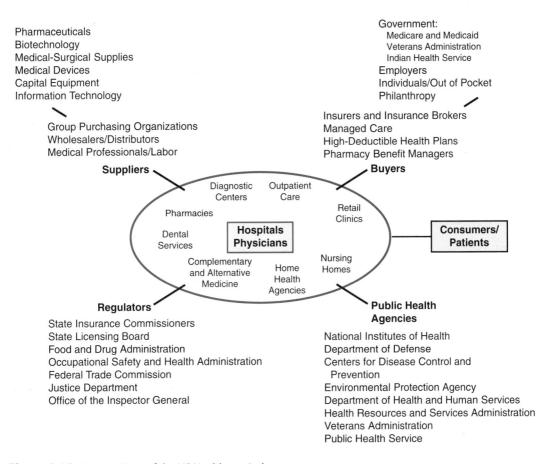

Pharmaceuticals
Biotechnology
Medical-Surgical Supplies
Medical Devices
Capital Equipment
Information Technology

Government:
  Medicare and Medicaid
  Veterans Administration
  Indian Health Service
Employers
Individuals/Out of Pocket
Philanthropy

Group Purchasing Organizations
Wholesalers/Distributors
Medical Professionals/Labor

Insurers and Insurance Brokers
Managed Care
High-Deductible Health Plans
Pharmacy Benefit Managers

**Suppliers**

**Buyers**

Diagnostic
Centers

Outpatient
Care

Pharmacies

Retail
Clinics

Dental
Services

**Hospitals
Physicians**

**Consumers/
Patients**

Complementary
and Alternative
Medicine

Home
Health
Agencies

Nursing
Homes

**Regulators**

State Insurance Commissioners
State Licensing Board
Food and Drug Administration
Occupational Safety and Health Administration
Federal Trade Commission
Justice Department
Office of the Inspector General

**Public Health
Agencies**

National Institutes of Health
Department of Defense
Centers for Disease Control and
  Prevention
Environmental Protection Agency
Department of Health and Human Services
Health Resources and Services Administration
Veterans Administration
Public Health Service

**Figure 3-10** • System View of the US Healthcare Industry.

move along the chain. This framework highlights the upstream (supplier) and downstream (buyer) trading partners of any firm operating in a healthcare system, the parties that may mediate these transactions, and the possible competitors and substitutes for the firm's product/service. An alternative representation is contained in Figure 3-10. The text below briefly describes what each of the 5 components of the value chain does.

**Payers.** The payer is "where the buck starts." There are 3 main sets of payers in the United States. First, most of the nonelderly get private insurance coverage through their employer. This is known as employer-based health insurance (EBHI; covered in Chapter 15). EBHI is part of the worker's total compensation (salary plus benefits); benefits are received in lieu of salary, making the employee the ultimate payer. Employer coverage is split between large accounts (large firms that tend to self-fund their insurance) and small accounts (smaller companies that

tend to be fully insured using an outside insurer). Second, the elderly and the nonelderly poor and unemployed get public health insurance coverage through Medicare and Medicaid (covered in Chapters 18 and 19). Other publicly insured portions of the population also receive public coverage through the various branches of the Department of Defense, the Veterans Administration, and the Public Health Service. Third, individual members of the population pay directly for healthcare via out-of-pocket payments, as well as through their municipal, state, and federal taxes.

**Insurers.** Insurers finance healthcare rather than paying for it. They thus serve as "fiscal intermediaries" between the payer and the provider (covered in Chapter 17). For fully insured firms, insurers collect the EBHI premiums from the employer, contract with providers, and process the providers' claims. For self-insured firms, insurers perform the latter 2 functions as part of "administrative services only" (ASO) contracts; the employer bears the risk and is on the hook for all claims. There can be different types of services covered by insurance: hospital, medical (ie, physician), vision, dental, and prescription drug. In recent years, the insurer space has been joined by high-deductible health plans and state-level insurance exchanges. Finally, many insurers also have an in-house pharmacy benefit manager that manages the pharmacy benefit for employers (covered in Chapter 16).

**Providers.** Providers include all parties that render healthcare services (primary, secondary, and tertiary). These parties are typically silos in the delivery system, operating independently of one another. They include inpatient hospitals, outpatient centers, physician offices, ambulatory surgery centers, post-acute care sites such as nursing homes and home healthcare agencies, and pharmacies (covered in Chapters 8 to 14). Providers account for roughly two-thirds of all healthcare spending in the United States. Other important providers include the Public Health Service, which usually manages public sector activities to monitor and control environmental quality (air, water, and sanitation), epidemics and contagions, and promote prevention.

**Distributors/Wholesalers.** Distributors serve as the logistics background to the healthcare system, ensuring the movement of products and supplies from manufacturers to providers. Their area is also known as supply chain management. Distributors typically take delivery of products from the manufacturer, hold them in inventory, and then distribute to providers as requested. This sector also includes mail-order distribution for drugs, as well as group purchasing organizations (GPOs), which act as centralized buying hubs for providers to purchase drugs, devices, and medical-surgical supplies. The distributors and GPOs are not covered in this text; other volumes examine them in depth.[22]

**Producers.** The producers, also known as product manufacturers, represent the key source of innovation in healthcare and its most profitable segment. This sector includes pharmaceutical, biotechnology, medical device, medical-surgical supply, and information technology companies (covered in Chapters 20 to 24). They sell their products to several sets of customers: hospitals, physicians, pharmacies, post-acute care sites, and patients.

Why is the value chain framework helpful? First, it reminds you that no matter what particular sector of the healthcare system you are studying or working in, "you are not alone." That sector rests inside a larger web of relationships with lots of stakeholders. As we argued earlier, healthcare is not so much a "system" of organized, interrelated parts as it is an ecosystem in which lots of species coexist.

Second, the value chain perspective reminds you of the enormous complexity of our healthcare system. There are 3 key sets of actors and 2 sets of intermediaries between them. The 3 key sets of actors are the individuals and institutions that purchase healthcare, provide healthcare services, and produce healthcare products (*purchasers*, *providers*, and *producers*). Two sets of intermediaries separate these key actors: those firms that finance healthcare (offer insurance to the purchasers and handle reimbursement to the providers) and those that distribute products (from the producers to the providers). This text is organized around the 3 key sets of actors.

Third, value chains are useful ways to describe other countries' healthcare systems and, thereby, to spot the differences with our own. In 2 other volumes, I have described the healthcare systems of China and India using such value chains (see Figure 3-11 for the value chain of the Indian state of Gujarat).[23] Compared to the United States, the systems in both of these countries lack the complex set of intermediaries between payers and providers (eg, private health insurers, pharmacy benefit managers, managed care organizations). India's system is focused heavily on primary care delivered by a large number of physician and nonphysician providers; China's system is focused heavily on its hospital sector because it lacks a primary care sector.

Fourth, the value chain distinguishes who innovates and who pays for innovation. All of the money that gets pumped into the healthcare system starts on the far-left side of Figure 3-9 (the *purchasers*) and flows to all of the boxes to the right. Conversely, much of the innovation in healthcare starts on the far-right side (the *producers*) and flows to the adjacent boxes on the left. This is portrayed in Figure 3-12.

## Gujarat—Healthcare Value Chain

**Hospitals**
- IKDRC, GCRI
  U.N. Mehta Heart Institute
- Shalby
- Apollo Hospital
- Krishna Heart Institute
- Wockhardt Hospital
- Sterling Addlife India Ltd.
- SAL Hospital
- Rajasthan Hospital
- Medisurge Hospital

**Pharmaceutical Companies**
- Zydus Cadila Healthcare Ltd.
- Claris Life Sciences Ltd.
- Cadila Pharmaceuticals Ltd.
- Intas Pharmaceutical Ltd.
- SUN Pharma
- Torrent Pharmaceuticals Ltd.
- Dishman Pharmaceuticals
- Abbott Laboratories
- Wyeth
- Jubilant Organosys

**Insurance Companies**
- Bajaj Allianz Health Insurance
  Company Ltd.
- TATA AIG General Insurance Company
- Vysya Life Insurance Company
- National Insurance Company Ltd.

| Producers | Purchasers | Fiscal Intermediaries -> Insurers / Providers | Payers |
|---|---|---|---|
| • Drug Manufacturers<br>• Device Manufacturers<br>• Surgical Manufacturers | • Wholesalers<br>• Mail-Order Distributors<br>• Group Purchasing Organizations | • Hospitals<br>• Pharmacies<br>• Physicians | • Government Employees<br>• Individuals<br>• Employer Coalition |

**Figure 3-11** • The Value Chain in the Indian State of Gujarat. GCRI, Gujarat Cancer & Research Institute; IKDRC, Institute of Kidney Diseases and Research Centre; PBM, Pharmacy Benefit Manager. (Source: Health and Family Welfare Department, Government of Gujarat.)

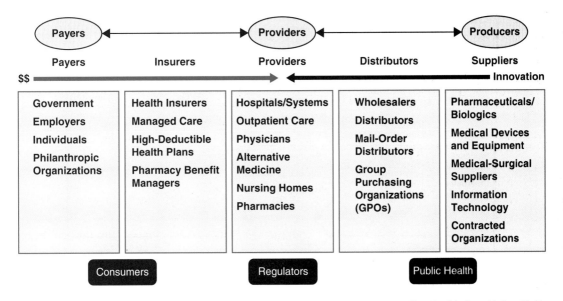

**Figure 3-12** • Balancing Funding and Innovation. (Source: Burns LR. 2002. *The Health Care Value Chain*. San Francisco: Jossey-Bass.)

Fifth, both Figures 3-9 and 3-10 place providers—especially physicians and hospitals—at the center of the system. Why are they central? The 2 flows of money and innovation discussed earlier collide in the middle among the *providers* of healthcare services—that is, doctors and hospitals—who then have to determine how much of the innovation from the right side they can afford to utilize in patient treatment given the limited supply of funds received from the left side. This is the point at which much of the spending on healthcare and the consumption of healthcare products takes place. These key providers are thus centrally involved in "rationing" the monies made available by payers to the seemingly endless flow of new technologies emanating from the producers.[24] Researchers suggest that physicians control, directly or indirectly, 85% of all monies spent in the system.[25]

Physicians and hospitals are central for another important reason. Collectively, they account for 53% of all healthcare spending: 33% of national health expenditure goes to hospitals, and 20% goes to physicians. That means that any effort to contain healthcare costs must,

almost by definition, curb the spending (and, thus, the incomes) of hospitals and physicians. Most cost-cutting efforts in the past—whether regulatory changes, reimbursement changes, or other efforts—have been focused on these 2 parties.

Hopefully, by now you should have asked, "What is the role of the patient?" In Figures 3-9 and 3-10, they are pushed off to the side. During much of the prior century, according to medical sociologists, patients were expected to play "the sick role" (ie, be totally dependent on their physician in a one-way exchange). Only since the turn of the millennium have patients been recast as "consumers" of healthcare; whether or not they play the part is taken up in other chapters. For now, we note that many of the major players in the value chain have made efforts to reach out to engage patients as consumers (Figure 3-13).

## NESTED ECOSYSTEMS

A final way to view a healthcare system is the nesting of ecosystems. What is nesting? Nesting means *embeddedness*, a term popularized

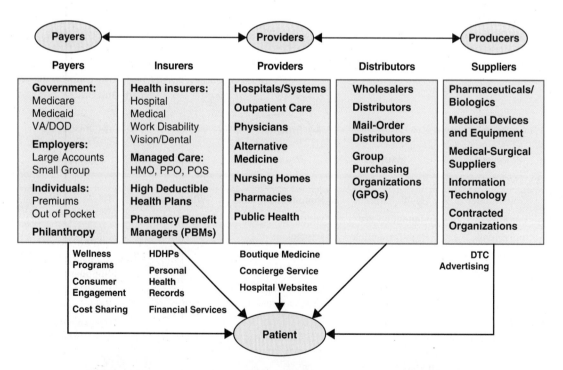

**Figure 3-13 •** Where Is the Patient in the Healthcare Value Chain? CAM, Complementary and Alternative Medicine; DOD, Department of Defense; DTC, Direct-to-Consumer; HDHPs, High-Deductible Health Plans; HMO, Health Maintenance Organization; POS, Point of Service; PPO, Preferred Provider Organization; VA, Veterans Administration. (Source: Lawton R. Burns, PhD, The Wharton School.)

by Mark Granovetter.[26] He used the term to capture the idea that the actions taken by individuals are importantly shaped by the social relations within which they function. The individual, thus, does not act alone but rather is shaped by a web of surrounding actions and social interactions. What is an ecosystem? An ecosystem is a community of organisms interacting in their environment, where everything touches everything else, and relationships between things matter. The emphasis here is not on structure as much as it is on process and interactions.

Innovation research provides an example of what a nested ecosystem looks like. Innovation occurs in a complex, multilevel ecosystem.[27] Relevant levels of analysis include the individual, team or department, organization, industry segment, and local environment.[28] Typically, different processes are at work at different levels, which contribute different resources that may impact innovation success. The involvement of multiple levels in healthcare innovation has been formalized in terms of "nesting."[29]

There are 3 levels of complexity in the US healthcare ecosystem, with each representing an ecosystem of relationships. These are the micro system, the macro system, and the societal system. These 3 levels roughly parallel the sub-framework, system framework, and supra-framework mentioned earlier in the chapter.

## Micro System

The *micro system* focuses on the patient-physician relationship, which represents the historical core of any healthcare system. This is where the treatment decisions are made and (hopefully) obeyed and ultimately impact the patient's health outcomes. Note that there are 3 primary elements to this relationship: the doctor, the patient, and their relationship. The first element encompasses what the physician does and does not do. This includes the physician's adherence to process measures of quality and practice guidelines and the physician's performance of high- or low-value care.

The second element encompasses what the patient does and does not do. This includes the patient's activation and engagement in their own care, understanding of the physician's orders, and adherence to medications prescribed. A recent national survey showed that 56% of the US population assigns low importance to their own personal health.[30] Data from Judith Hibbard and her associates suggest that a large percentage (35%-45%) of patients are low in terms of "activation": 15% to 20% are disengaged and overwhelmed, and another 20% to 25% aware but struggling.[31] These statistics are important because activation levels are inversely related to healthy behaviors, preventive behaviors, disease-specific self-care behaviors, and per-capita costs. Activation levels may be even lower among the Medicare population.[32] Physicians commonly report that only a minority of their patients are "highly engaged."[33] Nearly half (48%) of executives and clinicians surveyed in one study believe that patient engagement can impact quality, whereas only 27% believe it can impact cost.

The third element concerns the interactions between the 2 parties. Prior reviews of the literature suggest that the doctor-patient relationship is complex, spanning at least 3 different dimensions: longitudinal care (ie, seeing the same practitioner), the patient's consultation experience (eg, communication, expectations met), and depth (eg, the patient's trust in the physician, patient's knowledge of the physician and the physician's knowledge of the patient, patient loyalty, and respect).[34] Thus, the doctor-patient relationship has a *lot* of moving parts. Research suggests that the doctor-patient relationship impacts the efficiency and effectiveness goals discussed earlier (eg, cost, quality, access, patient experience, health outcomes)[35] and is considered central to the functioning of the healthcare delivery system.

The patient-physician relationship does not occur in a vacuum, however, but is encased in a larger network of players. Physicians practice in private clinics, often accompanied by nurse practitioners and schedulers; some may be affiliated with hospitals. They also practice in hospital outpatient departments and on inpatient floors, often as multidisciplinary teams or "clinical micro systems" surrounded by several different practitioners (eg, other physicians in the same or different specialties, nurse practitioners, pharmacists).[36] These clinical micro systems are also referred to as professional or interpersonal integration.[37] As a result, the patient-physician relationship often occurs under the umbrella of a hospital or hospital system. Many activities can be undertaken at the hospital organizational level to supplement the physician and clinical micro-system efforts, including

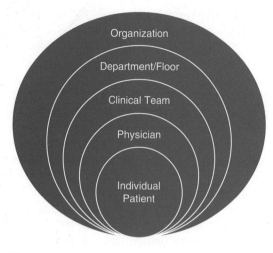

**Figure 3-14 •** Micro System.

several mechanisms to integrate care: functional, physician-system, clinical (or process), and normative.[38] This is represented in Figure 3-14.

## Macro System

The *macro system* consists of all of the players beyond the immediate provision of healthcare services. This is represented by the value chain in Figure 3-9. These players can have a significant impact on the micro system by virtue of (1) employers offering or not offering insurance coverage to their employees; (2) insurers covering or not covering specific services or including or excluding specific providers from their panels; (3) pharmacy benefit managers including or excluding specific drugs on their formularies; (4) providers consolidating horizontally or integrating vertically with one another; (5) distributors delivering supplies needed at the point of care on time; and (6) producers developing and supplying critical technologies at the point of care.

## Societal System

Finally, the *societal system* includes the social, economic, and physical environment in which all of the value chain players reside. It also includes the summation of health behaviors practiced by individuals within that society. The societal system came to prominence with the work of Princeton economists Anne Case and Angus Deaton.[39] They reported rising midlife mortality rates since the turn of the century for non-Hispanic, non-Black males lacking a college

education. They labeled this mortality "deaths of despair," reflecting a cumulative disadvantage accrued via broken familial background, loss of employment, and marital dissolution, all of which resulted in destructive behaviors (alcohol, drug abuse, suicide) and deterioration in their health status. This is represented by the left-hand side of Figure 3-5 and includes the following:

| Individual Behaviors | Socioeconomic Factors | Environment |
| --- | --- | --- |
| Caloric consumption per capita | Poverty/income inequality | Physical environment |
| Abuse of drugs and alcohol | Education | Food industry |
| Low use of seatbelts | Lack of safety net programs | Occupational stress |
| Driving under the influence accidents | Marital status | Housing |
| Firearms | Isolation/ loneliness | Pollution |
| Teen sexual activity | Employment | Transit |
| Social media use | Family and social support | Serious injury in family |
| Smoking/ vaping | Community safety | |
| Exercise | Food insecurity | |
| | Narrowing social networks | |
| | Corrections | |

## Three Nested Ecosystems

Figure 3-15 constitutes an attempt to combine the 3 ecosystems into 1 diagram. How these 3 ecosystems act, interact, and thereby shape what we observe in the healthcare system is a research area ripe for inquiry. Some suggest how the micro system (the doctor-patient relationship) is impacted by the macro system:

A series of organizational or system factors also affect the doctor–patient relationship. The accessibility of personnel, both administrative and clinical, and their courtesy level, provide a sense that patients are important and respected, as do reasonable waiting times and attention to personal comfort. The availability of covering

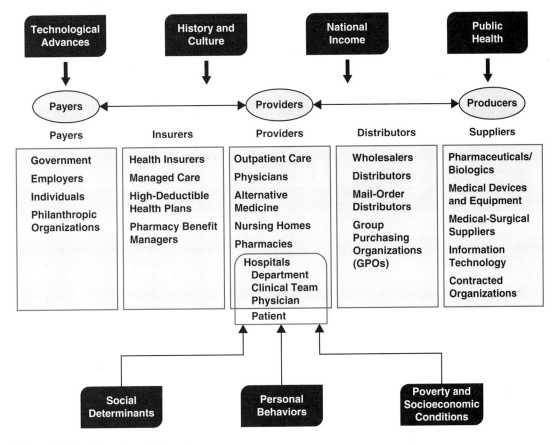

**Figure 3-15** • Three Nested Ecosystems.

nurses and doctors contributes to a sense of security. Reminders and user-friendly educational materials create an atmosphere of caring and concern. Organizations can promote a patient-centered culture, or one that is profit- or physician-centered, with consequences for individual doctor–patient relationships. Organizations (as well as whole health care systems) can promote continuity in clinical relationships, which in turn affects the strength of those relationships. For instance, a market-based system with health insurance linked to employers' whims, with competitive provider networks and frequent mergers and acquisitions, thwarts long-term relationships. A health plan that includes the spectrum of outpatient and inpatient, acute and chronic services has an opportunity

to promote continuity across care settings.[40]

At a minimum, the societal ecosystem that is concerned with population health must occasion a differentiated approach to patient care—one that tailors care to particular segments of the population. Figure 3-16 presents one approach to population health management developed by Cornerstone Health Care, an accountable care organization that once operated in North Carolina. In addition, producers of medical devices can develop wellness applications, health trackers, medication compliance products, virtual and telemedicine services, and biometric monitoring devices to promote greater patient activation and reinforce physician education. One can argue that the micro system is primary for issues dealing with efficiency measures (access, quality, and cost) and some dimensions of effectiveness (patient experience of care); conversely, the societal system is primary for issues dealing with population health and health outcomes.

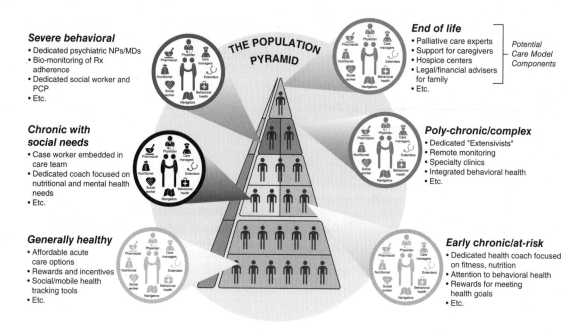

***Severe behavioral***
- Dedicated psychiatric NPs/MDs
- Bio-monitoring of Rx adherence
- Dedicated social worker and PCP
- Etc.

***End of life***
- Palliative care experts
- Support for caregivers
- Hospice centers
- Legal/financial advisers for family
- Etc.

*Potential Care Model Components*

***Chronic with social needs***
- Case worker embedded in care team
- Dedicated coach focused on nutritional and mental health needs
- Etc.

***Poly-chronic/complex***
- Dedicated "Extensivists"
- Remote monitoring
- Specialty clinics
- Integrated behavioral health
- Etc.

***Generally healthy***
- Affordable acute care options
- Rewards and incentives
- Social/mobile health tracking tools
- Etc.

***Early chronic/at-risk***
- Dedicated health coach focused on fitness, nutrition
- Attention to behavioral health
- Rewards for meeting health goals
- Etc.

**Figure 3-16** • Next-Generation Population Health Management. MD, Physician; NPs, Nurse Practitioners; PCP, Primary Care Physician. (Source: Presentation by Dr. Grace Terrell, *The Power of Primary Care Transformation.* http://www.ehcca.com/presentations/medhomesummit8/terrell_2.pdf. Used with permission from Oliver Wyman.)

## SUMMARY

This chapter has distinguished 3 key terms that get used together (often mindlessly): *health*, *care*, and *system*. The first 2 terms have distinct and precise meanings that need to be remembered. People often confuse health and healthcare; they are not the same. The former includes health status, functional status, life expectancy, and disease burden. The latter encompasses primary, secondary, and tertiary care and, thus, the provider sector of the healthcare system. By contrast, the term *system* is more elusive and harder to find in practice. Researchers have advanced several frameworks to depict the "system." Those interested in population health (the subject of Chapter 4) may be more interested in the "control knobs" view portrayed in Figure 3-5. Those interested in the transactions among the players in the healthcare system may be more interested in the "value chain" view portrayed in Figure 3-9.

## QUESTIONS TO PONDER

1. Are the various frameworks to describe a country's healthcare system that are described in this chapter consistent? Do some frameworks seem more useful than others?
2. How might the intermediate outcomes in Figure 3-5 (second column from the right) contribute to achieving the ultimate ends (last column on the right)?
3. In what ways do the boxes in Figure 3-9 add value for the boxes to the left of them? Does it make sense to refer to this figure as a value chain?
4. Why doesn't the patient play more of a central role in all of the frameworks described in this chapter?
5. Can you think of any country that has a well-organized, well-functioning healthcare system? In what ways does it work better? What might explain this?

# REFERENCES

1. Richard Smith and Kara Hanson. "What Is a 'Health System'?" in Richard Smith and Kara Hanson (Eds.), *Health Systems in Low- and Middle-Income Countries* (Oxford, UK: Oxford University Press, 2011). Chapter 1: pp. 3-19.
2. Daniel Callahan. "The WHO Definition of 'Health'," *The Hastings Center Studies* 1 (3) (1973): 77-87.
3. Amartya Sen. *Development as Freedom* (New York, NY: Alfred A. Knopf, 1999).
4. Lawton R. Burns. *The Health Care Value Chain: Producers, Purchasers, and Providers* (San Francisco, CA: Jossey-Bass, 2002).
5. Marc Roberts, William Hsiao, Peter Berman, et al. *Getting Health Reform Right* (New York, NY: Oxford University Press, 2003).
6. World Health Organization. *The World Health Report 2000–Health Systems: Improving Performance* (Geneva, Switzerland: WHO, 2000).
7. George Shakarishvili. "Building on Health Systems Frameworks for Developing a Common Approach to Health Systems Strengthening," Paper prepared for the World Bank, the Global Fund, and the GAVI Alliance Technical Workshop on Health Systems Strengthening (Washington, DC: June 25-27, 2009).
8. J.W. Hurst. "Reforming Health Care in Seven European Nations," *Health Aff.* 10 (3) (1991): 7-21.
9. Steven Hoffman, John-Arne Rottingen, Sara Bennett, et al. *Background Paper on Conceptual Issues Related to Health Systems Research to Inform a WHO Global Strategy on Health Systems Research.* Working Paper (February 29, 2012). Available online: https://www.who.int/alliance-hpsr/alliancehpsr_backgroundpaperhsrstrat1.pdf. Accessed on February 17, 2020.
10. Figures are taken from Lawton R. Burns and Gordon Liu. *China's Healthcare System and Reform* (Cambridge, UK: Cambridge University Press, 2017).
11. World Health Organization. *Guide to Producing National Health Accounts* (Geneva, Switzerland: WHO, 2003).
12. George Shakarishvili, Mary Ann Lansang, Vinod Mitta, et al. "Health Systems Strengthening: A Common Classification and Framework for Investment Analysis," *Health Policy and Planning* 26 (2011): 316-326.
13. World Health Organization. *The World Health Report 2000.* Available online: https://www.who.int/whr/2000/en/. Accessed October 26, 2020.
14. Anne J. Mills and M. Kent Ranson. "The Design of Health Systems," in Michael H. Merson, Robert E. Black, and Anne J. Mills (Eds.), *International Public Health: Diseases, Programs, Systems, and Policies* (Gaithersburg, MD: Aspen Publishers, 2001): Chapter 11.
15. World Health Organization. *The World Health Report 2000.* Available online: https://www.who.int/whr/2000/en/. Accessed October 26, 2020; Jane Menken and M. Omar Rahman. "Reproductive Health," in Michael H. Merson, Robert E. Black, and Anne J. Mills (Eds.), *International Public Health: Diseases, Programs, Systems, and Policies* (Gaithersburg, MD: Aspen Publishers, 2001): Chapter 3; Arthur L. Reingold and Christina R. Phares. "Infectious Diseases," in Michael H. Merson, Robert E. Black, and Anne J. Mills (Eds.), *International Public Health: Diseases, Programs, Systems, and Policies* (Gaithersburg, MD: Aspen Publishers, 2001): Chapter 4.
16. World Health Organization. *Strengthening Health Systems to Improve Health Outcomes* (Geneva, Switzerland: WHO, 2007).
17. William Hsiao. *What Is a Health System? Why Should We Care?* (Cambridge, MA: Harvard School of Public Health, August 2003).
18. Stuart Altman and Marc Rodwin. "Halfway Competitive Markets and Ineffective Regulation: The American Health Care System," *Journal of Health Politics, Policy and Law* 13 (2) (1988): 323-339.
19. Daniel C. Esty, et al. "State Failure Task Force Report: Phase II Findings," *Environmental Change and Security Project Report*, no. 5 (Washington, DC: Woodrow Wilson Center, Summer 1999): 49-72.
20. William Hsiao. *What Is a Health System? Why Should We Care?* (Cambridge, MA: Harvard School of Public Health, August 2003).
21. Lawton R. Burns. *The Health Care Value Chain* (San Francisco, CA: Jossey-Bass, 2002).
22. Lawton R. Burns. *The Health Care Value Chain* (San Francisco, CA: Jossey-Bass, 2002).
23. Lawton R. Burns. *India's Healthcare Industry: Innovation in Delivery, Financing, and Manufacturing* (Cambridge, UK: Cambridge University Press, 2014). Lawton R. Burns and Gordon Liu. *China's Healthcare System and Reform* (Cambridge, UK: Cambridge University Press, 2017).
24. Daniel Strech, Govind Persad, Georg Marckmann, et al. "Are Physicians Willing to Ration Health Care? Conflicting Findings in a Systematic Review of Survey Research," *Health Policy* 90 (2009): 113-124.

25. Alan Sager and Deborah Socolar. *Health Costs Absorb One-Quarter of Economic Growth, 2000–2005* (Boston, MA: Boston University School of Public Health, 2005).

26. Mark Granovetter. "Economic Action and Social Structure: The Problem of Embeddedness," *Am J Sociol.* 91 (3) (1985): 481-510.

27. Anil K. Gupta, Paul E. Tesluk, and Susan Taylor. "Innovation at and Across Multiple Levels of Analysis," *Organization Science* 18 (6) (2007): 885-897. Frank T. Rothaermel and Andrew M. Hess. "Building Dynamic Capabilities: Innovation Driven by Individual-, Firm-, and Network-Level Effects," *Organization Science* 18 (6) (2007): 898-921.

28. Lawton R. Burns and Philip Rea. "Organizing Discovery: Wild Ducks Nested in Multilevel Ecosystem," in Philip Rea, Mark Pauly, and Lawton R. Burns (Eds.), *Managing Discovery in the Life Sciences: Harnessing Creativity to Drive Biomedical Innovation* (Cambridge, UK: Cambridge University Press, 2018): pp. 449-489.

29. Lawton R. Burns and Philip Rea. "Organizing Discovery: Wild Ducks Nested in Multilevel Ecosystem," in Philip Rea, Mark V. Pauly, and Lawton R. Burns (Eds.), *Managing Discovery in the Life Sciences* (Cambridge, UK: Cambridge University Press, 2018): 449-489. Andrew Van de Ven and David Grazman. "Evolution in a Nested Hierarchy—A Genealogy of Twin Cities Health Care Organizations, 1853–1995," in Joel Baum and Bill McKelvey (Eds.), *Variations in Organization Science* (Thousand Oaks, CA: Sage, 1999): pp. 185-209.

30. Larry Bye, et al. "Datagraphic: Building a Culture of Health: What Americans Think," *Health Aff.* 35 (2016): 1982-1990.

31. Healthy Transitions Colorado. *The Patient Activation Measure and Care Transitions.* May 21, 2014.

32. Jessie L. Parker, Joseph F. Regan, and Jason Petroski. "Beneficiary Activation in the Medicare Population," *Medicare Medicaid Res Rev.* 4 (4) (2014): E1-E14.

33. Kevin Volpp and Namita Seth Mohta. "Patient Engagement Report: Improved Engagement Leads to Better Outcomes, but Better Tools Are Needed," *NEJM Catalyst* (May 12, 2016).

34. Matthew Ridd, Alison Shaw, Glyn Lewis, et al. "The Doctor-Patient Relationship: A Synthesis of the Qualitative Literature on Patients' Perspectives," *Br J Gen Pract.* (April 2009): e116-e133.

35. See the review by Timothy Hoff and Grace Collinson. "How Do We Talk About the Physician–Patient Relationship? What the Nonempirical Literature Tells Us," *Med Care Res Rev.* 74 (3) (2017): 251-285. Susan Ivey, Stephen Shortell, Hector Rodriguez, et al. "Patient Engagement in ACO Practices and Patient-Reported Outcomes Among Adults with Co-occurring Chronic Disease and Mental Health Conditions," *Med Care.* 56 (7) (2018): 551-556.

36. Eugene Nelson, Paul Batalden, Thomas Huber, et al. "Microsystems in Health Care: Part 1. Learning from High-Performing Front-Line Clinical Units," *Joint Commission Journal on Quality and Safety* 28 (2002): 472–93. Eugene Nelson, Paul Batalden, Karen Homa, et al. "Microsystems in Health Care: Part 2. Creating a Rich Information Environment," *Joint Commission Journal on Quality and Safety* 29 (2003): 5-15.

37. Sara Singer, Michaela Kerrissey, Mark Friedberg, et al. "A Comprehensive Theory of Integration," *Med Care Res Rev.* 77 (2) (2018): 196-207.

38. Stephen Shortell, Robin Gillies, David Anderson, et al. *Remaking Health Care in America: Building Organized Delivery Systems* (San Francisco, CA: Jossey-Bass, 1996).

39. Anne Case and Angus Deaton. "Mortality and Morbidity in the 21st Century," *Brookings Papers on Economic Activity* (Spring 2017): 397-476.

40. Susan Goold and Mack Lipkin. "The Doctor-Patient Relationship: Challenges, Opportunities, Strategies," *J Gen Intern Med.* 14 (January) (1999): S26-S33. Supplement 1.

# Population Health

# 4

## INTRODUCTION

There is no single, agreed-upon definition about what population health means and no single approach to implementing it. Some define population health broadly to mean taking accountability for a defined patient population in a community; others define it more narrowly in terms of managing wellness. These definitions appear to focus on population health *management* more than population *health*.

Two of the pioneers in this area, David Kindig and Greg Stoddart, defined population health as "the health outcomes of a group of individuals, including the distribution of such outcomes within the group."[1] They further argued that the subject encompasses not only health outcomes, but also the patterns of health determinants and the policies and interventions that link the two. Such policies and interventions might be considered their label for population health management. They view the determinants as independent variables and the outcomes as dependent variables. Their view is depicted in Figure 4-1.

Their definition is close to that popularized by Don Berwick and his colleagues, who defined population health as one angle of the "triple aim" (covered in the next chapter). It includes (1) disease burden (ie, incidence and/or prevalence of major chronic conditions); (2) health outcomes (eg, mortality, health and functional status, and health life expectancy); and (3) behavioral and physiological factors that affect both (1) and (2).[2]

Following the approach taken by Kindig and Stoddart, this chapter summarizes the evidence base on the health status indicators of the US population (including disease burden, chronic illness prevalence, functional status, and life expectancy), the distribution (including disparities) of health outcomes across the population, and the drivers of health status (behavioral factors, physiological factors, environmental factors, genetic factors). It then reviews some of the approaches that have been taken to managing population health.

## HEALTH DISPARITIES IN THE US POPULATION: ACCESS, UTILIZATION, AND HEALTH STATUS[3]

### There Is Good News and Bad News

Since the passage of the Patient Protection and Affordable Care Act (PPACA, also known as "Obamacare") in 2010, all racial and ethnic groups have experienced improvements in health coverage, access, and utilization compared to prior to the PPACA (Figure 4-2).[4] Hispanics and Blacks experienced improvements in the largest number of coverage, access, and utilization measures tracked by the Kaiser Family Foundation.[5] While these improvements helped narrow some disparities in health coverage, access, and utilization, nonelderly Blacks and Hispanics continued to fare worse than Whites across most examined measures after PPACA (Figure 4-3). Nonelderly Asians generally fared similar to Whites across measures. Across racial and ethnic groups, most measures of health status remained stable or improved compared to prior to the PPACA (see Figure 4-3).

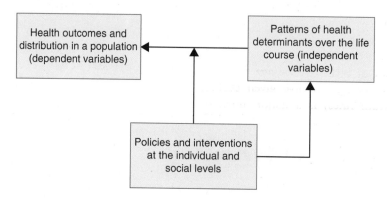

**Figure 4-1** • Population Health.

NUMBER OF MEASURES THAT IMPROVED, DID NOT CHANGE, OR GOT WORSE COMPARED TO BEFORE IMPLEMENTATION OF THE AFFORDABLE CARE ACT:

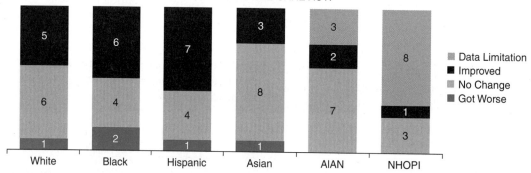

Note: Most measures compare data between 2013 and 2017; some use different years due to data availability. "Improved" or "Got Worse" indicates a statistically significant difference between years at the $p$ <0.05 level. "No change" indicates no statistically significant difference. "Data limitation" indicates no separate data for a racial/ethnic group, insufficient data for a reliable estimate, or comparisons not possible due to overlapping samples. AIAN refers to American Indians and Alaska Natives. NHOPI refers to Native Hawaiians and Other Pacific Islanders. Persons of Hispanic origin may be of any race but are categorized as Hispanic for this analysis; other groups are non-Hispanic.

**Figure 4-2** • Changes in Health Coverage, Access, and Use Since Implementation of the Affordable Care Act.

NUMBER OF MEASURES THAT IMPROVED, DID NOT CHANGE, OR GOT WORSE COMPARED TO BEFORE IMPLEMENTATION OF THE AFFORDABLE CARE ACT:

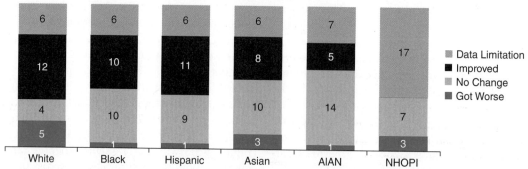

Note: Most measures compare data between 2013 and 2017; some use different years due to data availability. "Improved" or "Got Worse" indicates a statistically significant difference between years at the $p$ <0.05 level. "No change" indicates no statistically significant difference. "Data limitation" indicates no separate data for a racial/ethnic group, insufficient data for a reliable estimate, or comparisons not possible due to changes in measures or overlapping samples. AIAN refers to American Indians and Alaska Natives. NHOPI refers to Native Hawaiians and Other Pacific Islanders. Persons of Hispanic origin may be of any race but are categorized as Hispanic for this analysis; other groups are non-Hispanic.

**Figure 4-3** • Changes in Measures of Health Status Since Implementation of the Affordable Care Act.

## Health Status Indicators

### Life Expectancy

Life expectancy at birth (ie, the age to which a newborn is expected to live given current age-specific death rates) is a major indicator used to compare the health of countries. Life expectancy for the US population was 78.6 years in 2017, just 0.5 years higher than in 2007. Despite the slight rise over this 10-year period, life expectancy has decreased in recent years, falling 0.2 years between 2014 and 2015, with no change between 2015 and 2016, and then falling another 0.1 years between 2016 and 2017. The decline has been driven by increased mortality from several leading causes of death covered in Chapter 26, including injuries, suicide, and Alzheimer's disease, particularly among middle-aged White males with only high school education or less.[6]

Life expectancy and the gains or declines in life expectancy over time differ across gender and racial groups. Females exhibit longer life expectancy than males (81.1 vs 76.1 years in 2017) and did not experience the same decline in life expectancy as did males during the 2007 to 2017 period. Hispanics have higher life expectancy (81.8 years) than Whites (78.5 years) and Blacks (74.9 years). Both Hispanics and Blacks experienced larger gains in life expectancy during 2007 to 2017 (1.1 and 1.4 years, respectively) compared to Whites (0.1 years).

### Infant Mortality

Infant mortality is defined as the death of a baby before his or her first birthday. Infant mortality rate is considered a measure of the health status of a population because it can reflect living conditions, illness rates, access to healthcare, and maternal health. Although the rate has decreased sharply over the past 70 years, disparities remain according to race, socioeconomic status, and geography. Moreover, the United States typically compares unfavorably with other countries.

In 2017, the infant mortality rate was 5.79 deaths per 1,000 live births, which represented a 14% decline since 2007. However, although the rate declined across most racial groups, it remained much higher among Blacks and Native Americans. In 2017, the 5 leading causes of infant deaths were congenital malformations (119.2 infant deaths per 100,000 live births), preterm births and low birthweight (97.5), sudden infant death syndrome (35.3), maternal complications of pregnancy (37.2), and unintentional injuries (34.1).

### Mortality Rates

Death rates are an important summary measure of population health. Chapter 26 lists the top 10 causes of death in the United States, which have generally declined over the past decade. Death rates are often age-adjusted to remove the effects of changing age distributions over time or across population groups. The age-adjusted all-cause death rate was 731.9 deaths per 100,000 population in 2017, down from 775.3 in 2007. In 2017, the age-adjusted all-cause death rate among males was 864.5 deaths per 100,000 population, which represented a 6% decline since 2007. Females experienced a similar 6% decline but exhibited a much lower mortality rate in 2017 (619.7 deaths). Death rates were higher among males than females for all the selected causes of death except Alzheimer's disease, for which rates were lower among males.

One exception to the mortality decline statistics is death from drug overdose. From 2007 to 2017, the age-adjusted death rate for drug overdose increased from 11.9 to 21.7 deaths per 100,000. Drug overdose death rates were higher among males than among females throughout the period for all age groups, except for those aged 65 and older. Another exception is injuries. The age-adjusted death rate was stable for both genders from 2007 to 2013, but then increased for both genders from 2013 to 2017 (7.2% annually for males, 5.0% annually for females). The same pattern was observed for Alzheimer's disease for both genders. Another exception to the general decline in mortality is the rise in deaths from the COVID-19 virus in 2020. It is too early to discern any trend with the virus.

### Obesity

Obesity rates in the US population are high and rising. Among children and adolescents, excess body weight is associated with excess morbidity during childhood and obesity in adulthood. Children and adolescents with obesity are at higher risk of having other chronic health conditions, such as asthma, orthopedic joint problems, and type 2 diabetes. From the turn of the millennium to 2015-2016, obesity among males aged 2 to 19 increased from 14.0% to 19.1%, whereas obesity among females increased from 13.8% to 17.8%. In 2015-2016, 18.5% of children and adolescents were obese; there were no observed gender differences in obesity in this population.

Adult obesity (body mass index of ≥35.0) is also associated with excess morbidity, such as hypertension, high cholesterol, type 2 diabetes, and other conditions. Higher levels of obesity are correlated with increased mortality. During the 2000 to 2016 period, the age-adjusted prevalence of obesity increased from 27.4% to 38.1% among men and from 33.3% to 41.2% among women.

## Asthma

Asthma is a chronic lung disease that inflames and narrows the airways, causing recurring periods of wheezing, tightness in the chest, shortness of breath, and coughing. Asthmatic children are at increased risk of emergency department visits and hospitalizations. Those with continued, uncontrolled symptoms are at risk of activity limitation, decreased quality of life, and chronic obstructive pulmonary disease as adults. From 2007 to 2017, the prevalence of asthma among children under 18 decreased by an average of 0.1 percentage points per year, from 9.1% to 8.4%. Black children had a higher prevalence of asthma (12.6% in 2017) compared with Hispanics (7.7%) and Whites (7.7%) throughout this period.

## Diabetes

Diabetes is a chronic disease that affects the body's ability to produce and use insulin, a hormone that helps maintain blood sugar levels. High blood sugar levels can lead to long-term complications including heart disease, loss of vision, and kidney disease. In 2017, diabetes was the seventh leading cause of death in the United States. The age-adjusted prevalence of total diabetes (diagnosed and undiagnosed) among adults aged 20 or older increased from 10.0% in 2000 to 14.7% in 2016. The increase was driven by an increase in physician-diagnosed diabetes. There was no clear trend in the age-adjusted prevalence of undiagnosed diabetes throughout this period (4.7%). Older adults are more likely than younger adults to have diabetes. Diabetes prevalence ranged from 28.2%

among adults aged 65 and older, to 21.9% among adults aged 45 to 64, and to 5.6% among adults aged 20 to 44. The adult diabetes rate was higher among Blacks (11%) compared to Hispanics (9%) and Whites (7%).

## Hypertension

Hypertension is defined as having measured high blood pressure[7] or currently taking antihypertensive medication. Hypertension is a risk factor for cardiovascular disease, stroke, kidney disease, and other health conditions and is a leading preventable cause of cardiovascular deaths. The 2016 prevalence rate of hypertension was 31.3% among men and 28.7% among women. From 2000 to 2016, the age-adjusted prevalence of hypertension among men and women aged 20 or older showed no clear trend.

There are gender and age disparities, however, in the likelihood of *uncontrolled* high blood pressure (high blood pressure among those with hypertension). In 2016, among men with hypertension, 73.1% of those aged 20 to 44 had uncontrolled high blood pressure, compared with 50.1% of those aged 45 to 64 and 51.7% of those aged 65 or older. By contrast, uncontrolled high blood pressure was more likely among women with hypertension aged 65 or older (55.8%) compared with women aged 20 to 44 (37.9%) and aged 45 to 64 (42.1%). Although the percentage of uncontrolled high blood pressure was similar for men and women with hypertension aged 45 to 64 and 65 or older, men aged 20 to 44 with hypertension were more likely to have uncontrolled high blood pressure (73.1%) than women aged 20 to 44 (37.9%).

## Functional Status

Functional limitations reflect reported levels of difficulty (no difficulty, some difficulty, a lot of difficulty, or cannot do at all/unable to do) in 6 domains: seeing, hearing, mobility, communication, cognition, and self-care. Adults who report having "some difficulty" or "a lot of difficulty or cannot do at all" in at least 1 domain are classified as having difficulty in functioning. Such limitations are often caused by physical or mental impairments; in turn, they can result in lower educational attainment, higher unemployment, and reduced participation in other daily activities.

The age-adjusted percentage of adults aged 18 to 64 who report having "a lot of difficulty or cannot do at all" in at least 1 domain rose an average of 0.3 percentage points annually from 2010 to 2014, and then decreased by an average of 0.3 percentage points annually from 2014 to 2017. From 2010 to 2017, the age-adjusted percentage of adults aged 18 to 64 who reported having "some difficulty" in at least 1 domain rose an average of 0.3 percentage points annually. From 2010 to 2017, adults aged 18 to 64 were less likely to report having any difficulty than adults aged 65 or older. In 2017, 33.7% of adults aged 18 to 64 reported having a difficulty, 27.8% reported "some difficulty," and 5.9% reported having "a lot of difficulty or cannot do at all." From 2010 to 2017, the age-adjusted percentage of adults aged 65 or older reporting "some difficulty" or "a lot of difficulty or cannot do at all" showed no clear trend. In 2017, 61.1% of adults aged 65 or older reported having a difficulty, 41.6% reported "some difficulty," and 19.5% reported "a lot of difficulty or cannot do at all."

Among racial groups, Whites are more likely to report physical limitations (33%) compared to both Blacks (30%) and Hispanics (23%). The percentages reporting 14 or more "physically unhealthy" days are comparable across all 3 groups (11%-12%).[8]

## Health Access Indicators

### Health Insurance Coverage Among Children

Children and adolescents require regular, ongoing preventive care (eg, vaccinations and screenings), injury care, health and developmental guidance, and treatment of acute and chronic conditions. In recent decades, due to coverage expansions in Medicaid (see Chapter 19), children have enjoyed higher levels of insurance coverage than adults. Children with health insurance are more likely to have access to healthcare, a usual source of care, and a recent healthcare visit than those who are uninsured.

The percentage of children under age 18 years who were uninsured decreased by an average of 0.5 percentage points annually from 2007 to 2015 and then stabilized at 5.0% from 2015 to 2017 (5.0%). In 2018, 36.0% of children were covered by Medicaid; 54.7% of children had private coverage. In 2017, Hispanic children were more likely (7.7%) to be uninsured compared to Whites (4.1%), Blacks (4.0%), and Asians (3.8%). In 2017, White (69.0%) and Asian (70.8%) children were much more likely to have private insurance coverage relative to Blacks (36.3%) and Hispanics (34.8%). Conversely, Blacks (56.1%) and Hispanics (55.1%) were twice as likely to have Medicaid coverage as Whites (23.8%) and Asians (23.6%).

### Health Insurance Coverage Among Adults

Research shows that insurance coverage is associated with lower mortality rates and improved health outcomes, especially among those with chronic illnesses. Adults lacking insurance are more likely to delay or not receive needed medical care due to cost than those who are covered. The percentage of adults aged 18 to 64 lacking insurance increased by an average of almost 0.5% annually from 2007 to 2010, but then decreased by an average of 3.0% points annually from 2010 to 2015, due to passage of the PPACA. By 2018, 13.3% of adults were uninsured. The percentage of adults aged 18 to 64 with private insurance fell by an average of 1.3% annually from 2007 to 2010, and then rose by an average of 1.1% annually to 69.6% by 2017, reaching 68.9% in 2018. Due to PPACA, Medicaid coverage increased an average of 0.6% annually from 2007 to 2017, reaching 13.2% in 2017 and 12.8% in 2018.

In 2017, 27.5% of Hispanic adults aged 18 to 64 were uninsured, compared to 7.4% of Asians, 8.5% of Whites, and 14% of Blacks. By contrast, Whites (77.5%) and Asians (77.6%) were more likely to have private insurance relative to Hispanics (50.5%) and Blacks (57.5%). In 2017, White (9.4%) and Asian (12.2%) adults were less likely to be covered by Medicaid than Blacks (22.3%) and Hispanics (18.9%).

### Unmet Clinical Needs Due to Cost of Care

Failure to obtain needed healthcare can lead to delays in diagnosis or treatment and, as a consequence, poorer health outcomes. Underuse of medications is associated with poorer health, increased cardiovascular events, and increased use of healthcare services. From 2007 to 2017, lower-income adults aged 18 to 64 were more likely to delay or not receive needed care due to cost than those with higher incomes. Nevertheless, the percentage of those living below the federal poverty level (FPL)[9] with an unmet medical need due to cost decreased from 20.8% to 16.2% in 2017. For those living at 100% to 199% of FPL, the percentage with unmet need fell nearly the same amount to 15.3% by 2017. Adults living at 200% to 399% of FPL experienced a smaller decline in unmet need, falling to 11.6% in 2017. All of these declines occurred after passage of the PPACA. There was no change in the percentage with unmet medical needs among adults at or above 400% of the FPL.

From 2007 to 2017, adults aged 18 to 64 with lower incomes were less likely to receive needed prescription drugs due to cost than those with higher incomes. Nevertheless, among those living below the FPL, the percentage with unmet prescription drug need fell from 18.8% in 2007 to 11.9% in 2017, with improvements occurring after PPACA. For adults living at 100% to 199% of FPL, the percentage not receiving needed drugs fell from 17.2% in 2007 to 11.6% in 2017. For adults living at 200% to 399% of FPL, the percentage fell less, from 10.6% in 2007 to 7.0% in 2017. There was little change among adults at or above 400% of FPL.

## Healthcare Service Utilization Indicators[10]

### Vaccinations

Vaccination coverage is defined as the estimated percentage of the population who have received specific vaccines. The Advisory Committee on Immunization Practices recommends a series of vaccines for children aged 19 to 35 months. A summary index, the "combined 7-vaccine series," indicates whether children met the recommendations for 7 vaccinations.[11] In 2017, 70.4% of children had received the combined series, up from 56.6% in 2010. Black children were less likely to have received the series (66.5%) than Whites (71.5%); vaccination coverage for children in other racial groups did not differ significantly from Whites. Children living in nonmetropolitan areas (66.8%) were less likely to have received the series compared with those living in metro cities (71.9%). Vaccination coverage also varied by insurance status. Uninsured children were less likely to have received the series relative to those covered by private insurance (76.0%) or Medicaid (66.5%). Among insured children, vaccination coverage

was higher among those with private insurance (76.0%) than those with Medicaid (66.5%).

## Prescription Drugs

Prescription drugs help to reduce mortality, control disease, and prevent or delay the onset of chronic disease and disability. Greater use of prescription drugs is associated with an aging population, the rise in chronic illness, the availability of new prescription drugs, and enhancements to prescription drug coverage (eg, the Medicare Part D program; see Chapter 18). At the same time, increased use of prescription drugs has raised concerns about misuse (eg, overprescribing of antibiotics to treat viral infections) and adverse events resulting from inappropriate prescribing to the elderly.

The age-adjusted percentage of Americans taking 5 or more prescription drugs in the past 30 days increased from 6.5% in 2000 to 10.0% in 2004 and then stabilized at 11.0% between 2004 and 2016. The percentage who took 1 to 4 prescription drugs in the past 30 days decreased from 37.5% in 2000 to 34.4% by 2016. The percentage who took no drugs in the past 30 days decreased from 56.0% in 2000 to 52.1% in 2008 and then increased to 54.7% by 2016.

In 2016, 12.5% of children under age 18 took no prescription drugs in the past 30 days, compared with nearly 80% of adults aged 65 or older. Among adults, the percentage taking 5 or more drugs in the past 30 days increased from 3.9% (age 18-44) to 19.1% (age 45-64) to 39.8% (age ≥65).

## DISPARITIES IN HEALTH STATUS: UNITED STATES VERSUS THE WORLD

In 2013, the Institute of Medicine (IOM) published a report comparing the health status of the United States with that of 17 other Western nations. Their conclusions were shocking: the United States performed relatively poorly in 9 domains of health:

1. **Adverse birth outcomes:** For decades, the United States has had the highest infant mortality rate and also ranked poorly on other birth outcomes (low birthweight). American children are less likely to live to age 5 than children in other high-income countries.

2. **Injuries and homicides:** Deaths from motor vehicle crashes, non–transportation-related injuries, and violence occur at much higher rates in the United States and are a leading cause of death in children, adolescents, and young adults. Since the 1950s, US adolescents and young adults have died at higher rates from traffic accidents and homicide than their counterparts in other countries.

3. **Adolescent pregnancy and sexually transmitted infections:** Since the 1990s, US adolescents have had the highest rate of pregnancies and are more likely to acquire sexually transmitted infections.

4. **HIV and AIDS:** The United States has the second highest prevalence of HIV infection among Western countries and the highest incidence of AIDS.

5. **Drug-related mortality:** Americans lose more years of life to alcohol and other drugs than people in other countries, even when deaths from drunk driving are excluded.

6. **Obesity and diabetes:** For decades, the United States has had the highest obesity rate. High prevalence rates for obesity are seen in US children and in every age group thereafter. From age 20 onward, US adults have among the highest prevalence rates of diabetes.

7. **Heart disease:** The US death rate from ischemic heart disease is the second highest among peer countries. Americans reach age 50 with a less favorable cardiovascular risk profile; adults aged 50 or older are more likely to develop and die from cardiovascular disease than are older adults in other countries.

8. **Chronic lung disease:** Lung disease is more prevalent and associated with higher mortality in the United States than in the United Kingdom and other European countries.

9. **Disability:** Older US adults report a higher prevalence of arthritis and activity limitations than their counterparts in other countries.

According to the IOM report, several of these problems occur disproportionately among younger Americans. Deaths that occur before age 50 are responsible for about two-thirds of the difference in life expectancy between males in the United States and other countries and about one-third of the difference for females. Since 1980, the United States has had the first or second lowest probability of surviving to age 50 among 17 peer countries. Americans who do reach age 50 do so in poorer health and, as older adults, face greater morbidity and mortality from chronic diseases that arise from risk factors established earlier in life.

The "US health disadvantage" is more pronounced among socioeconomically disadvantaged groups, but even advantaged Americans fare worse than their counterparts in other countries. Americans with healthy behaviors or those who are White, insured, college educated, or in upper-income groups appear to be in worse health than those from other countries.

## DRIVERS OF HEALTH STATUS

According to the IOM report, there is no single or simple explanation for the US health disadvantage. Instead, it is driven by multiple factors that are now summarized by the phrase "population health." To quote the IOM report (p. 5):

> The U.S. health disadvantage probably has multiple explanations, some of which may be causally interconnected, such as unemployment and a lack of health insurance. Other explanations may share antecedents, especially those rooted in social inequality. Still others may have no obvious relationship, as in the very distinct causes of high rates of obesity and traffic fatalities. The relationships between some factors may develop over time, or even over a person's entire life course, as when poor social conditions during childhood precipitate a chain of adverse life events. Turmoil and risk-taking in adolescence can lead to subsequent setbacks in education or employment, fomenting life-long financial instability or other stresses that inhibit healthy life-styles or access to health care. In some cases, the explanation may simply be that the United States is at the leading edge of global trends that other high-income countries will follow, such as smoking and obesity.

In general, the IOM report concludes that the US health disadvantage is long-standing and pervasive across population segments and measures of health status and does not seem to be simply a function of uninsurance or poverty (although these are important factors). Instead, the drivers are multiple and located in diverse areas such as public health, medical care systems, individual behaviors, socioeconomic factors (education, income), and environmental factors. Many of these drivers interact with one another; they do not exert their influences in isolation of one another. Moreover, the major conclusion is that "health" is not determined solely or heavily by the healthcare system. Instead, health reflects the behavioral and biological consequences of income, occupation, education, and social and physical environments, which themselves are the product of public and private sector policies. Figure 4-4 portrays the IOM's ecological framework for explaining population health.

Other chapters in this book outline the role of public health and various sectors in the medical care system. Although the United States has a more fragmented public health sector than other countries, and although the United States fares poorly compared to other countries on some healthcare system indicators that may be important for health outcomes (eg, practicing

physicians per capita, access to primary care), the causal linkage between these sectors and health outcomes is modest at best (and often murky). As the IOM report notes, there is no consistent evidence that countries with better health outcomes have higher-performing healthcare systems. The sections that follow briefly review the role of the other factors in this ecological framework.

## Individual Behaviors

Individual health behaviors are the major contributor to the global burden of disease, especially in wealthier countries that have undergone the "epidemiologic transition" from acute care illness to chronic illness. Researchers long ago identified tobacco use, diet, physical inactivity, and other personal behaviors as the leading killers in the modern age.[12] These behaviors contribute significantly to each of the 9 domains of the US health disadvantage identified earlier. Smoking contributes to adverse birth outcomes, heart disease, and chronic pulmonary disease; unhealthy diet and low physical activity contribute to higher rates of obesity and diabetes; alcohol consumption, other drug use, and unsafe sexual practices

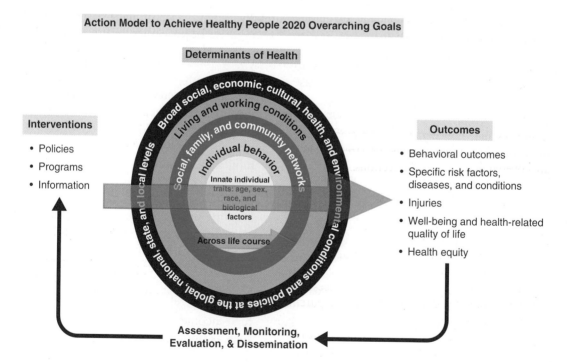

**Figure 4-4** • The Ecology of Population Health. (Reproduced from New York Department of Health. Action Model to Achieve Healthy People 2020 Goals. https://www.health.ny.gov/statistics/chac/improvement/hp2020_action_model.htm.)

contribute to drug-related mortality, HIV/AIDS, sexually transmitted infections, and adolescent pregnancies; substance abuse contributes to injuries (unintentional and intentional), as does the prevalence of firearms.

These conditions are causally interconnected. For example, obesity at a younger age can later on lead to diabetes and heart disease. Thus, health behaviors may play a critical role over the course of one's life in promoting health status or health disadvantage. However, whether or not such health behaviors in the United States differ significantly from other countries and explain the US health disadvantage cannot be determined without better cross-national data; research is needed to link specific behaviors with specific health status outcomes. Nevertheless, the IOM report concludes that although "no single behavior can explain the U.S. health disadvantage, the high prevalence of multiple unhealthy behaviors in the United States may play a large role."[13]

## Social Determinants

There is a growing recognition that health is largely driven by "social determinants." Such factors not only underlie disparities in health status in the United States, but may also explain the disparities between the United States and other countries. These determinants can be classified as *individual-level* characteristics (eg, income, wealth, household composition, education, occupation, social mobility, stressful events, and life circumstances linked to one's racial or ethnic background) and *community-level* characteristics (eg, housing, transportation, neighborhoods, and other sources of stress). These are covered in the following sections.

### Individual-Level Characteristics

At the same time that the United States began to diverge from other countries in terms of life expectancy, it also experienced a host of deteriorating social conditions. These included income inequality, affordable and accessible education, poverty, child poverty, single-parent households, divorce, and incarceration. There is no definitive evidence of causality here, but the data are both suggestive and alarming. Here are the conclusions reached by the IOM:

- Income inequality in a society has repeatedly been shown to be inversely associated with good health, but there is controversy about the health effects of relative income inequality apart from the effects of absolute poverty or economic hardship.
- Education and health outcomes are causally linked, and the linkages may be both direct and indirect. Education can improve one's health knowledge and coping skills and can also lead to better employment, health insurance coverage, and wealth.
- Employment positively influences health via income levels and social mobility, as well as negatively via exposure to toxic work environments and occupational injuries.
- Household composition (eg, low-income, single-parent families) can negatively impact health via poverty, food insecurity and nutrition, unstable housing, and adolescent pregnancy.
- Racial minorities may suffer health deficits from discrimination, such as reduced employment opportunities, material deprivations, and psychological stress. Such stressors can lead to destructive behaviors like smoking and substance abuse.

All of these factors play a role but are not totally determinative of the US health disadvantage. As noted earlier, health status problems exist at all socioeconomic levels in the United States and among all segments of the population. It is still unclear whether these co-occurring social trends, individually or in combination, are causally linked to the US health disadvantage.

### Community-Level Characteristics

#### Physical Environment
Physical environmental factors that impact health include exposure to harmful substances (eg, air pollution or proximity to toxic sites), access to various health-related resources (eg, healthy or unhealthy foods, recreational resources, medical care), and community design and the "built environment" (eg, land-use mix, street connectivity, transportation systems). One's physical working conditions can also impact health via exposure to dangerous substances (eg, lead, asbestos, mercury), the physical demands of work (eg, carrying heavy loads), and work safety conditions. Moreover, stressful

psychosocial work environments and "job strain" (high external demands on a worker with low levels of control) can lead to reduced levels of self-reported health.

### Social Environment

Social environmental factors that impact health include (1) general issues dealing with safety, violence, and social disorder; and (2) specific issues such as social connections, social participation, social cohesion, social capital, and the "collective efficacy" of the neighborhood environment. The former affect physical health; the latter appear to promote both mental and physical health. Social environment characteristics include solitary living, narrowing social networks, technology, and social media use, which can interact with one another. Recent evidence suggests that perceived social isolation and loneliness may harm health status. Such feelings can result from many factors, including divorce, death of a loved one, family separation, serious injury in the family, serious health problems, or a change in financial situation.

## Genetic Factors

Although many factors drive health status and morbidity, family history can be a strong risk factor for diseases such as cancer, cardiovascular disease, diabetes, autoimmune disorders, and psychiatric illness. A person's inherited genetic makeup can predispose one to certain types of cancer (eg, the role of the *BRCA* gene in breast cancer). One also inherits a vast array of cultural and socioeconomic experiences from their family, which can predict an individual's disease risk. In addition to genetic factors, there are also interactions between genes and environmental factors. For example, studies have found that genetic mutations are associated with differential response to cigarette smoke and its association with lung cancer.

## The Drivers, Overall

All of the factors reviewed earlier have a bearing on the health status of the population. What is not as well known is whether the disparities in health status between the United States and the rest of the Western world can be attributed to differences in these factors. To some degree, this is an issue in ecological analysis: That is, do relationships at one level of analysis hold at a higher, more aggregated level of analysis? To some degree, this is an issue in measurement and data collection.

To summarize the IOM report, current comparisons in the performance of health systems (that pertain to *medical care factors*) remain rudimentary. Validated indicators exist for delivery of specific performance measures but not for other dimensions of care important to outcomes. The only currently available, systematic data to compare the quality of health care in countries come from surveys of 7 to 11 countries conducted by the Commonwealth Fund. Moreover, any effort to compare the medical and public health systems across countries is confronted by the lack of established, validated measures of access or quality. Another problem is the availability of clearly defined and consistent data across countries on (1) *personal behaviors* (eg, physical activity, diet, sexual practices, drinking, driving practices, and violence), (2) *demographic and socioeconomic characteristics* (eg, race and ethnicity, income) that would facilitate valid cross-national comparisons (eg, comparing people at a given income level), (3) *physical environment characteristics* that allow comparisons of toxic exposure or built environments, and (4) *social environment characteristics* to compare countries in terms of social capital and social cohesion.

Overall, researchers recognize that all of these factors are associated with one's health status. However, one needs to be careful to identify the specific measures of health status (or health outcomes) of which one is speaking. The various determinants of health status may play very different roles (with very different weights in importance) in fostering different measures of health. For any given measure of health status, they may also play very different roles depending on the disparity one is trying to address (eg, urban vs rural, White vs non-White). One must also be careful to specify whether one is trying to explain cross-sectional variations (disparities) in health status or longer-term variations in health status. Economists suggest that social factors (eg, income, education, housing, nutrition) may be more important explanations in cross-sectional analyses or short-term studies, whereas advances in medical science and technology (ie, the medical care system) may be more important explanations longitudinally.[14] Finally, one must be cognizant that the different social factors are likely to be highly intercorrelated (eg, income and education), such that parsing their respective contributions may be difficult.

## THE BURDEN OF CHRONIC ILLNESS

The 20th century witnessed the supplanting of acute illness by chronic illness. The 2 types of illness are different but related. Acute conditions are severe, sudden in onset, and (when treated) resolved in the short term. Chronic conditions take a long time to develop, typically worsen over time, and can last months, years, or a lifetime, with little resolution despite medical treatment. Some chronic conditions (osteoporosis)

may cause an acute condition (broken bone); some acute conditions (eg, first acute asthma attack) may lead to a chronic condition if left untreated.

In 2014, 60% of the US adult population had at least 1 chronic condition; 42% had 2 or more such conditions.[15] The most prevalent of these conditions are presented in Figure 4-5. The presence of multiple chronic conditions is greatest among older adults. Women are also more likely than men to have multiple chronic conditions; the 2 most prevalent conditions among both genders are hypertension and lipid disorders. Whites are more likely than other racial and ethnic groups to have multiple chronic conditions. The latter may reflect differential access

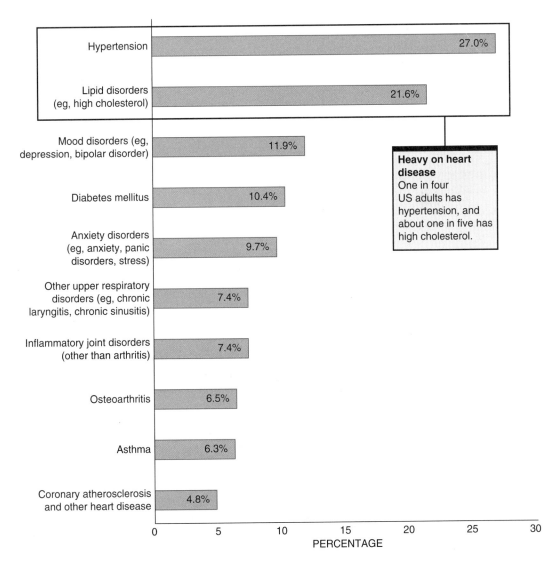

**Figure 4-5 •** Top 10 Chronic Conditions in 2014. (Source: Christine Buttorff, Teague Ruder, and Melissa Bauman, *Multiple Chronic Conditions in the United States*. Santa Monica, CA: RAND Corporation, 2017. https://www.rand.org/pubs/tools/TL221.html. Reproduced with permission from RAND Corporation.)

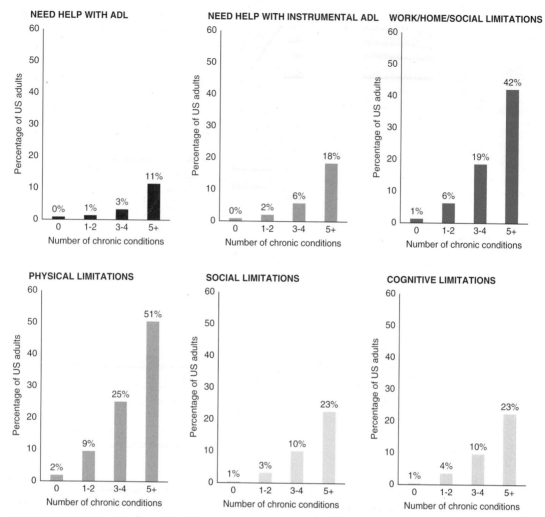

NOTES: ADL include such basic functions as being able to bathe, dress, eat, go to the bathroom, or do light activity—for example, walking up a flight of stairs. Instrumental ADL include light housework, preparing meals, paying bills, and shopping. We used the composite variables constructed in MEPS for the ADL and IADL, which indicate whether a person reported needing supervision to complete at least one ADL or instrumental ADL activity. A work/school/home limitation is defined as an impairment or a physical or mental health problem that limits a person's ability to work at a job, do housework, or go to school. A physical limitation is defined as having difficulties walking, climbing stairs, grasping objects, bending, or standing for long periods of time. MEPS defines social limitations as whether a person has trouble participating in social or family activities because of a physical or cognitive impairment. A cognitive limitation exists if the person has trouble with memory, is easily confused, has trouble making decisions, or needs to be supervised for his or her own safety.

**Figure 4-6** • Chronic Conditions and Limitations. (Source: Christine Buttorff, Teague Ruder, and Melissa Bauman, *Multiple Chronic Conditions in the United States.* Santa Monica, CA: RAND Corporation, 2017. https://www.rand.org/pubs/tools/TL221.html. Reproduced with permission from RAND Corporation.)

to care. Moreover, those with multiple chronic conditions are more likely to report more limitations in their functional, social, and cognitive status (Figure 4-6).

People with multiple chronic conditions are sometimes referred to as *poly-chronics.* Who are these individuals? They may consist of the following (this list is not encyclopedic): the elderly with multiple functional impairments, those with serious congenital anomalies, the morbidly obese, paraplegics and quadriplegics, trauma victims, cancer patients, and those with nonrecurring crises.

Data on the healthcare expenditures of the poly-chronics show that they account for the majority of US healthcare spending. A small proportion (12%) of poly-chronics—those with 5 or more chronic conditions—accounts for 41% of spending. Conversely, the 40% of the US population that does not have any chronic conditions accounts for only 10% of spending (Figure 4-7). This distribution seems to hold across segments of the insured population (commercially insured, Medicare beneficiaries, Medicaid beneficiaries). Those with 5 or more chronic conditions spend

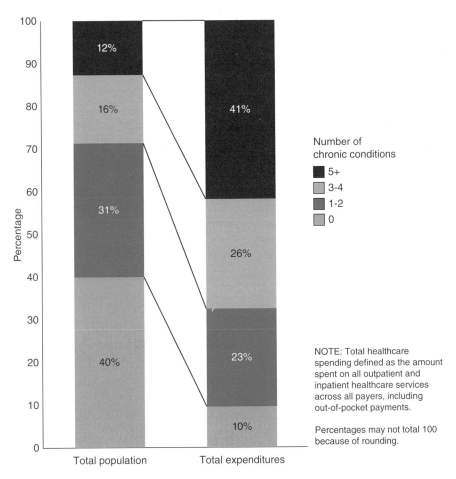

**Figure 4-7** • Poly-Chronics and Health Expenditures. (Source: Christine Buttorff, Teague Ruder, and Melissa Bauman, *Multiple Chronic Conditions in the United States*. Santa Monica, CA: RAND Corporation, 2017. https://www .rand.org/pubs/tools/TL221.html. Reproduced with permission from RAND Corporation.)

14 times more than those without any chronic issues; such spending is distributed across inpatient, outpatient, and drug utilization (Figure 4-8).

## POPULATION HEALTH MANAGEMENT

Healthcare providers and insurers (and, to some extent, self-insured employers) are all concerned with managing the utilization, spending, and health status of their populations. Thus, they are all involved in some way with population health. They are particularly interested in those who are heavy utilizers, since they account for more of the expenditures than others. As noted earlier, these high utilizers tend to have a lot of chronic conditions, which makes the management of their conditions challenging. Several

notable approaches are described in the following sections.

### Social Spending

Researchers at Yale University called attention to 2 types of spending that affect health status: medical care expenditures and social services expenditures.[16] Social services include education, transportation, environment, public safety, housing, corrections, income support, and public health. Globally, the United States spends more on medical care than it does on social services. The researchers found that when overall spending is adjusted for, countries with higher social services spending relative to medical spending had significantly better health outcomes. For example, in the United States, about $0.90 is spent on social services for every $1.00 spent on medical care; in Organisation for

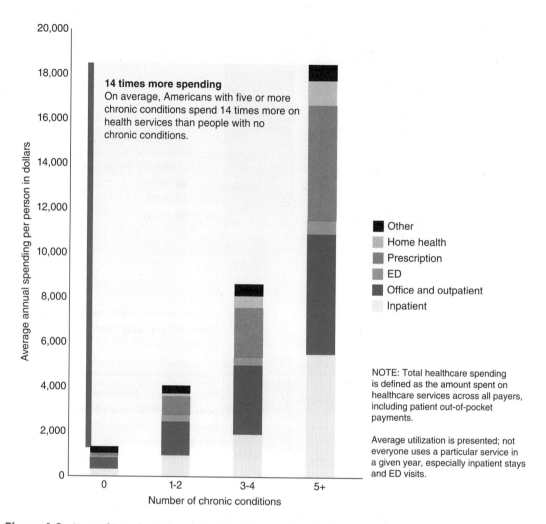

Figure 4-8 • Areas of Spending Among the Poly-Chronics. (Source: Christine Buttorff, Teague Ruder, and Melissa Bauman, *Multiple Chronic Conditions in the United States.* Santa Monica, CA: RAND Corporation, 2017. https://www.rand.org/pubs/tools/TL221.html. Reproduced with permission from RAND Corporation.)

Economic Co-operation and Development countries, about $2.00 is spent on social services for every $1.00 spent on medical care. The researchers also found that, within the United States, states that devoted proportionately more spending to social services and public health activities than to medical care (measured by the sum of Medicare and Medicaid spending) had significantly better health outcomes on 7 metrics: adult obesity, asthma, mentally unhealthy days, days with activity limitations, and mortality rates for 3 conditions (lung cancer, acute myocardial infarction, and type 2 diabetes).

However, when one studies social spending as a percentage of gross domestic product, the United States is on a par with other countries.[17] What differs between countries is the allocation of that spending across different social programs that support people at different stages of life (childhood, adulthood, and old age). The allocation chosen can impact population health because investments in younger populations may have greater marginal health benefits than investments in older populations. Research shows that the United States is an outlier on social spending for benefits to older populations (pensions, home help, and residential services) while spending relatively less on services benefitting younger populations (early childhood education, parental leave, and child allowances).

Such findings have led researchers to pose the question: If we spend more on social services, can we lower healthcare spending? The answer is neither simple nor clear-cut. Research shows that countries with high levels of social spending do not necessarily have lower levels of medical care spending.[18] In fact, the levels of spending in these 2 areas are positively correlated: Countries that increase their spending on one tend to increase their spending on the other. Moreover, the Yale researchers found that the United States spends about the same proportion of its gross domestic product on medical and social services as do most developed countries. It may be the case that there are trade-offs in spending in these 2 areas.

Moreover, although the ratio of social to medical spending is an attractive means to explain disparities in health outcomes across countries, we do not know whether and how such differences matter at the patient level.[19] Another important issue is that spending on social services (like public health, see Chapter 26) occurs largely at the state level in the United States. It is not clear that states have the capacity to invest more in such services beyond what they invest in their Medicaid programs (see Chapter 19).

## "The Hot Spotters"

In a famous article in *The New Yorker*, Atul Gawande described a program developed by the Camden Coalition of Healthcare Providers to identify patients from hospital admissions data with chronic conditions and complex medical needs.[20] Research suggested that 1% of the 100,000 users of Camden's medical facilities accounted for 30% of its costs. The program used an intensive, face-to-face model of team-based care, patient engagement, and referral management to facilitate the patient's navigation to the appropriate provider and types of care needed. The latter included "social services" that address nonmedical drivers of health status such as housing and food security. According to Gawande:

> The Camden Coalition has been able to measure its long-term effect on its first thirty-six super-utilizers. They averaged sixty-two hospital and E.R. visits per month before joining the program and thirty-seven visits after—a forty-per-cent reduction. Their hospital bills averaged $1.2 million per month before and just over half a million after—a fifty-six-per-cent reduction.

The Coalition's apparent success spawned an accountable care organization (ACO) demonstration project in 2011 that targeted the Medicaid population in New Jersey.

Despite the fanfare, the results have been less than advertised. The New Jersey ACO did not achieve any documented savings. More importantly, a randomized controlled trial of the Camden Coalition model found that it failed to impact hospital readmission rates.[21] The results observed by Gawande have been interpreted as "regression to the mean"—that is, super-utilizers in one period may be more normal utilizers during a subsequent period—a point that the Camden Coalition sponsors failed to consider. These findings have sparked an intense debate and conversation about similar programs to target high-utilizers and to alter the social determinants of health.[22]

## Chronic Care Management Programs

Providers and payers have developed a number of other chronic care management (CCM) programs to coordinate care for the high-cost, chronically ill populations for which they care. Such programs seek to reduce these populations' use of the 2 most expensive services in healthcare: hospital admissions and use of the emergency room. Techniques employed include (1) improved communications among providers and between providers and patients, (2) improved patient self-care, (3) early identification of exacerbations, (4) cycles of patient assessment/planning/implementing/monitoring, (5) disease management programs, and (6) care coordination. Prior research on care coordination and disease management has not found widespread, positive benefits from these CCM programs; typically, the benefits accrue only to small subsets of the patients, namely the high-risk patients.[23] This suggests that CCM programs need to be narrowly targeted rather than bluntly implemented across wide patient populations.

Moreover, CCM programs require other ingredients such as intensive in-person contacts with patients, access to timely information on acute care episodes, close interaction between primary care physicians and care coordinators, and sufficient registered nurse–trained coordinators and staff. For example, successful CCM programs that use "care coordinators" do the following: (1) have frequent face-to-face contact with patients, (2) build strong rapport with patients' physicians through face-to-face contact at hospital or office, (3) use behavior-change techniques to help patients increase adherence to medications and self-care, (4) know when

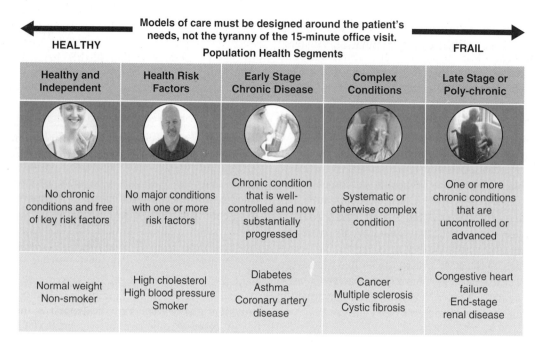

**Figure 4-9** • Population Segmentation Based on Chronic Conditions. (Source: Presentation by Dr. Grace Terrell, *The Power of Primary Care Transformation.* http://www.ehcca.com/presentations/medhomesummit8/terrell_2 .pdf. Used with permission from Oliver Wyman.)

patients are hospitalized and provide support for transition home, (5) act as a communications hub among providers and between patient and providers, and (6) have reliable information about patients' therapy and access to pharmacists or medical director.[24]

## Population Risk Segmentation

A common feature in population health management programs is the stratification or segmentation of their populations by level of health risk. Figures 4-9 and 4-10 illustrate 2 approaches: The first segments the population based on the number of chronic conditions, and the second highlights the different interventions that might be fashioned for each segment.

The Robert Wood Johnson Foundation took a different approach. They segmented the population based on their "culture of health"—that is, their beliefs about (1) the importance of health in daily life and (2) how active the government

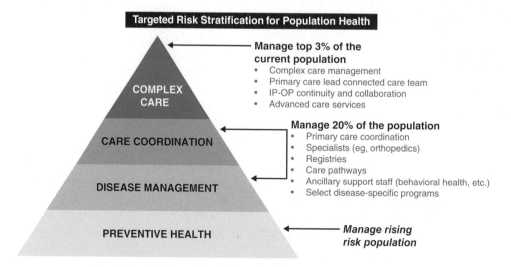

**Figure 4-10** • Targeted Interventions. IP, Inpatient; OP, Outpatient.

should be in health policy.[25] Cross-tabulating these 2 beliefs yielded 6 population clusters, including:

- "Committed activists" high on both dimensions
- "Private-sector champions" high on the first dimension but low on the second
- "Self-reliant individualists" also high on the first dimension but low on the second
- "Equity advocates" low on the first dimension but high on the second
- "Health egalitarians" also low on the first dimension but high on the second
- "Disinterested skeptics" low on both dimensions

The lesson here is that not all population segments can be mobilized, and not all are supportive of population health or the government's role in it.

Other researchers have segmented the population based on 4 levels of "patient activation."[26] This segmentation is important because controlling costs and achieving healthcare quality improvements require the participation of activated and informed consumers (patients). For example, the 4 activation levels exhibit different patterns of association with different, desired health behaviors (eg, take recommended prescription, monitor one's blood pressure). Patients at the highest level of activation have better health outcomes; they also have costs of roughly $2,000 less than those at the lowest activation level. The researchers conclude that some of the healthy behaviors we desire are only practiced by those at the highest activation level. Population health programs may need to focus on those who have higher levels of activation if we are to make progress and see some return on the investments in health. Practitioners may need to use different strategies to target patients at the different activation levels (eg, electronic resources, highly skilled care teams, peer support).[27]

## SUMMARY

One might conclude that in order to have a healthier population, we need to make greater investments in social services and public health, have more robust economic growth, more intact families, greater social cohesion, safer neighborhoods, a cleaner environment, less stressful environments, greater nutrition, healthier personal habits, and access to medical care. Public health would encompass both macro public health projects and micro public health behaviors (which are associated with education and socioeconomic status). Later chapters in this book suggest that key ingredients also include new medical technology and information, as well as the uptake of this technology and information. A more specific recommendation may not be possible.

### QUESTIONS TO PONDER

1. There are disparities in health status (a) between racial and ethnic groups in the United States, and (b) between the United States and other developed countries. Can either set of disparities be eliminated?
2. How might the different drivers of health status—individual behaviors, social determinants, genetic factors—be interrelated?
3. Why is the burden of chronic illness on the rise, both in the United States and in the rest of the world? What are the best ways to address this burden?
4. Given the increased attention paid to population health and its recognized importance, why hasn't the United States invested more in population health? In public health?

## REFERENCES

1. David Kindig and Greg Stoddart. "What Is Population Health?" *Am J Pub Health* 93(3) (2003): 380-383.
2. Donald Berwick, Thomas Nolan, and John Whittington. "The Triple Aim: Care, Health, and Cost," *Health Aff.* 27 (3) (2008): 759-769.
3. This section relies heavily on the following publication: Centers for Disease Control and Prevention (CDC). *Health—United States 2018.* National Center for Health Statistics. (Washington, DC: CDC, 2019).
4. This introductory section is based on: Samantha Artiga and Kendal Orgera. *Key Facts on Health and Health Care by Race and Ethnicity.* Chart Pack. November 2019. Kaiser Family Foundation. Available online: http://files.kff.org/attachment/Chart-Pack-Key-Facts-on-Health-and-Health-Care-by-Race-and-Ethnicity. Accessed on July 21, 2020.

5. For a listing of these measures, see Appendices 1 and 2 in: Samantha Artiga and Kendal Orgera. *Key Facts on Health and Health Care by Race and Ethnicity*. Chart Pack. November 2019. Kaiser Family Foundation. Available online: http://files.kff.org/attachment/Chart-Pack-Key-Facts-on-Health-and-Health-Care-by-Race-and-Ethnicity. Accessed on July 21, 2020.

6. Anne Case and Angus Deaton. "Mortality and Morbidity in the 21st Century." Available online: https://www.brookings.edu/wp-content/uploads/2017/08/casetextsp17bpea.pdf. Accessed on May 15, 2020.

7. High blood pressure is defined as systolic pressure of greater than or equal to 140 mm Hg or diastolic pressure of greater than or equal to 90 mm Hg.

8. Samantha Artiga and Kendal Orgera. *Key Facts on Health and Health Care by Race and Ethnicity*. Chart Pack. November 2019. Kaiser Family Foundation. Available online: http://files.kff.org/attachment/Chart-Pack-Key-Facts-on-Health-and-Health-Care-by-Race-and-Ethnicity. Accessed on July 21, 2020.

9. The Federal Poverty Level (FPL) for 2017 was $12,060 for an individual and $24,600 for a family of 4.

10. Another area of utilization is post-acute care (PAC). PAC providers serve those with chronic conditions and disabilities (see Chapter 11). PAC providers include home healthcare, skilled nursing facilities, hospices, adult day services centers, and residential care communities. Among adults aged 65 and older, home healthcare was the most-used PAC service in 2016, with 3.7 million users, followed by hospice services (1.3 million patients), nursing home residents (1.2 million), residential care community residents (0.8 million), and adult day services (0.2 million). There was little change in the number of users between 2012 and 2016 in each of these categories.

11. These include 4 or more doses of the diphtheria, tetanus toxoids, and pertussis vaccine (DTP), the diphtheria and tetanus toxoids vaccine (DT), or the diphtheria, tetanus toxoids, and acellular pertussis vaccine (DTaP); 3 or more doses of any poliovirus vaccine; 1 or more doses of a measles-containing vaccine (MCV); 3 or more doses or 4 or more doses of *Haemophilus influenzae* type b vaccine (Hib) depending on Hib vaccine product type (full series Hib); 3 or more doses of hepatitis B vaccine; 1 or more doses of varicella vaccine; and 4 or more doses of pneumococcal conjugate vaccine.

12. Michael McGinnis and William Foege. "Actual Causes of Death in the United States," *JAMA*. 270 (18) (1993): 2207-2212.

13. Institute of Medicine (IOM). *U.S. Health in International Perspective: Shorter Lives, Poorer Health* (Washington, DC: IOM, 2013): p. 159.

14. Victor Fuchs. "Social Determinants of Health: Caveats and Nuances," *JAMA*. 317 (1) (2017): 25-26.

15. Christine Buttorff, Teague Ruder, and Melissa Bauman. *Multiple Chronic Conditions in the United States* (Santa Monica, CA: RAND, 2017).

16. Elizabeth Bradley, Maureen Canavan, Erika Rogan, et al. "Variation in Health Outcomes: The Role of Spending on Social Services, Public Health, and Health Care, 2000–09," *Health Aff.* 35 (9) (2016): https://www.healthaffairs.org/doi/full/10.1377/hlthaff.2015.0814. Elizabeth H. Bradley, Benjamin R. Elkins, Jeph Herrin, et al. "Health and Social Services Expenditures: Associations with Health Outcomes," *Br Med J Qual Safety.* 20 (10) (2011): 826-831. Elizabeth Bradley and Lauren Taylor. *The American Health Care Paradox: Why Spending More Is Getting Us Less* (New York, NY: Public Affairs; 2013).

17. Roosa Tikkanen and Eric Schneider. "Social Spending to Improve Population Health: Does the United States Spend as Wisely as Other Countries?" *N Engl J Med.* 382 (10) (2020): 885-887.

18. Irene Papanicolas, Liani Woskie, Duncan Orlander, et al. "The Relationship Between Health Spending and Social Spending in High-Income Countries: How Does the U.S. Compare?" *Health Aff.* 38 (9) (2019): https://doi.org/10.1377/hlthaff.2018.05187.

19. Michelle Carlson, Brita Roy, and A. Stef Groenewould. "Assessing Quantitative Comparisons of Health and Social Care Between Countries," *JAMA*. 324 (5) (2020): 449-450.

20. Atul Gawande. "The Hot Spotters," *The New Yorker* (January 24, 2011).

21. Amy Finkelstein, Annetta Zhou, Sarah Taubman, et al. "Health Care Hotspotting: A Randomized Controlled Trial," *N Engl J Med.* 382 (2020): 152-162.

22. Joel Cantor. *Medicaid and the Future of Health Care Hot-Spotting*. Milbank Memorial Fund Issue Brief (April 2020). Shreya Kangovi and David Grande. "Don't Throw Cold Water on Health Care's Hot Spotters," *Health Affairs Blog* (February 11, 2020). Eric Schneider and Tanya Shah. "Cold Water or Rocket Fuel? Lessons From the Camden 'Hot-Spotting' Randomized Controlled Trial," *Health Affairs Blog* (February 11, 2020).

23. Deborah Peikes, Arnold Chen, Jennifer Schnore, et al. "Effects of Care Coordination on Hospitalization, Quality of Care, and Health Care Expenditures Among Medicare Beneficiaries: 15 Randomized Trials," *JAMA*. 301 (6) (2009): 603-618. David Bott, et al. "Disease Management for Chronically Ill Beneficiaries in Traditional Medicare," *Health Aff.* 28 (1) (2009): 86-98.

24. Randall Brown. "Lessons for ACOs and Medical Homes on Care Coordination for High-Need

Beneficiaries," Presentation to AcademyHealth Annual Research Meeting (June 2013).

25. Larry Bye, Alyssa Ghirardelli, and Angela Fontes. "Promoting Health Equity and Population Health: How Americans' Views Differ," *Health Aff.* 35 (11) (2016): 1982-1990.

26. Judith Hibbard, Jean Stockard, Eldon Mahoney, et al. "Development of the Patient Activation Measure (PAM): Conceptualizing and Measuring Activation in Patients and Consumers," *Health Serv Res.* 39 (4) (2004): 1005-1026.

27. Judith Hibbard. *Using the Patient Activation Measure to Improve Outcomes and Control Costs.* Available online: https://www.kingsfund.org.uk/sites/default/files/media/Judith%20H.%20Hibbard.pdf. Accessed on May 12, 2020.

# 5

# Goals of Healthcare

## MAJOR GOALS OF HEALTHCARE

The last 2 columns in Figure 3.5 (control knobs) represent "big, hairy, audacious goals" (BHAGs). Bill Hsiao, the author of this framework, likened them to the pursuit of efficiency (the intermediate outcomes) and effectiveness (the ultimate ends). They are more widely known today under different labels.

The first of these 2 columns constitutes one set of tripartite BHAGs known as "the iron triangle": access, quality, and cost. Within the past decade or so, that triangle has been supplanted by a new set of tripartite BHAGs (that parallel the second of these columns) known as "the triple aim": patient experience of care, population health, and cost per capita. Although there is nothing wrong with either set, it reinforces the observation made at the beginning of this book ("The Intro and the Outro" in Chapter 1): We have not only witnessed the continued introduction of new players, but we are also now witnessing the introduction of new goals. It raises the important question of whether or not these 2 sets of tripartite goals are synonymous and reinforcing, contradictory, or orthogonal. It also poses a dilemma for providers and the healthcare industry as a whole as to what they should focus on achieving. In business parlance, is this an instance of goal congruence, goal conflict, goal overload, or goal ambiguity?

## TRIANGLE 1: ACCESS, QUALITY, AND COST

Nothing better illustrates the opportunities and challenges we face than meeting the 3 goals of healthcare pursued by every country for decades: increase access, improve quality, and contain rising costs.[1] Public surveys frequently assess consumer satisfaction with achieving these 3 goals.[2] Attainment of these 3 goals is also baked into global frameworks of the functioning of every country's healthcare system.[3] They also define the strategic aim of major foundations like the Commonwealth Fund: *Affordable, quality health care. For everyone.* These tripartite goals have been widely acknowledged and studied for decades.

The 3 goals became embedded and embodied in geometric logic by Dr. William Kissick as "the iron triangle," depicted in Figure 5-1.[4] The logic of this triangle is that there are inevitable societal trade-offs in pursuing any of the goals (vertices) in the triangle. Often, these trade-offs are described as the tension between promoting access to care for everyone versus using price as a tool to ration healthcare services, or the tension between balancing equitable access and efficiency in the provision of services. If the triangle is an equilateral triangle, and thus each angle is 60 degrees, policy initiatives that expand 1 angle beyond 60 degrees force 1 or both of

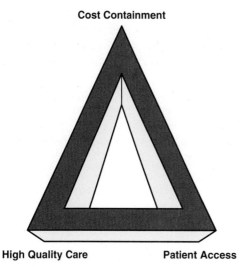

**Cost Containment**

**High Quality Care**          **Patient Access**

**Figure 5-1** • The Iron Triangle of Healthcare.

the other 2 angles to contract below 60 degrees. Thus, efforts to promote access to care (eg, via insurance coverage) will lead to higher demand for care, rising utilization, and higher costs. Similarly, efforts to promote quality by virtue of enabling access to modern technologies (drugs, medical devices, and equipment) will also likely raise costs. Determining the right thrust and mix among the 3 angles constitutes the balancing act in resource allocation faced by most countries.

And yet, despite the popularity and widespread mention of access, quality, and cost, remarkably few people can define what these 3 goals are. One reason is that they are all multidimensional. Let's look at them one at a time.

## Access

Access to care, studied by researchers for decades, has been linked to the availability of medical resources (physician and hospital supply), the ability to pay for care (family income, insurance coverage), travel distances to reach that care, and characteristics of the populations (eg, illness level, willingness to seek care, factors enabling care-seeking).[5] The literature subsequently distilled 5 dimensions of access that captured much of the initial access framework[6]:

1. Availability
   - Supply and demand mismatch
   - Rural and urban

2. Accessibility
   - Geography, infrastructure, transportation
3. Accommodation
   - Ability to accept patients when they need to be seen
   - Communication: e-mail, phone
4. Affordability
   - Lack of insurance
   - Underinsured
5. Acceptability
   - Cultural barriers and preferences

## Quality of Care

In the case *Jacobellis v. Ohio* before the Supreme Court in 1964, Justice Potter Stewart stated that although he could not define obscenity, "I know it when I see it." The same has been said in healthcare: Quality is like pornography—You can't define it, but you know it when you see it. But maybe you cannot even see it. There is the famous Indian parable about the 6 blind men and the elephant. Each one touches a different part of the elephant and claims it is something totally different. The man who touches the trunk says it is a thick snake; the man who touches the ear says that it is a fan; the man who touches the leg says it is a tree trunk.

Quality is even more multidimensional than access and less easy to define. In the 1960s, Dr. Avedis Donabedian characterized 3 dimensions of quality: structure, process, and outcome.[7] These encompassed the following:

*Structure:* the conditions under which care is provided
   - Material resources (facilities, equipment)
   - Human resources (ratios, qualifications, experience)
   - Organizational characteristics (size, volume, systems)

*Process:* the activities that constitute healthcare
   - Screening and diagnosis
   - Adherence to guidelines
   - Treatment and rehabilitation
   - Education and prevention

*Outcome:* changes attributable to healthcare
   - Mortality, morbidity (complications, readmissions), and functional status
   - Knowledge, attitudes, and behaviors
   - Satisfaction (including patient experiences)

In 2001, the Institute of Medicine (IOM) identified 6 domains of quality and outcomes known by the acronym STEEEP. These domains include care that is[8]:

- Safe
- Timely
- Effective
- Efficient
- Equitable
- Patient-centered

In parallel with these typologies, the National Committee for Quality Assurance (NCQA) developed performance measures to be used to assess the quality of care provided by health plans that contracted with employers. These measures are known as the Healthcare Effectiveness Data and Information Set (HEDIS). The HEDIS measures span 4 domains: effectiveness of care, access/availability of care, experience of care, and utilization and relative resource use. A subset of the HEDIS measures dealing with "effectiveness" are reproduced in the following box. Drawing on Donabedian's typology described earlier, most of the HEDIS measures are "process" measures of quality. The full list of HEDIS measures can be found online.[9]

The HEDIS measures do not begin to encompass the definition of quality or exhaust the compendium of quality measures. The federal government maintains several lists of quality measures—one for hospitals (Hospital Compare), another for accountable care organizations (ACOs; ACO Quality Measure Benchmarks), another for each type of post-acute care (PAC) provider (eg, home health, skilled nursing facility), one for Medicare Advantage plans (Star Ratings), and one for Medicaid managed care plans. Each private insurer also maintains its own list of quality metrics. Providers who treat both publicly and privately insured patients thus must report on a wide variety of quality measures that differ by insurer.

As of 2015, the comprehensive health measures database of the Agency for Healthcare Research and Quality, the National Quality Measures Clearinghouse, listed a total of 4,456 health measures. The Department of Health and Human Services' database indicated that its agencies used 3,801 measures. The Centers for Medicare and Medicaid Services (CMS) also maintained a Measures Inventory that listed 987 measures. Researchers have labeled this "The Quality Tower of Babble."[10] As in the

Biblical story about building a tower to reach the heavens, the quality effort has resulted in a cacophonous muddle of measures that don't talk to one another and that pile measures on top of other measures over time with no real central planning or integration, similar to "the intro and the outro." The result is also distracting clinicians, raising the cost of care delivery, and not helping consumers make better healthcare choices.

## Cost of Care

Cost of care can be measured several ways. At the national level, the CMS annually tracks national health expenditures (NHE), as well as NHE as a percentage of gross domestic product (GDP) and NHE per capita. The Kaiser Family Foundation annually tracks the rise in premiums (as well as the rise in deductibles) for employer-based health insurance. The Labor Department tracks the percentage of household spending on healthcare.

Cost can also be measured at the provider level. Hospitals can bill payers based on a percentage of billed charges. The billed charges are based on the hospital's list prices for every chargeable item, documented in the hospital's chargemaster. The chargemaster can include as many as 20,000 to 30,000 different items (and perhaps as many as 45,000). Hospitals frequently bill payers based on a small number of service lines, including pharmaceuticals, procedures, the laboratory, and hospital room charges.[11] Each hospital employs its own method to set chargemaster prices for drugs and other inputs. There is no standardized or mandated protocol.[12] As a result, chargemaster prices are based on a variety of factors. These can include the following: overall cost inflation, changes in the cost of specific services or procedures, competitive market forces, the influence of specific payers, community perception, and, to a lesser extent, indirect cost allocation.[13]

Chargemaster prices have so little to do with the input costs paid by hospitals or the reimbursement payments received by hospitals that they are often wildly inflated, on the order of several hundred percent relative to the acquisition cost. On average, chargemaster prices for drug administration typically equal a 3- to 4-fold multiple of average wholesale price. There is tremendous variation in chargemaster prices

## HEDIS Measures of "Effectiveness"

**Prevention and Screening**

- Adult BMI Assessment
- Weight Assessment and Counseling for Nutrition and Physical Activity for Children/Adolescents
- Childhood Immunization Status
- Immunizations for Adolescents
- Lead Screening in Children
- Breast Cancer Screening
- Cervical Cancer Screening
- Colorectal Cancer Screening
- Chlamydia Screening in Women
- Care for Older Adults

**Respiratory Conditions**

- Appropriate Testing for Children With Pharyngitis
- Use of Spirometry Testing in the Assessment and Diagnosis of COPD
- Pharmacotherapy Management of COPD Exacerbation
- Medication Management for People With Asthma and Asthma Medication Ratio

**Cardiovascular Conditions**

- Controlling High Blood Pressure
- Persistence of Beta-Blocker Treatment After a Heart Attack
- Statin Therapy for Patients With Cardiovascular Disease and Diabetes

**Diabetes**

- Comprehensive Diabetes Care

**Musculoskeletal Conditions**

- Disease-Modifying Anti-Rheumatic Drug Therapy for Rheumatoid Arthritis
- Osteoporosis Testing and Management in Older Women

**Behavioral Health**

- Antidepressant Medication Management

- Follow-Up Care for Children Prescribed ADHD Medication
- Follow-Up After Hospitalization for Mental Illness
- Follow-Up After Emergency Department Visit for Mental Illness
- Follow-Up After Emergency Department Visit for Alcohol and Other Drug Abuse or Dependence
- Diabetes and Cardiovascular Disease Screening and Monitoring for People With Schizophrenia or Bipolar Disorder
- Adherence to Antipsychotic Medications for Individuals With Schizophrenia
- Metabolic Monitoring for Children and Adolescents on Antipsychotics

**Medication Management and Care Coordination**

- Annual Monitoring for Patients on Persistent Medications
- Medication Reconciliation Post-Discharge
- Transitions of Care
- Follow-Up After Emergency Department Visit for People With Multiple High-Risk Chronic Conditions

**Overuse/Appropriateness**

- Non-Recommended Cervical Cancer Screening in Adolescent Females
- Non-Recommended PSA-Based Screening in Older Men
- Appropriate Treatment for Children With Upper Respiratory Infection
- Avoidance of Antibiotic Treatment in Adults With Acute Bronchitis
- Use of Imaging Studies for Low Back Pain
- Use of Multiple Concurrent Antipsychotics in Children and Adolescents
- Medication Management in the Elderly
- Use of Opioids at High Dosage
- Use of Opioids From Multiple Providers

---

ADHD, attention-deficit/hyperactivity disorder; BMI, body mass index; COPD, chronic obstructive pulmonary disease; PSA, prostate-specific antigen.

within, and particularly across, US hospitals. One study reported a mean hospital charge-to-cost ratio (defined as the chargemaster price divided by Medicare allowable cost) of 4.32 (ie, 432%). For this reason, the prices listed in the chargemaster are often referred to by people in the healthcare ecosystem as "funny money." They are not that funny, however, for those without insurance or those with high deductibles who are forced to pay the list price.

Then there is the hospital's reimbursement from the insurer, which represents a significant discount off the list price for most patients. These discounts vary according to the bargaining power of both the hospital and the payer. And then there are the real costs of what it took the hospital to provide the care, which are largely unknown (even to many hospitals) in the absence of sophisticated cost accounting systems. Hospitals nevertheless are required to submit their Medicare Cost Reports, which include cost and charges by cost center, to CMS at the national level, as well as their Medicaid Cost Reports to state agencies.

## Shifting Primacy of Access, Quality, and Cost Goals Over Time

Although these goals are global, emphasis on any one of them has varied over the past century. During the first part of the 20th century, the Flexner Report on medical education (1910) and the rise of The Joint Commission (1918) ostensibly focused on improving the quality of physician and hospital care (covered in Chapter 7). In the late 1920s, the Committee on the Costs of Medical Care in the United States obviously focused on cost. In the 1930s, due to the Depression and patients' inability to pay for healthcare, attention shifted to access and the introduction of insurance mechanisms to finance the care that hospitals and physicians rendered to patients. Labor shortages during the early 1940s (due to World War II) helped augment emphasis on access by encouraging employers to sponsor insurance coverage for their workers. In the 1960s, with the passage of Medicare and Medicaid, renewed emphasis was paid to access for 2 groups in the population not covered by employer-based health insurance:

the elderly and the poor. All of these insurance expansions increased demand for care, utilization of care, and (ultimately) the aggregate cost of care. Cost reclaimed primacy by the 1970s, which ushered in several decades of efforts to try to contain it—whether by regulation in the 1970s, budget remedies in the 1980s, or managed care, healthcare reform efforts (Clinton Health Plan), and budget cutting (eg, Balanced Budget Act) in the 1990s. During the 21st century, the Affordable Care Act (2010) tried to pursue all 3 goals simultaneously. During this time, policy makers have devoted more attention to quality via such initiatives as pay-for-performance (P4P), value-based purchasing (VBP), ACOs, and "never events" (reimbursement withheld for controllable adverse events in hospital episodes).

The dominant goal in the iron triangle not only varies over time but over space. The dominant goal in one state may not be dominant in another. In the early 2000s, Massachusetts became the first state to focus on nearly universal access to health insurance coverage by adopting a statewide insurance exchange—all at the expense of rising costs. The Massachusetts experiment served as the precursor to the state exchanges created under Obamacare (see Chapter 19). The dominant goal may not only vary across states but also across countries, as many countries have universal insurance coverage. Finally, the dominant goal may vary across stakeholders in the healthcare system.

## Is the Iron Triangle Generalizable?

The iron triangle can be found in other policy areas and corporate contexts. Countries like the United States face similar iron triangle trade-offs in sectors other than healthcare. For example, in the policy domain of energy, countries must balance their need for low-cost and efficient energy (cost angle) with low-emission and green energy (quality angle) and with rising demand and sustainable energy (access angle). Similarly, in corporate America, marketing executives believe that in order to position their product against the offerings of competitors, they must excel on 1 dimension (product cost, quality, or service) and seek parity on the other 2 dimensions. Optimization on all 3 is rarely considered (and is more rarely observed).[14]

| Critical Thinking Exercise | |
|---|---|

A multitude of innovations in provider payment and provider organization have been proposed as solutions to the iron triangle. That is, they purportedly help to improve quality and/or reduce cost of care, or they increase access to care without raising healthcare costs. Below is a "laundry list" of candidates for the "iron triangle award."

| | |
|---|---|
| Value-based payment (VBP) | Accountable care organization (ACO) |
| Pay-for-performance (P4P) | Patient-centered medical home (PCMH) |
| High-deductible health plan (HDHP) | Electronic medical record (EMR) |
| Medical tourism | Toyota production system (TPS) |
| Price transparency | Retail clinic |
| Consumerism | Urgent care center (UCC) |
| Analytics | Ambulatory surgery center (ASC) |

Do any of these innovations help to improve quality and/or reduce the cost of care? If not, can you think of other payment or provider organization innovations that are deserving of the award?

## TRIANGLE 2: CARE, HEALTH, AND COST

In 2008, the healthcare industry welcomed 3 "new goals on the block" to improve the US system: "the triple aim." Coined by Dr. Don Berwick and colleagues in an article in *Health Affairs*, the triple aim recast the goals of the iron triangle discussed earlier as care, health, and cost (Figure 5-2). Definitions of the new goals are as follows.

*Patient Experience of Care (Care).* The patient's experience of care drew heavily on the IOM's STEEEP measures for health system improvement, as well as on the Consumer Assessment of Healthcare Providers and Systems (CAHPS). The latter elicits

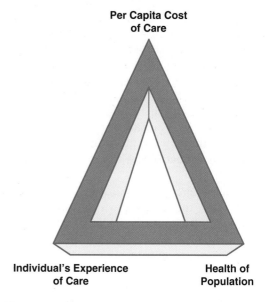

**Figure 5-2 •** The Triple Aim of Healthcare.

patient feedback on their providers, their health plans, nursing homes, surgical care, dental plans, and so on. For example, with regard to providers, CAHPS asks patients about (1) timeliness of appointments, care, and information; (2) how well providers communicate with patients; (3) providers' use of information to coordinate patient care; and (4) whether office staff are helpful, courteous, and respectful.[15]

*Population Health (Health).* Population health drew heavily on health outcome measures, such as life expectancy, health status, functional status, and mortality rates. It also drew on disease burden (ie, the incidence and prevalence of major chronic illness conditions), as well as on behavioral and physiological factors. Behavioral factors encompass lifestyle behaviors such as drinking alcohol, smoking, diet, and physical activity; physiological factors encompass blood pressure, body mass index, cholesterol, and blood glucose levels.

*Per Capita Cost (Cost).* Per capita cost included total cost for each member of the covered population per month, as well as the utilization rate and/or cost of hospitals and emergency rooms.

Shortly after publication, CMS baked many measures of the triple aim into its performance assessment of ACOs. The December 2014 cover of *Hospitals & Health Networks* included a picture of the new chair-elect of the American Hospital Association; the title accompanying the picture read, "It's All About the Triple Aim." The title conveys the industrywide embrace of the triple aim goals by hospitals.

Unlike Kissick's iron triangle, Berwick's triple aim downplayed (but still acknowledged) trade-offs among the 3 goals. Borrowing from organization theorists, the solution was no longer "satisficing" but now "optimizing" on all 3 dimensions.[16] Although there might be some tensions, the 3 goals could be harmonized and jointly pursued in the presence of (1) an "integrator" (whether an integrated delivery network like Kaiser or policy actors with political will who could alter provider incentives and structures); (2) "disruptive innovation"; (3) efficiency improvements; and (4) a population focus that included social services and preventive health.

Six years after its publication, the triple aim expanded into the "quadruple aim" to address the growing issue of physician burnout and dissatisfaction.[17] Care of the patient now also required care of the provider. Left unaddressed, physician burnout could torpedo the goals of the triple aim.

## DUELING TRIANGLES?

The 2 triangles depicted earlier—the iron triangle of access, quality, and cost, and the triple aim of care, health, and cost—dominate the deliberations of healthcare policy makers, regulators, payers, providers, and researchers. To become fluent in this industry, you *must* understand each triangle and what their constituent goals are. Every country's agenda for healthcare includes tackling access, quality, and cost; many now work toward achieving the triple aim as well.[18] Unfortunately, the 2 triangles are often confused, even by industry insiders who should know better.

Are the 2 triangles congruent? My students commonly think so. After all, they share the same geometric shape, and the goals of access/quality/cost sound a lot like care/health/cost. Moreover, if you read Kissick's book and Berwick's article, you will see that cost has primacy among the 3 goals—as evidenced by our historical preoccupation with that angle—and that the cost problem is ascribed to the same set of drivers (eg, fee-for-service medicine, the introduction of new expensive technology, the self-interest of the players in the industry). This

is covered in Chapter 6 of this book. Moreover, both Kissick and Berwick see the 3 goals as interdependent and interpenetrating, as well as central to a well-functioning health system.[19]

To harmonize the 2 triangles, my students sometimes get creative. First, they suggest that Kissick's iron triangle is the problem, while Berwick's triple aim is the solution. Never mind that Bill Hsiao referred to them as intermediate outcomes and ultimate ends. Second, they suggest that Kissick's model works at the micro level of individual actors seeking their own self-interest, whereas Berwick's model works at the level of a "covered population" (eg, like Kaiser).

One can also make the argument that the 2 triangle frameworks are incompatible and/or orthogonal. Kissick wrote in the early 1990s and took a historical look at our healthcare system; Berwick wrote in 2008 and took a more futuristic perspective. Kissick was descriptive and somewhat pessimistic about achieving all 3 goals; Berwick was prescriptive and optimistic about achieving all 3 goals. Kissick focused on the invisible hand, market forces (eg, individual actors pursuing their self-interest), and market failure; Berwick focused instead on the "visible hand" of coordinators and systems of care to pursue policy goals and avoid "the tragedy of the commons."[20] Kissick developed an analytic framework, whereas Berwick offered an action plan. Kissick focused on the cost and quality ramifications of biomedical advances, whereas Berwick concentrated on the benefits of integration and care coordination.

In sum, we seem to have 2 policy-oriented, physician thought-leaders coming up with very different frameworks, perhaps reflecting what one observer called "generational change."[21] Kissick's framework is zero sum, with trade-offs among the 3 angles; the advance of expensive innovation that increases cost must come at the expense of access and affordability.[22] More rationing of high-cost, high-tech healthcare is the result, with rationing occurring via a number of avenues: (1) the presence/absence of insurance coverage, (2) the ability/inability to make out-of-pocket payments required by cost sharing, (3) the physician's willingness to offer/not offer such services such as prescribing drugs or ordering diagnostic tests, and so on.[23] By contrast, Berwick's goal framework is synergistic and mutually attainable. Rationing is avoided by reducing waste and inefficiency, disruptive innovation, paying for "value," focusing on the social determinants of health, and having the visible hand of an integrator to help orchestrate it all.

To really answer the question of the compatibility of these 2 frameworks, one needs to "get into the weeds" on each of the 3 goals in these 2 triangles. In Kissick's model, "access" meant individual access to what patients *want*: free choice of provider in an open-network model. Here, the priority is on the individual. In Berwick's model, access meant population access to what patients *need*: a closed-network system of care. Here, the priority is on the health of a population. In Kissick's model, "quality" rests on access to high-tech medicine (eg, new biomedical advances and therapies); in Berwick's model, quality rests on access to social services, preventive services, and factors that promote population health (as defined earlier). In Kissick's model, "cost" referred to the cost of a specific therapy or societal-wide expenditures on healthcare; for Berwick, costs accrued at the population level in the systems of care taking care of defined patient populations.

Things get even more complicated when you try to equate the angles across the 2 triangles. Quality in Kissick's model does not easily translate into population health in Berwick's model; the latter includes a host of things (as noted earlier) such as health status, functional status, physiological measures, and self-behaviors. Quality and access in Kissick's model have some similarities with Berwick's patient experience of care (eg, consumer satisfaction, patient safety, HEDIS measures of effectiveness) but diverge in some ways as well (eg, no explicit mention of equity or patient-centered care). Cost, finally, is measured at different levels of analysis: the individual or society in Kissick's model; the population in Berwick's model.

So, what we are left with are 2 sets of tripartite goals with some overlaps, some divergences, and some totally different orientations. The contrast between the iron triangle and triple aim—and their dueling prognoses of the probability of achieving multiple goals simultaneously—surfaced at "The New Health Care Symposium" held at Yale University in early 2016.[24] The iron triangle has yielded the stage to the triple aim but is still quite relevant. The symposium considered but did not resolve the key question: If low cost and high quality are not synergistic (as the iron triangle suggests they are not), then is the triple aim really achievable? And are provider transformation efforts to simultaneously improve quality and reduce cost in vain?

Looking at the iron triangle and triple aim historically, one has been piled on top of the other. Berwick and colleagues do not reference Kissick, even though their article explicitly mentions access, quality, and cost. Like the ecosystem itself, healthcare goals are proliferating and becoming more muddled.

## SUMMARY

This chapter has outlined the 2 major sets of goals that policy makers and (some) providers seek to achieve. I qualify providers' pursuit of these goals because, as explained in later chapters, providers run businesses that seek growth, higher revenues, greater profits, and greater market power. This suggests that there is likely some disjunction between what policy makers want and what providers want and, thus, that it is important to wear 2 hats when studying healthcare: a health policy hat and a business school hat.

These 2 sets of goals are not the same but are not necessarily incompatible. You will likely hear healthcare executives espouse both, but it is not clear that executives understand the differences between them. You should understand them by now.

### QUESTIONS TO PONDER

1. Can you identify any healthcare system in another country that has successfully tackled the iron triangle? How do you know?

2. Avedis Donabedian's model of quality (structure, process, outcome) has been widely adopted in health services studies. However, research suggests it has some major limitations. In what ways is this model helpful and not so helpful?

3. Each of the 3 goals of the iron triangle is much more complex than most people realize. What should providers and policy makers do to help manage their way through this muddle?

4. The chapter argues that the iron triangle and the triple aim share some commonalities but also have major contrasts. Can you think of other similarities and differences between these 2 major goal frameworks?

# REFERENCES

1. John Hoadley. "Health Care in the United States: Access, Costs, and Quality," *PS (Political Science)* 20 (2) (1987): 197-201.
2. Robert Blendon, Mollyanne Brodie, John Benson, et al. "Americans' Views of Health Care Costs, Access, and Quality," *Milbank Q.* 84 (4) (2006): 623-657.
3. Marc Roberts, William Hsiao, Peter Berman, and Michael Reich. *Getting Health Reform Right* (New York, NY: Oxford University Press, 2008): Chapter 1. Eric Schneider, Dana Sarnak, David Squires, et al. *Mirror, Mirror 2017: International Comparison Reflects Flaws and Opportunities for Better U.S. Health* (New York, NY: Commonwealth Fund, 2017).
4. William Kissick. *Medicine's Dilemmas: Infinite Needs Versus Finite Resources* (New Haven, CT: Yale University Press, 1994).
5. Lu Ann Aday and Ronald Andersen. "A Framework for the Study of Access to Medical Care," *Health Serv Res.* Fall (1974): 208-220.
6. Roy Penchansky and J. William Thomas. "The Concept of Access: Definition and Relationship to Consumer Satisfaction," *Med Care.* 19 (2) (1981): 127-140.
7. Avedis Donabedian. "Evaluating the Quality of Medical Care," *Milbank Mem Fund Q.* 44(3) (1966): 166-203. Avedis Donabedian. *An Introduction to Quality Assurance in Health Care* (Oxford, United Kingdom: Oxford University Press, 2003).
8. Institute of Medicine. *Crossing the Quality Chasm: A New Health System for the 21st Century* (Washington, DC: Institute of Medicine, 2001).
9. NCQA. "HEDIS Measures and Technical Resources." Available online: https://www.ncqa.org/hedis/measures/. Accessed on February 8, 2020.
10. Elizabeth Teisberg and Scott Wallace. "The Quality Tower of Babble," *Health Affairs Blog* (April 13, 2015).
11. Allen Dobson, Joan DaVanzo, Julie Doherty, and Myra Tanamor. *A Study of Hospital Charge Setting Practices* (Washington, DC: Medicare Payment Advisory Commission, December 2005).
12. Allen Dobson, Joan DaVanzo, Julie Doherty, and Myra Tanamor. *A Study of Hospital Charge Setting Practices* (Washington, DC: Medicare Payment Advisory Commission, December 2005).
13. Allen Dobson, Joan DaVanzo, Julie Doherty, and Myra Tanamor. *A Study of Hospital Charge Setting Practices* (Washington, DC: Medicare Payment Advisory Commission, December 2005).
14. One global firm that came close to achieving all 3 simultaneously (at least in past decades) was the Swedish furniture maker Ikea. In the healthcare industry, Becton Dickinson also achieved strong performance on all 3 dimensions in prior decades.
15. Agency for Healthcare Research and Quality. "CAHPS Clinician and Group Survey Measures." Available online: https://www.ahrq.gov/cahps/surveys-guidance/cg/about/survey-measures.html. Accessed on February 9, 2020.
16. James March and Herbert Simon. *Organizations* (New York, NY: John Wiley & Sons, 1958).
17. Thomas Bodenheimer and Christine Sinsky. "From Triple to Quadruple Aim: Care of the Patient Requires Care of the Provider," *Ann Fam Med.* 12 (2014): 573-576.
18. Andy Slavitt. "The Triple Aim Must Overcome the Triple Threat," JAMA Forum (November 8, 2018). Available online: https://newsatjama.jama.com/2018/11/08/jama-forum-the-triple-aim-must-overcome-the-triple-threat/. Accessed on February 15, 2020.
19. William Sage. "New Health Care Symposium: Physicians and The New Health Care Industry—Benefits of Generational Change," Health Affairs Blog (March 1, 2016). Available online: https://www.healthaffairs.org/do/10.1377/hblog20160301.053479/full/. Accessed on February 15, 2020. More intriguingly, neither Kissick nor Berwick really defines the 3 goals. To arrive at Berwick's definition, one needs to visit the website for his Institute for Healthcare Improvement.
20. Alfred Chandler. *The Visible Hand: The Managerial Revolution in American Business* (Boston, MA: Harvard University Press, 1977).
21. William Sage. "New Health Care Symposium: Physicians and The New Health Care Industry—Benefits of Generational Change," Health Affairs Blog (March 1, 2016). Available online: https://www.healthaffairs.org/do/10.1377/hblog20160301.053479/full/.
22. Harvard economist David Cutler entitled chapter one of his book, *The Quality Cure,* as "Cost, Access, and Quality: The Three Horsemen of the Apocalypse." In an e-mail exchange, Professor Cutler espoused the belief that we are not likely to balance these 3 goals until "the end times."
23. Robert Sheeler, Tim Mundell, Samia Hurst, et al. "Self-Reported Rationing Behavior Among US Physicians: A National Survey," *J Gen Intern Med.* 31 (12) (2016): 1444-1451.
24. William Sage. "New Health Care Symposium: Physicians and The New Health Care Industry—Benefits of Generational Change," *Health Affairs Blog* (March 1, 2016). Available online: https://www.healthaffairs.org/do/10.1377/hblog20160301.053479/full/. Accessed on February 15, 2020.

# 6

# The 800-Pound Gorilla: Rising Healthcare Costs

## INTRODUCTION TO THE PROBLEM

As noted in Chapter 5, the United States has struggled with the problem of rising healthcare costs since (at least) the late 1920s. Indeed, the "cost" angle has dominated the iron triangle for attention in most decades since. That means we have an intractable problem—one going on for 90+ years. Of the 3 angles in the iron triangle or the triple aim, the cost angle has been particularly vexing. That is why this volume devotes an entire chapter to the topic.

So, what is "the problem," stated succinctly? The problem is manifold. First, rising costs are driven by *lots* of factors that can be classified according to supply, demand, price, and volume. Second, there have also been *lots* of efforts to control rising costs, whether via regulation, market-based remedies, changing how providers are paid, changing how providers are organized, reducing variations in care, reducing low-value and unnecessary care (eg, the downward-sloping part of the curve in Figure 2-4), using technological advances, promoting wellness and prevention, focusing on the chronically ill, and (more recently) using "big tech" to promote greater consumerism. This chapter examines these topics and draws some conclusions about what we can realistically expect to accomplish in controlling rising healthcare costs.

## EXAMINING THE TRENDS

Figure 6-1 shows the increase in national health expenditures (NHE) per capita in the United States between 1960 and 2019. The rate of increase accelerated between 1960 and 1970 (1.4x), accelerated even faster during 1970 to 1980 (2.1x) and 1980 to 1990 (1.6x), decelerated between 1990 and 2000 (0.7x) and 2000 and 2010 (0.7x), and then slowed down even further from 2010 to 2019 (0.4x). Figure 6-2 shows cost escalation data on an annualized basis.

There are several reasons why we need to understand this. *First*, rising healthcare costs now account for a growing share of the US government's federal budget due to spending on "entitlements" (eg, Medicare, Medicaid, Social Security). As noted in Chapter 2 (Figure 2-7), such entitlement spending begins to crowd out other (discretionary or nonhealthcare) spending. This is reflected in Figure 6-3. The majority of the federal government's budget of $4.1 trillion (2018) is devoted to Social Security ($982 billion, or 24%), Medicare/Medicaid ($971 billion, or 23.7%), and other mandatory spending programs ($570 billion, or 13.9%). Over time, federal spending on major health programs is projected to outstrip Social Security payments (Figure 6-4).

*Second*, inflationary healthcare spending has typically outpaced the growth in US gross domestic product (GDP) (Figure 6-5). This gives rise to the distinction between economy wide inflation and medical price inflation in excess of the economy; the delta between healthcare cost growth and GDP growth defines medical price inflation.

*Third*, as a result, such increased spending has also occasioned rising federal deficits and increased government borrowing to finance this spending. This was evidenced most recently by increased healthcare expansions authorized by the Bipartisan Budget Act of 2018. *Fourth*,

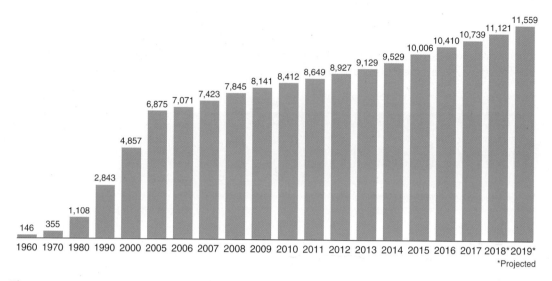

**Figure 6-1** • National Health Expenditures per Capita in the United States from 1960 to 2019 (in US Dollars). (Source: Centers for Medicaid and Medicare Services.)

increases in healthcare spending have outpaced growth in wages, making healthcare increasingly less affordable to the population (Figure 6-6).

There is a *fifth* reason why this accelerated spending is important. In the end, each of us pays for every single dollar spent on healthcare. If you have health insurance through your company, the employer is not really paying for it. To attract more and better-qualified labor, employers offer prospective employees a combination of salary and benefits. Together, salary and benefits are considered the employee's total compensation and the employee's money.[1] Employer payments for health insurance premiums ultimately come out of what would otherwise

have been paid to workers as money wages. As of the mid-1990s, consultants estimated that 88% of premiums were offset by money wage reductions.[2] Thus, it is the employee and not the employer who is paying for the health insurance premium. Employees have the discretion to accept the total compensation package in return for contributing their labor; however, it is financially disadvantageous for employees to forego the health insurance coverage since employer coverage helps them save on their income and payroll taxes, they would have to spend more on their own to obtain coverage without the group discount, and their wages would not rise.[3]

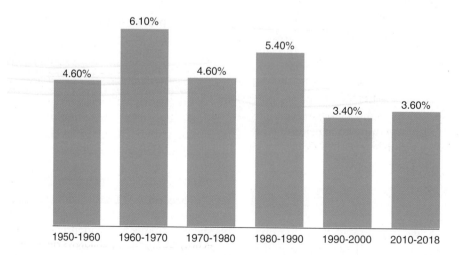

**Figure 6-2** • Average Annual Real Growth Rate in National Health Expenditures Per Capita. (Source: Centers for Medicaid and Medicare Services, https://www.healthaffairs.org/doi/full/10.1377/hlthaff.2019.01451.)

**Outlays, by Category**

Under current law, rising spending for Social Security and Medicare would boost mandatory outlays. Total discretionary spending is projected to fall as a share of gross domestic product as outlays grow modestly in nominal terms. At the same time, growing debt and higher interest rates are projected to push up net interest costs.

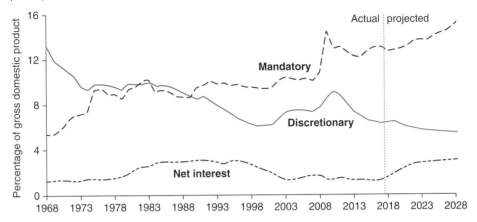

**Figure 6-3** • Entitlement Spending Crowds Out Discretionary Spending. (Source: Congressional Budget Office.)

Health insurers also do not really pay for healthcare; they are merely "financing" it (in some rather opaque and creative ways). If you have public insurance (eg, Medicaid, Medicare), the government is not really paying for it either. They "finance" healthcare costs through a maze of taxes (payroll taxes, general income taxes, sales taxes), as well as your premium contributions and cost-sharing obligations (deductibles, coinsurance), all of which go into various funds to pay for healthcare. Basically, it's your money that is being spent; you just don't know it or see it.

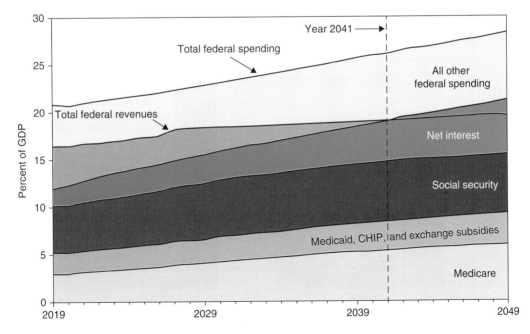

**Figure 6-4** • Health Program Spending Will Overtake Social Security Outlays. CHIP, Children's Health Insurance Program; GDP, Gross Domestic Product. (Reproduced from Medicare Payment Advisory Commission. March 2020 Report to the Congress: Medicare Payment Policy. http://medpac.gov/docs/default-source/reports/mar20_entirereport_sec.pdf.)

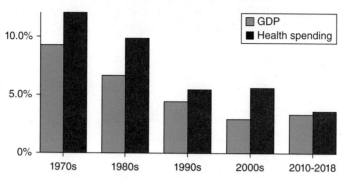

**Figure 6-5** • Per Capita Growth in Health Expenditures: Approximately 2% Growth Above Inflation for 50 Years. GDP, Gross Domestic Product. (Adapted from Peterson KFF Health System Tracker, December 20, 2019, https://www.healthsystemtracker.org/chart-collection/u-s-spending-healthcare-changed-time/#item start.)

Is the United States peculiar in this regard? Yes and no. Figure 6-7 shows the rise in healthcare expenditures in the United States compared to other countries in the Organisation of Economic Co-operation and Development (OECD). Although all countries face rising healthcare costs, Figure 6-7 suggests some divergence in spending between the United States and other countries. Critics of the US healthcare system point to such charts as evidence that the country is wasteful and inefficient. But the source of the difference between the United States and other countries may not lie so much in inefficiency as in higher input prices. Gerry Anderson and colleagues brought this to our attention in a 2003 article called, "It's the Prices, Stupid: Why the United States Is So Different From Other Countries."[4] Failure to control for higher prices in the United States exaggerates these differences. Indeed, adjusting for purchasing power parity (PPP), which takes a "market basket approach" to control for differences in standard of living, cost increases in the United States outstripped other countries in the 1980s, but not in subsequent decades (Figure 6-8).

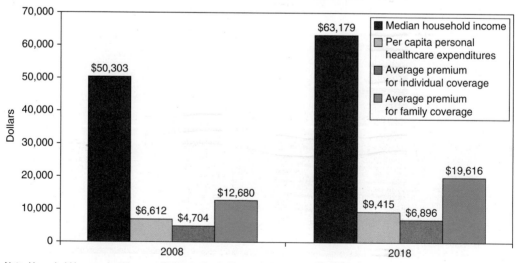

Note: Household income, health expenditures, and premiums are all measured in nominal dollars. Average premiums for individual and family coverage are for employer-sponsored health insurance and include contributions from workers and employers.

**Figure 6-6** • Growth in Healthcare Spending and Premiums Outpaced Growth in Household Income, 2008 and 2018. (Reproduced from Medicare Payment Advisory Commission. March 2020 Report to the Congress: Medicare Payment Policy. http://medpac.gov/docs/default-source/reports/mar20_entirereport_sec.pdf.)

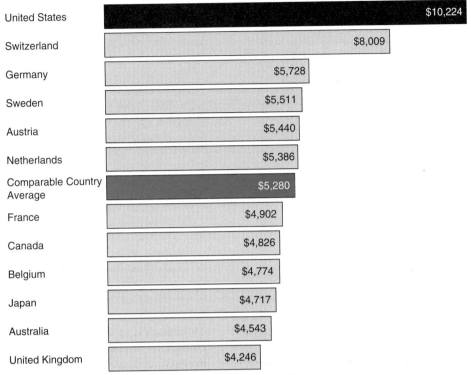

**Figure 6-7** • Health Consumption Expenditures Per Capita, US Dollars, Purchasing Power Parity Adjusted, 2017. (Reproduced from Peterson KFF Heath System Tracker, December 7, 2018, https://www.healthsystemtracker.org/chart-collection/health-spending-u-s-compare-countries/#item-average-wealthy-countries-spend-half-much-per-person-health-u-s-spends.)

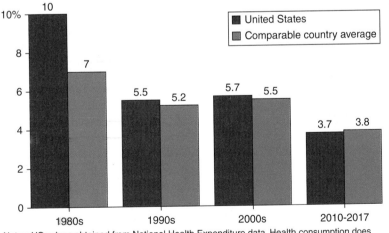

**Figure 6-8** • Health Spending Growth: United States Versus Comparable Countries. PPP, Purchasing Power Parity. (Reproduced from Peterson KFF Health System Tracker, December 7, 2018, https://www.healthsystemtracker.org/chart-collection/health-spending-u-s-compare-countries/#item-u-s-health-spending-growth-higher-1980s-similar-since.)

The similarity in spending growth rates holds for countries that have national health insurance and those that do not. Such similarities in spending growth rates suggest that there may be common drivers to rising costs across all countries. Institutional differences and different structural reforms may not be as important as economic cycle effects.[5] Such similarities also suggest that national health insurance (ie, single payer) may not be a home-run solution, as economists now note.[6]

---

### What Happened to US Healthcare Spending in the 1970s and 1980s?

Figures 6-2, 6-5, and 6-8 suggest that the escalation in US healthcare spending that both vastly exceeded GDP growth and distinguished us from the rest of the world occurred in the 1970s (especially) and 1980s. What happened? Historian Paul Starr pinpoints the Medicare and Medicaid programs.[7] Both programs were enacted as part of President Lyndon Johnson's "Great Society" agenda to deal with the war on poverty. The costs of both programs were grossly underestimated. For example, Robert Evans, the chief actuary for the government, estimated (using paper and pencil) that Medicare would cost $3 billion by 1970; it cost $6 billion. Medicare spending grew 28.6% annually from 1967 to 1973. Evans further forecasted Medicare spending in 1990 at $12 billion; it cost $129 billion. These discrepancies point out the fallacies of forecasts and show that the farther out you project, the more wrong you are likely to be.

According to Starr, the 2 programs "soaked up so much of the public budget at both the federal and state levels that other social programs were starved for funds."

Figure 6-9 shows the high growth rates in the cost of both programs during the 1970s relative to personal healthcare spending, compared to subsequent years.

A number of inflationary factors were at work during this era. The Social Security amendments in 1965 (passage of Medicare and Medicaid) and in 1971/1972 expanded enrollment in public insurance programs. Following the logic of the healthcare quadrilemma (see Chapter 2), expanded insurance coverage meant satisfying pent-up (previously unmet) demand; this meant enrollment growth, then higher utilization growth (due to the severity of illness among the elderly and poor populations now covered), and then cost growth. Additional amendments to Medicare expanded eligibility to the disabled population in 1972. Adding further fuel, there was strong price inflation across most provider categories (especially hospitals, which now enjoyed federal financing and generous reimbursement), abetted by high economy-wide inflation from 1974 to 1982 due to oil shocks, 3 recessions, and the removal of wage and price controls in 1974.

---

What this means is that the number one reason for higher costs in the United States is the higher prices we pay for labor and materials. Physicians and nurses get paid more than their counterparts in other countries. Hospitals get paid more per admission than their counterparts in other countries. Pharmaceuticals cost more in the United States than in other countries. The United States does not set (regulate) prices for these personnel and services across the board as is done in other countries. While some payers (eg, Medicare) have national, administratively set prices for hospitals, physicians, and post-acute care (PAC) providers, most payers do not.

Another reason for higher US costs is that this country does not ration expensive technology. Hospital and physician visits in the United States allow for use of more expensive inputs per service than in other countries, such as imaging tests, surgical procedures, and drugs. Studies of global technology diffusion show that Americans enjoy access to new technologies at a faster speed or at a higher take-up rate compared to citizens of other countries.[8] This is a macro version of the iron triangle: Americans get faster and broader access to new stuff, but we have to pay for it.

A third reason why the United States has higher costs is the proliferation of insurance companies and middlemen in the "healthcare value chain" (the second and fourth boxes in Figure 3-9). The United States has *lots* of intermediaries, including insurers, pharmacy benefit managers (PBMs), wholesalers, and group purchasing organizations (GPOs). This complexity

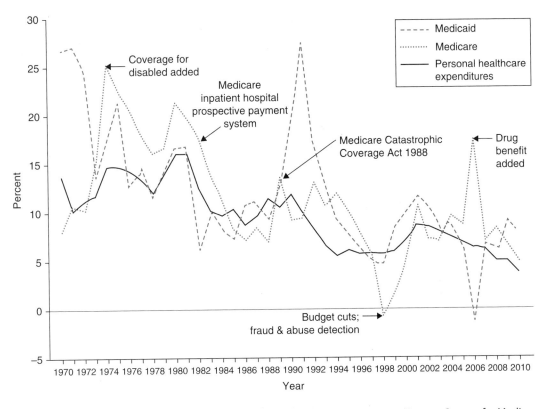

**Figure 6-9** • Growth Rate of Medicare and Total Medical Spending, 1970 to 2010. (Source: Centers for Medicare and Medicaid Services, Office of the Actuary, National Health Statistics Group.)

is summarized by some critics as a source of high "administrative costs" and by other critics as "administrative waste." A lower-bound estimate of these costs (7.9% of NHE in 2016) can be found in Figure 3-4 by summing the "net cost of health insurance" and "government administration." Harvard economist David Cutler offered an intermediate estimate of administrative spending in testimony before the US Senate in 2018, pegging it somewhere between 15% and 30%; other estimates place it slightly higher at 31%.[9] A great depiction of this administrative complexity with hordes of middlemen can be found in the pharmaceutical supply chain that extends from drug manufacturers to wholesalers, GPOs, and PBMs, down to hospitals and pharmacies, and down to insurers and employers (Figure 6-10).

A fourth reason why US healthcare spending outpaces the rest of the world is our country's higher ability to pay. As noted earlier, healthcare is a luxury good; societies with higher national incomes devote more of their wealth to spending on health. We spend more on healthcare because we can afford to do so.

## DRIVERS OF HEALTHCARE SPENDING

The important takeaway here is that healthcare costs are rising everywhere. Moreover, the drivers can be found in every country. These include population demographics (an aging population that uses more services), growing incidence of chronic disease (associated with both age and lifestyle), technological improvements and innovations, and rising public expectations from healthcare spurred by economic growth, rising national incomes, increased global travel, and immigration. Figure 6-11 compares the rate of increase in healthcare spending across countries during the periods 2003 to 2009 with 2009 to 2016. The United States is roughly average. No one country has fashioned "a better mousetrap" to deal with the problem of rising costs. Drawing on director Steven Spielberg's movie *E.T.,* "we are not alone." In the subsections that follow, we review the evidence on some of the "usual suspects" behind rising costs in the United States.

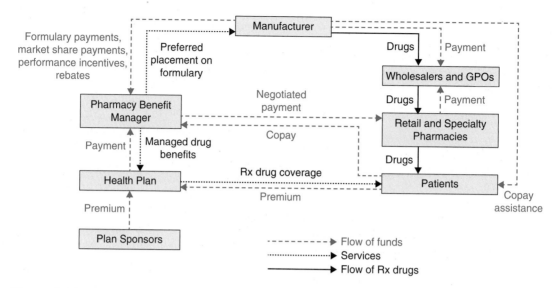

**Figure 6-10** • Retail Drug Product and Payment Flow. GPO, Group Purchasing Organization. (Source: Neeraj Sood, Tiffany Shih, Karen Van Nuys, and Dana P. Goldman. "Follow the Money: The Flow of Funds in the Pharmaceutical Distribution System," *Health Affairs Blog* 2017, https://www.healthaffairs.org/do/10.1377/hblog20170613.060557/full/.)

## Technological Advances

For much of the 20th century, technological improvements served as a major driver of rising healthcare costs in the United States. These improvements included surgical advances in the 1960s (eg, transplantation, coronary artery bypass with graft [CABG]), medical device advances in the 1970s to 1990s (eg, pacemakers, stents, implantable cardioverter-defibrillators [ICDs]), so-called "blockbuster" drugs in the 1990s to address chronic illnesses (eg, statins for cholesterol, angiotensin-converting enzyme [ACE] inhibitors for high blood pressure), and (more recently) biotechnology drugs. Economists cannot precisely estimate their contribution to rising costs due to difficulties in measurement. Instead, they take an indirect

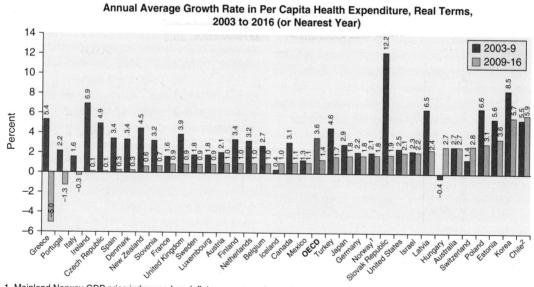

1. Mainland Norway GDP price index used as deflator.
2. CPI used as deflator.

**Figure 6-11** • Relative Slow Medical Spending Growth in Almost all Organisation of Economic Co-operation and Development (OECD) Countries, 2003 to 2016. (Source: OECD Health Statistics 2017.)

approach. They first estimate models to explain rising costs using what they can measure (eg, demographic transitions such as population growth and aging, rising national incomes, rising insurance coverage, economy-wide price inflation, medical price inflation) and then suggest that the "residual" (the error term in their models that cannot be explained) is likely the effect of technology.[10] While such modeling yields estimates that vary widely from 20% to 70%, the error term is often larger than the effects specified in their models.[11] Thus, they conclude that technology may be the primary driver.

A more nuanced version of this argument suggests that it is not technology per se that drives up NHE. Rather, it is patients with full insurance coverage that demand access to (and receive) this technology from their physicians, particularly those technologies that are not cost-effective or have uncertain clinical value. This includes greater utilization of magnetic resonance imaging (MRI) testing by orthopedic patients and greater use of intensive care units by the chronically ill.[12] This problem is alternatively labeled as "overuse" of care, unnecessary care, or "low-value care" (the downward-sloping portion of the curve in Figure 2-4). Thus, the spread of insurance coverage and the availability of new technologically based treatments combine to interact in a potent way to increase costs.

## Increased Prevalence of Chronic Illness

Since the 1990s, researchers suggest that technological drivers have been supplemented by the rise in chronic illness, the rising prevalence of treated (often chronic) disease, and the rise in spending per case treated. Following the Pareto principle (ie, 80-20 rule), a major share of healthcare spending is consumed by a small portion of the population with chronic conditions (Figure 6-12). Following up on the observation in Chapter 4 about the role of personal behaviors in determining one's health status, Figure 6-13 details which types of behaviors are involved. The chronically ill population includes people with hyperlipidemia (high blood cholesterol), hypertension, asthma, diabetes, chronic obstructive pulmonary disease (COPD), depression, and other conditions. Not only does a growing share of the US population have a chronic condition, but also a growing share has more than 1 chronic condition. People with 5 or more such conditions, known as "poly-chronics," account for a large share of spending under the Medicare program, the Medicaid program, and private insurance.[13]

## Increased Prevalence of Treated Disease

The rise in chronic (and acute) illness has been met by providers with more aggressive

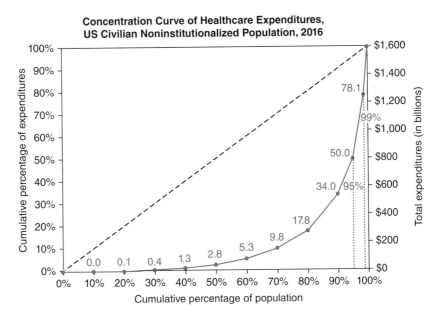

**Figure 6-12** • Top 1% of all Spenders Account for Greater Than 20% of all Spending. (Source: Agency for Healthcare Research and Quality, Medical Expenditure Panel Survey, Household Component, 2016.)

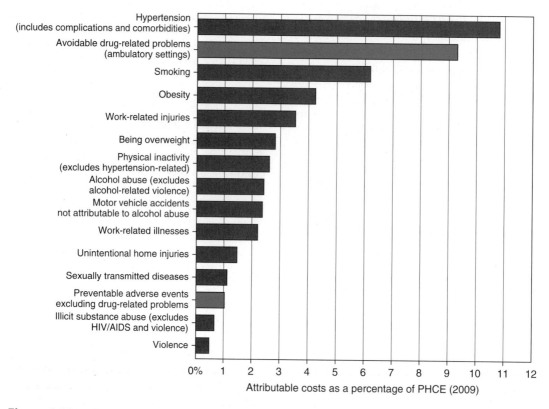

**Figure 6-13** • Fifty Percent or More of Health Spending Tied to Behavior and Lifestyle. PHCE, Personal Health Care Expenditures. (Source: Christopher Conover, "2.6 Half or More of Personal Health Spending Is Avoidable," Medical Industry Leadership Institute Open Education Hub, September 27, 2013, http://hub.mili.csom.umn.edu/content/m10014/latest/@collection=col10021_2f1.5.htm.)

management of these conditions. This includes a greater number and types of treatments, new therapies and combination therapies (including multiple medications), increased imaging tests, and improved detection and screening methods. Such increases in utilization have been abetted by changes in the clinical guidelines for treating such conditions, for example, by lowering the thresholds for treating patients and expanding the definitions of what is to be treated (eg, pain management). All of this has increased the number of cases treated and the cost per case treated.[14] This serves as a major contributor to what has been called overuse of care, low-value care, and unnecessary care.[15]

## Provider Consolidation

Provider consolidation (see Chapter 12) has emerged as the new "bad boy" in driving up healthcare costs. In recent years, we have witnessed growing "concentration" (ie, a smaller number of larger players) in hospital and physician markets. This consolidation has typically

taken 2 forms: horizontal integration and vertical integration. Horizontal integration (eg, linking up players within the *same stage* of the health-care value chain in Figure 3-9, such as the merger of several hospitals) can allow providers to increase their bargaining power with private insurers and thereby drive up their prices and, in turn, insurance premiums.[16] There have been several waves of consolidation in the hospital sector, beginning in the late 1960s, the 1970s, the 1990s, and most recently since 2010.[17] Vertical integration, by contrast, involves linking up players *across stages* in the healthcare value chain. Their combination allows physicians to obtain higher reimbursement by virtue of being linked to the hospital.

## Systemic View of Rising Costs

There is a voluminous research literature on the cost drivers in the US healthcare system, and they are too voluminous to review here. Suffice it to say that both *supply* and *demand* side factors are at work (Figure 6-14).[18] On the supply side

| Supply Side Factors | Demand Side Factors |
|---|---|
| Imperfect information on price and quality | Tax treatment of healthcare benefits<br>1) Purchase of more insurance<br>2) Use of more care |
| Large price differentials | |
| Nonprice competition (technology wars) | |
| Technological change and diffusion | Broader health insurance coverage |
| Technology complements (not substitutes) | Government financing of healthcare |
| Medical practice variations | Third-party reimbursement |
| Excess capacity | Rising national income |
| Resource focus on acute over preventive | Rising expectations about value<br>of healthcare |
| Malpractice fears and pressures | |
| Consumer choice | Poor health behaviors |

**Figure 6-14** • Supply and Demand Factors.

are some factors already discussed here (market failure, technological change, add-on technologies that supplement rather than replace old technologies, malpractice fears, consumer choice), as well as others we have not discussed, including provider inefficiency, price variations, nonprice competition among providers (eg, "technology wars"), and excess provider capacity. On the demand side are many factors we have already touched on, including the tax treatment of health benefits (which spurs moral hazard),

expansions in insurance coverage (which fuel the healthcare quadrilemma), third-party reimbursement, rising national incomes, lack of price controls, and underemphasis on prevention.

An alternative way to classify the cost drivers is to separate those that drive *price* from those that drive *volume* (or quantity). Healthcare costs are a function of price times quantity. Figure 6-15 presents a "fishbone diagram" of these 2 sets of drivers. Among all of these, many observers suggest that "fee-for-service"

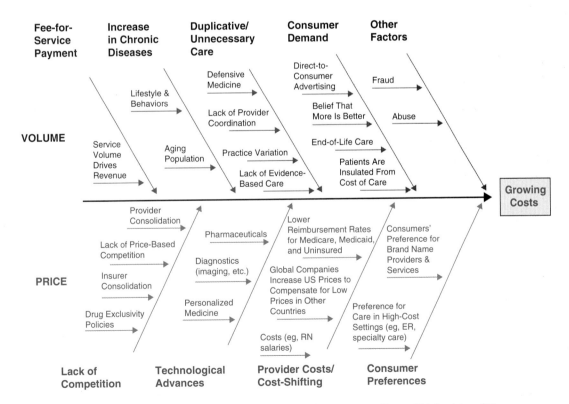

**Figure 6-15** • Volume and Price Drivers of Growing Costs. ER, Emergency Room; RN, Registered Nurse.

(FFS) reimbursement is the root cause, because it incentivizes higher volume and utilization to increase the provider's income.

One should also recognize that the cost drivers identified earlier vary in magnitude over time, even in the short term. Use and intensity of services played a larger role during the period of 1990 to 2007 than during the period of 2008 to 2013. The obverse was true for the age/sex mix of the population.[19]

## Implications

Given the plethora of healthcare cost drivers, what is the likelihood of gaining any control over spending? Before answering that question, it is important to note that a boatload of solutions have been proposed over time to tame rising costs. These include:

- Build an "escape fire" from FFS payment
- Bundled payments for different types of providers
- Pay-for-performance (P4P)
- Value-based purchasing (VBP)
- Risk-based contracts (RBCs)
- Accountable care organizations (ACOs)
- Patient-centered medical homes (PCMHs)
- Health information technology (HIT)
- Reduced care variations
- Wellness and prevention

Note that many of these solutions have a 3-letter acronym (TLA). TLAs unfortunately lend themselves to becoming "buzzwords" (see Chapter 2) that are repeated so often that everyone thinks they are not only well understood but also true. Sometimes they are neither.

It is important to observe that singular solutions are not likely to succeed and that any effort to "crack the code" on healthcare costs is likely to be too simplistic.[20] Indeed, as noted elsewhere, what is needed is not so much a "silver bullet" as a *lot* of "bronze buckshot" to hit all of the drivers of costs.[21] This is why, in recent years, policy makers and researchers have advocated 2-pronged solutions, such as changing how providers are paid *and* changing how providers are organized.[22]

The overarching strategy, at least since the early 2000s, has been to "bend the trend" (or, alternatively, "bend the curve"). What the "trend" is may vary, depending on who you talk to. In an early version, Stuart Altman plotted NHE per capita (adjusted for inflation) over 1966-2004, and found a fairly linear, upward-sloping line. Others portray it as the upward trend in Medicare spending as a percentage of US GDP. Either way, bending this trend would mean finding some way to reduce spending to reduce the slope of the line. Note that the goal is not to stop spending but rather to reduce its rate of growth.

Some observers thought that the 2010 Patient Protection and Affordable Care Act (PPACA, or "Obamacare") succeeded in bending the trend. In a famous article published in 2013, David Blumenthal and colleagues considered if the 800-pound gorilla of rising costs might have been tamed.[23] Other researchers similarly cited trend data between 2010 and 2012, following PPACA's passage, showing roughly equivalent rates of growth in GDP per capita and health expenditures per capita. Subsequent research showed that this was not true, however. The downturn in healthcare spending was caused by cyclical, economic factors common to all countries, not any structural changes undertaken in the United States.[24] Moreover, Victor Fuchs found that 2-year downturns in spending typically forecast future spending increases.[25]

## DEGREE OF PAST SUCCESS IN COST CONTAINMENT

Several of the earlier figures (Figures 6-1 and 6-5) suggest we have not been that successful in controlling the rising cost of healthcare. The titles of 3 articles confirm this dour conclusion. In 2012, Timothy Jost published an article entitled, "Eight Decades of Discouragement: The History of Health Care Cost Containment in the USA."[26] In December 2017, Joseph Antos and James Capretta published an article entitled, "National Health Expenditure Report Shows We Have Not Solved the Cost Problem," while David Cutler published the article, "Rising Medical Costs Mean More Rough Times Ahead."[27] Cutler concluded that addressing costs in a meaningful way is difficult, partly due to the fact that money is spent on both valuable services and less valuable services. To control costs therefore requires identifying lower-value services and then disincentivizing their use. The corrective needed will necessarily involve difficult trade-offs (see Chapter 2) such as cutting prices for some services and charging consumers more (eg, higher cost sharing) for others. In sum, to quote the subtitle of a book on waging war with insurgents, cutting costs resembles "eating soup with a knife."[28]

An examination of Figure 6-9 suggests there have been periodic moments in the history of the US healthcare system when the rate of increase in health spending approximated (rather than exceeded) the rate of increase in US GDP. Such moments occurred in 1973, 1979, and 1993. What explains these anomalies? President Nixon imposed wage and price controls in late 1971; they were lifted within 3 years and healthcare spending increases resumed. President Carter threatened regulation of the healthcare industry in 1979; following his defeat for reelection the following year, healthcare spending increases resumed. Finally, President Clinton threatened the pharmaceutical industry with price controls in 1993, which restrained drug price hikes; after the demise of the Clinton Health Plan in 1994, healthcare spending increases resumed. The lesson? Federal regulation, if not sustained, has few lasting salutary effects (when it does work).

## CYCLES IN HEALTHCARE SPENDING

One observation that readers should bear in mind is that healthcare spending increases wax and wane over time, much in the way of a cycle. This is somewhat evident from Figure 6-9 discussed earlier. Another way to depict this is in Figure 6-16, which charts the ups and downs in private health insurance premiums between 1991 and 2019.

Premium increases decelerated between 1991 and 1997 as employers shifted (or incentivized their workers to shift) to cheaper managed care plans, like health maintenance organizations (HMOs). Employee dislike of HMOs and their restricted networks and restrictive policies—the iron triangle trade-off—occasioned a "managed care backlash" and a switch to more expensive plans like preferred provider organizations (PPOs). This led to an increase in insurance premiums between 1997 and 2003. Higher premiums also resulted from provider consolidation efforts to "strike back" against the insurers. Beginning around 2004, premium increases again decelerated as employers began to offer their employees cheaper, high-deductible health plans (HDHPs).

Why is the chart in Figure 6-16 important? Industry observers and participants should recognize whether premium increases (and thus cost increases) are on the rise or on the decline. If they are on the rise, healthcare is becoming more expensive, putting greater pressure on consumers' ability to afford care and greater pressure on their employers to do something about it. Conversely, if premium (cost) increases are on the decline, healthcare may be more affordable but employers may become less watchful.

## TARGETS FOR CUTTING COSTS

If one were to target areas for cost cutting, where should you start? The discussion of national health accounts in Chapter 3 provides one clue. Data in Figure 3-4 describe the

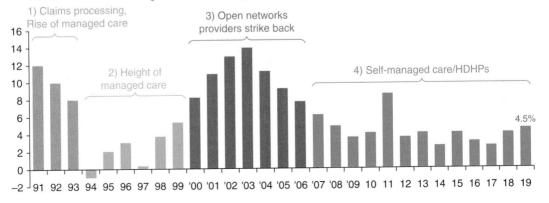

**Figure 6-16** • Cycles in Health Spending. HDHP, High-Deductible Health Plan. (Source: Kaiser Family Foundation, Employer Health Benefits Annual Surveys. Slide Courtesy of Sean Nicholson. Cornell University.)

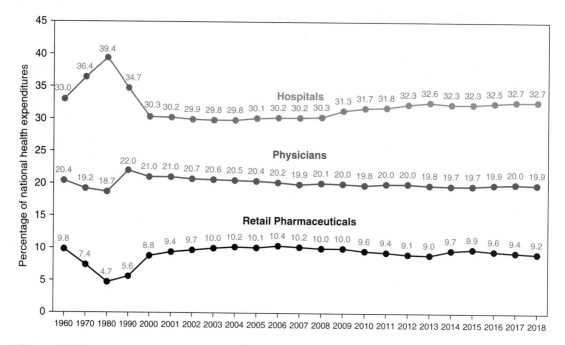

**Figure 6-17** • Hospital, Physician, and Retail Pharmaceutical Spending, 1960 to 2018, in the United States (as Percentage of National Health Spending).

destination of all NHE in the United States over time (ie, who gets the money). The proportion of NHE going to the major destinations varies over time, as depicted graphically in Figure 6-17. Hospitals were the major recipient of spending (35%-40%) between 1975 and 1980 and then experienced a declining share through 2005 (to 30%), and thereafter a slightly increasing share of total spending (now roughly 32%). Physician spending has been relatively constant at 20%. By contrast, pharmaceuticals consumed a small share of national spending during 1975 to 1995 (5%-6%) and then increased their share thereafter to 11% to 12% due to the advent of drug benefit coverage, blockbuster drugs, and then biologics. These are the 3 main sources of spending, accounting for roughly two-thirds of NHE. That is why a lot of cost-cutting efforts are directed their way, such as the "boatload of solutions" itemized earlier.

Of course, there are other, smaller cost-cutting targets hidden in the data in Figure 3-4. One is insurance ($258.5 billion in 2018). Proposals for economizing here include cutting out the insurance middlemen altogether via national health insurance and reducing how much the federal government pays private insurers who enroll Medicare and Medicaid patients in risk plans.

Another target is PAC. PAC providers include the array of home health agencies (HHAs), long-term care hospitals (LTCHs), intermediate rehabilitation facilities (IRFs), skilled nursing facilities (SNFs), and hospices. Researchers suggest that the greatest variations in care occur in the PAC sector, making this a potentially important arena to address.[29] However, although these PAC settings all treat similar types of patients, they are all paid differently, resisting efforts to control PAC spending (see Chapter 14).

## PROGNOSIS FOR CUTTING COSTS[30]

So what are the options and prospects for managing costs? One possibility is to anticipate *resignation* to a future in which spending continues to outpace income and any effort made to transform our healthcare system fails to make an impact. That this result is heartily undesired by all does not make it impossible. Spending can continue to grow at its current pace (with at least the dividend of better new technology) as long as real income grows. The doomsday prophecy that medical care costs are increasing so fast that no one can afford them is mildly preposterous, because, if no one can or will spend more, spending cannot rise. There will, following Stein's law, eventually be a slow-down, even if at a higher share of spending on medical care and a lower share on other things than at present.

The challenges in this scenario are 2-fold. One is that the intense desire to change things quickly that cannot be changed may lead to regulation, frustration, false promises and the associated waste, and political turmoil that a more realistic evaluation of the prospects could avoid. Rather than grasping at straws, a policy of keeping an open door for new inno-vations (whatever the source) may be supe-rior to planning what cannot be successfully planned. One feature of such a policy would be to permit, even encourage, insurers to develop new methods for allocating resources and organizing physicians without handicap-ping one form or another; let consumer choice in the insurance market work it out. The other challenge is that we do not yet know the mech-anism by which the inevitable slowdown will be accomplished, with attendant worry and impatience, until it appears.

Another more optimistic view is that a *bet-ter targeted strategy* than current policy might work. Rather than focus on replacing FFS payment to organizations (which has not been shown to accelerate spending despite its poor reputation), one might focus on (1) getting physicians to change behavior and (2) shifting focus to new technology (rather than fixating on old but stubborn waste that has been around for years). Here, again, current evidence does not endorse a particular strategy to deal with these problems, but greater focus on them, while avoiding prohibitions on rationing or contracting (with physicians or consumers), might be wise.

A third strategy is to *count on small steps*. That seems to be all that can be expected from current transformation models, but perhaps 1 percentage point lower cost from ACOs, added to a couple of points from bundled pay-ment, might someday add up to real money. The challenge here is the limited bite these measures can take out of the "one-third of all spending is waste." If these changes could shave percentage points off spending growth rates rather than levels (what the HMOs of the 1990s failed to do), that would amount to something over time.

The final strategy is to *hope for the big one*. We do not know yet what it might be, but there is always the possibility that someone, somewhere, will invent a method of payment or manage-ment that can slow spending growth appreciably without harming quality. We suspect that it will have to affect physicians and technology.

Are there more concrete ways to pursue these options? As part of the first option, given its prevalence and popularity among physicians, we may need to stop bashing FFS models and look for ways to retool this payment method. With the rapid growth of HDHPs that almost all pay FFS and require patient consent to bear-ing the cost, FFS may get a new lease on life. As part of the second and third options, provider reorganization is likely a gradual, even glacial, process that gives physicians time to get used to the idea; it is not a recent, radical change. Trends in larger practice size and hospital sys-tem formation have been occurring slowly for decades. The problem is that, so far, such con-solidation is associated with higher costs and doubtful improvements in quality, contrary to what transformation advocates envision.

## STAKEHOLDERS: MY EXPENSE IS YOUR INCOME

Another set of considerations regarding the prognosis for controlling healthcare costs is that (1) healthcare has become such a large per-centage of our GDP, and partially as a result, (2) many people's incomes and livelihoods derive from healthcare spending. Over 14% of US employment is in healthcare; in 2017, healthcare surpassed both manufacturing and retail as the largest employment sector.[32] That means lots of wages and salaries are dependent on healthcare spending. Healthcare is a driver of both rising employment and rising GDP—things we value. There is recent evidence that during periods of high economy-wide unem-ployment, the growth in medical spending increases medical sector employment and reduces the rate of unemployment.[33] Thus, any attempt to control healthcare costs "gores someone's ox" and invites pushback from lots of constituencies.

In their article on the triple aim, Don Berwick and colleagues propose that one solution to rising healthcare costs is the use of an "integrator."[31] According to them, the integrator replaces the invisible hand of the market with the visible hand of management.

An "integrator" is an entity that accepts responsibility for all three components of the Triple Aim for a specified population.... That role might be within the reach of a powerful, visionary insurer; a large primary care group in partnership with payers; or even a hospital, with some affiliated physician group, that seeks to be especially attractive to payers.... In crafting care, an effective integrator, in one way or another, will link health care organizations (as well as public health and social service organizations) whose missions overlap across the spectrum of delivery. It will be able to recognize and respond to patients' individual care needs and preferences, to the health needs and opportunities of the population (whether or not people seek care), and to the total costs of care. The important function of linking organizations across the continuum requires that the integrator be a single organization (not just a market dynamic) that can induce coordinative behavior among health service suppliers to work as a system for the defined population.

What does the integrator do to achieve these ends?

**Involve Individuals and Families:** Pursuit of the Triple Aim requires that the population served become continually better informed about both the determinants of their own health status and the benefits and limitations of individual health care practices and procedures. An effective integrator would work persistently to change the "more-is-better" culture through transparency, systematic education, communication, and shared decision making with patients and communities, rather than by restricting access, shifting costs, or erecting administrative hurdles to care....

**Redesign of Primary Care Services and Structures:** We believe that any effective integrator will strengthen primary care for the population. To accomplish this, physicians might not be the sole, or even the principal, providers. Recently, physicians and other clinicians have proposed principles for expanding the role of primary care under the title of the medical home....

**Population Health Management:** The integrator would be responsible for deploying resources to the population, or for specifying to others how resources should be deployed. Segmentation of the population, perhaps according to health status, level of support from family or others, and socioeconomic status, will facilitate efficient and equitable resource allocation....

**Financial Management System:** ... An effective integrator would assure that payment and resource allocation support the Triple Aim. An important first step for a systems approach to cost control would be defining, measuring, and making transparent the per capita cost of care for a defined population.

Just how feasible is the use of a visible hand to accomplish all of this? What visionary organizations have performed these functions? Are there enough to them to do the job?

During the past few years, there has been a serious effort to control rising drug costs. As noted earlier, those costs are borne by the patients at the pharmacy (and by taxpayers ultimately). At the same time, rising drug costs translate into rising revenues for all of the players in the pharmaceutical distribution channel (see Figure 6-10): drug manufacturers, drug wholesalers, pharmacies, PBMs, and insurers. These companies all employ people in decent-paying jobs.

What is important here is that policy efforts to "bend the trend" may overlook human agency. As Stuart Altman and colleagues noted, the US political system has lacked the will to stay in the background when the negative consequences of reduced healthcare spending growth became apparent and has been pressured by consumers and other interest groups to ease off brakes on spending.[34] In a similar vein, Joseph White stated[35]:

> Policies do not simply play out and have predictable effects. People who object to the planned effects fight back. Health care costs at any time are the result of, among other things, efforts by people who earn their incomes from the system to extract money from it. If prices are lowered, providers may try to increase volume; if volume is constrained they may try to raise prices; if employers and insurers demand better prices the providers consolidate to increase their market power; if regulation is successful the providers claim the public is being denied quality care or campaign to create parallel markets where people can pay more for more "choice." Whatever policy-makers do in Year One, the health care industry will seek to undo by Year Five or Year Ten. The metaphor of "bending the curve" ignores the fact that health care spending is a political/economic struggle. Either there is no function, or policy-makers are not the only ones who get to manipulate the terms of the function.

In addition, the drug manufacturers use their revenues to invest in research and development (R&D), which involves high-paying jobs and also attracts highly trained workers from other countries and their drug companies to come set up their R&D operations here. Cost-cutters should keep in mind that pharmaceutical companies (and the life sciences sector in general) are a major contributor to employment.[36] Finally, the R&D conducted here in pharmaceutical research can translate into discovery of new drugs that become available here in the United States before other countries, thereby improving our access to high-tech care (albeit at a higher cost). Research suggests that the United States has enjoyed value (benefits that exceed costs) from technology advances and medical spending.[37]

To the above, we might add the following corollary: My expense is my health benefit. Much of the rising cost of care has come in the form of new technologies that address unmet medical needs. Cost containment may thus not be what consumers really want, if the new technology is worth the cost.[38] It is hard to prospectively discern high-value from low-value healthcare. It is also hard to get both physicians and consumers to "choose wisely" among them.[39] Physicians report that they feel pressure from malpractice as well as from their patients to render what some view as unnecessary services.[40] At the same time, physicians are also slow to abandon practices that are contradicted by the medical literature.[41] The persistence of highly cited observational research findings despite their contradiction by randomized controlled trials does not help.[42] The savings here could be enormous, if we can collect enough "nickels and dimes" from avoiding a lot of low-cost, high-volume services.[43] This approach is consistent with the third strategy above of "count on small steps."

## SUMMARY

The rising cost of healthcare is an intractable problem. It is not just a US issue, but rather a global problem. No one has come up with a better mousetrap to solving this (see Figure 6-11). One reason is the variety of cost drivers that encompass supply, demand, price, and volume. These are all targets that can and should be addressed, but without a seriously *multipronged* approach, our efforts are likely to yield limited success. This may be all we can hope for at present.

## QUESTIONS TO PONDER

1. What seems to be the biggest obstacle to reducing healthcare costs?
2. What seem to be the most promising avenues to try to reduce healthcare costs?
3. If a combination of approaches (eg, multiple levers) is needed to control costs, what approaches should be tried together?
4. Can we really cut healthcare costs? Or are we resigned to just slowing down its rate of increase?
5. Are healthcare costs "out of control," as many casual observers claim?
6. Does the US "ration" healthcare?
7. Are rising healthcare costs necessarily a bad thing?

## REFERENCES

1. Mark V. Pauly. *Health Benefits at Work* (Ann Arbor, MI: University of Michigan Press, 1997).
2. Lewin-VHI. *The Financial Impact of the Health Security Act* (Fairfax, VA: Lewin-VHI, 1993).
3. Mark V. Pauly. *Health Benefits at Work* (Ann Arbor, MI: University of Michigan Press, 1997).
4. Gerard Anderson, Uwe Reinhardt, Peter Hussey, et al. "It's the Prices, Stupid: Why the United States Is So Different From Other Countries," *Health Aff.* 22 (3) (2003): 89-105.
5. David Dranove, Craig Garthwaite, and Christopher Ody. "Health Spending Slowdown Is Mostly Due to Economic Factors, Not Structural Change in the Health Care Sector," *Health Aff.* 33 (8) (2014): 1399-1406.
6. Sherry Glied. "Single Payer as a Financing Mechanism," *J Health Polit Policy Law.* 34 (4) (2009): 593-615.
7. Paul Starr. "The Health-Care Legacy of the Great Society," in Norman J. Glickman et al. (Eds.), *Reshaping the Federal Government: The Policy and Management Legacies of the Johnson Years.* Chapter 8. Forthcoming.
8. Technological Change in Health Care (TECH) Research Network. "Technological Change Around the World: Evidence From Heart Attack Care," *Health Aff.* 20 (3) (2001): 25-42.
9. Laura Tollen, Elizabeth Keating, and Alan Weil. "How Administrative Spending Contributes to Excess US Health Spending," *Health Affairs Blog* (February 20, 2020). Available online: https://www.healthaffairs.org/do/10.1377/hblog20200218.375060/full/. Accessed November 3, 2020.
10. Sheila Smith, Joseph Newhouse, and Mark Freeland. "Income, Insurance, and Technology: Why Does Health Spending Outpace Economic Growth?" *Health Aff.* 28 (5) (2009): 1276-1284.
11. Joseph Newhouse. "An Iconoclastic View of Health Cost Containment," *Health Aff.* 12 (No. Suppl. 1) (1993). Available online at: https://www.healthaffairs.org/doi/full/10.1377/hlthaff.12.suppl_1.152. Accessed on March 27, 2020.
12. Amitabh Chandra and Jonathan Skinner. "Technology Growth and Expenditure Growth in Health Care," *J Econ Lit.* 50 (3) (2012): 645-680.
13. Christine Buttorff, Teague Rudorf, and Mellissa Bauman. *Multiple Chronic Conditions in the United States* (Santa Monica, CA: Rand Corporation, 2017). Susan Hayes, Claudia Salzberg, Douglas McCarthy, et al. *High-Need High-Cost Patients: Who Are They and How Do They Use Health Care?* (New York, NY: Commonwealth Fund, August 29, 2016).
14. Kenneth Thorpe, Curtis Florence, David Howard, et al. "The Rising Prevalence of Treated Disease: Effects on Private Health Insurance Spending," *Health Aff.* (Web Exclusive) (June 27, 2005): W5, 317-325. Available online: https://www.healthaffairs.org/doi/pdf/10.1377/hlthaff.W5.317. Accessed on February 27, 2020.
15. PerryUndem Research/Communication. *Unnecessary Tests and Procedures in the Health Care System: What Physicians Say About the Problem, the Causes, and the Solutions* (The ABIM Foundation, May 1, 2014). Available online: https://www.choosingwisely.org/wp-content/uploads/2015/04/Final-Choosing-Wisely-Survey-Report.pdf. Accessed November 3, 2020.
16. Massachusetts Division of Health Care Finance and Policy. *Massachusetts Health Care Cost Trends: Trends in Health Expenditures* (June 2011). McKinsey. *Accounting for the Cost of U.S. Health Care* (McKinsey Center for U.S. Health System Reform, December 2011).
17. Gregory Kruse, Lawton R. Burns, and Ralph Muller. "Health Care Inc.," in James Schaefer, Richard M. Mizelle, Jr., and Helen K. Valier (Eds.), *Oxford Handbook of American Medical History* (Oxford, United Kingdom: Oxford University Press, Forthcoming): Chapter 16.
18. Henry Aaron and Paul Ginsburg. "Is Health Spending Excessive? If So, What Can We Do About It?" *Health Aff.* 28 (5) (2009): 1260-1275.
19. Andrea Sisko, Sean Keehan, John Poisal, et al. "National Health Expenditure Projections, 2018-27: Economic and Demographic Trends Drive Spending and Enrollment Growth," *Health Aff.* 38 (3) (2019): 491-501.

20. See, for example, Miller Center. *Cracking the Code on Health Care Costs*. A Report by the State Health Care Cost Containment Commission (Charlottesville, VA: University of Virginia, The Miller Center, 2014). Available online: http://www.cms.org/uploads/HealthcareCommission-Report.pdf. Accessed on February 27, 2020.

21. Lawton R. Burns and Mark V. Pauly. *Detecting BS in Health Care* (Philadelphia, PA: Leonard Davis Institute, 2018). Available online: https://ldi.upenn.edu/brief/detecting-bs-health-care. Accessed on February 28, 2020.

22. Lawton R. Burns and Mark V. Pauly. "Transformation of the Healthcare Industry: Curb Your Enthusiasm?" *Milbank Q.* 96 (1) (2018): 57-109.

23. David Blumenthal, Kristof Stremikis, and David Cutler. "Health Care Spending: A Giant Slain or Sleeping?" *N Engl J Med.* 369 (2013): 2551-2557.

24. David Dranove, Craig Garthwaite, and Christopher Ody. "Health Spending Slowdown Is Mostly Due to Economic Factors, Not Structural Change in the Health Care Sector," *Health Aff.* 33 (8) (2014): 1399-1406.

25. Victor Fuchs. "The Gross Domestic Product and Health Care Spending," *N Engl J Med.* 369 (2013): 107-109.

26. Timothy Stoltzfus Jost. "Eight Decades of Discouragement: The History of Health Care Cost Containment in the USA," *Forum for Health Economics and Policy* 15(3) (2012): 53-82.

27. Joseph Antos and James Capretta. "National Health Expenditure Report Shows We Have Not Solved the Cost Problem," *Health Affairs Blog* (December 6, 2017). Available online: https://www.healthaffairs.org/do/10.1377/hblog20171205.607294/full/. Accessed on February 27, 2020. David Cutler. "Rising Medical Costs Mean More Rough Times Ahead," *JAMA.* 318 (6) (2017): 508-509.

28. John Nagl. *Learning to Eat Soup With a Knife: Counterinsurgency Lessons From Malaya and Vietnam* (Chicago, IL: University of Chicago Press, 2002).

29. Joseph Newhouse and Alan Garber. "Geographic Variation in Medicare Services," *N Engl J Med.* 368 (2013): 1465-1468.

30. This section draws on Lawton R. Burns and Mark V. Pauly. "Transformation of the Healthcare Industry: Curb Your Enthusiasm?" *Milbank Q.* 96 (1) (March 2018): 57-109.

31. Donald M. Berwick, Thomas W. Nolan, and John Whittington. "The Triple Aim: Care, Health, and Cost," *Health Aff.* 27 (3) (2008): 759-769.

32. Derek Thompson. "Health Care Just Became the U.S.'s Largest Employer," *The Atlantic* (January 9, 2018).

33. Mark Pauly and Vivek Nimgaonkar. "Medical Employment Growth, Unemployment, and the Opportunity Cost of Health Care," *Int J Health Econ Manage.* 16 (2016): 387-396.

34. Stuart Altman, Christopher Tompkins, Efrat Eilat, et al. "Escalating Health Care Spending: Is It Desirable or Inevitable?" *Health Aff.* 22 (Web Exclusives) (2003). Available online: https://www.healthaffairs.org/doi/full/10.1377/hlthaff.W3.1. Accessed on February 28, 2020.

35. Joseph White. "The Mixed (De)Merits of 'Bending the Cost Curve,'" *Health Affairs Blog* (June 17, 2011). Available online: https://www.healthaffairs.org/do/10.1377/hblog20110617.011786/full/. Accessed on February 28, 2020.

36. Archstone Consulting and Lawton R. Burns. *The Biopharmaceutical Sector's Impact on the U.S. Economy: Analysis at the National, State, and Local Levels.* Report issued by PhRMA, 2009.

37. David Cutler and Mark McClellan. "Is Technological Change in Medicine Worth It?" *Health Aff.* 20 (5) (2001): 11-29. David Cutler, Allison Rosen, and Sandeep Vijan. "The Value of Medical Spending in the United States, 1960-2000," *N Engl J Med.* 355 (2006): 920-927.

38. Mark Pauly. "The Business of Healthcare and the Economics of Healthcare: Shall Ever the Twain Meet?" *Int J Econ Business.* 25 (1) (2018): 181-189.

39. American College of Cardiology. *Choosing Wisely: Five Things Physicians and Patients Should Question* (April 4, 2012). Available online: https://www.choosingwisely.org/societies/american-college-of-cardiology/. Accessed on February 28, 2020.

40. PerryUndem Research/Communication. *Unnecessary Tests and Procedures in the Health Care System* (ABIM Foundation, 2014). Available online: https://www.choosingwisely.org/wp-content/uploads/2015/04/Final-Choosing-Wisely-Survey-Report.pdf. Accessed on February 28, 2020.

41. David Epstein and ProPublica. "When Evidence Says No, but Doctors Say Yes," *The Atlantic* (February 22, 2017).

42. Athina Tatsioni, Nikolaos Bonitsis, and John Ioannidis. "Persistence of Contradicted Claims in the Literature," *JAMA.* 298 (21) (2007): 2517-2526.

43. John Mafi, Kyle Russell, Beth Bortz, et al. "Low-Cost, High-Volume Health Services Contribute the Most to Unnecessary Health Spending," *Health Aff.* 36 (10) (2017): 1701-1704.

# Managing Quality: Another 800-Pound Gorilla?

## INTRODUCTION

What is "quality"? Back in the 1970s, it meant avoiding negative patient outcomes such as death, disease, disability, discomfort, and dissatisfaction. More recently, quality has meant achievement of positive objectives such as care consistent with knowledge, maximization of the quality of life, maximization of duration of life, achievement of desired health outcomes, and maximization of population health.[1]

There is no single, agreed-upon definition of quality. As noted in Chapter 5, it is a construct with multiple dimensions on which different stakeholders place different emphases. Chapter 5 introduced the reader to the plethora of quality measures that providers are subjected to and held accountable for. These include Donabedian's structure, process, and outcome measures; the STEEEP measures advocated by the Institute of Medicine (IOM); the Healthcare Effectiveness Data and Information Set (HEDIS) measures used by health plans; the 4,456 measures listed by Agency for Healthcare Research and Quality (AHRQ); and the 2,266 measures listed by the Centers for Medicare and Medicaid Services (CMS) in its Inventory Tool, of which 788 have been implemented or finalized for use in a CMS program. Chapter 2 described the "murky relationships" among these quality measures, as well as between the angles of the iron triangle (eg, cost and quality). These observations set the stage for this chapter: the challenge of managing quality when "quality" is a multidimensional vector of measures that may not be highly correlated with one another. You can build an entire career working in this area.

## QUALITY MANAGEMENT VERSUS MEDICAL MANAGEMENT

Before proceeding, it is important to distinguish 2 terms that are easily confused: quality management and medical management. *Quality management* includes tools that payers and providers use to inform the decisions that doctors and patients make to improve quality of care (usually focused on changes to process or outcome measures). *Medical management* includes tools that payers and providers use to reduce expensive types of healthcare utilization (eg, inpatient days, hospital admissions, emergency room visits). These tools include prior authorization, provider credentialing, hospitalists, disease management, case management, physician profiling, provider education, patient education, disease registries, patient-centered medical homes, and health promotion and wellness programs. Researchers suggest that medical management tools are expensive to operate and often have low payoffs; they are most efficacious when targeted narrowly to small, high-cost patient populations (eg, the top 3% of plan members who account for 47% of health plan costs).[2] Quality management may help with medical management, and vice versa. This chapter focuses more on the former than the latter.

## WHY THE NEED FOR QUALITY MANAGEMENT?

There is no doubt that quality of care delivered in the United States has improved over time. For example, the rate of Americans dying annually

| | 1984 | 2011 |
|---|---|---|
| HIV | Dead in 18 months | Chronic disease |
| Cholecystectomy | 10-12 inpatient days<br>3-6 months of restrictions | Home that evening<br>Back to work in 1 week |
| Acute mylogenous leukemia (AML) | Dead in 18 months | Gleevec |
| HPV | Cervical cancer | Vaccine available |
| Cataract surgery | 3 days inpatient | 20-minute surgery |

**Figure 7-1** • Improvement in Healthcare Outcomes Since Medical School Graduation. (Source: Jeffrey Levin-Scherz.)

has fallen from 1 in 40 in 1900 to 1 in 140 by 2013. The number of deaths from heart disease has markedly declined from 589 per 100,000 population in 1950 to 170 per 100,000 by 2013. Other improvements are also noticeable, such as the decline in the infant mortality rate and the increase in life expectancy at birth from 47 years to 79 years between 1900 and 2013.[3] According to Dr. Jeffrey Levin-Scherz, who lectures at Wharton, the outcomes of care are much better today than when he attended medical school (Figure 7-1).

Nevertheless, quality of care in the United States still has lots of room for improvement. In 1998, researchers reported that "contraindicated" (ie, the wrong) care was frequently provided to patients suffering from both acute and chronic conditions (Figure 7-2). In 1999, the IOM reported that medical errors in hospitals caused anywhere from 44,000 to 98,000 deaths annually.[4] Others have reported that as many as 974,000 medical errors occur in hospitals each year, costing the system anywhere from $17 to $29 billion.[5] The Office of the Inspector General (OIG) reported that 13.5% of Medicare beneficiaries experienced an adverse event during their hospital stays, nearly half of which were avoidable.[6]

Similar statistics have been reported regarding the failure to provide appropriate care. The National Committee on Quality Assurance noted that more than 57,000 patients die needlessly each year because they do not receive the appropriate healthcare, mostly for common,

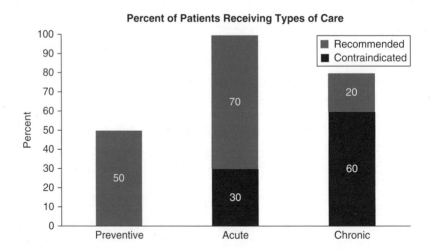

**Figure 7-2** • Quality in America. (Source: Mark A. Schuster, Elizabeth A. McGlynn, and Robert H. Brook. "How Good Is the Quality of Health Care in the United States?" https://www.ncbi.nlm.nih.gov/pmc/articles/PMC2690270/pdf/milq0083-0403.pdf, page 884.)

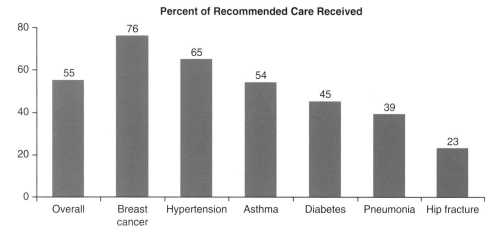

**Figure 7-3 •** Overall, Only 55% of Evidence-Based Care Is Delivered to Patients. (Source: Elizabeth McGlynn, Steven M Asch, John Adams, et al. "The Quality of Health Care Delivered to Adults in the United States," *N Engl J Med*. 348 (2003): 2635-2645.)

chronic conditions such as high blood pressure and high cholesterol levels. RAND Corporation researchers conducted a survey of adults in 12 cities to gauge their receipt of appropriate care measured on 439 indicators covering 30 acute and chronic conditions. They reported that, on average, only 55% of evidence-based care was delivered to US patients (Figure 7-3), suggesting a massive "underuse" of appropriate care.[7] There was no difference in receipt of recommended care depending on whether it was preventive, acute, or chronic. The AHRQ subsequently reported progress in patients' receipt of recommended care, rising from 66% in 2005 to 70% by 2010.[8]

Not only are there gaps in the quality of care provided, but evidence that documents quality improvement over time is decidedly mixed, with painstakingly slow progress.[9] On the *positive* front, AHRQ released its *2015 National Healthcare Quality and Disparities Report* assessing progress on 191 quality metrics over the period from 2001 to 2013. Of the 191 metrics studied, 110 showed progress, whereas 62 showed no improvement and 19 showed declines (Figure 7-4). Speed of improvement varied considerably across priority areas targeted by AHRQ. Great progress was observed in reducing the incidence of hospital-acquired conditions (HACs; Figure 7-5); there was also some improvement in certain measures of care coordination (Figure 7.6).

On the *negative* front, an analysis of outpatient care delivered to adults between 2002 and 2013 revealed no consistent improvement.[10] Of the 9 composite measures of clinical quality (representing both underuse and overuse of care, which reflect the upward- and downward-sloping portions of the curve in Figure 2-4), 4 showed improvement, 3 were unchanged, and 2 worsened. Improvements were found among the underuse measures, while declines occurred more among the overuse measures. Among the underuse measures, improvements were noted in recommended counseling (smoking cessation) and recommended treatments (use of statins for stroke and use of β-blockers for heart failure). Among the overuse measures, improvements were found in avoiding inappropriate cervical cancer screening; other overuse measures worsened over time. Many of the clinical measures exhibited low absolute levels and only small absolute improvements over time. Patient experience measures did show improvement.

What explains the slow improvement among these somewhat lackluster statistics? Researchers have ascribed the tepid results to the failure of pay-for-performance (P4P) programs (covered later), the lack of investment in primary care, the unfelt effects expected from the Patient Protection and Affordable Care Act (PPACA), and the role of social determinants of health. Slow improvement may also reflect problems with the specific quality improvement initiatives undertaken. The following sections review the historical record of quality improvement efforts and the evidence for their impacts.

**Quality of healthcare improved generally through 2013, but the pace of improvement varied by the NQS priority.**

Number and percentage of all quality measures that are improving, not changing, or worsening through 2013, overall and by NQS priority

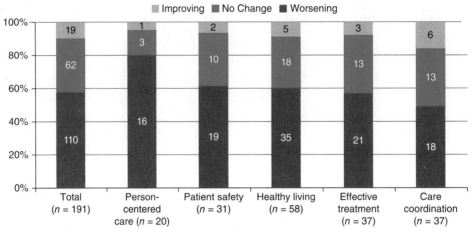

**Key:** *n* = number of measures.
**Note:** For the majority of measures, trend data are available from 2001 to 2013. Measures of Care Affordability are included in the Total but not shown separately.
For each measure with at least 4 estimates over time, log-linear regression is used to calculate average annual percentage change relative to the baseline year and to assess statistical significance. Measures are aligned so that positive change indicates improved care.

- **Improving** = Rates of change are positive at 1% per year or greater and are statistically significant.
- **No Change** = Rates of change are less than 1% per year or not statistically significant.
- **Worsening** = Rates of change are negative at −1% per year or greater and are statistically significant.

**Figure 7-4** • Improvement in Quality of Healthcare. NQS, National Quality Strategy. (Source: Agency for Healthcare Research and Quality. National Healthcare Quality and Disparities Report and 5th Anniversary Update on the National Quality Strategy, 2015. https://www.ahrq.gov/sites/default/files/wysiwyg/research/findings/nhqrdr/nhqdr15/2015nhqdr.pdf.)

## HISTORICAL PROGRESSION OF QUALITY MANAGEMENT EFFORTS

### American College of Surgeons and The Joint Commission

As noted in prior chapters, initial quality management efforts focused on standardizing the medical school training of physicians and the provision of proper equipment by hospitals, both "structural" measures of quality. The latter effort began with the 1912 formation of the American College of Surgeons (ACS), which was concerned with the ability of physicians to perform surgery in hospitals that lacked the proper infrastructure. The ACS's initiative, the Committee on the Standardization of Hospitals, mirrored earlier efforts by the American Medical Association (AMA) to standardize medical training based on the Flexner Report of 1910.

The ACS Committee undertook quality reviews of hospitals (beginning in 1918), expanding its focus on minimum standards for surgery to all aspects of hospitals' operations. The standards included the medical staff organization (see Chapter 11), patient medical records, and provision of clinical laboratory and x-ray facilities. The ACS initiative later came under the aegis of the Joint Commission for Accreditation of Hospitals (JCAH) in 1951, subsequently renamed the Joint Commission for Accreditation of Healthcare Organizations (JCAHO) in 1987 to account for a greater diversity of provider organizations it reviewed, and now known as The Joint Commission.

### Accreditation: The Joint Commission and the National Committee for Quality Assurance

External agencies today accredit both hospitals and health plans. The previous section describes how hospital accreditation via

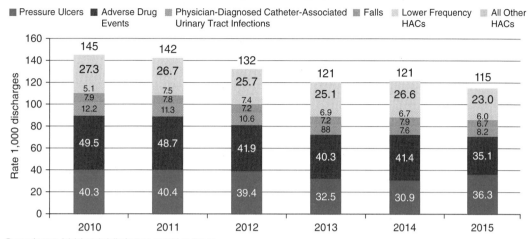

**Distribution of Hospital-Acquired Conditions, Based on National Rates Per 1,000 Adult Hospital Discharges, 2010-2015**

Denominator: Adult hospital discharges, age 18 and over.

**Note**: Lower Frequency HACs (<3/1,000 discharges) include central line-associated bloodstream infections, venous thromboembolisms, surgical site infections, obstetric adverse events, and ventilator-associated pneumonia. All Other Hospital-Acquired Conditions includes: inadvertent femoral artery puncture for catheter angiographic procedures, adverse events associated with hip joint replacement, adverse events associated with knee joint replacement, contrast nephropathy associated with catheter angiography, methicillin-resistant *Staphylococcus aureus* (MRSA), vancomycin-resistant *Enterococcus* (VRE). *C.difficile*, mechanical complications associated with central venous catheters, postoperative cardiac events for cardiac and noncardiac surgeries, postoperative pneumonia, iatrogenic pneumothorax, postoperative hemorrhage or hematoma, postoperative respiratory failure, and accidental puncture or laceration. For more information on methods, see https://www.ahrq.gov/professionals /quality-patient-safety/pfp/index.html. The 2015 data on this graph reflect interim results. Prior analysis suggest that the (pending) final data should be very similar.

**Figure 7-5 •** Distribution of Hospital-Acquired Conditions (HACs). (Source: Agency for Healthcare Research and Quality. National Healthcare Quality and Disparities Report, 2016. https://www.ahrq.gov/sites/default/files/ wysiwyg/research/findings/nhqrdr/chartbooks/patientsafety/qdr2016-ptschartbook.pdf.)

The Joint Commission originated. CMS requires that hospitals gain accreditation or pass state inspection in order to be reimbursed by the Medicare program. Most US hospitals (88%) seek accreditation by The Joint Commission. But is accreditation associated with quality of care rendered by hospitals? Earlier studies found that accredited hospitals are more likely to adhere to process measures of quality and show improvements on these measures[11]; other studies also found that accredited hospitals score slightly higher on patient outcome measures. The question of causation was not addressed, however: Does accreditation lead to quality, or does quality lead hospitals to seek accreditation?[12] A more recent study found no significant relationship between The Joint Commission accreditation and hospital mortality rates. While accredited hospitals had lower rates of readmission for 15 medical conditions, the differences were modest; there was no difference in readmission rates for 6 surgical conditions. Moreover, accredited hospitals exhibited modestly worse patient experience (ie, Hospital Consumer Assessment of Healthcare Providers and Systems [HCAHPS]) scores than hospitals

undergoing state surveys.[13] The researchers concluded that accrediting bodies are not focused on measures that matter to patients (eg, health, safety, patient experience), but rather on administrative issues (eg, documentation of processes).

Health plans can also be accredited. Accreditation by the National Committee for Quality Assurance (NCQA) uses consistent criteria to evaluate health plans at the national level. NCQA's assessment uses measures of clinical process performance (ie, HEDIS measures) and consumer experience (ie, HCAHPS measures). NCQA accredits plans that cover 136 million people (43%) in the US population. NCQA has 3 levels of accreditation status: (1) "accredited" status, the lowest level, is accorded to plans that meet basic requirements for consumer protection and quality improvement; (2) "commendable" status is accorded to plans that satisfy rigorous requirements for consumer protection and quality improvement; and (3) "excellent" status, the highest level, is accorded to plans that meet or exceed rigorous requirements for consumer protection and quality improvement, with HEDIS results in the highest range of national performance. According to one

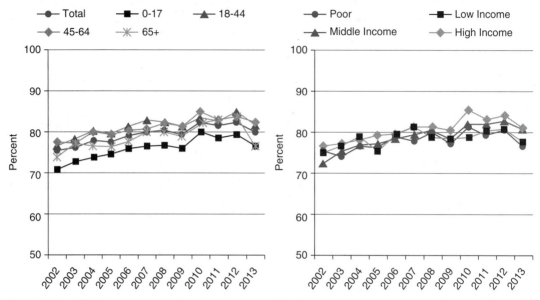

**Care Coordination: People who report that their usual source of care usually asks about prescription medications and treatments from other doctors, by age and income, 2002-2013**

From 2002 to 2013, the percentage of people who reported that their usual source of care usually asked about prescription medications and treatments from other doctors increased overall and among all age and income groups.

**Figure 7-6** • Care Coordination. (Source: Agency for Healthcare Research and Quality. National Healthcare Quality and Disparities Report, 2015. https://www.ahrq.gov/sites/default/files/wysiwyg/research/findings/nhqrdr/nhqdr15/2015nhqdr.pdf.)

research study of 351 plans in 2015, the level of accreditation was positively associated with patient satisfaction, monitoring and prevention activities, and appropriate care; level of accreditation was not associated with the ratio of observed-to-expected readmissions or degree of appropriate care.[14]

## Role of the Medicare Program

The Medicare program (1965) wanted to ensure that the care that it financed was of sufficient quality. One organization it relied on was The Joint Commission: Accreditation became a prerequisite for reimbursement under the Medicare program. This set the stage for later efforts to impose "conditions of participation" (CoPs) on providers of Medicare services. The 1972 Social Security Amendments established professional standard review organizations (PSROs) to assess the appropriateness of inpatient care rendered to Medicare and Medicaid beneficiaries via peer review by physicians in that hospital. According to a government evaluation, PSROs did reduce Medicare days of hospitalization,

but their effect on Medicaid use was unclear. PSROs did reduce Medicare spending, but the federal government saved little more than the cost of the review itself.[15]

The ineffectiveness of PSROs led to their replacement in 1982 by peer review organizations (PROs), external bodies that contracted with the government. The PROs randomly sampled hospital records looking for deficient care in an "inspect and detect" approach. They were viewed with great suspicion by providers, suffered from poor reliability of peer assessments of quality, and developed adversarial relationships with providers. Moreover, the government was unable to document any improvement in the quality of care delivered to Medicare beneficiaries as a result of the PRO "inspect and detect" efforts.

The PROs were subsequently renamed in 2001 as quality improvement organizations (QIOs). At this time, the QIO program encompassed 41 organizations that contracted with CMS to offer technical assistance to and collaborate with providers to improve the quality of care they provided to Medicare beneficiaries.

According to an evaluation conducted by the IOM,[16] the quality of the care received by Medicare beneficiaries improved over time, but there was insufficient evidence to show the extent to which QIOs contributed directly to those improvements. While the QIO program provided some potentially valuable nationwide infrastructure to promote quality, the IOM was unable to tell whether individual QIOs or the program as a whole had a positive impact, a negative impact, or no impact.

Another evaluation examined whether hospitals that voluntarily participated with QIOs had higher quality of care.[17] The investigators looked at 15 process indicators of quality care associated with improved outcomes for treatment and prevention in 5 clinical areas prevalent among Medicare beneficiaries: atrial fibrillation, acute myocardial infarction, heart failure, pneumonia, and stroke. Participating hospitals showed significantly greater improvement than nonparticipating hospitals on only 1 of the 15 measures. Nevertheless, the CMS cites statistics that seek to demonstrate the contribution of the QIOs, including adverse drug event screenings for more than 2.3 million beneficiaries, a 26% reduction in antipsychotic medication at nursing homes, and more than 47,800 beneficiaries completing diabetes self-management education and support programs.[18]

Medicare also authorized utilization review (UR) programs to reduce unnecessary care, as well as the OIG (see Chapter 25) to root out fraud and abuse (see Chapter 24). UR was introduced in the 1960s to reduce overutilization of resources and identify waste. The UR function was initially performed by registered nurses in hospitals, but then spread to use by health insurers who reviewed provider claims for medical necessity. The 3 UR activities included (1) *prospective review* (review of medical necessity for the performance of services or scheduled procedures before admission), (2) *concurrent review* (review of medical necessity decisions made while the patient is currently in an acute or post-acute setting), and (3) *retrospective review* (review of coverage after treatment is provided).

How well did UR programs fare in quality management? An early review of the literature by the IOM found that they tended to cut utilization and costs in the short term; there was no rigorous evidence regarding quality or the provision of unnecessary care.[19] Despite widespread use, such programs have sparked debate and controversy, particularly among physicians who feel UR programs eroded their clinical autonomy. By the late 1990s, some health plans began to abandon UR in favor of disease management programs.[20]

## Total Quality Management/Continuous Quality Improvement

During the 1980s, US industry embraced the work of W. Edwards Deming, Joseph Juran, and others on quality improvement. They had pioneered these approaches decades earlier by helping Japan rebuild its industrial base after World War II. Japan institutionalized their approaches in their manufacturing industries and began to outcompete their US counterparts during the 1970s; ironically, US firms learned of these approaches from Japan and imported them back home.

A panoply of related approaches can be grouped under the quality improvement banner, including total quality management (TQM), continuous quality improvement (CQI; plan-do-study-act [PDSA]), Zero Defects, Six Sigma, root cause analysis, failure modes and effects analysis (FMEA), the Toyota Production System (TPS), and lean management. Such efforts seek to remove waste from organizational processes, standardize work and reduce variability in process performance, and reduce defects and errors in production. The overall aim of several of these approaches, such as the TPS, is to constantly reduce cost, increase quality, and improve customer service, somewhat representing an amalgam of the iron triangle and the triple aim.

TQM rested on the efforts of frontline workers offering suggestions on how to improve the work processes they were both knowledgeable about and responsible for. Such suggestions were continuously incorporated into work process improvements. The goals of TQM were 2-fold: (1) reduce variations in the work process and (2) raise the average level of performance in that process.

TQM and CQI were widely embraced in the healthcare industry during the 1990s as possible solutions to low performance in both clinical and nonclinical areas. Researchers studied TQM implementation in both hospital and nonhospital settings using rigorous empirical methods, publishing their findings in leading academic journals.[21] Unfortunately, the findings were mixed. For example, in a cross-sectional study of hospitals in 1997, clinical quality was positively associated with the participation of hospital senior managers and nonmedical staff in quality improvement teams but was not associated with higher participation by physicians in such teams. Moreover, quality was negatively associated with broader participation of hospital units in quality improvement efforts. At the same time, a literature review of the few randomized studies suggested no impact of CQI on clinical outcomes and no evidence to date of organization-wide improvement in clinical performance.[22] Twenty-two years later, another review concluded the impact of CQI remains equivocal.[23]

The TPS has also been applied to healthcare delivery, usually to reduce several sources of "waste."[24] TPS gained national visibility at Virginia Mason Medical Center, where it was used to eliminate the following types of waste: patients waiting to be treated in the emergency room, patients waiting to be admitted, hospital rooms waiting to be cleaned, procedure and test rooms waiting for patients to arrive, doctors waiting for test results, patients waiting for test results, and patients waiting for discharge. Such waste was reportedly associated with higher cost and lower quality (eg, longer hospital stays, slower turnover in hospital beds, higher risk of hospital-acquired infections, and lower patient satisfaction).

Qualitative analyses suggest that TPS could successfully tackle these problems[25]; empirical confirmation in peer-reviewed journals is unfortunately still largely lacking, however. One recent study shows that adoption of lean management is associated with lower Medicare spending per beneficiary but is not significantly associated with 8 other performance measures of cost and quality.[26] Literature reviews of the impact of TPS and lean management likewise indicate weak results. One review reported that lean management had no impact on health outcomes or patient satisfaction.[27] Another review concluded that the scientific evidence was limited and inconsistent. Outcomes varied considerably across studies, making it impossible to draw conclusions about the impact on overall quality of care or quality dimensions.[28] Physicians deride systems like TPS as "medical Taylorism" (ie, efforts to apply assembly-line standardization methods to healthcare that

cannot be easily or successfully done). In contrast to TPS and Taylorism, "people" come first, not the system.[29]

## Business Process Reengineering

Another earlier approach to quality improvement related to TQM was business process reengineering (BPR). BPR emphasized a radical redesign and improvement of work. The approach, popularized by Michael Hammer, enunciated several principles[30]:

1. Organize around outcomes and compress tasks: Enlarge the worker's job and have them perform all tasks in a process; eliminate the assembly line.
2. Have those who use the output of a process also perform it: Reduce specialization, reduce centralized staff departments, and reduce the use of interfaces and liaisons.
3. Have those who gather and produce information also process it: Process information at the local level where the information is gathered.
4. Have those who do the work make the decisions and operate the controls: Let those who perform the work also make the decisions about planning and controlling the work.

This approach swept across US industry in the late 1980s, much in the manner of a fad or bandwagon, and was heralded as the cure for every organizational problem. BPR was often used to just cut jobs in order to cut costs, however, rather than make substantive improvements. Moreover, the BPR failure rate reached 70%, and perhaps as high as 85%, due to its association with layoffs and the fear and resistance such layoffs generated. Workers were reluctant to recommend process efficiencies that could cut their jobs.

Despite the emerging poor track record, BPR was embraced by the hospital industry. Academic research showed that it did not fare much better in a healthcare context.[31] One set of studies found that hospitals gained little or no economic value from adopting BPR or doing more of it than others. Moreover, implementation of BPR during the period from 1988 to 1996 could actually damage a hospital's cost position and thus its competitiveness. BPR was not a silver bullet solution: It required other concomitant changes to make it work.

Research also showed that hospitals adopted BPR in the presence of other hospitals adopting it, suggesting it may indeed have been a bandwagon movement.

## Scorecards and Transparency: Leapfrog Group and Hospital Compare

During the past 2 decades, hospitals have sometimes sought public recognition by voluntarily participating in surveys of their quality of care, which are subsequently published as performance "scorecards." Many report cards have been published (Figure 7-7). Such efforts are designed to promote transparency of results and enhance consumerism and shopping behavior. These efforts began with involuntary efforts during the 1980s when the Health Care Financing Administration (now CMS) published "raw data" (ie, no adjustment for patient severity of illness) on each hospital's mortality rates. The IOM provided a major stimulus to these efforts in the late 1990s and early 2000s with its publications on healthcare errors and patient safety (covered later).

Both the public sector and private sector responded with transparency initiatives. In 2005, CMS launched a public website (Hospital Compare) containing data on 7 domains of hospital quality and safety. Studies have found that its "5-star" rating of hospitals based on patient experience (using HCAHPS data) is associated with favorable patient outcomes such as lower mortality and readmission rates.[32] It is unclear, however, how much assistance such data provided to patients in choosing their hospital providers. Researchers note that there is low overlap in the scores derived by Hospital Compare with other scorecards, perhaps reflecting differences in their ratings methods and measures, which may sow confusion among those they are designed to inform.[33]

Moreover, studies indicated that patients rarely used this information in their choice of hospital; some suggested the problem lay in poor dissemination of the findings (eg, patients' awareness of hospital quality scores did not improve).[34] One problem was the sheer number of measures (64) included on the Hospital Compare website. A second was the crude scoring metrics ("star ratings"), which represent composite scores of the 64 measures that lack severity-adjustment, do not take patient sociodemographic characteristics into account, and

reflect only a fraction of inpatient care.[35] A third problem was that measures *within* some of the quality domains captured by Hospital Compare were only modestly correlated, whereas measures across the domains were not correlated.[36] In 2019, the American Hospital Association and the Association of American Medical Colleges both called on CMS to take the website down until it had improved the precision and consistency of the measures.

In the private sector, several large employers (along with a foundation) founded the Leapfrog Group in 2000. The Leapfrog Group launched a survey in 2001 to ascertain and report on hospital performance on 3 indicators: (1) whether the hospital had computerized physician order entry (CPOE); (2) whether their intensive care units (ICUs) were staffed appropriately with intensivists; and (3) whether the hospital had enough surgical volume to safely perform certain high-risk procedures. These 3 measures were chosen because the Leapfrog Group believed they were supported by research, their adoption could lead to measurable "leaps" in improved safety, and the leaps had intuitive appeal to the general public. The Leapfrog Group added more measures over time: safe practices to reduce patient harm in 2004; "never events" (serious reportable events) in 2007; patient safety in 2012; and ambulatory surgery centers and hospital outpatient care in 2019. According to one evaluation, the Leapfrog Group's efforts led to greater publication of hospital performance on the Leapfrog Group's indicators and elevated the conversation on how hospitals might improve patient safety. However, there was no evidence of hospitals' reported improvement on the Leapfrog Group's measures.[37] One study found that the safety practices score was not associated with patient outcomes reported by Hospital Compare or Medicare penalties for readmissions or complications.[38]

In general, research suggests that hospital scorecards and quality reports are not associated with improved outcomes (eg, mortality, readmissions, complications, surgical outcomes).[39] Such reporting may provide hospitals feedback on their outcome performance and assist with benchmarking with other hospitals, but does not by itself lead to outcomes improvement. What may be required are complex, sustained, multifaceted interventions to change the practice behaviors of physicians, which most hospitals lack the resources and expertise to launch.[40]

| REPORT CARD | ORGANIZATION BIO | DATA SOURCE | SCORING METHODOLOGY | ADVANTAGES | DISADVANTAGES |
|---|---|---|---|---|---|
| CMS Hospital Star Ratings (Hospital Compare) | Published by the Centers for Medicare and Medicaid Services (CMS) | CMS's Hospital Inpatient Quality Reporting (IQR) and Outpatient Quality Reporting (OQR) programs | 1-5 stars based on performance on 57 measures | Draws on measures from required reporting programs (so no additional reporting required)<br><br>Star rating may be easier to understand than individual measure scores<br><br>Medicare is the single largest payer of healthcare services and many programs tie a significant amount of dollars to quality | Recent studies have raised serious questions on validity of methodology<br><br>The list of selected measures may not be fully representative of hospital quality, providing a misleading picture |
| Leapfrog Hospital Survey | Non-profit organization representing employers and insurance purchasers | Unvalidated survey data reported by hospitals; additional data from secondary sources including AHA Health IT (HIT) supplement and annual survey, Hospital Compare, HAC Reduction program, AHRQ Patient Safety Indicators (PSI) | Grade A-F based on composite score from evaluation on performance in ensuring "Freedom from harm": Process/structure (how often a hospital gives patients recommended treatment for given condition/procedure), and Outcomes | Measures focused on patient safety issues, which are a key priority for hospitals | Use of deeply flawed claims-based safety measures in methodology<br><br>Measure data may be up to 3 years old and not show more recent improvements in care<br><br>VA, critical access hospitals, specialty, children's, mental health hospitals not included; arbitrary weighting of measures in composite score |
| US News and World Report Best Hospitals | For-profit company | AHA Annual Survey (volume), Medicare Provider Analysis and Review (MedPAR) (mortality); Medicare Standard Analytic File (SAF); survey of physician specialists | Ranking by specialty and by state based on performance on structure (volume, staffing, other resources), process (reputation among physicians, patient safety indicators), outcomes (mortality) | No application of data submission required<br><br>Assesses multiple aspects of care | Reputational data alone may not fully reflect quality of care |
| Truven Top 100 Hospitals | For-profit healthcare research and consulting firm | MedPAR, Medicare hospital cost reports (all-payer), CMS Hospital Compare | List of 100 hospitals with highest achievement in scores on 11 measures including inpatient outcomes, process of care, extended outcomes, process efficiency, cost efficiency, financial health, and patient experience | Variety of types of measures provides more nuanced picture of quality than just mortality or infection<br><br>Compares hospitals in groups with similar characteristics (bed size, teaching status, extent of residency/fellowship program) | Bases risk-adjustment model on proprietary methodology that projects discharge data, so results of scoring are not replicable and internal methodology is speculative<br><br>VA, critical access hospitals, specialty, children's, mental health hospitals not included |

| REPORT CARD | ORGANIZATION BIO | DATA SOURCE | SCORING METHODOLOGY | ADVANTAGES | DISADVANTAGES |
|---|---|---|---|---|---|
| Consumer Reports Hospital Safety Ratings | Non-profit organization supported by subscriptions | Hospital Compare, Leapfrog, specialty societies, AHA annual survey | Score between 1 and 100 (higher is better) based on Performance on outcomes (infections, mortality, readmissions, adverse surgical events); Experience (communication about discharge, drug information); Practices (appropriate use of scanning, avoiding C-sections) | Numerical score may be easier for consumers to understand | Overall score not fully reflective of overall hospital quality<br><br>Some underlying measures (CT imaging, mortality, readmission) have reliability and validity problems; uses unvalidated Leapfrog survey data |
| Healthgrades | For-profit company providing information to consumers | MedPAR, all-payer state data | List of top 50 (top 1%) and top 100 (top 2%) performers on mortality and in-hospital complications by procedure who have received the Healthgrades Distinguished Hospital Award for Clinical Excellence for a specific number of consecutive years | Rewards consistent, year-over-year quality<br><br>Listing hospitals that have reached performance threshold avoids confusing, arbitrary grading or rating system. What does "list system" mean? | Limited measures used to calculate scores; only risk-adjusted for comorbid diagnoses, age and gender, and source of admission; inaccuracy of claims data<br><br>23 states have no hospital receiving award; to be eligible for Distinguished Hospital Award for Clinical Excellence, hospital has to have evaluations in at least 21 of the 32 Healthgrades procedures and conditions using Medicare inpatient data |
| ProPublica Surgeon Scorecard | Independent, non-profit newsroom that produces investigative journalism in the public interest. | Medicare Standard Analytic File (SAF) | Low, medium, or high "Adjusted complication rate": hospital readmissions for conditions plausibly related to surgery and mortality within 30 days for eight surgical procedures, exclamation point symbol shown with rate for hospitals with at least one surgeon with a high adjusted complication rate | Uniquely focuses on surgeons, provides insight on specific specialties that might be more relevant for patients interested in those procedures | Masks hospital-to-hospital performance differences; questionable accuracy of methodology (doesn't include) complications beyond those accompanied with 30-day readmission, patient risk doesn't affect score<br><br>Claims data are notoriously inaccurate in individual provider assignments |

**Figure 7-7 •** Quality Performance Scorecards. AHA, American Hospital Association; CT, Computed Tomography; VA, Veterans Administration. (Source: American Hospital Association. "A Comparison of External Quality and Safety Scorecards," https://trustees.aha.org/sites/default/files/trustees/trustee-toolkit-scorecards-grid.pdf.)

## Guidelines and Checklists

### Clinical Practice Guidelines

Clinical practice guidelines (CPGs) advise practitioners regarding the most appropriate treatment for a given patient condition. They generally include (1) statements of expected practice; (2) benchmarks or standards against which individuals can audit, compare, and potentially improve their practices; and (3) guidance regarding undertaking particular tasks.

CPGs have existed for many decades but spread rapidly during the 1970s and 1980s—anticipating the movement toward evidence-based medicine. In 1989, the AHRQ formed to explicitly develop CPGs and helped to create the National Guidelines Clearinghouse in 1990.[41] In 1992, the IOM defined CPGs as "systematically developed statements to assist practitioner and patient decisions about appropriate healthcare for specific clinical circumstances." Over time, numerous sets of CPGs have been developed by multiple medical societies as well as the federal government. By 2006, AHRQ listed over 2,000 such guidelines. The process undertaken to develop these guidelines usually includes assembling an expert panel of clinicians in the relevant medical area, assessing the available clinical evidence, and developing recommendations on the best manner of treatment.

CPGs can have several purposes: improve effectiveness and quality of care, decrease practice variations and preventable mistakes, and reduce adverse events. There are several problems, however. First, there are discrepancies among the different CPGs issued for treating the same condition. Second, the process of guideline development is unregulated, and the quality of many guidelines is low. Third, the few tools available to assess the quality of guidelines are time consuming and designed for researchers rather than clinicians. Fourth, few guidelines are evaluated before or after dissemination regarding their impact on patient outcomes. Fifth, although CPGs were once used to support physicians' clinical decisions, they have morphed to serve broader purposes such as informing insurance coverage, setting institutional policies, and serving medicolegal liability standards.[42] Sixth, adherence to CPGs may not improve outcomes, not because they are invalid but because they do not take into account patient lifestyles (see Chapter 4).[43]

Research has shown that CPGs are modestly effective in changing physicians' practices: The changes are statistically significant but rather small in magnitude. Moreover, many practitioners do not follow them. One reason may be that only 6% to 33% of CPG recommendations have a strong evidence base. Other reasons include the following: (1) CPGs don't take account of variations in patient preferences for outcomes or variations in patient comorbidities; (2) it is hard to determine the applicability of CPGs to specific patients; (3) CPGs focus little on diagnosis (eg, diagnostic testing); and (4) it is hard to develop a "checklist" for the complexity of patient diagnoses. As a result, much of the CPG effort involves strategies to improve physician compliance.

The CPG effort thus relies on effective dissemination. In the past, hospitals and medical societies simply mailed CPGs to physicians; most of this mail is never read. The most heavily utilized strategies include educational outreach, reminders, and feedback on guideline compliance. When used independently, the latter 2 strategies seem to improve outcomes; multipronged approaches are also important and perhaps more important than single interventions. However, the number of strategies employed was not associated with improved outcomes, nor were interventions that incorporated patient-directed strategies.[44]

### Checklists

Checklists have long been used by cockpit crews in airplanes to ensure full adherence to safety measures prior to takeoff. These entail a set of different tasks the pilot must perform or verify in order to configure the aircraft and prepare the crew for certain macro-tasks such as engine start, taxi, and takeoff. For each one of these macro-tasks, there are several "items" to be accomplished and verified by the flight crew. The improper use or nonuse of checklists by flight crews is often cited as the probable cause or a contributing factor to aircraft accidents.

Atul Gawande suggested this approach be applied to healthcare delivery in his highly publicized volume, *The Checklist Manifesto.* He argued this approach could improve clinicians' performance of appropriate tasks in an uncertain, complex, and demanding environment. Literature reviews indicate this approach has been most widely applied to the work of anesthesiologists, radiologists, surgeons, and intensive care units. Some reviews find benefits of using checklists in the form of adherence to processes that should be performed; others report mixed impacts on patient outcomes.[45] Empirical research suggests that the introduction of checklists does not improve patient outcomes (mortality, complications).[46] Literature reviews suggest that documenting the performance of checklists is made difficult by virtue of their inconsistent use, which results from the lack of effective, standardized methodologies for designing, developing, and implementing them.[47] Commentators note that checking off a list may improve communication but does not improve quality; the latter relies on performance of the tasks on the list, an exercise in which physicians and hospitals may need assistance.[48]

## Errors and Systems of Care

The 2000 IOM publication *To Err Is Human: Building a Safer Health System* suggested that as many as 98,000 deaths occurred in US hospitals as a result of medical "errors." The report emphasized that these errors were not a function of provider incompetence, bad intentions, or sloppy work. Rather, they were a "system property" that required attention to well-designed processes of care that could prevent, recognize, and quickly recover from errors to minimize harm to patients. By "system," analysts depicted errors as the result of many simultaneous factors: complex care processes, multiple staff handoffs of work, staffing discontinuities (eg, nursing shifts), the presence of multiple professions and languages of work, the nature and uncertainty of the technology, and the pursuit of research and patient education objectives in addition to patient care (Figure 7-8).

The organizational culture of hospitals also played a major role, including a presumption of excellence (eg, "only the best and brightest work here"), the resulting failure to implement error systems, the failure to attend to and collect data on errors, the tendency to attribute errors to screwups or the high severity of illness among patients, the sentiment that providers are working "at the frontier" where there is already a high risk of failure, and limited oversight from above.

This IOM publication instigated the movement to improve patient safety. Hospitals pursued a multiprong strategy that included at least 6 elements: (1) leadership (honesty, accountability, and transparency); (2) vigilance (seek out and root out error); (3) patient-centered and family-centered care (share information with patients and families); (4) fairness and openness to the victims (disclose and explain errors); (5) systems (adopt new technologies [CPOE] to help flag errors); and (6) interdisciplinary practice, teamwork, and a team-based culture of safety and responsibility.

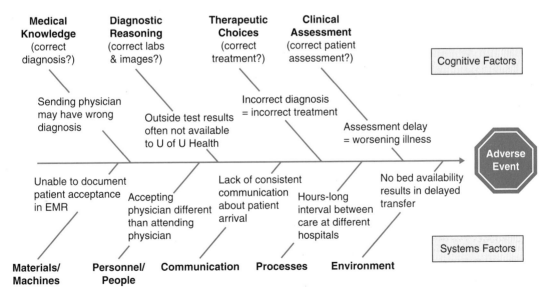

**Figure 7-8** • Systems Framework of Medical Errors. EMR, Electronic Medical Record; U of U, University of Utah. (Source: Dr. Darlene Tad-Y, Department of Medicine, University of Colorado Anschutz Medical Campus. https://pubmed.ncbi.nlm.nih.gov/26983075/.)

What has been the long-term impact of this movement? As noted in Chapter 26, adverse events and preventable errors are the third leading cause of death in the United States. Researchers suggest that while the industry has conducted research and developed initiatives to improve patient safety, progress has been slow.[49] According to one study, between 2005 and 2016, only 21% of hospitals showed a sizable improvement (>10%) in work environment measures tied to safety, while 7% had worse scores.[50] Indeed, compared to the 1999 IOM report, patient deaths resulting from medical errors may have risen by a factor of 3 to 5 times.[51] Some suggest that this flows from a myopic preoccupation with specific indicators, such as HACs (eg, central line–associated bloodstream infections) and preventable hospital readmissions, where the United States has made considerable improvement. This may reflect a siloed approach to quality rather than a comprehensive, all-cause approach to patient safety.

## Clinical Variations

Variations in medical practice came to researchers' attention during the 1970s. John Wennberg documented wide variations across hospital service areas in Vermont in terms of their manpower, facilities, spending, and utilization (number of surgical procedures per 10,000 population).[52] He concluded such variations reflected differences in the behaviors of physicians and patients across these areas. This work inaugurated the analysis of "small area variations." During the 1980s, while at Dartmouth Medical School, Wennberg compared utilization levels between Boston and New Haven.[53] Despite demographic similarities, the 2 cities differed markedly in their spending and utilization levels for certain surgical services. This effort culminated in the publication of The Dartmouth Atlas in 1993.[54] The Atlas described the distribution and utilization of medical resources across the United States, as well as the differences across geographic areas in terms of their use of medical resources, mostly based on Medicare data.

The Atlas made 2 contributions to the analysis of variations. First, the Atlas distinguished 3 categories of medical services: effective care, preference-sensitive care, and supply-sensitive care.

*Effective care* is based on strong medical science (eg, randomized controlled trials) and clear treatment paths, where the treatment works as advertised and where physician

and patient preferences are aligned. For such care, variations in hospitalization are linked to underlying illness rates, not to the supply of hospital capacity or the physician's practice style. Examples of effective care included surgery for hip fracture and colorectal cancer, as well as use of β-blockers following acute myocardial infarction. According to Wennberg, there is systematic "underuse" of such care.

*Preference-sensitive care* includes cases where there are trade-offs among alternative types of treatments for a given condition (eg, prostate cancer) because the doctor and patient are not sure what the outcomes are or what is the best thing to do. In such cases, physician and patient preferences may conflict; this situation calls for shared decision-making programs to bring patient preferences up to the physician. Wennberg considered this area subject to "misuse of care."

*Supply-sensitive care*, finally, includes situations where clinical theories regarding treatment efficacy are absent (eg, hospitalization for medical conditions, ICU stays, physician office visits, specialist referrals). In these cases, capacity supply often drives utilization rather than illness levels. This type of care is akin to "overuse."

Second, the Atlas documented that the "system" of care in the United States is not a system at all, but a largely unplanned and irrational sprawl of resources (see Chapter 1). Moreover, there were enormous variations in the distribution of hospital resources and inpatient hospital spending in contiguous geographic areas. These findings led Wennberg to conclude that "geography is destiny." The Atlas reported that, echoing Milt Roemer's earlier observation, the supply of acute care hospital beds exerted a substantial influence on rates of hospitalization for medical (nonsurgical) conditions. In addition, hospital capacity was strongly linked to rates of hospitalization for "ambulatory care sensitive conditions" (eg, chronic obstructive pulmonary disease, asthma).[55]

Wennberg drew different conclusions regarding variations in medical versus surgical services. Variation in hospitalization for medical conditions was driven by variations in acute care bed capacity, whereas variation in surgical procedures was driven by physician practice style—what Wennberg called the "surgical signature" (ie, propensity to operate). Surgical variations may also reflect (1) variations in diagnostic intensity (how hard physicians look for surgically treatable disease; eg, prostate-specific antigen testing), (2) professional uncertainty reflecting gaps in medical science (radical prostatectomy vs radiation vs watchful waiting), and (3) failure to incorporate patient preferences into treatment decisions where trade-offs are present (eg, prostate cancer, herniated disk).

Wennberg identified the possible problem as one of physician uncertainty, which exerts a huge impact on supplier-induced demand. Geographic variations in quality of surgical care reflected the poor quality of clinical decision making, whereby patients received treatments they didn't want or need. In addition, the poor quality of the scientific basis for clinical practice fostered uncertainty about outcomes of care.[56]

Wennberg concluded that "more is not always better." Greater levels of spending were not associated with less underuse of effective care, improved patient safety (surgical death rates), population illness levels, patient health status, or life expectancy. Moreover, there was no evidence that variations in physician distribution were linked to variations in population health and no evidence that bed capacity was linked to mortality rates. On the other hand, greater spending levels were associated with physician supply, hospital bed supply, and supply-sensitive services. Based on these results, Wennberg surmised that quality, rather than access or cost, might be the real problem.

Since publication of *The Dartmouth Atlas*, healthcare leaders have sought ways to reduce practice variations observed within medical groups, within hospitals, and among providers contracting with health plans. One approach has been to show physicians in the same specialty empirical data on how they practice in comparison with their colleagues or to show physicians in one group how they stack up against physicians in the same specialty in other groups (as has been done in the Alternative Quality Contract in Massachusetts; see Chapter 17). This approach relies on the competitiveness of physicians and their desire not to deviate in "a negative way" relative to their peers. Research evidence confirms that quality performance feedback to physicians that includes comparisons with their peers helps to improve clinicians' quality of care.[57] A related approach is to decompose the spending of such physicians into its components (eg, length of stay, admission rates, referrals, use of branded vs generic drugs) to identify the root drivers of the cost variations observed. In such exercises, it is important to severity-adjust all comparisons to account for physicians having sicker patients to treat. It is also important that such comparisons include enough cases (ie, patients) per physician to make the comparisons statistically powerful. There are a host of other approaches to attack the issue of variation, depending on whether the interventions are applied by a provider or a health plan (Figure 7-9).

| | Overuse | Underuse |
|---|---|---|
| **Provider Delivery Network** | • EMR decision support<br>• Provider education<br>• Profiling/reporting<br>• Disease management<br>• Lower compensation for overutilized procedures | • EMR decision support<br>• Physician education<br>• Patient engagement<br>• Disease management<br>• Registries<br>• Raise compensation for underutilized procedures |
| **Health Plan** | • Prior authorization<br>• Disease management<br>• Case management<br>• Provider education<br>• Benefit design<br>• Profiling and reporting<br>• Lower reimbursement for overutilized procedures<br>• Pay for performance to penalize continued overutilization | • Disease management<br>• Registries<br>• Provider education<br>• Patient education<br>• Raise reimbursement for underutilized procedures<br>• Pay for performance to reward increasing utilization |

**Figure 7-9 •** Interventions to Decrease Variation. EMR, Electronic Medical Record.

A researcher at the University of Pennsylvania pushed back on *The Dartmouth Atlas* findings based on analysis of commercial as well as Medicare data (which Wennberg relied on). He found that geographic areas with greater physician supply (both generalists and specialists) exhibit higher quality of care.[58] He also found that areas with higher levels of spending also have higher quality of care.[59] To explain why these results diverged from Wennberg's, he argued that (1) many states in the South had high Medicare spending per enrollee but low healthcare spending per capita and (2) their poor quality correlated with their overall low levels of healthcare spending. He also reported that quality levels not only correlated with spending but also with sociodemographic characteristics, such as income, race, and spending for K-12 education. This suggests that although healthcare spending is an important contributor to quality, the determinants of quality reach more deeply into the sociodemographic fabric of the community.

## Clinical Integration

Another approach to quality management, and one that does not get much attention, is clinical integration. The term *clinical integration* was developed by the Department of Justice (DOJ) and the Federal Trade Commission (FTC) to decide when to challenge certain provider combinations (eg, physician-hospital joint ventures) that were conducting joint contracting with payers. The DOJ and FTC were concerned that such joint contracting might be anticompetitive. The DOJ and FTC criteria were initially set forth in *Statements of Antitrust Enforcement Policy in Health Care* (Statement 6 in 1993, Statement 8 in 1996),[60] and subsequently appended in FTC advisory letters to specific joint ventures. Anticompetitive contracting might still be allowed if it promoted clinical integration.

Joint ventures deemed to be sufficiently clinically integrated include the following features. First, joint contracting should achieve benefits ancillary to the operation of the venture. Such benefits constitute a "new product" generated by the venture. This new product should entail some change in services offered to payers and/or some change in physicians' provision of services to patients. It should not entail simply joint contracting on price with payers. Second, the "new product" should entail clinical integration across physicians in the joint

venture. At a general level, clinical integration entails interaction and interdependence among physicians in their provision of medical services. The joint venture should thus develop an active, ongoing process to facilitate cooperative activity among physicians, a process in which physicians are actively involved. Third, at a more granular level, physicians should be actively engaged in the following list of activities:

- Form clinical committees to develop and apply CPGs
- Develop performance benchmarks and physician scorecards as clinical goals
- Engage in quality measurement and management programs
- Develop transitional care programs
- Engage in medical management practices
- Conduct practice audits to monitor the performance of their peers in using CPGs
- Issue performance reports on a regular basis to physicians
- Invest in computer systems and information training
- Integrate all physicians using a common electronic medical record (EMR)
- Exchange clinical information using the EMR to coordinate patient care
- Increase patient referrals among physicians to increase information captured on EMR
- Develop disease registries
- Develop population health programs
- Develop data analytics programs
- Develop tools to risk-stratify patients according to severity of illness
- Develop programs to actively manage the highest-risk, highest-cost patients
- Develop quality assurance councils to review physicians' performance
- Participate in physician education programs to improve adherence to CPGs
- Develop criteria to selectively recruit physicians who can practice cost-effective care

A series of antitrust cases brought by these federal agencies (and their local counterparts, state attorney generals) revealed that most activities were sadly absent or seriously underdeveloped. Too often, the providers in these joint ventures combined to do joint contracting in order to extract higher reimbursement fees (ie, higher prices) from payers but postponed the clinical integration work to a later date.

**Critical Thinking Exercise**

Among all healthcare provider organizations, the Mayo Clinic in Rochester, Minnesota, is typically mentioned as a "paragon of virtue" when it comes to quality of care. Mayo physicians attribute their reputed quality advantage to a multipronged approach (depicted below). This includes (1) a *culture* of safety, outcomes, and service that has been built up over time (since the late 19th century) and is embedded in its salaried, integrated, multispecialty group practice model with an emphasis on collaborative teams and team communication; (2) supportive *infrastructure*, including an EMR and point-of-care information; (3) an emphasis on both systems and human factors *engineering*, including many of the quality approaches identified earlier (lean management, PDSA); and (4) disciplined, effective *execution*, including quality dashboards to monitor performance and diffusion of best practices.[61]

The Mayo approach seems much more encompassing than the quality improvement approaches profiled earlier. Is that what it takes? How can anyone tell whether the 4 components of the Mayo approach are both necessary and sufficient to improve quality?

**Mayo Quality Approach**

Source: Stephen J. Swensen, James A. Dilling, Dawn S. Milliner, et al, "Quality: The Mayo Clinic Approach", *American Journal of Medical Quality* 24 (2009): 428-440. Adapted from Bisognano, Pisek. 10 More Powerful Ideas for Improving Patient Care. Chicago: Health Administration Press & Institute for Healthcare Improvement, 2006.

## PROGNOSIS FOR QUALITY IMPROVEMENT

There is no shortage of recommended strategies to improve quality of care. Many of these have been reviewed earlier, with several found "seriously wanting." There are many others, to be sure, and some are covered in other chapters of this volume. These strategies can be classified according to whom they target (eg, physicians, patients, or health organizations). AHRQ has summarized them as follows[62]:

**Physician Focused**
- Provider reminder systems
- Data audit, reporting, and feedback
- Provider education
- Continuing medical education
- Provider incentives and reimbursement
- Local opinion leaders
- Physician engagement programs

- Enabling clinician-led teams for performance improvement
- Total cost contracting with payers (Alternative Quality Contract in Massachusetts)
- Patients as agents of social change

**Patient Focused**
- Patient reminder systems
- Patient education
- Self-care management
- Behavioral economics

**Organization Focused**
- Regulation
- P4P
- No-pay-for-no-performance (never events)
- Shared savings approach with accountable care organizations (bonus once you hit quality metrics)
- Reorganization around clinical areas/patient groupings
- Micro systems of care
- Organizational change efforts

There is certainly not a lack of effort. Indeed, some researchers suggest that some of the biggest progress that has been made is "cultural": the growing recognition that errors and problems in quality are systemic in nature rather than the fault of the individual clinician. There has also been some notable progress in addressing infection rates (HACs). These items reflect healthcare "misuse"; other issues may be more important (eg, underuse) or more stubborn (eg, overuse), as well as underaddressed.[63]

One effort underway to address overuse is the "Changing Wisely" campaign, sponsored by the American Board of Internal Medicine (ABIM). The ABIM encourages frank dialogue between physician and patient to reduce unnecessary tests, procedures, and treatments. For a variety of physician specialties, the campaign lists 5 types of care that physicians and patients should question. Forgoing these types of care can reportedly save the healthcare system billions of dollars in waste; as such, they represent "low-value" healthcare (ie, low quality divided by high cost). One issue, however, is *who* is to choose wisely? Between 2000 and 2010, imaging and tests were 2 areas with high expenditures and rapid volume growth. Often, these can be ordered by residents in teaching hospitals for a wide variety of reasons: duplicate the role-modeled behavior of the attending physician,

ensure thoroughness, reduce anxiety stemming from diagnostic uncertainty, satisfy one's curiosity, practice defensive medicine, satisfy patient requests, and reflect a lack of knowledge about the costs and harms of testing.

There are other barriers confronting this campaign. Recent research suggests that only half of physicians are aware of "Choosing Wisely," with primary care physicians being most aware (47%), medical specialists less aware (37%), and surgical specialists least aware (27%).[64] Fewer than half of physicians absolutely feel that the campaign is a legitimate source of guidance, with specialties falling along the same gradient as described earlier. Moreover, less than one-fifth of physicians report they feel empowered by the campaign to reduce their use of unnecessary tests (again, along the same gradient).

Other research on unnecessary tests and procedures points to additional barriers to change. One survey found that only 29% of physicians believe this issue is a serious problem; 44% say it is somewhat serious, and 21% say it is not serious. Moreover, nearly one-third of physicians report that their patients request unnecessary tests and procedures every day or several times a week. When asked about the major reasons for ordering such tests and procedures, physicians articulated the following familiar list: malpractice concerns (52%), "just to be safe" (36%), want more information to reassure myself (30%), patients insist on tests (28%), and "want to keep patients happy" (23%).[65]

Nevertheless, despite all of these efforts, quality improvement still comes up short. Some suggest that the efforts chronicled in this chapter reflect strategies pursued by health plans, employers, and the government—parties far removed from the frontline of healthcare delivery. Their strategies to increase transparency, focus on measurement and reporting, invest in EMRs, and marginally increase payment incentives for providers (eg, P4P programs) do not necessarily resonate with frontline providers, who may not respond to them. Effective approaches may require the active input, effort, and collaboration among these providers (as well as change in their clinical behaviors), which will involve time, money, and effort that may be in short supply among very busy and stressed out physicians (and nurses). Unless (1) the organizations in which these clinicians work make the needed investments to improve quality and safety and (2) the physicians buy into these efforts, progress is likely to remain slow. Such investments and efforts may only be forthcoming when the healthcare providers face a huge chunk of their reimbursement tied to quality measures and error rates, which is not yet the case.[66] Moreover, as noted in Chapters 11 and 12, most hospital executives emphasize goals of "growth" and "expansion," not goals of quality and safety.

Making things even more complicated, patients' views of "high value" versus "low value" also need to be considered. This perspective underlies the movement to patient-centered care and patient-reported outcome measures (PROMs). These approaches may be congruent with the other quality initiatives profiled earlier, but they may not always be so. Patients' views of quality are often about timely access to care than about technical quality or health outcomes. Moreover, there is currently an ongoing trend to see orthodontists, have one's teeth straightened, and replace lost teeth to have a nice smile. This craze is partially driven by media advertising by dental professionals and partly driven by patients' desires for aesthetics. Such treatments are expensive; it is not clear how much "value" (in terms of quality outcomes or health status) they deliver.[67]

It may also be the case that many of the approaches described in this chapter, such as BPR and TPS, that were borrowed from industry do not fit well into the delivery of healthcare. As one observer noted, the work of medical professionals is not well suited to standardization and programing (eg, guidelines, care paths, reduced variations) due to the craft nature of patient treatment and the enormous complexity and uncertainty confronting physicians.[68] Moreover, just as there may be few opportunities to borrow innovative ideas from industry, there may be few opportunities to borrow innovative ideas from other countries. Healthcare observers opine that all developed countries face the same quality issues, and none have produced effective, long-lasting solutions.[69]

One underlying problem may lie in diagnostic uncertainty. According to the IOM, diagnostic error represents the failure to (1) establish a timely and accurate explanation of the patient's health problems or (2) communicate that explanation to the patient. Such errors occur among 5% of adults getting outpatient care, among 10% of patient deaths, and among 6% to 17% of adverse events.

Diagnostic error constitutes one of the many sources of errors and quality problems. Researchers estimate that as many as 30 or more causes may lie behind a given problem or event failure. Moreover, multiple interventions may be required to deal with the multitude of causes. While it may be common for 5 or 6 causes to explain most of the reasons for a particular problem at a given hospital, a different group of drivers may be responsible at other hospitals, thus making any generalizations difficult.[70]

Figure 7-10 illustrates the sequence of the diagnostic process. Diagnosis is complicated by many factors, including the lack of a rigorous evidence base for an estimated 80% to 85% of

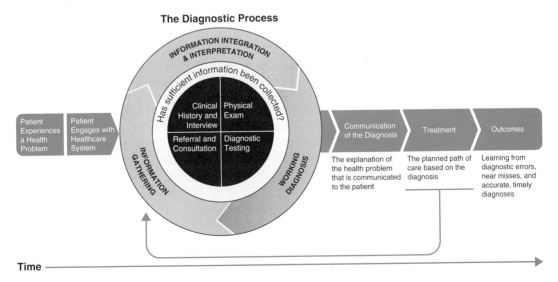

Figure 7-10 • The Committee's Conceptual Model of the Diagnostic Process. (Source: National Academies of Sciences, Engineering, and Medicine. 2015. *Improving Diagnosis in Health Care*. https://doi.org/10.17226/21794. Reproduced with permission from the National Academy of Sciences, Courtesy of the National Academies Press, Washington, D.C.)

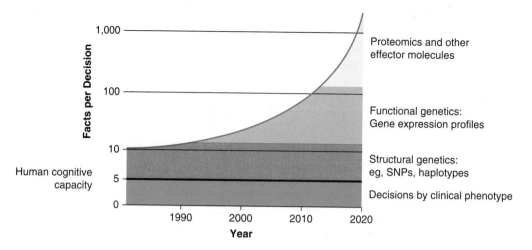

**Figure 7-11** • Volume of Medical Information to Synthesize. (Source: Institute of Medicine. 2013. *Best Care at Lower Cost: The Path to Continuously Learning Health Care in America.* https://doi.org/10.17226/13444. Reproduced with permission from the National Academy of Sciences, Courtesy of the National Academies Press, Washington, D.C.)

medicine, the resulting uncertainty in medicine, the complexity and accelerating volume of new medical information that physicians must embrace, the fact that diseases manifest themselves and evolve over time, the fact that diagnosis occurs in multiple clinical settings, the presence of ongoing population trends (need to consider comorbidity, polypharmacy), the copresence of mental health diagnoses that are hard to detect, and variations in health literacy across population segments. Physicians are confronted by an increasing volume of medical science reported in the medical and science literature (encompassing both biomedical and clinical knowledge) that they have limited cognitive capacity to manage, let alone synthesize (Figure 7-11). This makes it hard to apply the extant evidence base at the point of care delivery. Moreover, physicians may not be fully adept at or receptive to using the extant evidence. There can be breakdowns all along the "diagnostic process."

An additional set of problems concerns the measures of quality. Physicians and hospitals are bombarded by a plethora of quality measures issued by different payers with multiple formats that do not necessarily align. The proliferation of measures imposes a huge cost and reporting burden on physicians, which may dilute their focus on more important issues that do impact quality.[71] They may also detract from quality, since a recent analysis found that only 37% of the ambulatory care measures of quality were valid.[72] Researchers have advocated for a much shorter and simplified set of measures.[73] Moreover, the measures they need to report on cover both the process and outcomes of care—2

sets of measures that are not highly correlated, which leads some physicians to discount the former. This has led to debate over which is better to use. Process measures are easier to collect and are more prevalent than outcome measures (66% vs 20%) in 6 prominent quality programs.[74] Outcomes data are more expensive to collect and require a lot of severity adjustment (with only a limited amount of measures to do it).[75,76]

The Congressional Budget Office (CBO) has highlighted several other issues with quality measurement and management that will need to be addressed.[77] First, most efforts focus on conditions that are easily measured or on clinical processes for which there is consensus regarding what is "appropriate." Where efforts run into difficulties are physician decisions about how to manage patients with multiple chronic conditions, or physicians' interpretation of diagnostic images, or the possible need to risk-adjust quality measures to take account of differences in the health status of patients, or the possible need to adjust these measures for differences in the patients' sociodemographic characteristics. The quality measures providers have been subjected to, such as hospital readmission rates for medical conditions, are driven more by the patient's severity of illness and home situation (ie, the ability of the family to act as caregivers) than by quality of care considerations.

Beyond these issues are the importance of long-term observation of patients to gauge some outcomes of interest (cancer survival) and the importance of weighing the contribution of providers versus the contribution of social determinants (which providers have little control over).

There are also organizational factors, such as medical uncertainty, specialization, professional hierarchies, suboptimal hospital-physician relationships, and the lack of good performance measures, that predispose hospitals to "innovation implementation failure" with the initiatives reviewed earlier and in Chapter 24 (CPGs, error reporting EMRs).[78] Finally, it may be the case that the medical profession still does not know how to define evidence-based medical practice.[79]

## SUMMARY

Quality of care means a lot of different things to a lot of different stakeholders. That may explain why there are so many quality metrics. Little wonder that researchers refer to this topic as the "new tower of babble." And no wonder that the plethora of quality metrics serves as a huge annoyance to providers who have increasingly seen their compensation tied to performance on such metrics. You might forgive providers for being just a bit jaded or skeptical of quality measurement and quality improvement efforts given the "many shots taken on goal" over the past several decades. This topic, like the topic of rising healthcare costs covered in the prior chapter, clearly qualifies as an 800-pound gorilla that needs to be mastered. As I mentioned in an earlier chapter, healthcare presents you with a lifetime of work to pursue.

### QUESTIONS TO PONDER

1. Why is it so hard to improve the quality of healthcare?
2. What improvements can you suggest that would make current efforts more successful?
3. Which of the historical approaches to quality improvement chronicled in this chapter seem to have worked the best? Why?
4. Why is such a low percentage of recommended care actually delivered to patients, as suggested by Figure 7-3?
5. Figure 2-4 suggests that the quality problem is 3-fold: underuse, misuse, and overuse of care. Do the quality improvement approaches analyzed in this chapter address this problem fully?
6. Why don't providers devote much attention and effort to the "clinical integration" activities itemized earlier?

## REFERENCES

1. Sanford Schwartz. "U.S. Health Care System: Quality," *Presentation to the Wharton School*, 2007.
2. Jeffrey Levin-Scherz. "Medical Management in Managed Care," *Presentation to the Wharton School*, February 24, 2004.
3. Gary Claxton, Cynthia Cox, Selena Gonzales, et al. "Measuring the Quality of Healthcare in the U.S.," *Health System Tracker* (September 10, 2015). Available online: https://www.healthsystemtracker.org/brief/measuring-the-quality-of-healthcare-in-the-u-s/. Accessed on May 27, 2020.
4. Institute of Medicine. *To Err Is Human: Building a Safer Health System* (Washington, DC: IOM, 1999).
5. Steven Spear. "Fixing Health Care From the Inside, Today," *Harvard Business Review*. 83(9) (2005): 78-91.
6. Daniel R. Levinson. *Adverse Events in Hospitals: National Incidence Among Medicare Beneficiaries* (Washington, DC: Office of the Inspector General, November 2010).
7. Elizabeth McGlynn, Steven Asch, John Adams, et al. "The Quality of Health Care Delivered to Adults in the United States," *N Engl J Med.* 348 (2003): 2635-2645.
8. Gary Claxton, Cynthia Cox, Selena Gonzales, et al. "Measuring the Quality of Healthcare in the U.S.," *Health System Tracker* (September 10, 2015). Available online: https://www.healthsystemtracker.org/brief/measuring-the-quality-of-healthcare-in-the-u-s/. Accessed on May 27, 2020.
9. Mark Chassin. "Improving the Quality of Health Care: What's Taking So Long?" *Health Aff.* 32 (10) (2013): 1761-1765. Leah Binder. "Progress in Health Care Is Still 'Excruciatingly Slow' Says Harvard Expert," *Forbes* (February 20, 2014). Austin Frakt. "Why Is Improvement in the Quality of Health Care So Slow?" *The Incidental Economist* (October 18, 2016). Available online: https://theincidentaleconomist.com/wordpress/why-is-improvement-in-the-quality-of-health-care-so-slow/. Accessed on May 25, 2020.
10. David Levine, Jeffrey Linder, and Bruce Landon. "The Quality of Outpatient Care Delivered to Adults in the United States, 2002 to 2013," *JAMA.* 176 (12) (2016): 1778-1790.
11. Stephen Schmaltz, Scott Williams, Mark Chassin, et al. "Hospital Performance Trends on National Quality Measures and the Association With Joint Commission Accreditation," *J Hosp Med.* 6 (8) (2011): 454-461.
12. Ashish Jha. "Accreditation, Quality, and Making Hospital Care Better," *JAMA.* 320 (23) (2018): 2410-2411.
13. Miranda Lam, Jose Figueroa, Yevgeniy Feyman, et al. "Association Between Patient Outcomes and Accreditation in US Hospitals: Observational

Study," *Br Med J.* 363 (2018). doi: https://doi.org/10.1136/bmj.k4011.

14. Jason Richter and Brad Beauvais. "Quality Indicators Associated With the Level of NCQA Accreditation," *Am J Med Qual.* 33 (1) (2018): 43-49.

15. Congressional Budget Office. *The Impact of PSROs on Health-Care Costs: Update of CBO's 1979 Evaluation* (Washington, DC: CBO, 1981). Available online: https://www.cbo.gov/sites/default/files/97th-congress-1981-1982/reports/doc03-entire_2.pdf. Accessed on May 22, 2020.

16. Institute of Medicine. *Medicare's Quality Improvement Organization Program: Maximizing Potential* (Washington, DC: IOM, 2006).

17. Claire Snyder and Gerard Anderson. "Do Quality Improvement Organizations Improve the Quality of Hospital Care for Medicare Beneficiaries?" *JAMA.* 293 (23) (2005): 2900-2907.

18. Maria Castellucci. "CMS Delays Funding Renewal for Quality Improvement Organizations," *Modern Healthcare* (August 2, 2019).

19. Bradford Gray and Marilyn Field (Eds.). *Controlling Costs and Changing Patient Care? The Role of Utilization Management* (Washington, DC: Institute of Medicine, 1989).

20. Thomas Wickizer and Daniel Lessler. "Utilization Management: Issues, Effects, and Future Prospects," *Annu Rev Public Health.* 22 (2002): 233-254.

21. Stephen Shortell, Robert Jones, A.W. Rademaker, et al. "Assessing the Impact of Total Quality Management and Organizational Culture on Multiple Outcomes of Care for Coronary Artery Bypass Graft Surgery Patients," *Med Care.* 38 (2) (2000): 207-217. Bryan Weiner, Jeffrey Alexander, Laurence Baker, et al. "Quality Improvement Implementation and Hospital Performance on Patient Safety Indicators," *Med Care Res Rev.* 63 (1) (2006): 29-57.

22. Stephen Shortell, Charles Bennett, and Gayle Byck. "Assessing the Impact of Continuous Quality Improvement on Clinical Practice: What It Will Take to Accelerate Progress," *Milbank Q.* 76 (4) (1998): 593-624.

23. James Hill, Anne-Marie Stephani, Paul Sapple, et al. "The Effectiveness of Continuous Quality Improvement for Developing Professional Practice and Improving Health Care Outcomes: A Systematic Review," *Implement Sci.* 15 (2020): 23.

24. Roger Bush. "Reducing Waste in US Health Care Systems," *JAMA.* 297 (8) (2007): 871-874.

25. C. Craig Blackmore, Robert Mecklenburg, and Gary Kaplan. "At Virginia Mason, Collaboration Among Providers, Employers, and Health Plans to Transform Care Cut Costs and Improved Quality," *Health Aff.* 30 (9) (2011): 1680-1687.

26. Thomas Rundall, Stephen Shortell, Janet Blodgett, et al. "Adoption of Lean Management and Hospital Performance: Results from a National Survey," *Health Care Manage Rev.* 47 (2) (2020). doi: 10.1097/HMR.0000000000000287.

27. John Moraros, Mark Lemstra, and Chijoke Nwankwo. "Lean Interventions in Healthcare: Do They Actually Work? A Systematic Literature Review," *Int J Qual Health Care.* 28 (2) (2016): 150-165.

28. Janneke E. van Leijen-Zeelenberg, Arianne M.J. Elissen, Kerstin Grube, et al. "The Impact of Redesigning Care Processes on Quality of Care: A Systematic Review," *BMC Health Serv Res.* 16 (2016): 19.

29. Pamela Hartzband and Jerome Groopman. "Medical Taylorism," *N Engl J Med.* 374 (2016): 106-108.

30. Michael Hammer. "Reengineering Work: Don't Automate, Obliterate," *Harvard Business Review* 68 (4) (1990): 104-112. Michael Hammer and James Champy. *Reengineering the Corporation: A Manifesto for Business Revolution* (New York, NY: HarperBusiness, 1993).

31. Stephen Walston, Lawton R. Burns, and John Kimberly. "Does Reengineering Really Work? An Examination of the Context and Outcomes of Hospital Reengineering Initiatives," *Health Serv Res.* 34 (6) (2000): 1363-1388. Stephen Walston, John Kimberly, and Lawton R. Burns. "Institutional and Economic Influences on the Adoption and Extensiveness of Managerial Innovation in Hospitals: The Case of Reengineering," *Med Care Res Rev.* 58 (2) (2001): 194-228.

32. David Wang, Yusuke Tsugawa, Jose Figueroa, et al. "Association Between the Centers for Medicare and Medicaid Services Hospital Star Rating and Patient Outcomes," *JAMA Intern Med.* 176 (2016): 848-850.

33. J. Matthew Austin, Ashish Jha, Patrick Romano, et al. "National Hospital Ratings Systems Share Few Common Scores and May Generate Confusion Instead of Clarity," *Health Aff.* 34 (3) (2015): 423-430.

34. Dennis Scanlon, Yunfeng Shi, Neeraj Bhandari, et al. "Are Healthcare Quality 'Report Cards' Reaching Consumers? Awareness in the Chronically Ill Population," *Am J Manag Care.* 21 (3) (2015): 236-244.

35. Karl Bilimoria and Cynthia Barnard. "The New CMS Hospital Quality Star Ratings–The Stars Are Not Aligned," *JAMA.* 316 (17) (2016): 1761-1762.

36. Jianhui Hu, Jack Jordan, Ilan Rubinfeld, et al. "Correlations Among Hospital Quality Measures: What 'Hospital Compare' Data Tell Us," *Am J Med Qual.* 32 (6) (2017): 605-610.

37. Dennis Scanlon, Jon Christianson, and Eric Ford. "Hospital Responses to Leapfrog in Local Markets," *Med Care Res Rev.* 65 (2) (2008): 207-232.

38. Shawna Smith, Heidi Reichert, Jessica Ameling, et al. "Dissecting Leapfrog: How Well Do Leapfrog Safe Practices Scores Correlate With Hospital Compare Ratings and Penalties, and How Much Do They Matter?" *Med Care.* 55 (6) (2017): 606-614.

39. Nicholas Osborne, Lauren Nicholas, Andrew Ryan, et al. "Association of Hospital Participation in a Quality Reporting Program With Surgical Outcomes and Expenditures for Medicare Beneficiaries," *JAMA.* 313 (5) (2015): 496-504. David Etzioni, Nabil Wasif, Amylou Dueck, et al. "Association of Hospital Participation in a Surgical Outcomes Monitoring Program With Inpatient Complications and Mortality," *JAMA.* 313 (5) (2015): 505-511.

40. Donald Berwick. "Measuring Surgical Outcomes for Improvement – Was Codman Wrong?" *JAMA.* 313 (5) (2015): 469-470.

41. George Weisz, Alberto Cambrosio, Peter Keating, et al. "The Emergence of Clinical Practice Guidelines," *Milbank Q.* 85 (4) (2007): 691-727.

42. Sheldon Greenfield. "Clinical Practice Guidelines: Expanded Use and Misuse," *JAMA.* 317 (6) (2017): 594-595.

43. John Ioannidis. "Diagnosis and Treatment of Hypertension in the 2017 ACC/AHA Guidelines and in the Real World," *JAMA.* 319 (2) (2018): 115-116.

44. Jennifer Tomasone, Kaitlyn Kauffeldt, Rushil Chaudhary, et al. "Effectiveness of Guideline Dissemination and Implementation Strategies on Health Care Professionals' Behaviour and Patient Outcomes in the Cancer Care Context: A Systematic Review," *Implement Sci.* 15 (June 2020): 41.

45. Heidi Kramer and Frank Drews. "Checking the Lists: A Systematic Review of Electronic Checklist Use in Health Care," *J Biomed Inform.* 71 (2017): S6-S12. Henry Ko, Tari Turner, and Monica Finnigan. "Systematic Review of Safety Checklists for Use by Medical Care Teams in Acute Hospital Settings: Limited Evidence of Effectiveness," *BMC Health Serv Res.* 11 (2011): 211.

46. David Urbach, Anand Govindarajan, Refik Saskin, et al. "Introduction of Surgical Safety Checklists in Ontario, Canada," *N Engl J Med.* 370 (2014): 1029-1038.

47. Brigette Hales, Marius Terblanche, Robert Fowler, et al. "Development of Medical Checklists for Improved Quality of Patient Care," *Int J Qual Health Care.* 20 (1) (2008): 22-30.

48. Lucian Leape. "The Checklist Conundrum," *N Engl J Med.* 370 (2014): 1063-1064. Dante Conley, Sara Singer, Lizabeth Edmondson, et al. "Effective Surgical Safety Checklist Implementation," *J Am Coll Surg.* 212 (5) (2011): 873-879.

49. Stan Pestotnik and Valere Lemon. "How to Use Data to Improve Quality and Patient Safety," *Health Catalyst* (April 30, 2019).

50. Linda Aiken, Douglas Sloane, Hilary Barnes et al. "Nurses' and Patients' Appraisals Show Patient Safety in Hospitals Remains a Concern," *Health Aff.* 37 (11) (2018): 1744-1751.

51. Johns Hopkins Medicine. "Study Suggests Medical Errors Now Third Leading Cause of Death in the U.S.," May 3, 2016. Available online: https://www.hopkinsmedicine.org/news/media/releases/study_suggests_medical_errors_now_third_leading_cause_of_death_in_the_us. Accessed on May 24, 2020.

52. John Wennberg and Alan Gittelsohn. "Small Area Variations in Health Care Delivery: A Population-Based Health Information System Can Guide Planning and Regulatory Decision-Making," *Science.* 182 (4117) (1973): 1102-1108.

53. John Wennberg, Jean Freeman, and William Culp. "Are Hospital Services Rationed in New Haven or Over-Utilised in Boston?" *Lancet.* 329 (8543) (1987): 1185-1189.

54. The Dartmouth Institute of Health Quality and Clinical Practice. "Dartmouth Atlas Data." Available online: https://atlasdata.dartmouth.edu/long_data/new. Accessed on May 24, 2020.

55. Ambulatory care–sensitive conditions (ACS) initially comprised 28 medical conditions/diagnoses "for which timely and effective outpatient care can help to reduce the risks of hospitalization by either preventing the onset of an illness or condition, controlling an acute episodic illness or condition, or managing a chronic disease or condition." The Dartmouth Institute of Health Quality and Clinical Practice. "Dartmouth Atlas Data. Concept: Ambulatory Care Sensitive (ACS) Conditions." Available online: http://mchp-appserv.cpe.umanitoba.ca/viewConcept.php?printer=Y&conceptID=1023. Accessed on May 27, 2020.

56. Another important finding of the *Atlas* was the lack of evidence that hospital referral regions substitute outpatient and home health services for inpatient services: The correlation between inpatient and outpatient spending was low ($r = 0.12$), as was the correlation between inpatient and physician spending ($r = 0.19$) and between inpatient and home health spending ($r = 0.24$).

57. Amol Navathe, Kevin Volpp, Amelia Bond, et al. "Assessing the Effectiveness of Peer Comparisons as a Way to Improve Health Care Quality," *Health Aff.* 39 (5) (2020): 852-861.

58. Richard Cooper. "States With More Physicians Have Better-Quality Health Care," *Health Aff.* 27 (2008): 91-102.

59. Richard Cooper. "States With More Health Care Spending Have Better-Quality Health Care: Lessons About Medicare," *Health Aff.* 27 (2008): 103-115.

60. Department of Justice and Federal Trade Commission. *Statements of Antitrust Enforcement*

*Policy in Health Care* (Washington, DC: USDOJ and FTC, 1996).

61. Stephen Swenson, James Dilling, Dawn Milliner, et al. "Quality: The Mayo Clinic Approach," *Am J Med Qual.* 24 (5) (2009): 428-440.

62. Agency for Healthcare Research and Quality. "AHRQ Review of Quality Improvement Approaches." Available online: https://www.ahrq.gov/ncepcr/tools/pf-handbook/mod4.html. Accessed on November 24, 2020.

63. Mark Chassin. "Improving the Quality of Health Care: What's Taking So Long?" *Health Aff.* 32 (10) (2013): 1761-1765.

64. Carrie Colla, Elizabeth Kinsella, Nancy Morden, et al. "Physician Perceptions of Choosing Wisely and Drivers of Overuse," *Am J Manag Care.* 22 (5) (2016): 337-343.

65. American Board of Internal Medicine. *Unnecessary Tests and Procedures in the Health Care System* (Philadelphia, PA: ABIM Foundation, 2014).

66. Leah Binder. "Progress in Health Care Is Still 'Excruciatingly Slow' Says Harvard Expert," *Forbes* (February 20, 2014).

67. Isobel Whitcomb and Undark. "Americans Are Spending Billions on Unnecessary Dental Treatments," *The Atlantic* (July 25, 2020).

68. Austin Frakt. "Why Is Improvement in the Quality of Health Care So Slow?" *The Incidental Economist* (October 18, 2016). Available online: https://theincidentaleconomist.com/wordpress/why-is-improvement-in-the-quality-of-health-care-so-slow/. Accessed on May 25, 2020. See also: Institute of Medicine. *Improving Diagnosis in Health Care* (Washington, DC: IOM, 2015).

69. Mark Chassin. "Improving the Quality of Health Care: What's Taking So Long?" *Health Affairs* 32 (10) (2013): 1761-1765.

70. Mark Chassin. "Improving the Quality of Health Care: What's Taking So Long?" *Health Affairs* 32(10) (2013): 1761-1765.

71. Lawrence Casalino, David Gans, Rachel Weber, et al. "US Physician Practices Spend More Than $15.4 Billion Annually to Report Quality Measures," *Health Aff.* 35 (3) (2016): 401-406.

72. Rishi Wadhera, Jose Figueroa, Karen Joynt Maddox, et al. "Quality Measure Development and Associated Spending by the Centers for Medicare and Medicaid Services," *JAMA.* 323 (16) (2020): 1614-1616.

73. Gail Wilensky. "The Need to Simplify Measuring Quality in Health Care," *JAMA.* 319 (23) (2018): 2369-2370.

74. Eric Kessel, Vishaal Pegany, Beth Keolanui, et al. "Review of Medicare, Medicaid, and Commercial Quality of Care Measures: Considerations for Assessing Accountable Care Organizations," *J Health Polit Policy Law.* 40 (4) (2015): 759-794.

75. Karl Bilimoria. "Facilitating Quality Improvement: Pushing the Pendulum Back Toward Process Measures," *JAMA.* 314 (13) (2015): 1333-1334.

76. An additional issue is the inconsistent association among quality measures. Measures used by the Medicare program to incentivize hospitals (eg, readmission rates) have been found to be more closely associated with other quality metrics (eg, complication rates) for surgical cases than for medical cases. Ryan Merkow, Mila Ju, Jeanette Chung, et al. "Underlying Reasons Associated With Hospital Readmission Following Surgery in the United States," *JAMA.* 313 (5) (2015): 483-495. Justin Dimick and Amir Ghaferi. "Hospital Readmission as a Quality Measure in Surgery," *JAMA.* 313 (5) (2015): 512-513.

77. Tanara Hayford and Jared Maeda. *Issues and Challenges in Measuring and Improving the Quality of Health Care* (Washington, DC: Congressional Budget Office, December 2017).

78. Ingrid Nembhard, Jeffrey Alexander, Timothy Hoff, et al. "Why Does the Quality of Health Care Continue to Lag? Insights From Management Research," *Acad Manag Perspect.* 23 (1) (2009): 24-42.

79. Aaron Carroll. "What We Mean When We Say Evidence-Based Medicine," *New York Times* (December 27, 2017).

# SECTION II

## Provider Sectors in the Ecosystem

# Healthcare Providers

## WHAT IS A PROVIDER?

What is a "provider"? It is a generic, umbrella term under which 2 main classes of players in the middle of the healthcare value chain (Figure 3-9) fall: professionals and institutions. These are defined below:

Under federal regulations, a "healthcare provider" is defined as a doctor of medicine or osteopathy, podiatrist, dentist, chiropractor, clinical psychologist, optometrist, nurse practitioner, nurse-midwife, or a clinical social worker who is authorized to practice by the state and performing within the scope of their practice as defined by state law. They are collectively known as *professionals*.

*Health care institution* means an organization within the state that provides healthcare and related services, including but not limited to the provision of inpatient and outpatient care, diagnostic or therapeutic services, laboratory services, medicinal drugs, nursing care, assisted living, elderly care and housing, including retirement communities, and equipment used or useful for the provision of healthcare and related services as defined by state law. They are collectively known as *professionals*.

Chapter 9 analyzes perhaps the most important sector of providers: the medical profession. Following this, Chapter 10 examines nurses, pharmacists, and other paraprofessionals. The volume then turns its attention to the major institutional providers, including hospitals (Chapters 11 and 12), ambulatory care sites and pharmacies (Chapter 13), and post-acute care sites (Chapter 14).

## NUMBER AND DIVERSITY OF PROVIDERS

The US healthcare system employs a *lot* of providers in many different settings. According to the North American Industry Classification System (NAICS) kept by the US Bureau of Labor Statistics (BLS), these settings include hospitals, ambulatory care, nursing and residential care facilities, and social assistance. The NAICS lists 99 different occupations working in these settings, accounting for more than 20.7 million workers (as of January 2020). Ten-year rates of growth in healthcare employment (over varying intervals between 1992 and 2014) have ranged anywhere from 20% to 28% (Figure 8-1).[1] This made healthcare the economic sector with the fastest rate of growth in employment!

This growth has been focused in health-specific occupations, not jobs found in health settings that were not health related (eg, food service, maintenance). There is heavy, but not complete, overlap between healthcare occupations and employment in healthcare settings (Figure 8-2). Over time, since the 2008-2009 recession, more of the employment in healthcare settings is accounted for by healthcare-specific occupations. The 2 largest settings accounting for the majority of healthcare employment are hospitals and the offices of healthcare practitioners such as physicians, dentists, and other ambulatory care (Figure 8-3).

BLS projections for 2018 to 2028 suggest that healthcare job growth will continue to outstrip the rest of the economy (14% vs 5.2%,

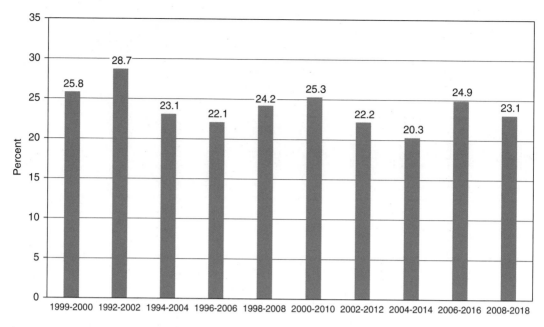

**Figure 8-1** • Growth in Healthcare Employment 1992 to 2018. (Source: Bureau of Labor Statistics, Employment Projections.)

respectively; 1.6% vs 0.5% annual change). Moreover, 6 of the 10 fastest-growing occupations nationally will be in healthcare, including occupational therapy assistants (33.1%), physician assistants (31.1%), home health aides (36.6%), personal care aides (36.4%), nurse practitioners (28.2%), and speech-language pathologists (27.3%).[2] Federal government data released in January 2020 show that nearly 1 in 5 newly created jobs have been in healthcare, increasing from 350,000 jobs in 2018 to 399,000 jobs in 2019.[3] This spanned both ambulatory care (269,000) and hospital settings (102,000).

Healthcare is thus becoming the largest employer in the United States—what journalists describe as "the new steel" in the country's labor market.[4] Between 2000 and 2017, healthcare surpassed both manufacturing and retail in terms of the number of workers in these sectors. Aging and chronic illness are not the only drivers. So, also, is expanding insurance coverage (eg, Patient Protection and Affordable Care Act [PPACA]), growing administrative burdens in responding to new quality and payment models (leading to perhaps one-fifth of healthcare workers in administrative roles), and the recession-proof nature of healthcare demand. Moreover, median

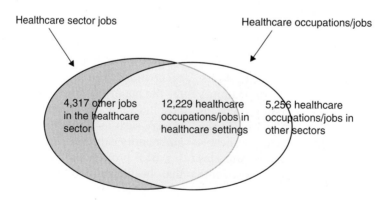

**Figure 8-2** • Overlap Between Healthcare Occupations and Employment in Healthcare Settings (in 1,000s). (Source: Centers for Disease Control and Prevention, Center for Health Workforce Studies.)

| | |
|---|---|
| **Hospitals** | Industries in the Hospitals subsector provide medical, diagnostic, and treatment services that include physician, nursing, and other health services to inpatients and the specialized accommodation services required by inpatients. Hospitals may also provide outpatient services as a secondary activity. Establishments in the Hospitals subsector provide inpatient health services, many of which can only be provided using the specialized facilities and equipment that form a significant and integral part of the production process. |
| **Offices of physicians** | This industry comprises establishments of health practitioners having the degree of M.D. (Doctor of Medicine) or D.O. (Doctor of Osteopathy) primarily engaged in the independent practice of general or specialized medicine (eg, anesthesiology, oncology, ophthalmology, psychiatry) or surgery. These practitioners operate private or group practices in their own offices (eg, centers, clinics) or in the facilities of others, such as hospitals or managed care organizations. |
| **Offices of other health practitioners** | This industry group comprises establishments of independent health practitioners (except physicians and dentists). |
| **Medical and diagnostic laboratories** | This industry comprises establishments known as medical and diagnostic laboratories primarily engaged in providing analytic or diagnostic services, including body fluid analysis and diagnostic imaging, generally to the medical profession or to the patient on referral from a health practitioner. |
| **Nursing and residential care facilities** | Industries in the Nursing and Residential Care Facilities subsector provide residential care combined with either nursing, supervisory, or other types of care as required by the residents. In this subsector, the facilities are a significant part of the production process, and the care provided is a mix of health and social services with the health services being largely some level of nursing services. |
| **Offices of dentists** | This industry comprises establishments of health practitioners having the degree of D.M.D. (Doctor of Dental Medicine), D.D.S. (Doctor of Dental Surgery), or D.D.Sc. (Doctor of Dental Science) primarily engaged in the independent practice of general or specialized dentistry or dental surgery. These practitioners operate private or group practices in their own offices (eg, centers, clinics) or in the facilities of others, such as hospitals or managed care organizations. They can provide either comprehensive preventive, cosmetic, or emergency care, or specialize in a single field of dentistry. |
| **Outpatient care centers** | This industry group comprises establishments with medical staff primarily engaged in providing a range of outpatient services, such as family planning, diagnosis and treatment of mental health disorders and alcohol and other substance abuse, and other general or specialized outpatient care. |
| **Home healthcare services** | This industry comprises establishments primarily engaged in providing skilled nursing services in the home, along with a range of the following: personal care services; homemaker and companion services; physical therapy; medical social services; medications; medical equipment and supplies; counseling; 24-hour home care; occupation and vocational therapy; dietary and nutritional services; speech therapy; audiology; and high-tech care, such as intravenous therapy. |

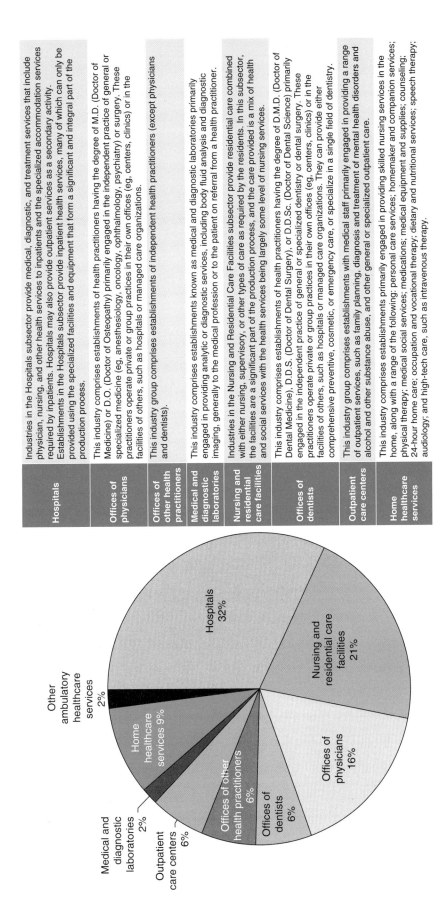

Hospitals 32%

Nursing and residential care facilities 21%

Offices of physicians 16%

Offices of dentists 6%

Offices of other health practitioners 6%

Home healthcare services 9%

Other ambulatory healthcare services 2%

Medical and diagnostic laboratories 2%

Outpatient care centers 6%

**Figure 8-3 •** Healthcare Employment by Healthcare Sector. (Source: US Bureau of Labor Statistics, classcodes.com.)

| Provider Category | No. of Providers |
|---|---|
| Hospitals | 5,198[a] |
| Physicians | 1,005,295[b] |
| | 953,695[c] |
| Nurses | 4,029,400[b] |
| Ambulatory surgery centers[b] | 5,446 |
| Urgent care clinics | 7,100 |
| Imaging centers[a] | 6,740 |
| Diagnostic labs[c] | 35,866 |
| Retail clinics[b] | 1,914 |
| Hospices[a] | 4,092 |
| Home health agencies | 12,400 |
| Nursing homes[a] | 15,634 |
| Pharmacies | 62,145[d] |
| Pharmacists | 314,000[b] |
| Dentists | 155,000[b] |

[a]Community hospitals 2018 data from American Hospital Association.
[b]Bureau of Labor Statistics (2018 data).
[c]Data for 2016.
[d]Drug Channels Institute, data for 2019.

**Figure 8-4 •** Provider Statistics.

annual wages in healthcare are almost double those found in other sectors.

Not only does the United States have a lot of providers, but it has a lot of providers operating in a *lot of different categories and settings*. These categories are depicted in Figure 8-4. One important observation is the sheer number of categories represented, each with a cast of

| | Spending (billions) | | | Distribution | | | Growth | | |
|---|---|---|---|---|---|---|---|---|---|
| | 1997 | 2016 | 2017 | 1997 | 2016 | 2017 | 1997-2017 | 2016 | 2017 |
| National Health Expenditures | $1,135.20 | $3,361.10 | 3,492.10 | 100% | 100% | 100% | 5.90% | 4.80% | 3.90% |
| Hospital Care | 363.4 | 1092.8 | 1,142.60 | 32% | 33% | 33% | 5.90% | 5.60% | 4.60% |
| Physician and Clinical Services | 238.9 | 666.5 | 694.3 | 21% | 20% | 20% | 5.50% | 5.60% | 4.20% |
| Dental Services | 50.3 | 125.1 | 129.1 | 4% | 4% | 4% | 4.80% | 5.20% | 3.20% |
| Other Professional Services | 31.3 | 92.4 | 96.6 | 3% | 3% | 3% | 5.80% | 5.10% | 4.60% |
| Nursing Care Facilities | 74.1 | 163 | 166.3 | 7% | 5% | 5% | 4.10% | 3.10% | 2.00% |
| Home Health Services | 36.9 | 93.1 | 97 | 3% | 3% | 3% | 5.00% | 4.30% | 4.30% |
| Other Healthcare | 50 | 173.4 | 183.1 | 4% | 5% | 5% | 6.70% | 5.30% | 5.60% |
| Prescription Drugs | 77.6 | 332 | 333.4 | 7% | 10% | 10% | 7.60% | 2.30% | 0.40% |
| Other Medical Products | 46.8 | 113.6 | 118.5 | 4% | 3% | 3% | 4.80% | 4.40% | 4.30% |
| Net Cost of Health Insurance | 48.5 | 220.7 | 229.5 | 4% | 7% | 7% | 8.10% | 6.20% | 4.00% |
| Government Administration | 12.3 | 44.7 | 45 | 1% | 1% | 1% | 6.70% | 4.80% | 0.50% |
| Public Health Activities | 34.8 | 85.6 | 88.9 | 3% | 3% | 3% | 4.80% | 2.70% | 3.90% |
| Investment | 70.4 | 158.2 | 167.6 | 6% | 5% | 5% | 4.40% | 2.40% | 6.00% |

**Figure 8-5 •** National Health Expenditures by Provider Category. (Source: Centers for Medicare and Medicaid Services.)

**Hospital Care:**
Covers all services provided by hospitals to patients. These include room and board, ancillary charges, services of resident physicians, inpatient pharmacy, hospital-based nursing home and home healthcare, and any other services billed by hospitals in the United States. The value of hospital services is measured by total net revenue, which equals gross patient revenues (charges) less contractual adjustments, bad debts, and charity care. It also includes government tax appropriations as well as non-patient and nonoperating revenues. Hospitals fall into NAICS 622-Hospitals.

**Physician and Clinical Services:**
Covers services provided in establishments operated by Doctors of Medicine (M.D.) and Doctors of Osteopathy (D.O.), outpatient care centers, plus the portion of medical laboratories services that are billed independently by the laboratories. This category also includes services rendered by a doctor of medicine (M.D.) or doctor of osteopathy (D.O.) in hospitals, if the physician bills independently for those services. Clinical services provided in freestanding outpatient clinics operated by the US Department of Veterans' Affairs, the US Coast Guard Academy, the US Department of Defense, and the US Indian Health Service are also included. The establishments included in Physician and Clinical Services are classified in NAICS 6211-Offices of Physicians, NAICS 6214-Outpatient Care Centers, and a portion of NAICS 6215-Medical and Diagnostic Laboratories.

**Other Professional Services:**
Covers services provided in establishments operated by health practitioners other than physicians and dentists. These professional services include those provided by private-duty nurses, chiropractors, podiatrists, optometrists, and physical, occupational, and speech therapists, among others. These establishments are classified in NAICS 6213-Offices of Other Health Practitioners.

**Dental Services:**
Covers services provided in establishments operated by a Doctor of Dental Medicine (D.M.D.) or Doctor of Dental Surgery (D.D.S.) or a Doctor of Dental Science (D.D.Sc.). These establishments are classified as NAICS 6212-Offices of Dentists.

**Other Health, Residential, and Personal Care:**
This category includes spending for Medicaid home and community-based waivers, care provided in residential care facilities, ambulance services, school health, and worksite healthcare. Generally these programs provide payments for services in non-traditional settings such as community centers, senior citizens centers, schools, and military field stations. The residential establishments are classified as facilities for the intellectually disabled (NAICS 62321), and mental health and substance abuse facilities (NAICS 62322). The ambulance establishments are classified as ambulance services (NAICS 62191).

**Home Healthcare:**
Covers medical care provided in the home by freestanding home health agencies (HHAs). Medical equipment sales or rentals not billed through HHAs and nonmedical types of home care (eg, Meals on Wheels, chore-worker services, friendly visits, or other custodial services) are excluded. These freestanding HHAs are establishments that fall into NAICS 6216-Home Healthcare Services.

**Nursing Care Facilities and Continuing Care Retirement Communities:**
Covers nursing and rehabilitative services provided in freestanding nursing home facilities. These services are generally provided for an extended period of time by registered or licensed practical nurses and other staff. Care received in state and local government facilities and nursing facilities operated by the US Department of Veterans Affairs is also included. These establishments are classified in NAICS 6231-Nursing Care Facilities and NAICS 623311-Continuing Care Retirement Communities with on-site nursing care facilities.

**Figure 8-6** • Provider Category Definitions.

thousands (and, in some cases, millions). The fact that these categories serve as the destination for the vast majority of the US national health expenditures (Figure 8-5; definitions of categories shown in Figure 8-6) suggests that cost containment efforts will have to be a multipronged approach. Moreover, because these categories are professionals and institutions licensed at the state level, some portion of the cost containment efforts may need to be decentralized rather than centralized.

These categories and settings have, historically, operated independently of one another as "silos." This fact underlies the importance, and the challenge, of integrating healthcare delivery across sites and silos. Integration efforts are further challenged by the fact that each category may have a different "revenue model" based on (1) who their major payers are, (b) the unit

of service on which they are paid, and (c) the reimbursement method used to pay them. This diversity is presented in Figures 8-7 and 8-8. Such diversity in payment methods and units of service makes it difficult to provide comprehensive coverage across related sites of care, such as in post-acute care, even though these sites see many of the same patients for the same conditions. This problem keeps fragmentation intact. Moreover, as silos, several of these categories have engaged in "turf protection" to restrict the scope of practice and rebuff encroachments on their business by others—sometimes using quality of care rationales.

Another important observation is that these categories are both individuals and institutions. This means that any effort to integrate healthcare and coordinate their efforts will need to span lots of sites of care of very different sizes at different geographic loci (eg, concentrated or

| Year | Provider Type | Prior Method | New Method | Classification System for the New Method |
|------|---------------|--------------|------------|-------------------------------------------|
| 1983 | Hospital inpatient | 7. Per dollar of cost | 4. Per episode | Diagnosis-Related Group (DRG) |
| 1984 | Clinical laboratory | 8. Per dollar of charges | 6. Per service | Clinical Laboratory Fee Schedule (CLFS) |
| 1992 | Physician | 8. Per dollar of charges | 6. Per service[d] | Resource-Based Relative Value Scale (RBRVS) |
| 1997 | Critical access hospital | 4. Per episode | 7. Per dollar of cost | |
| 1998 | Nursing facility | 7. Per dollar of cost | 5. Per day | Resource Utilization Group (RUG) |
| 2000 | Hospital outpatient | 7. Per dollar of cost | 6. Per service[e] | Ambulatory Payment Classification (APC) |
| 2000 | Home healthcare | 7. Per dollar of cost | 4. Per episode | Home Health Resource Group (HHRG) |
| 2002 | Long-term care hospital | 7. Per dollar of cost | 4. Per episode | Long-Term Care DRG (LTC DRG) |
| 2002 | Rehabilitation facility | 7. Per dollar of cost | 4. Per episode | Case-Mix Group (CMG) |
| 2002 | Ambulance | 8. Per dollar of charges[a] | 6. Per service | |
| 2005 | Psychiatric hospital | 7. Per dollar of cost | 5. Per day | |
| 2008 | Ambulatory surgical center | 5. Per day | 5. Per day[e] | Ambulatory Payment Classification (APC) |
| 2012 | ACO | 4. Per episode[b] | Same as prior method except with savings incentives most similar to method 2 | |
| | | 6. Per service[c] | | |

[a]Before 2002, ambulance services were typically, but not always, paid at a percentage of charges.
[b]Hospital inpatient.
[c]Physician and hospital outpatient.
[d]Physician surgical services are commonly paid per episode.
[e]In practice, the incentives of the Medicare APC-based method align more closely with payment per day for ambulatory surgical centers and with payment per service for hospital outpatient care.

**Figure 8-7 •** Medicare Initiatives to Change Basic Payment Methods. ACO, Accountable Care Organization; APC, Ambulatory Payment Classification. (Source: Adapted from Kevin Quinn.)

| Provider Type | 1. Per Time Period | 2. Per Beneficiary | 3. Per Recipient | 4. Per Episode | 5. Per Day | 6. Per Service | 7. Per Dollar of Cost | 8. Per Dollar of Charges |
|---------------|------|------|------|------|------|------|------|------|
| Managed Care Organization | | P | O | | | | | |
| Hospital Inpatient | O | | | P | O | | O | O |
| Hospital Outpatient | O | | | | O | P | O | O |
| Ambulatory Surgical Center | | | | | P | | | O |
| Physician | O | O | O | O | | P | | O |
| Dentist | | | | | | P | | O |
| Therapy (outpatient) | | | | | | P | | O |
| Clinical Laboratory | | | | | | P | | O |
| Ambulance | | | | | | P | | O |
| Drugs (pharmacy) | | | | | | P | | O |
| Nursing Facility | | | | | P | | O | O |
| Home Healthcare | | | | P | | O | | O |
| Hospice | | | | | P | | | O |
| HCBS* | | | | | | | O | O |
| ICF/DD** | | | | | O | | O | O |

P = Predominant method used by Medicare
O = Other methods commonly used in the United States
*Typically provided to persons requiring personal assistance and funded by Medicaid programs per 15 minutes service unit.
**Typically funded by Medicaid programs per day or at a percentage of cost.

**Figure 8-8 •** Payment Methods Commonly Used in the United States by Payment Type. HCBS, Home and Community-Based Services; ICF/DD, Intermediate Care Facility for People With Developmental Disabilities. (Source: Adapted from Kevin Quinn.)

dispersed). Many of these sites of care are organized around individuals or small groups of providers, giving rise to the adage that healthcare is a "cottage industry." This is important for several reasons. The large number of small care sites signals that healthcare is more a "labor-intensive" industry than a "capital-intensive" industry. This limits the efficiencies to be gained by consolidating them all into larger aggregates. Nevertheless, the large number of small sites lends itself to efforts by (1) larger providers to conduct "mergers and acquisitions" and (2) private equity firms to try to consolidate them via "roll ups."

These few observations about providers suggest several other challenges facing the US healthcare industry. First, they illustrate that our country's approach to healthcare delivery has focused on fragmented specialty care for acute illness, not coordinated care for primary conditions, chronic illness, or prevention. Second, they illustrate the potential importance of developing interdisciplinary teams of practitioners that span these silos. Third, they reflect our failure to address the growing importance of population health, the social determinants of health, and inequities and disparities in the treatment of illness.

The challenges will likely grow even bigger. According to researchers, an aging population and growing disease burden, outlined in Chapters 4 and 26, will require a large and specialized workforce by 2025.[5] To be sure, primary care providers (covered in Chapters 9 and 10) will play an important role in providing preventive services and caring for this growing elderly population. However, the expanding medical knowledge base and armamentarium of treatment options for these (and other) diseases will also contribute to a proliferation of medical and surgical specialties and subspecialties. More than one-third of patients get specialty referrals annually, which serve an important role in the diagnosis, treatment, and monitoring of patients afflicted with chronic illness and adverse medical events.

More specialists will be needed along with more primary care physicians and other providers. They will all need to be trained in the art of teamwork and collaboration, something medical schools have only begun to address in recent decades.[6] They will also need to be trained in how to treat "poly-chronics"—those with multiple chronic conditions. Currently, the evidence base for their treatment is underdeveloped, since most biomedical research and most evidence-based medicine focuses on individual conditions. Students in medicine and other health professions will all require such training and education on these difficult patients and will need to work together on developing guidelines to follow in their treatment (as well as how to divide up the tasks).

Such efforts are necessary not only to ensure quality of care but also to control the rising cost of healthcare. Policy analysts suggest that the poly-chronics over the age of 65 are responsible for 96% of all spending! People with multiple chronic conditions are responsible for half of all patient encounters.

As Chapters 9 and 10 describe, the 3 largest occupations in healthcare delivery—physicians, nurses, and pharmacists—are already feeling the stress of taking care of a growing population of elderly, chronically ill, and disease-burdened people. It is not just the task at hand that causes the stress ("burnout" is the current phrase) but also the conditions under which these occupations work. These conditions include growing bureaucratization of professional labor, in the form of salaried employees working in large chains with less control over the content of their work. The challenges going forward are not only to provide care to the sick but also to take care of the caregivers (ie, moving from the triple aim to the quadruple aim; see Chapter 5). Their dilemma is compounded by the growing demands of those who pay for healthcare (government, insurers) for more transparency of results, demonstrated impacts on quality and cost-effectiveness of the care delivered, and increased productivity.

The problem is further compounded by the silos in the healthcare value chain (see Figure 3-9). Each player in the value chain competes against the others for their share of national healthcare expenditures (ie, the "budget pie"). Each player sets its own operating rules in how it recruits, trains, and motivates its workers—subject to professional licensure requirements, usually at the state level. And, sadly, each professional group along this value chain feels that it should control the content of its own work and protect this turf, rather than develop norms emphasizing collaboration with other players. Finally, each player along this value chain may be well versed about its own sector but is usually less knowledgeable and, thus, less respectful of the roles played by others. We have a lot of work ahead of us.

## Critical Thinking Exercise

A key problem facing healthcare is overcoming the divisions (ie, silos) among providers. One of my colleagues at the Harvard Business School has written about methods to "break down silos."[7] He wrote about MedTech companies (see Chapter 23) like General Electric (GE) that pioneered ways to combine both their products and their services to satisfy customer needs. In particular, GE followed the following 4 principles:

**Coordination:** Establishing structural mechanisms and processes that allow employees to improve their focus on the customer by harmonizing information and activities across units.
**Cooperation:** Encouraging people in all parts of the company—through cultural means, incentives, and the allocation of power—to work together in the interest of customer needs.
**Capability development:** Ensuring that enough people in the organization have the skills to deliver customer-focused solutions and defining a clear career path for employees with those skills.
**Connection:** Developing relationships with external partners to increase the value of solutions cost-effectively.

Other researchers have also written extensively on this same topic. A team of European researchers identified the following 5 factors that serve to break down silos and promote collaboration[8]:

1. **Value** placed on collaboration as part of company culture to bring people and units in an organization together
2. A **collaborative operating model** that refers to how the organization's social, knowledge, and management infrastructure itself is organized and aligned in such a way that collaboration across units is facilitated and thus made easier
3. A **collaborative environment** that relates to fostering a collaborative mindset, focus, behavior, and culture in the organization, and ensures all units are treated equally so there is no distrust between them
4. **Leadership** as evidenced by managers taking the lead in showing and promoting collaborative behavior
5. Emphasis on **people reward and development** that focuses on rewarding people for collaborative behavior and making sure they are capable of actually cooperating across unit boundaries

Such frameworks were not necessarily developed for improving coordination in healthcare delivery by providers. How useful do they seem?

## SUMMARY

*Providers* is a catch-all term that encompasses a lot of people working in a lot of different occupational categories at a lot of different sites that deliver care. Such differentiation drives much of the fragmentation in our healthcare system, which complicates efforts to integrate care and foster provider collaboration. As noted in Chapter 1, there is no rational design to the provider sprawl. These players in the healthcare value chain have evolved over time and now crowd the stage. The next 6 chapters dive into many of these players.

## QUESTIONS TO PONDER

1. Healthcare has lots of individuals and organizations serving as providers of care. Can you think of other US industries with this diverse mix?
2. What might be good ways to coordinate the work performed by this mix of individuals and organizations?
3. Is "professionalism" at odds with the goal of integrating and coordinating healthcare?

## REFERENCES

1. Center for Health Workforce Studies. *Health Care Employment Projections, 2014-2024: An Analysis of Bureau of Labor Statistics Projections by Setting and by Occupation* (Albany, NY: School of Public Health, SUNY, April 2016).
2. US Bureau of Labor Statistics. *Employment Projections—2019-2029.* Available online: https://www.bls.gov/news.release/pdf/ecopro.pdf. Accessed on March 9, 2020.
3. US Bureau of Labor Statistics. *Employment Situation Summary.* Available online: https://www.bls.gov/news.release/empsit.nr0.htm. Accessed on March 9, 2020.
4. Derek Thompson. "Health Care Just Became the U.S.'s Largest Employer," *The Atlantic* (January 9, 2018).
5. Timothy Dall, Paul Gallo, Ritasree Chakrabarti, et al. "An Aging Population and Growing Disease Burden Will Require a Large and Specialized Workforce by 2025," *Health Aff.* 32 (11) (2013): 2013-2020.
6. Kathryn Roethel. "Medical Schools Push Teamwork," *US News and World Report* (March 19, 2012). Available online: https://www.usnews.com/education/best-graduate-schools/top-medical-schools/articles/2012/03/19/medical-schools-push-teamwork. Accessed on March 10, 2020. See also: Susan Lerner, Diane Magrane, and Erica Friedman. "Teaching Teamwork in Medical Education," *Mt Sinai J Med.* 76 (4) (2009 Aug): 318-329. Available online: https://www.ncbi.nlm.nih.gov/pubmed/19642146. Accessed on March 10, 2020.
7. Ranjay Gulati. "Silo Busting: How to Execute on the Promise of Customer Focus," *Harvard Business Review* (May 2007). Available online: https://hbr.org/2007/05/silo-busting-how-to-execute-on-the-promise-of-customer-focus. Accessed on August 5, 2020.
8. André de Waal, Michael Weaver, Tammy Day, et al. "Silo-Busting: Overcoming the Greatest Threat to Organizational Performance," *Sustainability* 11 (2019). Available online: https://www.researchgate.net/publication/337714303_Silo-Busting_Overcoming_the_Greatest_Threat_to_Organizational_Performance. Accessed on August 5, 2020.

# 9

# The Medical Profession

## THE CENTRAL ROLE OF PHYSICIANS

Earlier chapters depict the centrality of physicians in the US healthcare ecosystem. There are many reasons for ascribing them this central role. Put simply, physicians control 85% to 90% of all personal healthcare spending, either directly (through their professional incomes) or indirectly (through their orders and oversight of others).[1] How do they exercise such discretion? Physicians have a monopoly or virtual monopoly over most major decisions that drive healthcare spending. These decisions include:

- Admitting to a hospital
- Discharging from a hospital
- Referring to a specialist (for those enrolled in a narrow network plan)
- Authorizing home healthcare
- Performing a surgical procedure
- Performing a diagnostic test
- Using expensive equipment and technologies
- Writing a prescription for a drug

Such discretion did not come the medical profession's way via legislative fiat. Rather, it came about through a series of political negotiations between the emerging professional organizations (eg, American Medical Association [AMA] and its state medical societies) and state governments. Such negotiations with professional groups were perceived during the progressive era of the late 19th century not only as a vehicle to improve quality amid a range of unregulated practitioners, but also to mitigate and regulate the harmful impacts of competition on the public interest.[2] To a limited extent, some nonphysicians like nurse practitioners (NPs) and other advanced practice registered nurses (APRNs) have been allowed some clinical autonomy (eg, to write prescriptions); these exceptions are driven by state-level scope of practice regulations (see Chapter 10).

Physicians occupy central roles for other reasons. Due to their "power of the purse" in controlling healthcare spending and utilization, they are courted by many of the other players in the healthcare ecosystem. Hospitals have courted the physicians on their medical staffs for years since the advent of the Inpatient Prospective Payment System (IPPS) in 1983 to help them control inpatient spending and succeed financially under (1) diagnosis-related groups (DRGs) and then (2) risk-based contracts (RBCs) and value-based payments (VBPs). Pharmaceutical firms have long courted physicians, particularly those treating chronic conditions, to prescribe the drugs they make to treat these conditions. Medical device firms have long courted certain types of specialists (eg, cardiovascular surgeons, electrophysiologists, orthopedists) to select their instruments and implants for surgery. Medical technology firms that make imaging equipment have long courted radiologists to use their scanners. Group purchasing organizations (GPOs) that purchase many of these products on behalf of the hospitals they represent also court the hospitals' physicians to ascertain and then perhaps shape their preferences for these technologies (in order to concentrate buying and thereby obtain lower unit prices).

Physicians are, thus, squarely in the middle of the healthcare value chain (see Figure 3-9) and occupy the most influential role in most decision making. They are also the only ones who wear white coats around the hospital, physically distinguishing themselves from all other workers.

## THE BIG DISCONNECT: PHYSICIANS DON'T FEEL CENTRAL

And, yet, physicians typically feel powerless and at "the bottom of the food chain." What's up with this? Physicians can be characterized by a number of paradoxes that need to be explained:

- They are all-powerful and yet they feel powerless.
- They are highly paid healthcare professionals and yet their incomes are stagnant.
- They work long hours and yet are less productive.
- They have specialized medical knowledge and yet are business challenged.
- They are organized members of medical societies and yet are disorganized.
- They are members of care teams and yet are autonomous.

Physicians wield considerable power as individual practitioners, both in doctor-patient relationships and in care teams they participate in (usually as team leaders). This is reflected in the "micro ecosystem" portrayed in Figure 3-14. However, consolidation has taken place across much of the macro ecosystem, starting with hospitals in the 1960s and 1970s (see Chapter 12). Physicians have been latecomers to the consolidation party, and thus face off (usually as individuals or small groups) in their negotiations with huge corporations and hospital systems.[3] Moreover, both public and private sector payers (Medicare on the public side, managed care plans on the private side) have confronted physicians with a bewildering array of quality metrics to adopt, electronic medical records (EMRs) that need to be filled out, and quality performance systems tied to new forms of compensation called "alternative payment models" (APMs).

All of these developments have contributed to what observers call "physician burnout,"

"compassion fatigue," and disgruntlement with their profession.[4] In October 2019, the National Academy of Medicine released a 312-page report on the impacts of such changes on the US health labor force.[5] The following is a list of sentiments from physicians that have been reported in the popular press and trade literature:

- Declining professional status
- Diminished respect from patients and managers
- Sense of blame for rising costs and questionable quality
- Pressured by public payers and managed care companies
- Lots of paperwork to deal with reimbursement from payers
- Second-guessed by everyone
- Stagnant incomes
- Administrative tasks that leave insufficient time with patients
- Increasing chronic illness among patients to be managed
- Asked to do more and get less

This has led to newspaper articles that report, "Why Doctors Are Sick of Their Profession," and professional journal articles that analyze "Dissatisfaction With Medical Practice."[6] Surveys indicate that physicians feel "like cogs in a machine" and face too many bureaucratic tasks, an increasing computerization of their practices, too many hours at work without commensurate compensation, too many patient appointments in a day, and too many difficult patients.

According to 2019 survey data, for example, 33.4% of physicians reported working 41 to 50 hours; 18.5% reported working 51 to 60 hours; and 12.3% reported working 61+ hours a week.[7]

Delivering safe, patient-centered, high-quality, and high-value healthcare (eg, the 6 quality domains of the Institute of Medicine, aka STEEEP [see Chapter 5]) requires a clinical workforce that is functioning at the highest level, which may be eroding. Burnout may also contribute to rising healthcare costs, perhaps as much as $4.6 billion annually, due to reduced motivation, reduced physician health status, reduced hours, and turnover from the medical profession.[8] Before discussing how we have arrived at this point, the next 2 sections outline how physicians are trained and what their age and gender composition looks like.

## HOW PHYSICIANS ARE TRAINED

US physicians undergo the most extensive training in the world. In other countries like Germany, India, and China, medical education may begin right out of high school; in the United States, the prerequisite for medical training is a 4-year college degree. Following college, there is a 4-year medical school curriculum that culminates with each student taking a state medical licensing examination. This entitles them to practice medicine in that state. The majority of medical school graduates continue their medical training in a postgraduate, specialty-oriented (rather than primary care–oriented) residency program, which, depending on the specialty, lasts another 3 to 7 years. Following residency training and successful passage of an examination hosted by that specialty society, physicians become "board certified" in that specialty. Some may continue for another couple of years to complete a clinical fellowship in an applied branch of practice in their specialty (eg, electrophysiology).

There are 2 major types of physicians: allopaths and osteopaths. Allopathic medicine, also commonly known as Western medicine, mainstream medicine, or biomedicine, refers to a system that treats symptoms and diseases using drugs, radiation, or surgery. Training in allopathic medicine occurs in schools of medicine, which confer the MD degree and are overseen by the Liaison Committee on Medical Education (LCME) which is co-sponsored by the AMA and the Association of American Medical Colleges (AAMC). By contrast, osteopathic medicine complements the allopathic approach with the added benefits of a holistic philosophy and a system of hands-on diagnosis and treatment known as osteopathic manipulative medicine. Osteopaths are trained in schools of osteopathic medicine and receive the degree of DO (doctor of osteopathy). Over time, the distinction between these 2 types of practitioners has narrowed, and both are typically found on the medical staffs of hospitals.

One feature of medical education needs to be emphasized: its cost. Consultants estimate that the cost of 1 year of medical school tuition during the 2019-2020 academic year ranged from $37,556 (public, in state) to $62,194 (public, out of state). Average private school figures were $60,665 and $62,111, respectively.[9]

Students graduate with a median of nearly $200,000 debt.[10] This debt load can be relieved over time by entering residency programs in higher-paying specialties; it can also be avoided entirely by attending a handful of medical schools that now make medical education tuition-free (eg, New York University); finally, such debt can be relieved through loan-repayment and -forgiveness programs (eg, National Health Service Corps).[11]

There are growing issues with placement in residency programs, however. First, the growth in medical school graduates without a commensurate growth in residency slots has resulted in more students applying to residency programs, flooding them with applications (at a cost of $26 per application, not to mention the cost of travel to interview). Across specialties, students now apply to an average of 50 or more programs. Between 2010 and 2015, the average number of applications to otolaryngology programs rose from 47 to 64 per student and from 200 to 275 per program. Second, the increasing competition has meant a lower "match rate" between students applying and programs accepting. In 2018, 32,232 residency positions were offered to a total of 43,909 registrants—both all-time highs. In 2019, 1.7 US medical school graduates applied for each open residency slot in orthopedics.[12] This has led to a second round of matching known as "SOAP" (Supplemental Offer and Acceptance Program). Matching rates may be lower for trainees in schools of osteopathy, for US citizens graduating from overseas medical schools, and for international medical graduates (IMGs) of foreign schools.

## DEMOGRAPHY OF THE MEDICAL PROFESSION

The AMA halted their annual publication of statistics on the medical profession several years ago. One must rely here on other national surveys to describe the physician landscape.

Figure 9-1 provides some recent statistics on the size and distribution of the medical profession using data from state licensing boards.[13] There are roughly 1 million actively licensed physicians in the United States. Of these, roughly three-quarters are graduates of US and Canadian medical schools, with the remainder as IMGs; the latter include US citizens

| | 2010 | | 2018 | |
|---|---|---|---|---|
| | Counts | Percentages | Counts | Percentages |
| Doctor of Medicine (MD) | 789,788 | 92.9% | 892,583 | 90.6% |
| Doctor of Osteopathic Medicine (DO) | 58,329 | 6.9% | 89,764 | 9.1% |
| Unknown | 1,968 | 0.2% | 2,679 | 0.3% |
| **Medical School** | | | | |
| US and Canadian Graduates (MD or DO) | 649,736 | 76.4% | 748,398 | 76% |
| International Graduates | 188,598 | 22.2% | 222,708 | 22.6% |
| Unknown | 11,751 | 1.4% | 13,920 | 1.4% |
| **Age** | | | | |
| <30 years | 16,519 | 1.9% | 16,250 | 1.6% |
| 30-39 years | 184,120 | 21.7% | 219,711 | 22.3% |
| 40-49 years | 214,595 | 25.2% | 233,192 | 23.7% |
| 50-59 years | 215,541 | 25.4% | 213,860 | 21.7% |
| 60-69 years | 138,815 | 16.3% | 191,794 | 19.5% |
| 70+ years | 75,627 | 8.9% | 106,349 | 10.8% |
| Unknown | 4,868 | 0.6% | 3,870 | 0.4% |
| **Gender** | | | | |
| Male | 583,315 | 68.6% | 630,598 | 64% |
| Female | 252,861 | 29.7% | 346,005 | 35.1% |
| Unknown | 13,909 | 1.6% | 8,423 | 0.9% |
| **Certified by an ABMS/AOA Specialty Board** | | | | |
| Yes | 633,733 | 74.5% | 807,451 | 82% |
| No | 216,352 | 25.5% | 177,575 | 18% |
| **Number of Active Licenses** | | | | |
| 1 | 657,208 | 78.4% | 767,978 | 78% |
| 2 | 142,423 | 15.7% | 152,422 | 15.5% |
| 3 or more | 50,454 | 5.8% | 64,626 | 6.6% |

**Figure 9-1** • Licensed Physicians in the United States and the District of Columbia, 2010 and 2018. ABMS, American Board of Medical Specialties; AOA, American Osteopathic Association. (Source: Adapted from Aaron Young, Humayun J. Chaudhry, Xiaomei Pei, et al. 2018 FSMB Census of Licensed Physicians in the United States, 2018. https://www.fsmb.org/siteassets/advocacy/publications/2018census.pdf.)

and non–US citizens trained overseas, both of whom nevertheless go through the US medical licensing process. Over 90% of physicians have an MD degree, whereas less than 10% are osteopaths (DOs). Over three-quarters of physicians are board certified. Demographically, roughly half are aged 50 and over. Between 2010 and 2016, the largest increase has been among physicians aged 60+ years old (from 25.2% to 29.2%) and the largest decrease among physicians aged 50 to 59 years old (from 25.4% to 22.5%). There is little change in the distribution among physicians less than 40 years old. However, there has been an enormous increase in the percentage of female physicians (from 29.7% to 33.5%), with the biggest increase observed among physicians under 40 (from 18.6% to 33.6%) followed by physicians between 40 and 49 (from 21.7% to 29.2%). At the same time, the percentage of physicians who are male and 60+ years has

remained quite high (35.9%). We thus have a bifurcated physician workforce composed of doctors who are either (1) young and female or (2) old and male.

Why is the issue of physician age important? Some studies show that patients treated by older physicians have higher mortality rates than patients treated by younger physicians. The age effect is muted if the older physician sees a high volume of patients; however, data show that the average number of patient care hours per week falls over the physician's life span. Physician age is also associated with slightly higher costs of care.[14] This may require hospitals to assess both the physical and mental agility of the older members on their medical staffs for quality assurance purposes.

Data from 2018 from the Association of American Medical Colleges (AAMC) further reveal that half of all physicians are white

(56.2%), followed by Asian (17.1%), Hispanic (5.8%), and Black (5.0%); extant surveys are unable to identify the race of nearly one-fifth of physicians. The vast majority of physicians (89%) practice in urban rather than rural settings (11%; with only 9% of specialists in rural practice) and are office-based (75%) rather than hospital-based (25%). The latter are roughly split between full-time hospital staff and residents/fellows. In terms of specialty mix, roughly two-thirds (68%) are specialists, whereas nearly one-third (32%) are primary care physicians (PCPs; defined as general and family practitioners, general internists, and general pediatricians). Among the specialists (68%), 16% are medical subspecialists, 20% are surgeons, and 32% are in other specialties.

## TRENDS IN PHYSICIAN SUPPLY AND DEMAND

A major, ongoing issue has been the adequacy of physician supply. The Flexner Report of 1910 and the Commission on Medical Education Report of 1932 both concluded the country had too many physicians. However, no action was taken by the federal government. Following World War II, there was great concern about the supply of medical professionals to meet the

needs of returning veterans and to harness the growing number of discoveries in biomedical science uncovered during the war. By the end of the 1950s, 2 reports suggested an imminent shortage.[15]

These concerns sparked federal assistance to construct new schools of medicine as well as subsidize graduate training of physicians. The Health Professions Education Assistance Act of 1963 provided funds for new medical school construction. The legislation was subsequently reinforced by several national reports that concluded that the country must train more physicians as quickly as possible.[16] The President's National Advisory Committee on Health Manpower (1967) also called for rapid growth in medical education, and by 1968, both the AAMC and the AMA had committed to the goal of medical school expansion. Between 1972 and 1982, the number of medical schools had grown from 89 to 127, whereas the number of graduates doubled (Figure 9-2).[17]

Twenty years after it began, the physician expansion party was over. In 1980, the Graduate Medical Education National Advisory Council (GMENAC) concluded the country had overshot the mark and was now facing a surplus of 70,000 physicians by the end of the millennium.[18] This raised concerns due to academic research that physicians can (and might) induce demand for their own services, which can

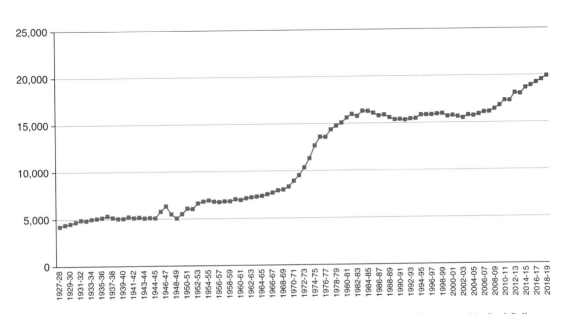

**Figure 9-2** • U.S. Medical School Graduates, 1927 to 2019. (Source: Association of American Medical Colleges. Longitudinal Applicant, Matriculant, Enrollment, and Graduation Tables. https://www.aamc.org/media/37816/download.)

lead to higher healthcare costs. In a 1994 report to both Congress and the Secretary of Health and Human Services, the AMA's College of Graduate Medical Education argued that with a shift to managed care and greater use of outpatient care, the country now faced a shortage of 35,000 PCPs and a surplus of 115,000 specialists by 2000 and recommended that the United States reduce physician production by one-quarter. A 1996 report from the Institute of Medicine recommended the country reduce the size of the entering class of medical schools and construct no new medical schools.[19] The medical schools responded to these recommendations and held constant the size of their graduating classes from 1980 to 2005; physician supply nevertheless continued to increase due to expansion in the prior 20-year period.

It should be evident that forecasting supply and demand in the medical workforce (just like forecasting Medicare spending) is more of an art than a science; it is not unusual to over- and underestimate what is actually required. This is because the manpower supply is shaped by a host of public policies and private sector activities, the latter of which can be either institutionally or individually driven. Some suggest the task is also complicated by the inability to forecast the productivity of individual physicians.[20]

Perhaps the biggest public policy initiative impacting physician supply has been the Balanced Budget Act (BBA) of 1997. To curb federal spending, BBA capped the number of residency and fellowship positions that the Medicare program would fund in graduate medical education (GME). This was significant, because Medicare was the largest source of GME funding. During the decade prior to BBA (1987-1997), the number of residents in training grew 20.6%; after BBA, residency growth slowed to 8.0%. In the presence of US population growth of 12.6% from 1997 to 2007, the country experienced a net decrease in the ratio of resident physicians to 100,000 population from 36.7 (1997) to 35.1 (2007).[21]

The debate nevertheless continues, as witnessed by 2 competing viewpoints in a recent issue of the *Journal of the American Medical Association*.[22] In 2020, however, the AAMC issued a report projecting physician supply through 2033.[23] They estimated a shortfall of anywhere from 54,100 to 139,000 physicians, encompassing 21,400 to 55,200 PCPs and 33,700 to 86,700 specialists.

Figure 9-3 shows the increase in total physician supply between 1975 and 2015. Note that the rate of increase has slowed since 2005. Figure 9-4 shows the supply of the physician workforce standardized by the size of the US population between 1980 and 2012. Note the negligible increase in supply after 2003. This suggests that medical manpower is barely keeping pace with population growth.

Why is this of potential concern? An undersupply of physicians means potential problems facing patients in accessing needed care. This

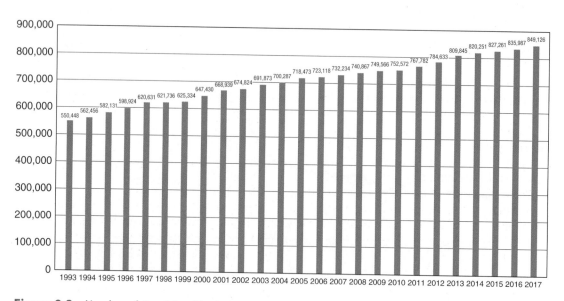

**Figure 9-3 •** Number of Practicing Physicians in the United States, 1993 to 2017. (Source: Organisation for Economic Co-operation and Development statistics.)

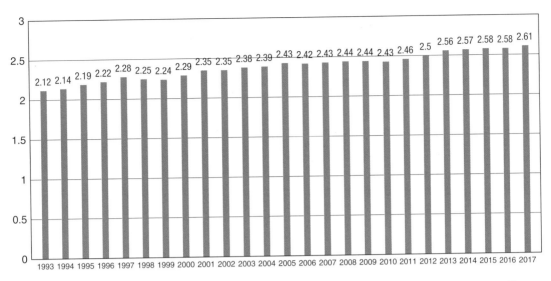

**Figure 9-4 •** Number of Practicing Physicians Per 1,000 People in the United States, 1993 to 2017. (Source: Organisation for Economic Co-operation and Development statistics.)

includes finding a PCP with a patient panel that is still open and accepting new patients, as well as waiting time for an appointment, waiting time in the office, and time spent with the physician. This issue has been exacerbated by expansions in insurance coverage (eg, the Patient Protection and Affordable Care Act [PPACA]), which results in more people looking for physicians but unable to find them. An undersupply also exacerbates difficulties in providing rural health, population health, dealing with the growing scourge of chronic illness, and dealing with an aging population.

What are the major drivers of this shortage (to the degree that it really exists)? One problem is the aging of the (particularly male) physician workforce. Since 2000, the number of physicians retiring has grown to approximate the number of new physicians entering the workforce. Another issue is an observed fall in physician productivity. Research shows that physicians reduced the average number of hours they worked by 7.2% between 1996 and 2008 (from 54.9 to 51.0).[24] Part of this is attributed to the stagnation in physician incomes. Controlling for inflation, physician hourly earnings barely increased from the period 1996 to 2000 ($65.4) to 2005 to 2010 ($67.3); taking into account their reduced productivity, physician annual earnings fell from $166,773 to $157,751.[25] There are many reasons for this income decline; most stem from the rise of managed care in the 1990s, rising bargaining power of commercial insurance companies,

slow growth in Medicare reimbursement, and cuts in Medicaid reimbursement.

Of course, there are other reasons for the fall in physician productivity. Among the growing cohort of younger physicians, there is greater interest in "work-life balance." In one survey, physicians under 50 years of age cited the following factors as "very important" in a desirable medical practice: time for family/personal life (71%), flexible scheduling (37%), and no or limited on-call responsibility (31%); by contrast, practice income was cited as very important by only 39% of respondents.[26] These figures are much higher among female physicians than among male physicians. Given the growth in the female composition of the medical workforce and the stated intention of female physicians to retire earlier than their male counterparts, this may spell trouble for physician access going forward.

## ADDRESSING THE PHYSICIAN SHORTAGE

There are several avenues available to address the shortage of physicians. One is to increase supply by increasing the number of medical schools and their students. Indeed, from 2002 to mid-2019, 29 new accredited medical schools and 17 new schools of osteopathic medicine opened.[27] Medical school enrollments have increased 31% over this time period; considering both medical and osteopathic schools, enrollment has risen 52%. Nevertheless, residency positions are still capped following the BBA of 1997; such positions have increased only 1% a year. Thus, expansions in medical school capacity and enrollments must be matched with expansions in residency positions, which will require bipartisan support for new Medicare funding.

Two pieces of proposed 2019 legislation in the US Congress sought to add (1) 15,000 residencies over the next 5 years, known as the Resident Physician Shortage Reduction Act, as well as (2) 1,000 residency slots to fund training in opioid-related specialties (addiction medicine, pain management). Of course, hospitals might establish their own residency programs without federal support; however, hospitals report that each residency position costs them $150,000 annually, perhaps making this option untenable.

Other strategies to deal with the shortage are to bolster the productivity of current physicians in practice. Attempts here include the use of "scribes" to enter patient information on the EMR while the physician attends directly to the patient. Other initiatives include off-loading other nonclinical tasks, using lean management techniques to reduce wasted time, and teaching patients more self-care techniques to reduce the demand on physician time.

Another set of strategies includes attracting more students into medical school. This can include free tuition, tuition loan-forgiveness programs, and other compensation incentives to reduce the high burden of student debt. Still other strategies include complementing

the physician workforce with nonphysicians; Chapters 7 and 9 describe some of the options. They include NPs, physician assistants (PAs), retail clinics, telemedicine, and greater use of IMGs; the IMG approach is somewhat dependent on US immigration policy.

## WHERE DO PHYSICIANS PRACTICE?

Physicians historically worked independently in solo practices on a fee-for-service basis. Group practice was officially opposed by the AMA, which viewed it as a form of communism and "collectivism."[28] This opposition subsided by the late 1950s, partly due to antitrust actions taken against the AMA and state medical associations, when group models began to emerge and grow.

According to national census data collected by the AMA, group practices grew in prevalence from 6,371 (in 1969) to nearly 30,000 by 2012, accounting for roughly one-third of all physicians (Figure 9-5).[29] This latter statistic may be a middle-range estimate. The Medicare Payment Advisory Commission (MedPAC), Congress's watchdog over the Medicare program, suggests that 23% of physicians practice in groups, while 16% practice in solo practice. AMA data based on benchmark surveys suggest that the percentage in group practice may be as high as 68%, while the percentage of physicians in solo practice has dropped to less than 15% (2018 data).[30] Physicians in single-specialty

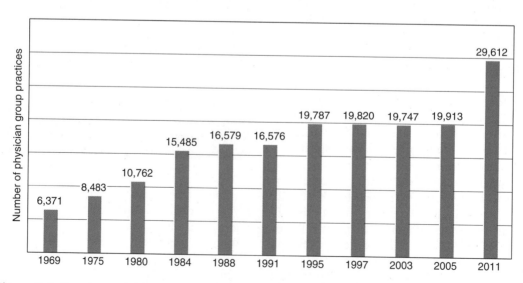

**Figure 9-5** • Prevalence of Physician Group Practices. (Source: American Medical Association.)

groups outnumber physicians in multispecialty groups by a roughly 2:1 ratio, whereas the number of single-specialty groups outnumbers multispecialty groups by a roughly 3:1 ratio. The difference is explained by the much larger size of multispecialty groups.

Much has been written and said about the more recent trend toward "physician employment," so much so that these estimates are (also) all over the map. The MedPAC data suggest that 39% of physicians are employed by a hospital or health system (as of 2014); American Hospital Association data for 2017 estimate the percentage is much lower at 15%, whereas AMA survey data provide an intermediate estimate of 27% of physicians (2018 data). Some of this employment comes in the form of working as spokes of ambulatory care for a hospital hub; some of this employment comes in the form of working as employed specialists for the hospital out in the community (eg, oncologists). Some of this employment comes in the form of working as "hospitalists": for example, in-house hospital specialists in surgical units (surgicalists), labor units (laborists), intensive care units (intensivists), and internal medicine units that obviate the need for community-based physicians to attend to their hospital patients.

Finally, there has been a slow movement toward "concierge medicine" in which a physician contracts directly with consumers on a monthly or annual fee and eliminates the health insurer as a middleman. Such an approach appeals to physicians with large patient panels who feel constrained in how much time they can spend with a patient (up to 20 minutes), tight patient scheduling, and lots of paperwork to satisfy third-party payers. Such an approach can reduce patient workload from 30 to 6 patients per day. The approach resembles the older model of physicians working in solo practice on a fee-for-service basis. It appears to be limited to 3% of family physicians, according to a 2018 survey conducted by the American Academy of Family Physicians, with another 3% planning to transition to this model.[31] Barriers to further diffusion of this model may be patients' willingness to pay the physician a retainer fee (estimated to range from $900 to $2,500 annually) on top of their regular insurance premium. The physicians surveyed reported that their current patient panels are only 345 patients, short of their target of 596 patients. This is far lower than the normal patient panel of 2,000 to 2,500 patients of a PCP.

## THE ECONOMICS OF PHYSICIAN PRACTICE

Physicians have traditionally been self-employed in small practices. Their revenues consist of reimbursements from a range of public and private insurers, patient copayments (that need to be collected at the clinic visit) that insurers require in many managed care plans, and out-of-pocket payments for those patients without insurance (see Figure 11-10). This sets up a dynamic where office-based physicians must employ staff to manage "accounts receivables" not only from insurers but also from patients, contributing to the administrative burden of medical practice. It also creates the potential for physicians to close their practices and screen out patients who lack certain types of insurance coverage (eg, "Medicare patients-only" practice in some specialties).

Similar to hospitals, insurer reimbursements are a fraction of what the physician "charges," usually based on the insurer's bargaining power. Physician practice expenses are listed in Figure 9-6.[32] The largest include wages and benefits for office staff (eg, nursing), as well as medical supplies. Collectively, these expense categories account for anywhere from 50% to 60% of practice revenues; after subtracting these overhead expenses from revenues, physicians in the practice split the remainder as their incomes. The bottom panel of Figure 9-7 shows the expenses and net incomes for practices of different sizes; note that there do not appear to be any major economies of scale.

Figure 9-8 shows that these practice expenses have grown over time (data for multispecialty groups). The costs are growing for a number of reasons: growing administrative burden of EMRs, growing demands by insurers for documentation of quality, growing need to respond to APMs, and so on. According to researchers, US physician practices in 4 common specialties spend, on average, 785 hours per physician and more than $15.4 billion dealing with the reporting of quality measures.[33]

All of this requires physicians to become more able "managers" of their practices—a skill not taught in medical school or residency training. Traditionally, physicians relied on their spouses to help manage their practices. In recent decades, physicians have resorted to outside help in the form of "management services

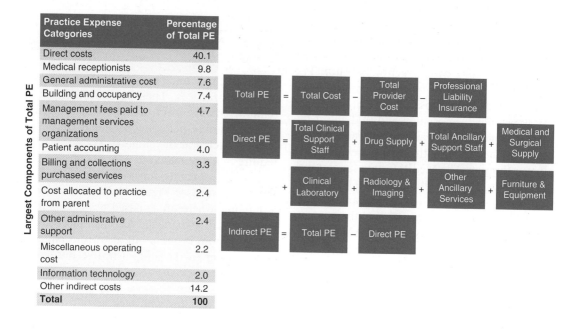

| Practice Expense Categories | Percentage of Total PE |
|---|---|
| Direct costs | 40.1 |
| Medical receptionists | 9.8 |
| General administrative cost | 7.6 |
| Building and occupancy | 7.4 |
| Management fees paid to management services organizations | 4.7 |
| Patient accounting | 4.0 |
| Billing and collections purchased services | 3.3 |
| Cost allocated to practice from parent | 2.4 |
| Other administrative support | 2.4 |
| Miscellaneous operating cost | 2.2 |
| Information technology | 2.0 |
| Other indirect costs | 14.2 |
| **Total** | **100** |

*Largest Components of Total PE*

**Figure 9-6** • Practice Expense (PE). Construction of Total PE, Direct PE, and Indirect PE Using Medical Group Management Association Survey Data. (Source: Rand Analysis of Centers for Medicare and Medicaid Services Data; Adapted from Lane F. Burgette, Jodi L. Liu, Benjamin M. Miller, et al. Practice Expense Methodology and Data Collection Research and Analysis. https://www.rand.org/content/dam/rand/pubs/research_reports/RR2100/RR2166/RAND_RR2166.pdf.)

organizations" (MSOs) or employment contracts with hospitals (and other owners) to help them. It should be noted that free-standing practices do not retain earnings at the end of the year—unlike other businesses—because to do so would expose them to double taxation (tax on personal take-home income and tax on group income). Thus, office physicians are dependent not only on managing their cash flow carefully in the current year but also on seeking

| | Median | Mean | Range |
|---|---|---|---|
| Charges | $1,000,000 | $1,173,743 | $50,000-$5,144,630 |
| Collections | $714,896 | $780,495 | $32,389-$3,264,948 |
| Expenses | $400,000 | $464,523 | $16,667-$1,862,121 |
| Profit | $291,198 | $356,263 | $73,525-$1,402,827 |

| | Solo (n = 29) | Group of 2-3 (23 groups/52 physicians) | Groups >4 (14 groups/103 physicians) |
|---|---|---|---|
| Charges | $1,355,533 | $1,037,963 | $1,145,560 |
| Collections | $915,272 | $697,367 | $709,162 |
| Expenses | $588,484 | $359,282 | $446,052 |
| Profit | $394,332 | $338,086 | $326,140 |

**Figure 9-7** • Physician Practice Financial Profile Data from the American Academy of Allergy, Asthma, and Immunology, 2007 (Per Physician Per Year for 57 Practices). (Source: Adapted from Marshall Grodofsky. Using Simple Bookkeeping Principles and Reports to Analyze Allergy Practice Performance. https://www.aaaai.org/Aaaai/media/MediaLibrary/PDF%20Documents/Practice%20Management/PM%20Resource%20Guide/Chapter-12-Using-simple-bookkeeping-principles-and-reports.pdf.)

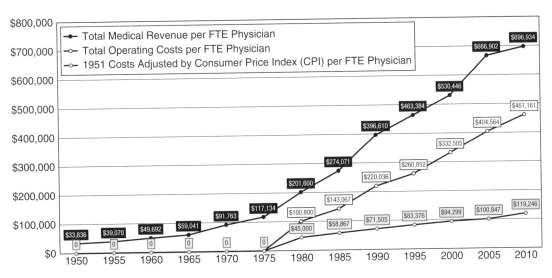

**Figure 9-8 •** Key Operating Indicators for Multispecialty Practices, 1951 to 2010. FTE, Full-Time Equivalent. (Source: Medical Group Management Association Cost Survey reports.)

outside capital to support future growth and expansion of their practices.

## How Physicians Are Paid

Physicians are compensated by any number of mechanisms, as noted in the prior chapter (see Figures 8-7 and 8-8). Solo practice physicians typically work in a fee-for-service environment where their income depends entirely on their productivity. According to AMA data (for 2014), 61.2% of nonsolo physicians receive at least some portion of their compensation in the form of salary, although this may paradoxically need to be earned on a fee-for-service basis.[34] As testimony to this, 53.3% report they are compensated on a personal productivity basis. Nearly one-third (32.2%) report working under financial incentives for their practice, and another one-third (30.5%) report receiving a bonus. When queried about the use of multiple payment methods, nearly one-half of physicians (49%) are compensated under 1 mechanism, nearly one-third (29.6%) are paid using 2 mechanisms, and the remainder (22%) are compensated using 3 or more methods.

The use of these different methods varies by physician specialty. Physicians in pediatrics, emergency medicine, psychiatry, and general surgery are more likely than others to be compensated using only or primarily salaried methods; other surgical and internal medicine subspecialists are more likely to be compensated using productivity models. Few specialists (<10%) report

receiving more than half of their compensation from financial performance arrangements.

## Physician Incomes

Research evidence cited earlier indicates the "flatlining" of real physician incomes over time. This may help to explain why some specialties jealously guard their "turf" against intrusion from other physician specialties looking for more patients and revenues. Such turf wars were evident in the 1960s when general surgeons, ear/nose/throat surgeons, and oral maxillofacial surgeons each competed for head and neck patients to train their residents. In the 1990s, more conflicts surfaced when electrophysiologists began to implant coronary stents in patients with coronary artery disease and took patients away from cardiac surgeons who performed coronary artery bypass with graft procedures (CABGs). More recently, interventional (or vascular) radiologists, interventional cardiologists, and endovascular surgical (interventional) neuroradiologists compete for volumes in stenting procedures. The rapid new development of imaging technologies, mechanical devices, and treatment methods, while certainly beneficial to the patient, can also lead to ambiguity regarding specific specialty claims on certain techniques and devices. Even more recently, physician incomes have been hammered by COVID-19 and the ensuing recession in the US economy (see box titled "Impact of COVID-19 Crisis on Physician Incomes").

### Impact of COVID-19 Crisis on Physician Incomes

COVID-19 is impacting both demand and supply of healthcare services. On the *demand side*, patients have reduced physician visits, with sharp declines in volumes (~60%) and revenues (~55%) since the crisis began.[35] Simulations suggest that PCPs will lose $67,774 (or 13%) in gross revenues per full-time physician in 2020.[36] On the *supply side*, physicians report concerns with staff layoffs and furloughs and higher expenditures on Personal Protective Equipment (PPE) supplies and technology to support telemedicine visits. Nearly half report they have enough cash on hand to remain open for the next 4 weeks.[37] Paycheck Protection Program (PPP) and Small Business Administration (SBA) loans may not sustain them in a prolonged crisis and may lead to permanent closure.

Here are some Spring 2020 headlines from the frontline of healthcare delivery:

- Between March 10th and March 15th, the percentage of nephrologists reporting the virus was having a high impact on their practices rose from 22% to 58%. A March 20th survey of multiple specialties showed that this rate was 97%![38]
- Patient "no-show" rates jumped from 5% to 75%.[39]
- Physicians compensated on productivity models suffered sudden income shocks.[40] Those in private practice who do not retain earnings have little financial buffer.
- Patients have struggled to pay their cost sharing, while providers have struggled with collection efforts.[41]
- Patient appointments have migrated to telemedicine consultations, which aggravate the problem. Although the Centers for Medicare and Medicaid Services recently expanded reimbursement to cover telehealth, it is

unclear if private insurers will follow suit and if such telehealth payments can substitute for office visit payments. PCPs have cut back on nonurgent and preventive visits (most of their appointments).

- The complexity of COVID-19 patients has further stressed already strained nurse staffing ratios, which can lead to even greater provider burnout, absenteeism, illness, and the need to hire *locum tenens*.

There is even greater cause for concern downrange. The US economy has entered a recession likely to impact provider operations going forward. Analyses of the fallout from the 2008 recession suggest that patient volumes decline, cash flow slows down, days in cash shorten, unemployment increases, insurance coverage falls, service mix and payer mix deteriorate, charitable donations fall, revenue and profitability fall, and bad debt rises.[42]

One should remember that small physician practices are also small businesses that have been adversely affected by COVID-19.[43] The United States has relied upon small primary care practices to serve as the frontline in responding to such health crises. Many have been forced to turn to telehealth and remote visits to treat patients and stay afloat financially, although the telehealth reimbursement model is uncertain (see Chapter 24). Perhaps in addition to stockpiling ventilators and PPE, the United States also needs to think about either stockpiling or restructuring primary care capacity. This subject is taken up in Chapter 10. Another approach is to move physicians to value-based purchasing models that replace fee-for-service with capitation approaches; this subject is taken up in Chapter 12.

Nevertheless, physicians earn substantial incomes, according to various surveys. The 2019 Medscape Physician Compensation Report indicates that PCPs earn $237,000, while specialists earn $341,000.[44] Among the specialties covered in the report, public health and prevention physicians and pediatricians earn the lowest ($209,000 and $225,000, respectively), while orthopedic surgeons and plastic surgeons earn the most ($482,000 and $471,000, respectively).

Self-employed (independent) physicians earn much more than their employed counterparts ($359,000 vs $289,000), as do solo physicians (see Figure 9-7).

Incomes of US physicians are much higher than their counterparts around the world. McKinsey data from 2006, controlling for purchasing parity power (PPP), suggest that US generalist physician incomes are a 4.1-fold multiple of gross domestic product (GDP) per capita, while the average physician in Organisation of Economic Co-operation and Development (OECD) countries earns a 2.8-fold multiple. The gap is even greater for specialists, who earn a 6.5-fold multiple in the United States versus a 3.9-fold multiple in OECD countries. It should be noted, however, that although physicians in other countries like Germany earn less, they have the advantage of tax-subsidized medical education (and no tuition debt) that US physicians don't have.

## PHYSICIAN PRACTICE CHALLENGES

The Medscape survey queries physicians about the most challenging and most rewarding parts of their job. Not surprisingly, the former is extrinsic, while the latter is intrinsic. In rank order, physicians report that the biggest challenges are rules and regulations (26%), working with the EMR (15%), working long hours (14%), dealing with difficult patients (14%), reimbursement from insurers (13%), and being sued (8%). Conversely, the most rewarding parts of their jobs are gratitude and relationships with patients (29%), being good at what they do and finding the diagnoses (24%), and making the world a better place (22%).

Another Medscape report charts the sources of growing burnout among physicians. The sources of some of these feelings are itemized at the beginning of this chapter.[45] Physicians report being on a "treadmill" in their hospital practice: forced to be more productive to avoid stagnating incomes but also faced with rising patient complexity that demands more of their time. They also feel that quality metrics from payers are (1) "the bane of their existence" and/or (2) what managers want to extract from EMRs rather than what doctors or their patients perceive as quality care (eg, listening to patients). With the growing size and bureaucracy of hospital systems, physicians feel that the C-suite is increasingly detached from the reality of frontline medicine and is increasingly focused on data, metrics, and policies (eg, standardization, in-house referrals). Some medical groups also have reportedly ditched clinical integration mechanisms (see Chapter 7) designed to improve quality due to perceived ineffectiveness and the disruption caused to their practices.

There are also reports of growing physician "burnout" at the frontline of care delivery caused by the above. This dissatisfaction may increase even further as APMs receive greater impetus and the physician supply shortage worsens. Recently, 10 health system executives labeled physician burnout as a "public health crisis." Some analysts have called for an extension of Berwick's triple aim to encompass "the quadruple aim" of improving the work lives of providers. This is discussed in the next section.

---

### Critical Thinking Exercise

One oft-mentioned solution to the issue of physician burnout (covered earlier) and physician engagement (covered later) is leadership. Specifically, researchers argue that what physicians and healthcare provider organizations need are physicians in charge as the chief executive officer (CEO).[46] How does physician (as opposed to lay) leadership help? Consider the following comments:

Physicians may create a more sympathetic and productive work environment for other clinicians, because they are "one of them." Being a physician can inform leadership through a shared understanding about the motivations and incentives of other clinicians. Dr. Toby Cosgrove, former CEO of the Cleveland Clinic, stated that physician CEOs have "credibility . . . peer-to-peer credibility." In other words, it signals that they have "walked the walk" and thus have earned credibility and insights into the needs of their fellow physicians.

The website for the Mayo Clinic notes that it is physician-led because, "This helps ensure a continued focus on our primary value, the needs of the patient come first." Having spent their careers looking through a patient-focused lens, physicians moving into executive positions might be expected to bring a patient-focused strategy that other physicians find reassuring.

Does putting physicians in charge of our provider organizations solve the problems identified in this chapter? How strong is the evidence base for the assertion that physician CEOs are the answer?

## PHYSICIAN ENGAGEMENT

At the same time that physicians are reporting "burnout," other parties are seeking their "engagement" in a host of endeavors.[47] These include controlling healthcare costs, using quality metrics to assess their performance, collaborating with nonphysician practitioners, working with hospitals and health systems on integration, and helping with the (so-called) "transformation from volume to value." Burnout can perhaps be addressed by bolstering 5 factors of engagement that (according to survey research) are correlated with it: organizational support for the physician's desired work-life balance, the organization's responsiveness to the physician's input, professional autonomy to manage one's individual practice, executive actions that reflect the goals and priorities of clinicians, and the organization's recognition of excellent clinical work.[48]

Needless to say, suffering from stagnant incomes and the psychological stress of burnout, physicians may be "late to the engagement." For example, a national survey revealed that only a minority of physicians (36%) feel a major responsibility for reducing healthcare costs. Instead, physicians believe that other parties need to shoulder that responsibility, including trial lawyers (60%), health insurers (59%), hospitals and health systems (56%), drug and medical device manufacturers (56%), and patients (52%).[49]

Similarly, PCPs are not generally positive about the impact of using NPs and PAs on their own ability to provide quality of care. Data gathered by the Commonwealth Fund reveal that only 29% are positive about the quality impact of NPs and PAs; 41% are negative, whereas 18% report no impact and 12% are unsure. PCPs are more likely to be satisfied if they have an NP or PA in their office. Although the vast majority (81%) of PCPs are satisfied with their collaboration with NPs and PAs, more are somewhat satisfied (46%) than very satisfied (35%). Of greater concern is that PCPs are less satisfied with this collaboration than are the NPs and PAs (89%).[50]

PCPs are also not entirely positive about the impact of patient-centered medical homes (PCMHs), which embellish the PCP's office with an NP, EMR, and linkages to help coordinate care with other practitioners. Only 33% of PCPs believe the PCMH helps to improve the quality of care they provide; 14% report it has a negative impact; 26% report no impact; and 27% are unsure. Similarly, only 14% of PCPs report that

accountable care organizations (ACOs) have a positive impact on the quality of care they provide to their patients; 26% report that ACOs exert a negative impact; 21% report no impact; and 38% are unsure. Finally, only 22% of PCPs believe that the use of quality metrics as a vehicle to assess their performance has a positive impact on the quality of care they provide; 50% believe these metrics have a negative impact!

What else might improve the physician experience? One recent approach is to bolster primary care delivery with organizational supports. Another suggested approach is to place physicians back in control over healthcare quality and quality improvement—a task ceded over time to the health insurance and managed care companies. This is because burnout is thought to be linked to a loss of "control"—a major hallmark of a profession.[51] These 2 alternatives are discussed in the next 2 sections.

## NEW KID ON THE BLOCK: THE PATIENT-CENTERED MEDICAL HOME

There is widespread consensus that primary care (in some form) is good for patients and for the healthcare system overall (see Chapter 10). All that is needed is to put into place policies and incentives to achieve a high-functioning primary care system. Over the past decade, health plans and other stakeholders have pursued a new avenue: the patient-centered medical home (PCMH). These efforts seek to use alternative primary care payment models to create an environment that supports the transformation of primary care practices to PCMHs. This environment includes multidisciplinary teams of PCPs and NPs, enhanced use of health information technology (eg, EMR) and chronic disease registries for population health management, data to inform care management, online patient portals for proactive management of acute and chronic conditions, and a focus on patient care transitions across sites and care coordination.

To assist PCPs in this transition, new resources are made available to them, including technical assistance, coaching, and enhanced payments that can take many possible forms (per-member-per-month supplemental payments, shared savings, or fee-for-service rate hikes). PCMHs face new requirements to receive this assistance. PCPs must engage in practice transformation by

**Principal Characteristics of PCMH (Promised)**

- Personal Physician
- Physician-Directed Practice
- Whole-Person Care Orientation
- Coordinated Care
- More Time for Patients
- Better Care Continuity
- Improved Care Transitions
- Simplified and Coordinated Healthcare Experience

- Improved Clinical Indicators
- Lower Per-Capita Costs
- Increased Patient Participation in Healthcare Decisions and Adherence to Care Plans
- Quality and Safety
- Enhanced Care Access
- Optimization Through HIT Integration
- Increase in Practice Profitability and Satisfaction

**Figure 9-9** • Patient-Centered Medical Home (PCMH). HIT, Health Information Technology.

adopting new capabilities, developing engaged physician leadership, and demonstrating "medical homeness" by meeting National Committee on Quality Assurance (NCQA) requirements: obtain NCQA medical home recognition (level 1 or higher) within first 12 months, participate in learning collaborative activities, and report registry-based performance data. Structure alone, however, does not drive outcomes; PCMHs must also adopt and sustain processes to realize clinical and operational efficiency improvements.

To date, unfortunately, the promise of PCMHs (Figure 9-9) exceeds their performance. RAND researchers studied 32 pilot PCMH practices in southeastern Pennsylvania. The practices successfully achieved NCQA recognition and adopted new structural capabilities such as registries to identify patients overdue for chronic disease services. Pilot participation was associated with statistically significantly greater performance improvement, relative to comparison practices, on only 1 of 11 investigated quality measures. Pilot participation was not associated with statistically significant changes in utilization or costs of care. Pilot practices accumulated average bonuses of $92,000 per PCP during the 3-year intervention. The researchers concluded that medical home interventions may need further refinement if we are to make progress on solving the 3 angles of the iron triangle.[52]

## GETTING PHYSICIANS TO CHANGE THEIR BEHAVIOR[53]

One mantra of healthcare delivery bears repeating: Physicians control (directly and indirectly) 85% of all spending. It stands to reason that if

you want to change the healthcare system, you have to change how physicians use their pens. More than anything else, this is where megaproviders have failed. Although large institutional providers (hospital systems, ACOs) seem ready to take on financial risk, through shared savings and provider-sponsored plans, they seem unable to get physicians to act as if they bear the same financial responsibility. This problem is hardly exclusive to hospital systems; all organizations face the same problem. It is a simple fact about human nature that workers will place their own parochial interests above those of their organization. An important challenge for all managers is to create a team-first mentality.

This challenge is magnified in hospital systems, where physicians are the most important contributors to organizational success, yet often feel that their "physician team" stands in opposition to management or is at best indifferent. Among all the stakeholders of large hospital systems, physicians are the least satisfied and play little part in administration. This is not how things work in other businesses that are dependent on their frontline professional staff. The most obvious comparison is with law firms, which are invariably run by lawyers, or high-tech engineering firms where the C-suite and rank-and-file share the same occupational training, language, and culture. Boeing and 3M's leadership teams are packed with engineers and scientists. Data scientists and engineers hold most of the top positions at Apple and Google. Large research universities are largely run by academics, although their influence (like that of doctors) is on the wane.

The general principle of involving the professional staff in strategic decision making applies to businesses across the economy. Yet, if we look at the biggest hospital systems, it is difficult to find physicians or nurses in leadership positions.[54] This is another example of the pendulum swinging too far back. Four decades ago, physicians were at the helm of many poorly run hospitals. Hospital boards replaced them with MHAs and MBAs, hospital finances improved, and the business ethos became more entrenched. What choice do hospitals have? Physicians who have the desire and skills to manage a healthcare enterprise are few and far between. Given the often adversarial relationship that exists between many system C-suites and their medical staffs, it is difficult to imagine that there is much enthusiasm among physicians to enter management. Even so, there is some evidence (albeit not very rigorous) that healthcare organizations run by physicians are more successful.[55]

Regardless of whether MBAs, MDs, or RNs are at the helm, they must grapple with a fundamental problem: Physicians are the dominant medical decision makers and are willing to address the issue of waste in the healthcare system. Yet they see waste as someone else's fault and not necessarily under their individual control. This may explain why physicians are (1) averse to contracting for risk they feel they cannot control and (2) skeptical about new organizational models to improve quality or reduce cost. Beyond these sentiments, physician behaviors may undermine both APMs and new organization models. A recent case study highlighted the high rate of physician turnover in the Partners HealthCare ACO.[56] Only 52% of physicians were on contract over the first 3 years, with many physicians coming and going each year. The downside here is that departing physicians sometimes take their patients (the ACO beneficiaries) with them. This partly explains why ACOs also experience high patient turnover. Both types of turnover likely undermine quality, cost, and population health efforts. After one accounts for the nonrandom exit of physicians from ACOs, the evidence that they improve quality or reduce costs becomes almost nonexistent.[57]

Some ACO advocates now suggest that financial incentives currently offered inside new organizational models may be too weak to motivate physicians to change their behaviors and deliver more cost-effective care. One problem is that the amount of compensation at risk in pay-for-performance (P4P) programs is too low, an issue considered later. Another problem is that risk-bearing provider organizations frequently avoid passing the risk down to their rank-and-file practitioners. Still others argue that financial incentives for physicians usually change their behavior—just not always in the desired direction leading to desired outcomes. The health economics literature is rife with studies of how payment reforms that focus on a piece of the healthcare pie led to harmful unintended consequences. P4P encourages providers to skimp on valuable services that are not included in the performance metrics.[58] Medicare's Hospital Readmissions Reduction Program, introduced with much fanfare a decade ago, may have discouraged readmissions that would have saved lives.[59] These examples are just the tip of the iceberg. Instead of (or in addition to) financial incentives, according to advocates, hospital systems and ACOs must employ robust nonfinancial motivational strategies to change (in turn) PCPs' behaviors, PCPs' care delivery (eg, using teams, physician champions, data sharing, care coordination), and hopefully their costs, quality, and patient outcomes. Others suggest that only a large-scale shift to capitation can prevent the kind of financial games that providers play. The unanswered question is whether enough physicians will accept such a change at a low enough price.

A totally opposite view is that financial incentives are the entirely wrong solution. Management research has shown that extrinsic rewards (eg, monetary incentives) can undermine intrinsic motivation. These unanticipated consequences may occur particularly among professionals who perform complex tasks calling for cognitive flexibility, creativity, and problem solving.[60] By contrast, reviews suggest that "autonomous motivation"—linked to intrinsic motivation and self-determination—is directly and positively tied to patient-centeredness, safety, and quality of care.[61]

A more fundamental issue with physician engagement in transformation is the downward-sloping gradient from the hospital C-suite to clinician leaders to rank-and-file clinicians in their favorable views of transformation. When asked about the impact of value-based care delivery on quality, more executives responded favorably compared to clinician leaders and rank-and-file clinicians. A similar gradient was observed when asked about the impact of APMs or the value of Medicaid demonstration programs. Executives and physicians also differ in their views about how to reduce costs. The divide separating the C-suite from practicing physicians is based in part on geographic location (hospital system headquarters vs a hospital-specific clinical department), hierarchical level, and professional training (eg, MHA/MBA vs MD). The multiple fault lines suggest that alignment and engagement are likely to be difficult and even deteriorating. Surveys show a decrease in physicians reporting intellectual stimulation, collegial interaction, financial rewards, and the prestige of medicine as most satisfying about their practice. These issues may, in turn, cause downstream problems with quality improvement and cost control: Disengaged physicians are reportedly a cause of poor quality and medical errors.

Moreover, despite payer efforts to promote value-based purchasing, physicians continue to deliver the wrong care in the wrong place at the wrong time. Part of the problem is staying current with the growing scientific literature. Medical practices that have diffused are often contradicted by recently published evidence, but physicians lag in altering their practice patterns. Physicians also make low use of quality or cost data in their referrals.

What is needed, then? At a minimum, putting more physicians and nurses in C-suites might engender greater trust between the executive office and clinical staff, thereby improving corporate culture and facilitating the use of informal incentives. This is no panacea, as rank-and-file clinicians can be just as distrustful of MD and RN leaders as MBAs. Some call for investing in the "capabilities" of clinical staff (eg, physicians, nurses, social workers, discharge planners) with additional support from their organizations.[62] What capabilities might be desired? One might be the ability to deal with the stress associated with treating complex, severely ill patients as a way to deal with the burnout

issue. It would also include more autonomy delegated to the frontline staff in managing such patients and the ability to tailor the work environment (including the EMR and data reporting requirements) to the needs of the professionals doing the work. Surveys mention the importance to physicians of innovative clinical roles, team-based support, and autonomy in the face of (externally imposed) performance goals. The overall goal, drawn from decades of research in organizational behavior, is to increase the intrinsic satisfaction and fulfillment of professionals in carrying out work on the frontline and to foster more productive professional cultures.[63]

## MULTIPLE AGENCY ROLES

Perhaps we are placing too many demands on our physicians. John Eisenberg long ago noted the difficulty that physicians face in performing and balancing multiple agency roles (Figure 9-10).[64] First, physicians act as the *patient's agent*, doing no harm and promoting the patient's welfare. Second, physicians act as their own self-interested *economic agent*, maximizing their own income and professional satisfaction. Third, physicians act as *society's agent*, allocating scarce and valuable medical and technological resources to those in need and, hopefully, improving population health while also minimizing healthcare spending. Fourth, physicians are increasingly being employed and thereby acting as the *organization's agent*, helping to improve revenues and maintain profitability.

Some industry analysts have likened the physician's agency dilemma to the iron triangle discussed in Chapter 5. They call it "the iron triangle of conflicting expectations."[65] These include what is best for the patient (prevention,

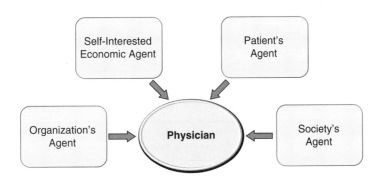

**Figure 9-10** • Multiple Agency Roles Influence Physician Decision Making.

care, information, guidance, value), what is best for medicine (professionalism, autonomy, technology), and what is best for society (measured effectiveness, access, cost).

This dilemma has not diminished the importance of the doctor-patient relationship. This can still be a rewarding interaction. However, many physicians experience a great deal of anger, inadequacy, and frustration, and much of the actual practice of medicine may become a burden rather than a source of satisfaction. Physicians may encounter a subset of patients who engender strong negative feelings, despair, and even downright malice—what some researchers have (unfortunately) labeled the "hateful patient."[66] Part of the issue may be patients who demand doctors do something versus doctors who wish to remain cautious and conservative in their treatment.[67] Physicians report that a major source of unnecessary, low-value care is demanding patients.

The decline in the public's trust of physicians—whether deserved or not—has not helped. According to researchers, the proportion of Americans who "had great confidence in medical leaders" dropped from more than 75% in 1966 to just 34% by 2018. Moreover, Americans are less likely than those in other developed nations to trust their physicians, with just 25% of Americans overall saying they feel confident about the healthcare system.[68] Such distrust can manifest itself in lack of patient compliance with physician orders

and recommendations (eg, taking medications, engaging in preventive behaviors).

This decline has been attributed in part to "consumerism" (eg, leveling of the playing field in the doctor-patient relationship) and recognition of possible "conflicts of interest" on the part of doctors in dealing with pharmaceutical and medical device companies. It has also been attributed to the "commercialization" of healthcare (eg, financing via out-of-pocket payment or private insurance, production of services by physicians acting as self-interested economic agents, and reliance on market mechanisms and ability to pay to access care) found in some Western countries like the United States.[69]

The decline does not appear to be driven by a rise in malpractice, however. Over a 10-year period, from 2007 to 2016, the rate of medical professional liability claims declined 27% from 5.1 cases per 100 physicians to 3.7 cases per 100 physicians.[70] Nevertheless, the average expense incurred in managing these cases increased on average 3.5% annually.

## SUMMARY

US physicians are the most powerful profession in the healthcare ecosystem and yet are besieged on all fronts. Drawing on Figure 9-10 regarding multiple roles and expectations, their position is one of pressure on all fronts. As Figure 9-11

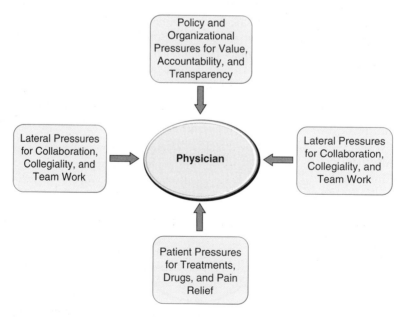

**Figure 9-11** • Pressures on Physicians.

suggests, they are pressured from above by public policy and payer (both public and private) demands for accountability, transparency, and "value" (high quality at a reasonable cost). They are pressured from below by increasingly demanding patients who (1) expect more and ask more, (2) present more challenging conditions to be treated (the poly-chronics), (3) present with more drug-related conditions, and (4) may be hostile as well. Malpractice, by contrast, does not appear to be as big of a factor as in the past. Finally, they are pressured from the side by other healthcare providers (and the systems in which they work) to be more collaborative and collegial and to be team players—skills in which most older physicians were not trained in medical school.

---

### QUESTIONS TO PONDER

1. This chapter concludes that one solution to the issues of physician burnout and low engagement is to give physicians more autonomy over their work in the frontline of healthcare delivery. This is what the work of physicians used to look like for most of the 20th century. Do you think we need to "move back to the future"?

2. If we do indeed move back to the future and cede physicians more autonomy, does this help with the issue of "silo busting" and collaboration discussed at the end of Chapter 8?

3. Why is it so hard to forecast the number of physicians our country needs? Is there any way to improve our forecasts?

4. How might the growing diversity of the medical profession along gender and racial/ethnic lines be good for care delivery? Are there any consequences of increasing diversity that we need to watch out for?

5. There is an ongoing trend of physicians working in organized settings (eg, large physician groups, hospitals). How will this trend influence our ability to solve the iron triangle or address the triple aim?

6. Finally, are we asking too much of our doctors?

---

### REFERENCES

1. John Eisenberg. *Physician Utilization: The State of Research About Physicians' Practice Patterns*, Med Care. 40 (11) (2002): 1016-1035. Alan Sager and Deborah Socolar. *Health Costs Absorb One-Quarter of Economic Growth, 2000-2005*, Boston University School of Public Health, Data Brief no. 8 (2005). Alan Sager estimated the mix of direct and indirect spending to be 21% and 66%, respectively, in 2003.

2. Carl Ameringer. *The Health Care Revolution: From Medical Monopoly to Market Competition* (Berkeley, CA: University of California Press, 2008).

3. Lawton R. Burns and Douglas R. Wholey. "Responding to a Consolidating Healthcare System: Options for Physician Organizations," in *Advances in Health Care Management*, Volume 1 (New York, NY: Elsevier, 2000): 273-335.

4. Carol Peckham. "Medscape Lifestyle Report 2016: Bias and Burnout," *Medscape*, January 13, 2016. Available online: https://www.medscape.com/slideshow/lifestyle-2016-overview-6007335. Accessed on July 27, 2020.

5. National Academy of Medicine. *Taking Action Against Clinician Burnout: A Systems Approach to Professional Well-Being* (Washington, DC: Institute of Medicine, 2019).

6. Sandeep Jauhar. "Why Doctors Are Sick of Their Profession," *Wall Street Journal*, August 29, 2014. Available online: https://www.wsj.com/articles/the-u-s-s-ailing-medical-system-a-doctors-perspective-1409325361. Accessed on July 27, 2020. Abigail Zuger. "Dissatisfaction With Medical Practice," *N Engl J Med.* 350 (2004): 69-75.

7. The Medicus Firm. *2019 Physician Practice Preference and Relocation Survey.* The data for 2019 suggest physicians are working fewer total hours than they did just 2 years earlier, though.

8. Arlen Moller, Andrew Jager, Geoffrey Williams, et al. "US Physicians' Work Motivation and Their Occupational Health: A National Survey of Practicing Physicians," *Med Care.* 57 (5) (2019): 334-340.

9. Shemassian Academic Consulting. "Tuition at Every Medical School in the United States." Available online: https://www.shemmassianconsulting.com/blog/medical-school-tuition. Accessed on March 10, 2020.

10. Daniel Barron. "Why Doctors Are Drowning in Medical School Debt," *Scientific American*, July 15, 2019. Available online: https://blogs.scientificamerican.com/observations/why-doctors-are-drowning-in-medical-school-debt/. Accessed on March 10, 2020.

11. David Asch, Justin Grishkan, and Sean Nicholson. "The Cost, Price, and Debt of Medical Education," *N Engl J Med.* 383 (1) (2020): 6-9.

12. Alison Volpe Holmes and Mona M. Abaza. "Ideas for Easing Medical Students' Match Day 'Frenzy,'" *Stat*, March 16, 2019. Available online: https://www.statnews.com/2019/03/15/easing-medical-students-match-day-frenzy/. Accessed on March 10, 2020.

13. Aaron Young, Humayun Chaudhry, Xiammei Pei, et al. "A Census of Actively Licensed Physicians in the United States, 2016," *J Med Regul.* 103 (2) (2017): 7-21.

14. Yusuke Tsugawa, Joseph Newhouse, Alan Zaslavsky, et al. "Physician Age and Outcomes in Elderly Patients in Hospital in the US: Observational Study," *Br Med J.* 357 (2017): j1797.

15. US Department of Health, Education, and Welfare, Office of the Secretary. *The Advancement of Medical Research and Education Through the Department of Health, Education, and Welfare. 1958. Final Report of the Secretary's Consultants of Medical Research and Education.* Stanhope Bayne-Jones Report (Washington, DC: Government Printing Office, June 27, 1958). Frank Bane. *Physicians for a Growing America: Report of the Surgeon's General's Consultant Group on Medical Education* (Washington, DC: US Public Health Service, Publication No. 709, 1959).

16. Lowell T. Coggeshall. *Planning for Medical Progress Through Education: A Report Submitted to the Executive Council of the Association of American Medical Colleges* (Evanston, IL: Association of American Medical Colleges, 1965).

17. Michael Dill and Edward Salsberg. *Complexities of Physician Supply and Demand: Projections Through 2025* (Washington, DC: Center for Workforce Studies, Association of American Medical Colleges, November 2008).

18. US Graduate Medical Education National Advisory Committee. *Summary Report of the Graduate Medical Education National Advisory Committee: To the Secretary, Department of Health and Human Services, Volume 1* (Washington, DC: US Department of Health and Human Services, Public Health Service, Health Resources Administration, Office of Graduate Medical Education, 1980).

19. Kathleen N. Lohr, Neal A. Vanselow, and Don E. Detmer (Eds.). *The Nation's Physician Workforce: Options for Balancing Supply and Requirements.* Institute of Medicine Committee on the US Physician Supply (Washington, DC: National Academy Press, 1996).

20. Emily Gudbranson, Aaron Glickman, and Ezekiel Emanuel. "Reassessing the Data on Whether a Physician Shortage Exists," *JAMA.* 317 (19) (2017): 1945-1946.

21. Edward Salsberg, Paul Rockey, Kerri Rivers, et al. "US Residency Training Before and After the 1997 Balanced Budget Act," *JAMA.* 300 (10) (2008): 1174-1180.

22. Darrell Kirch and Kate Petelle. "Addressing the Physician Shortage: The Peril of Ignoring Demography," *JAMA.* 317 (19) (2017): 1947-1948. Emily Gudbranson, Aaron Glickman, and Ezekiel Emanuel. "Reassessing the Data on Whether a Physician Shortage Exists," *JAMA.* 317 (19) (2017): 1945-1946.

23. Association of American Medical Colleges. *The Complexities of Physician Supply and Demand: Projections From 2018 to 2033* (Washington, DC: AAMC, June 2020).

24. Douglas Staiger, David Auerbach, and Peter Buerhaus. "Trends in the Work Hours of Physicians in the United States," *JAMA.* 303 (8) (2010): 747-753.

25. Seth Seabury, Anupam Jena, and Amitabh Chandra. "Trends in the Earnings of Health Care Professionals in the United States, 1987-2010," *JAMA.* 308 (20) (2012): 2083-2085.

26. Michael Dill and Edward Salsberg. *Complexities of Physician Supply and Demand: Projections Through 2025* (Washington, DC: Center for Workforce Studies, Association of American Medical Colleges, November 2008).

27. Association of American Medical Colleges. "U.S. Medical School Enrollment Surpasses Expansion Goal" (July 25, 2019). Available online: https://www.aamc.org/news-insights/press-releases/us-medical-school-enrollment-surpasses-expansion-goal. Accessed on March 6, 2020.

28. Morris Fishbein. "The Report of the Committee on the Costs of Medical Care," editorial, *JAMA.* 99 (December 10, 1932): 2034-2035.

29. Lawton R. Burns, Jeff C. Goldsmith, and Aditi Sen. "Horizontal and Vertical Integration of Physicians: A Tale of Two Tails," *Adv Health Care Manag.* 15 (2013): 39-117. Available online: https://ldi.upenn.edu/publication/horizontal-and-vertical-integration-physicians-tale-two-tails. Accessed on July 27, 2020.

30. Carol Kane. *Updated Data on Physician Practice Arrangements: For the First Time, Fewer Physicians Are Owners Than Employees* (Chicago, IL: AMA, 2019).

31. Results available online at: American Academy of Family Physicians. "AAFP Survey Reveals DPC Trends" (June 19, 2018). Available online: https://www.aafp.org/news/blogs/inthetrenches/entry/20180619ITT_DPC.html. Accessed on March 9, 2020. See also Matthew Perrone. "Some Family Doctors Ditch Insurance for Simpler Approach," *The Washington Post* (December 10, 2018).

32. Reed Tinsley. "The 12-Step Way to Reduce Practice Expenses: Part 1, Staffing Efficiencies," *Fam Pract Manag.* 17 (2010): 38-43. Available online: https://www.aafp.org/fpm/2010/0300/p38.html. Accessed on March 9, 2020.

33. Lawrence Casalino, David Gans, Rachel Weber, et al. "US Physician Practices Spend More Than

$15.4 Billion Annually to Report Quality Measures," *Health Aff.* 35 (3) (2016): 401-406.

34. Carol Kane. *How Are Physicians Paid? A Detailed Look at the Methods Used to Compensate Physicians in Different Practice Types and Specialties* (Chicago, IL: AMA, 2015).

35. Medical Group Management Association. "Covid-19 Financial Impact on Medical Practices." Available online: https://mgma.com/getattachment/9b8be0c2-0744-41bf-864f-04007d6adbd2/2004-G09621D-COVID-Financial-Impact-One-Pager-8-5x11-MW-2.pdf.aspx?lang=en-US&ext=.pdf. Accessed on April 20, 2020.

36. Sanjay Basu, Russell Phillips, Robert Phillips, et al. "Primary Care Practice Finances in the United States Amid the COVID-19 Pandemic," *Health Aff.* 39 (9) (2020). Available online: https://www.healthaffairs.org/doi/full/10.1377/hlthaff.2020.00794. Accessed on August 28, 2020.

37. David Raths. "Survey: Primary Care Practices Endangered by Steep Declines in Revenue, Staff," *Healthcare Innovation* (April 17, 2020). Available online at: https://www.hcinnovationgroup.com/policy-value-based-care/practice-management/news/21134503/survey-primary-care-practices-endangered-by-steep-declines-in-revenue-staff. Accessed on April 29, 2020.

38. P&T Community. "COVID-19 Wreaking Havoc in Specialty Practices and the Vast Majority of Physicians Expect It to Get Worse in the Next Two Weeks, According to a New Report by Spherix Global Insights" (March 24, 2020). Available online: https://www.ptcommunity.com/wire/covid-19-wreaking-havoc-specialty-practices-and-vast-majority-physicians-expect-it-get-worse. Accessed on April 29, 2020.

39. Knowledge Leader. "From the Eyes of the Independent Practice: How Physicians and Smaller Practices Are Coping With COVID-19" (April 1, 2020). Available online: https://knowledge-leader.colliers.com/editor/how-physicians-and-smaller-practices-are-coping-with-covid-19/. Accessed on April 29, 2020.

40. Neal Barker, Eric Andreoli, and Terrence McWilliams. "COVID-19 and Its Impact on Physician Compensation," *Becker's Hospital Review* (April 6, 2020). Accessed on April 29, 2020. Available online: https://www.beckershospitalreview.com/covid-19-and-its-impact-on-physician-compensation.html. Accessed on April 29, 2020.

41. Markian Hawryluk. "High-Deductible Plans Jeopardize Financial Health of Patients and Rural Hospitals," *Kaiser Health News* (January 10, 2020). Available online: https://khn.org/news/high-deductible-plans-jeopardize-financial-health-of-patients-and-rural-hospitals/ Accessed on May 2, 2020.

42. Nora Kelly, Dan Majka, and Dawn Samaris. "Monitoring the Financial Implications of COVID-19 on Hospitals and Health Systems," *KaufmanHall* (March 2020). Available online: https://www.kaufmanhall.com/ideas-resources/article/monitoring-financial-implications-covid-19-hospitals-health-systems. Accessed on April 29, 2020. Jeremy B. Sussman, Lakshmi K. Halasyamani, and Matthew Davis. "Hospitals During Recession and Recovery: Vulnerable Institutions and Quality at Risk," *J Hosp Med.* 5 (5) (2010): 302-305. Available online: https://onlinelibrary.wiley.com/doi/abs/10.1002/jhm.654. Accessed on April 29, 2020.

43. Donna Shelley, Ji Eun Chang, Alden Lai, et al. "Independent Primary Care Practices Are Small Businesses, Too," *Health Affairs Blog* (May 21, 2020). Available online: https://www.healthaffairs.org/do/10.1377/hblog20200518.930748/full/. Accessed on November 5, 2020.

44. Medscape. *Physician Compensation Report 2019.* Available online: https://www.medscape.com/slideshow/2019-compensation-overview-6011286#3. Accessed on March 5, 2020.

45. Medscape. *Bias and Burnout: Lifestyle Report 2016.* Available online: https://www.medscape.com/slideshow/lifestyle-2016-overview-6007335. Accessed on March 6, 2020.

46. James K. Stoller, Amanda Goodall, and Agnes Baker. "Why the Best Hospitals Are Managed by Doctors," *Harvard Business Review* (December 27, 2016). Available online at: https://hbr.org/2016/12/why-the-best-hospitals-are-managed-by-doctors. Accessed on August 5, 2020.

47. Thomas Lee and Toby Cosgrove. "Engaging Doctors in the Health Care Revolution," *Harvard Business Review* (June 2014). Available online: https://hbr.org/2014/06/engaging-doctors-in-the-health-care-revolution. Accessed on July 27, 2020.

48. Jackie Kimmell. "The 5 Biggest Risk Factors for Physician Burnout, According to Our 13,371-Physician Survey," *Advisory Board* (October 30, 2018). Available online: https://www.advisory.com/daily-briefing/2018/10/30/burnout. Accessed on July 27, 2020.

49. Jon Tilburt, Matthew Wynia, Robert Sheeler, et al. "Views of U.S. Physicians About Controlling Health Care Costs," *JAMA.* 310 (4) (2013): 380-388.

50. Commonwealth Fund. *Primary Care Providers' Views of Recent Trends in Health Care Delivery and Payment.* August 2015 Issue Brief. Available online: https://www.issuelab.org/resources/25044/25044.pdf. Accessed on March 6, 2020.

51. Lisa Rotenstein and Amanda Johnson. "Taking Back Control—Can Quality Improvement Enhance the Physician Experience?" *Health Aff.* (January 14, 2020). Available online: https://www.healthaffairs.org/do/10.1377/hblog20200110.543513/full/. Accessed on July 27, 2020.

52. Mark Friedberg, Eric Schneider, Meredith Rosenthal, et al. "Association Between

Participation in a Multipayer Medical Home Intervention and Changes in Quality, Utilization, and Costs of Care," *JAMA*. 311 (8) (2014): 815-825.

53. This section is adapted from David Dranove and Lawton R. Burns. *Big Med: Megaproviders and the High Cost of Health Care in America* (Chicago, IL: University of Chicago Press, 2021).

54. According to Bloomberg, there are 4 physicians among the top 25 executives at Sutter Health. At the University of Pittsburgh Medical Center, 2 of the 11 top executives are doctors. Northshore has 4 doctors and 1 nurse among its top 20 executives. New York Presbyterian does a bit better, with 7 physicians and 2 nurses among the top 30 leadership positions. Cf. "UPMC Leadership." Available online: https://www.upmc.com/about/why-upmc/mission/leadership. Accessed on July 27, 2020.

55. Amanda Goodall. "Physician-Leaders and Hospital Performance: Is There an Association?" *Soc Sci Med*. 73 (4) (2011): 535-539. James Stoller, Amanda Goodall, and Agnes Baker. "Why the Best Hospitals Are Managed by Doctors," *Harvard Business Review* (December 27, 2016).

56. John Hsu, Christine Vogeli, Mary Price, et al. "Substantial Physician Turnover and Beneficiary 'Churn' in a Large Medicare Pioneer ACO," *Health Aff*. 36 (4) (2017): 640-648.

57. Adam Markovitz, John Hollingsworth, John Ayanian, et al. "Performance in the Medicare Shared Savings Program After Accounting for Nonrandom Exit," *Ann Intern Med*. 171 (1) (2019): 27-36.

58. Kathleen J. Mullen, Richard G. Frank, and Meredith B. Rosenthal. "Can You Get What You Pay For? Pay-for-Performance and the Quality of Healthcare Providers," *Rand J Econ*. 41 (1) (2010): 64-91.

59. Robert Pearl. "The Deadly Consequences of Financial Incentives in Healthcare," *Forbes* (January 28, 2019). Available online: https://www.forbes.com/sites/robertpearl/2019/01/28/financial-incentives/#6b36d9365eb9. Accessed on June 14, 2019.

60. Marylene Gagne and Edward Deci. "Self-Determination Theory and Work Motivation," *J Organization Behav*. 26 (2005): 331-362.

61. Gepke Veenstra, Kirsten Dabekaussen, Eric Molleman, et al. "Health Care Professionals' Motivation, Their Behaviors, and the Quality of Care: A Mixed-Methods Systematic Review," *Health Care Manag Rev*. (April 2020). doi: 10.1097/HMR.0000000000000284.

62. Jessica Sweeney-Platt. "The Business Case for Physician Capability," *Athena Insight* (October 6, 2017). Available online: https://www.athenahealth.com/insight/physician-capability-leads-long-term-success. Accessed on June 14, 2019.

63. Katharina Janus. "The Effect of Professional Culture on Intrinsic Motivation Among Physicians in an Academic Medical Center," *J Healthcare Manag*. 59 (4) (2014): 287-303.

64. John M. Eisenberg. *Doctors' Decisions and the Cost of Medical Care* (Ann Arbor, MI: Health Administration Press, 1986).

65. Hamilton Moses III, David Matheson, E. Ray Dorsey, et al. "The Anatomy of Health Care in the United States," *JAMA*. 310 (18) (2013): 1947-1963.

66. Rael Strous, Anne-Marie Ulman, and Moshe Kotler. "The Hateful Patient Revisited: Relevance for 21st Century Medicine," *Eur J Int Med*. 17 (6) (2006): 387-393.

67. Sandeep Jauhar. "A Patient's Demands Versus a Doctor's Convictions," *The New York Times* (April 3, 2007). Available online: https://www.nytimes.com/2007/04/03/health/03essa.html. Accessed on March 10, 2020.

68. Dhruv Khullar, "Do You Trust the Medical Profession?" *The New York Times* (January 23, 2018). Available online: https://www.nytimes.com/2018/01/23/upshot/do-you-trust-the-medical-profession.html. Accessed on March 10, 2020.

69. Ellery Chih-Han Huang, Christy Pu, Yiing-Jenq Chou, et al. "Public Trust in Physicians—Health Care Commodification as a Possible Deteriorating Factor: Cross-sectional Analysis of 23 Countries," *Inquiry* 55 (Jan-Dec 2018). Available online: https://www.ncbi.nlm.nih.gov/pmc/articles/PMC5843089/. Accessed on March 10, 2020.

70. Cision. "Insights From New CRICO Strategies CBS Report, Medical Malpractice in America: A 10-Year Assessment With Insights" (February 12, 2019). Available online: https://www.prnewswire.com/news-releases/insights-from-new-crico-strategies-cbs-report-medical-malpractice-in-america-a-10-year-assessment-with-insights-300794160.html. Accessed on March 10, 2020.

# Primary Care: Physicians, Nurses, and Pharmacists

10

Chapter 3 distinguished primary from secondary and tertiary care. Primary care has been defined as core functions that patients receive from their usual source of care. The World Health Organization (WHO) recognized the important role played by primary care. Similar to the Institute of Medicine's 6 dimensions of quality (STEEEP, see Chapter 5), the WHO stated that primary care should be comprehensive, integrated, continuous, team-based, patient empowering, health promoting, and bridging of personal and family and community health.[1]

Other researchers have distilled 5 elements of primary care that, when collectively present, distinguish it from specialty-oriented care: first-contact accessibility, continuity, comprehensiveness, coordination, and whole-person accountability.[2] The definitions for these 5 elements are presented in Figure 10-1. Research has shown the positive impact on important patient outcomes by (1) *accessibility*: hospitalization rates, emergency department (ED) visits, and patient satisfaction; (2) *continuity*: hospitalization rates, complication rates, ED visits, total costs, and adherence to provider recommendations; (3) *comprehensiveness*: hospitalization rates, better health outcomes at lower cost, and self-reported health outcomes; (4) *coordination*: less duplication of services, better patient outcomes, and greater satisfaction; and (5) *accountability*: patient self-management for chronic conditions and adherence to provider recommendations.

Primary care has long been viewed as essential to maintaining and promoting the health status of the population, improving the patient's experience of care, and controlling per-capita costs (ie, the triple aim). Historically, it has also been viewed as critical to improving access to care and quality of care and lowering the cost of care (ie, the iron triangle).[3] Analysts suggest that primary care benefits both population and personal health by improving health status, lowering utilization of care, increasing use of preventive services, reducing disease and death rates, and reducing the negative health effects of income inequality on health and mortality, especially in areas where income inequality is greatest.[4]

Two recent studies published in the medical literature lend credence to these claims. They indicate that the availability of primary care is associated with higher health status (as measured by patient mortality), higher quality of care (as measured by clinical process measures), and higher patient experience measures.

One study used an epidemiological approach and found a positive association of primary care physician (PCP) supply (ie, number of PCPs per 100,000 in a region) with changes in life expectancy between 2005 and 2015. Every additional 10 PCPs were linked to an increased life expectancy of 51.5 days, as well as reduced rates of mortality from cardiovascular, respiratory, and cancer conditions. By contrast, the supply of specialist physicians had weaker, but still positive associations with the same outcomes.[5]

The other study used a national population survey approach and found that adults with a "usual source of primary care" (defined as a physician) were more likely to fill their

1. **Accessible first-contact care**
   Primary care clinicians make their services available and easily accessible to patients with new medical needs or ongoing health concerns. This includes shorter waiting times for urgent needs, enhanced in-person hours, around-the-clock telephone or electronic access to a member of the care team who has access to the patient's medical record, and alternative methods of communication including patient portals. This also includes providers who speak the language of the population served.

2. **Continuous care**
   Primary care clinicians have a personal and uninterrupted caring relationship with their patients, with continuous exchange of relevant information about healthcare and health needs.

3. **Comprehensiveness of care**
   Primary care clinicians, working with the interprofessional primary care team, meet the large majority of each patient's physical and mental healthcare needs, including prevention and wellness, acute care, chronic and comorbid care, and discussing end-of-life care.

4. **Coordinated care**
   Primary care practices coordinate care across all elements of the broader healthcare system, including specialty care, hospitals, home healthcare, and community services and support.

5. **Accountable whole-person care**
   Primary care clinicians and teams are knowledgeable about and oriented toward the whole person, understanding and respecting each patient's unique needs, culture, values, and preferences in the context of their family and community. "Accountability" refers to caring for the whole person, not just an isolated body system.

**Figure 10-1 •** Elements of Primary Care.

prescriptions, have preventive office visits, and have higher-value (and often under-used) care such as cancer screening, counseling, and recommended diagnostic and preventive testing. However, they had the same levels of inpatient, outpatient, and ED utilization and similar levels of low-value care; indeed, those with a usual source of primary care were slightly more likely to report more low-value care for some conditions. Those with a usual source of primary care also reported higher patient access and experience scores as well.[6]

There are, nevertheless, some important caveats and some disquieting findings in these (and other recent) studies. *First*, although the number of PCPs has increased over time, it has not kept up with population growth. From 2005 to 2015, the ratio of PCPs per 100,000 fell from 46.6 to 41.4. This is due not only to a larger population but also physician migration and loss of physician supply in certain (ie, rural) areas. In 2017, the United States had an estimated 223,125 office-based direct PCPs. Among these, the 3 biggest specialties were family practitioners (39.5%), general internal medicine practitioners (34.5%), and general pediatricians (21.3%). The number of physician graduates from primary care residency programs peaked in the late 1990s and (through 2014) had not risen above that level.

*Second*, Americans' use of primary care appears to be both low and falling. At the aggregate level, the percentage of healthcare spending devoted to primary care fell from 6.5% in 2002 to 5.4% by 2016.[7] The survey data just reviewed indicate that roughly one-quarter of the adult population lacks a usual source of primary care (ie, a PCP), despite the fact that two-thirds of them have health insurance coverage. This may reflect geographic access issues (ie, low supply in some areas), or it may reflect a lower perceived need for primary care, as has been reported recently among the Millennial population. Empirical research also shows declining use of PCPs between 2008 and 2016: The proportion of adults with no medical visits rose from 26.1% to 32.5%, and the percentage with no PCP visits rose from 38.1% to 46.4%.[8] By contrast, visits to specialists did not change. Declines were greatest for younger, healthier adults, those with lower-acuity conditions, and those in low-income communities. These patterns may thus reflect several dynamics at work: preference for convenience care among Millennials, a decline in unnecessary visits, growing financial barriers to care, a shift within PCP practices to offering preventive services, and/or substitution of PCP visits by specialist visits.

Regardless of the cause, the decline in PCP use may lead to fewer medical school graduates going into primary care specialties, leading to a vicious cycle that fosters even greater medical specialization and perhaps lower care continuity. Recent research suggests that PCPs' practice styles have long-lasting effects on the quality and quantity of healthcare patients receive and thus potentially on their health outcomes.[9] The direction of these effects partly depends on the practice styles of those PCPs who remain versus leave the field. This decline needs to be closely monitored.

*Third*, the beneficial effects of primary care availability are not seen across the board. They do not appear to affect utilization of expensive services (eg, hospital admissions, ED use) and do not appear to lower all forms of low-value (unnecessary) care. In most studies, the association between primary care utilization and spending is static (rather than dynamic) and often based on observational studies (ie, areas with proportionately more PCPs have lower spending).[10] There is some question as to whether increasing the amount of primary care spending by a state or country would bend the trend in healthcare spending over time. Rhode Island passed a statute that required commercial insurers to increase the percentage of spending on primary care by 1%, raising spending on primary care statewide from $47 million to $74 million over 7 years. The underlying "theory of action" is that such spending will be devoted to prevention and care coordination, which can lead to healthier lives and lower need for acute care utilization. Overall, the thesis is that primary care can substitute for secondary and tertiary care. Unfortunately, the evidence supporting this theory is mixed.

*Fourth*, empirical evidence is mixed regarding whether primary care and specialty care are substitutes or complements.[11] There are 3 reasons why primary care might be a *substitute*: prevention and detection in the PCP setting that may avoid need for specialty care, prevention or delay of specialty care by managing chronic conditions, and gatekeeping performed by the PCP (referral to specialist is needed). There are 3 reasons why primary care might be a *complement*: need for specialty diagnostic tests following a PCP visit, detection of illness by a PCP that cannot be treated in that office, and identification of acute episodes that need specialty treatment.

*Fifth*, efforts by the Patient Protection and Affordable Care Act (PPACA) to foster 2 new care delivery models in primary care have met with only limited success. The Comprehensive Primary Care (CPC) and CPC Plus (CPC+) initiatives embedded care managers in PCP offices to enhance their management of chronic conditions, linked patients to a single PCP to promote continuity and follow-up after hospitalization, and included integration with behavioral healthcare. However, practices found it difficult to find the time and resources to implement these changes fully (eg, hire and integrate staff) as well as make the necessary changes in their care processes. Moreover, the models left the volume-based, fee-for-service incentives largely intact and did not pay the practices a large bump in reimbursement to make changes. Needless to say, the initiatives exerted little impact on cost, quality, and utilization of either the hospital or the ED.[12] Overall, the added payments to providers for "care management fees" outweighed any savings on utilization. It may be that more primary care improves health status, but it may also cost more and will not bend the trend.[13]

*Sixth*, the presence of PCPs may not be the same as the provision of primary care. Researchers suggest that the constellation of all 5 elements of primary care identified at the start of this chapter are needed. Initiatives that focus on manpower levels and other *structural* interventions neglect the *process* dimensions of the care that is delivered. PCP practices likely vary in their capabilities regarding these 5 elements, and their patients likely vary in terms of their need for all of these elements. Some of these 5 elements (continuity of care) are prerequisite for some others (coordination of care).

*Seventh*, PCPs are under siege, according to one ethnographic study.[14] Since the 1970s, most PCPs transitioned from a traditional professional role to a primarily business role, where they now see themselves as performing a job rather than fulfilling a vocation. This transition reflects the dictates of maximizing patient volume and productivity targets in the face of constrained reimbursement. Moreover, PCPs have undergone a "deskilling" and narrowing of their scope of work whereby they delegate all facility-based visits to hospitalists and cede responsibility for procedures to subspecialists. PCPs have thus lost technical skills and medical knowledge as a consequence of not following their patients across office and hospital settings and have become isolated from other specialties.

More may be needed—perhaps investments in nursing and pharmacists. One needs to be cautious here. One of the studies cited earlier performed supplementary analyses that included nurse practitioners and physician assistants in its measure of primary care supply. Greater supply was positively associated with increased life expectancy, but the results were not statistically significant.[15] Greater investments in nonphysician primary care providers and virtual care delivery models (aided by telemedicine) may also replace the "one-to-one" patient-physician relationship with a "one-to-many" relationship.[16] The impacts of such a shift will also need to be closely monitored, particularly on coordination, continuity, follow-up, and patient trust.

## NEW MODELS OF PRIMARY CARE DELIVERY BY PRIMARY CARE PHYSICIANS

Over the past few decades, private sector entrepreneurs have developed new models to deliver organized ambulatory care centered around PCPs. These include CareMore, Iora Health, One Medical, and direct primary care. These models and their experience are briefly chronicled in the following sections.

### CareMore

CareMore was founded in 1993 in southern California by Dr. Sheldon Zinberg, a gastroenterologist in his 60s. He recruited and merged together 28 practices of nonemployed physicians to contract with HMO plans on a capitated basis. In 1997, CareMore developed its own in-house health plan to serve the Medicare Advantage population.

The goal was to develop high-quality, coordinated, high-touch care for a small base of elderly with a focus on preventing progression of chronic conditions, keeping patients healthy, and keeping them out of hospital. To do so, his model included 4 elements: (1) a small network of PCPs; (2) an "extensivist" physician, directly employed by CareMore, and (similar to a hospitalist) stationed at community hospitals to serve as the principal provider for frail and medically complex patients to coordinate care and transitions across care sites; (3) neighborhood care centers, similar to outpatient facilities, to serve chronically ill patients using patient engagement and disease

management strategies; and (4) nurse case managers who would coordinate all aspects of care, serve as the principal point of contact for enrollees, monitor enrollees' health in disease-specific registries, reach out to patients who miss appointments, and lead the daily patient telephone rounds with the extensivists.

It took CareMore 7 years to make a profit. Growth in patient enrollment was slow, reaching only 22,000 enrollees. By 2006, despite expansion to neighboring states, enrollment still totaled only 55,000. CareMore was acquired by JP Morgan in 2006 and then subsequently sold to Wellpoint/Anthem in 2011. When growth in CareMore's Medicare Advantage market stalled, the company shifted to Medicaid managed care.

CareMore has received a lot of attention for its Tennessee and (more recently) Iowa Medicaid operations. However, enrollment still remains low (8,000 in Tennessee, 10,000 in Iowa). This has challenged its ability to apply a resource-rich, comprehensive model of care initially developed for seniors in California to a population of poor women and children in the Midwest that is not well reimbursed by Medicaid and may need more behavioral health and attention paid to "super-utilizers."

### Iora Health

Iora Health was launched in 2010 in Massachusetts as a for-profit firm with the help of venture capital funding. It cares for 30,000 patients (mostly enrolled in Medicare Advantage) at 48 practice locations (as of early 2020). Iora contracts on a monthly capitated basis (rather than fee-for-service) that requires no fees, no coinsurance, and no copays. Iora contracts with large self-insured companies and health plans to provide primary care for employees (enrollees), endeavoring to keep both out of the hospital and the hospital ED. Iora takes a percentage of the savings on these costly services as profit. How does it seek to manage utilization? Iora markets its advantages as lower doctor-to-patient ratios, 4 coaches for every PCP who engage with patients, the use of an information technology platform to allow patient engagement and track all patient data, around-the-clock availability, excellent customer service, and unlimited visits per patients. Iora also contracts with specialists as consultants to the primary care practice, basically empowering the PCPs to see the majority of patients who might otherwise be referred to the specialists (with their telephonic or online advice). In this manner, they claim they can effectively manage most chronic illness before it progresses. Iora claims to have achieved 35% to 40% drops in hospitalization and 12% to 15% lower healthcare costs. They also claim that their goal is not to provide healthcare but rather to empower patients to take charge of their own health.

Two features of Iora's model are unusual. First, they have been supported by a lot of venture capital money ($381 million total, including $100 million raised in 2018 and $126 million raised in early 2020), which likely limits any replicability of Iora's model and its service-rich offering. Second, Iora serves patients with insurance; it does not serve the uninsured or Medicaid patients.

## One Medical

One Medical was founded in 2007 in San Francisco to bring a "hospitality-minded approach" to primary care. It offers 24/7 access to virtual care via voice, text messaging, or video visits. It also offers in-person care via a network of 70+ private clinics with short office waits. One Medical contracts with more than 1,000 employers (Uber, Lyft, Airbnb) to provide healthcare benefits to their employees. It has been described as a tech-enabled, on-demand primary care model for yuppies. Patient testimonials mention the convenience and the "vibe" of being at a boutique clinic.[17]

Like Iora Health, it has heavy funding from venture capitalists ($350 million raised in 2018 from the Carlyle Group) as well as backing from Google's parent, Alphabet. The investment will be used to expand One Medical's physical footprint of clinics around the United States. It charges a $199 annual concierge fee to employers to belong, which does not cover visits or services; the latter must be covered by the enrollee's health plan. Unlike Iora, they still operate in the fee-for-service environment. Like Iora, they too claim to reduce overall costs of care by 4% to 5%.

One Medical went public in January 2020 but experienced a sharp decline in office visits in March due to COVID-19. The company responded by launching COVID-19 care and billable remote visits, as well as on-demand symptom assessment, testing, and follow-up. It has since reported a 25% increase in membership year-over-year, with 475,000 members by mid-2020. In August 2020, One Medical announced it had beat Wall Street expectations on earnings and revenues during the second quarter. The positive lift resulted from COVID-19 and stay-at-home orders, which boosted its virtual care business. The company also rolled out a virtual care option for patients living in areas where it had no physical locations.

## Direct Primary Care

Direct primary care (DPC) models, finally, differ from the previous models by omitting the third-party payer from the patient-doctor relationship, and instead feature direct contracting between patients and PCPs. Patients pay a recurring out-of-pocket fee to the PCP (ranging from $50 to $200 per month) in exchange for a defined set of primary care benefits. The benefits include acute care, long-term care, and discounted prescriptions; they do not include more expensive subspecialist fees and hospitalizations, for which patients need wrap-around insurance coverage such as through a high-deductible health plan.[18]

The model's appeal rests on the continuity of the patient-doctor relationship—basically a "return to the womb" or "ground zero" of healthcare, where the microcosm of care (see Figure 3-14) is paramount. Because physicians are capitated, they are not incentivized by volume or fee-for-service, but rather by focusing on the patient, developing patient intimacy, and coordinating their care needs. The typical DPC practice has 1 to 2 doctors, 600 patients per physician, and 10 visits per doctor per day. There are few staff and low overhead costs, and there is minimal office space. Moreover, the model fits with the frequently mentioned assertion that 80% of a patient's needs can be met in such a practice.[19]

Researchers suggest that, like the other models discussed earlier, DPC may be hard to scale up. This is due to the small number of patients in each DPC doctor's panel—perhaps only one-third or one-quarter of what a typical PCP has in their panel. The DPC physician may also have incentives to limit the amount of care they deliver, given the capitated risk they bear to deliver defined services for the monthly capitated fees received.

| **Critical Thinking Exercise: Oak Street Health** |
|---|

Oak Street Health (OSH) was founded in 2012 with funding (>$105 million) from angel investors and then private equity. OSH opened its first primary care clinics in northern Chicago the following year. The clinic grew rapidly in just a few short years, reaching 7 sites by 2014, 19 sites by 2016, and then 50 or more sites in multiple states (Illinois, Indiana, Michigan, Ohio, Pennsylvania, and North Carolina), with 2020 plans to expand into Tennessee and Texas. The majority of their 80,000 enrollees were Medicare Advantage members (see Chapter 18), while some were dually eligible for both Medicare and Medicaid (see Chapter 19).

As part of its claimed competitive advantage, OSH touts its consumer friendliness and goal of providing a better user experience than is typically found in traditional settings (similar to One Medical). Its clinics reportedly offer a more personalized experience, where PCPs spend more time with patients, and services include expanded mental health and a focus on "whole body health." OSH also provides transportation to the centers and a 24/7 call line for support. OSH claims its regular clients are 41% less likely to require hospitalization compared to the average Medicare enrollee and 49% less likely to visit a hospital ED.[20] To deal with the challenge of COVID-19, OSH quickly developed a remote care program to see 93% of their 2,200 daily patients by phone or video.[21]

At face value, the OSH strategy seems to be focused on rapid growth in a rapidly growing segment of the insurance market (Medicare Advantage). Based on what you have already learned from the 3 other primary care delivery models profiled earlier, what do you need to know to evaluate the prospects of OSH? What might be your concerns about OSH?

## NURSING

### The Important Role of Nursing

Anyone who has ever been unfortunate enough to be hospitalized overnight knows this one fact: The only people you can count on are the nursing staff. Nurses provide care in the hospital on a 24/7 basis, usually in the form of three 8-hour shifts. Studies show an association between lower nurse workloads (eg, higher nurse-to-patient staffing ratios) and a higher proportion of nurses with baccalaureate degrees with better patient outcomes (including lower hospital mortality).[22]

Nurses are also in heavy demand, as more healthcare shifts from inpatient to outpatient and, increasingly, home-based settings. Indeed, the occupations with the greatest demand for the period of 2018 to 2028, listed in Chapter 8, are heavily represented by nurse practitioners (NPs) and physician assistants (PAs). Prior forecasts for the period of 2014 to 2024 also mention the need for more medical assistants, licensed practical nurses, and licensed vocational nurses.[23]

### History of Nursing Training

Historically, hospitals developed nurse training programs after the Civil War and then expanded them rapidly through the end of the 19th century to handle the rising number of inpatients cared for. Most programs involved anywhere from 6 months to 2 years of training (with little standardization) and produced "hospital diploma" nurses. By the early 1900s, the first university-based training programs at the baccalaureate level were established as part of an effort to raise the educational standards. Similar to the Flexner Report in medicine, the Goldman Report of 1923 (*Nursing and Nurse Education in the United States*) called for strengthening the link between nurse education and university affiliations for schools of nursing. Over time, many nonaffiliated schools closed, whereas those with university affiliations increased.

After World War II, 2 reports urged a 2-tiered system of nurse training, one based in a 4-year university curriculum for professional nurses and another based in 1- to 2-year training programs for practical nurses. The latter became enshrined in "associates degree" programs offered by the burgeoning programs of community colleges that sprang up after the war to provide adult and continuing education. At the same time, the newly formed (1952) National League of Nursing promulgated higher standards for nursing school accreditation, which included fewer hours of hospital experience.

| Nursing Category | No. Employed | No. Total (NCSBN) |
|---|---|---|
| • RNs | 3,059,800 | 4,015,000 |
| • LPNs/LVNs | 728,900 | 922,196 |
| • NAs/orderlies | 1,564,200 | |
| • APRNs | 240,700 | |

**Figure 10-2** • Distribution of Nursing Personnel (2018). APRNs, Advanced Practice Registered Nurses; LPNs, Licensed Practical Nurses; LVNs, Licensed Vocational Nurses; NCSBN, National Council of State Boards of Nursing; NAs, Nursing Assistants; RNs, Registered Nurses. (Source: US Bureau of Labor Statistics. Available online: https://www.bls.gov/ooh/home.htm.)

This change caused higher tuitions in hospital diploma programs and made them more expensive than the community colleges. As a result, the latter began to supplant the diploma programs as training sites. In 1965, the American Nurses Association issued a controversial (at the time) position paper calling for nurse education to occur in institutions of higher learning. By 1973, there were 1,373 registered nurse (RN) training programs, distributed as follows: 494 (36%) diploma programs, 574 (42%) associate degree programs, and 305 (22%) baccalaureate programs.[24]

## Types and Training Levels

Nursing personnel can be classified as follows: RNs, licensed practice nurses (LPNs), licensed vocational nurses (LVNs), nursing assistants (NAs), and advanced practice registered nurses (APRNs). APRNs, in turn, can be subclassified into NPs, certified nurse midwives (CNMs), certified registered nursing anesthetists (CRNAs), and clinical nurse specialists (CNSs). These categories are briefly defined in the following paragraphs. The number of personnel across all of these categories is presented in Figure 10-2; the distribution of APRNs is depicted in Figure 10-3.[25]

*Registered nurses* (RNs) come through 3 routes of training. They can be trained at the university level, the community college level, or the hospital (diploma programs). Their training can last anywhere from 1 to 4 years. The most popular programs at the undergraduate level are the 2-year associate degree in nursing (ADN),

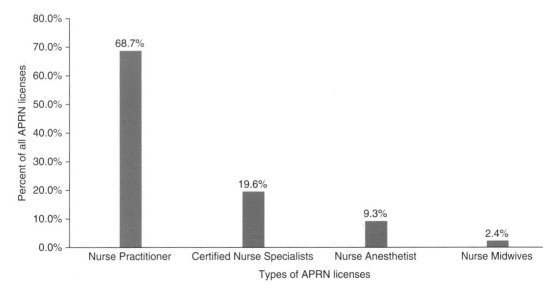

**Figure 10-3** • Distribution of Advanced Practice Registered Nurse (APRN) Licenses. (Source: Health Resources and Services Administration. *2018 National Survey Sample of Registered Nurses: Brief Summary of Results* [Washington, DC: HRSA, 2019]. https://data.hrsa.gov/DataDownload/NSSRN/GeneralPUF18/2018_NSSRN_Summary_Report-508.pdf.)

found in community colleges, and the 4-year bachelor degree in nursing (BSN), found in universities and nursing schools. The ADN degree can serve as the stepping stone to the BSN degree; some 4-year nursing schools also offer a 2-year ADN. The hospital diploma programs last anywhere from 1 to 3 years and focus primarily on patient/clinical practice rather than theory.

*Licensed practice nurses and licensed vocational nurses* (LPNs and LVNs) receive 9 to 12 months of training in practical nurse programs, which serve as entry-level licensure routes more than degree-conferring programs. LPNs and LVNs are subject to restricted scope of practice and typically are supervised by RNs. Like many nurses receiving ADN degrees, they are trained in local community colleges. The only difference between LPNs and LVNs is the state in which the training is received: California and Texas use the LVN rather than the LPN title.

*Nursing assistants* (NAs)—or certified nursing assistants (CNAs)—work under the supervision of either an RN or an LPN/LVN. They typically work in home healthcare settings, long-term care residential settings, rehabilitation centers, and adult senior day care centers to assist patients with activities of daily living (ADLs; eg, bathing and grooming). NAs lack both a formal degree and formal training. They do need to be certified at the state level, which only requires them to take classes.

*Nurse practitioners* (NPs) are RNs who have obtained additional training at either the master's or doctoral level. Such training began during the 1960s and became more mainstream by the 1980s. They pursue this training to acquire specialized knowledge and clinical competency for practice in ambulatory, acute, or post-acute care settings. NPs are also distinguished by their focus on health promotion, disease prevention, patient counseling, and education, much in the manner of promoting population health.

*Certified nurse midwives* (CNMs) are trained in master's degree programs to provide specialized care in pregnancy, labor, and postpartum care. A small but growing percentage of mothers are choosing CNMs over obstetricians to help deliver their babies. In contrast to nurse midwives, CNMs can legally practice in all states, can prescribe medications, and are considered primary care providers.

*Certified registered nurse anesthetists* (CRNAs) are also trained at the master's level (although some receive doctoral training). They administer anesthesia and other medications, as well as monitor patients in postoperative recovery. They work with patients in operating rooms, surgical facilities, EDs, and intensive care units. CRNAs differ from anesthesiologists by virtue of where they train (nursing schools vs medical schools) and for how long (1-2 years postgraduate vs 7-8 years). Although their job responsibilities overlap to a significant degree, they differ in their patient care orientation (treat vs diagnose and treat disease). Only one state (New Jersey) requires that CRNAs work under the direction and supervision of a physician anesthesiologist. Nevertheless, there are 4 different models governing their working relationship: CRNA-only, anesthesiologist supervision, anesthesiologist direction, and anesthesiologist only.

*Clinical nurse specialists* (CNSs) also have training at the master's or doctoral level. They obtain advanced education and specialized training in specific areas such as the patient population (pediatrics, geriatrics, women's health), clinical setting (critical care or ED), disease or medical subspecialty (diabetes or oncology), type of care (psychiatric or rehabilitation), or patient problem (pain, wounds, stress).

## Trends in Nursing Personnel Training

The nursing profession has witnessed an upskilling in their training. Between 2013 and 2017, the percentage of nurses with bachelor degrees increased from 40% to 45%, whereas those with master's degrees increased from 14% to 17%. Conversely, those with ADNs decreased from 33% to 29%, and those with diplomas decreased from 13% to 8%.[26] The distribution of nursing graduates by highest level of training is presented in Figure 10-4.

## Scope of Practice Issues

NPs typically staff the retail clinics found in local pharmacies. A mix of NPs, PAs, and physicians can be found in urgent care centers. Might the large numbers of NPs and PAs, which together nearly total the number of PCPs, alleviate the PCP shortage noted at the outset of this chapter? One barrier is the state-level practice environment for NPs. States vary in their "scope-of-practice" regulations that govern what NPs can and cannot do. The 3 categories of these regulations fall under (1) full practice

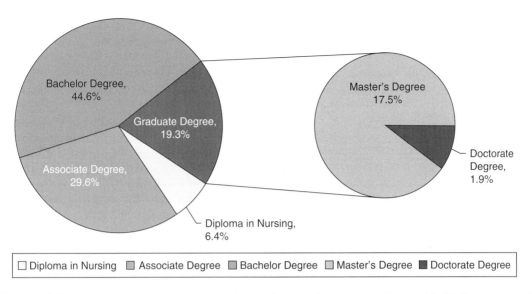

**Figure 10-4** • Highest Nursing and Nursing-Related Educational Attainment. (Source: Health Resources and Services Administration. *2018 National Survey Sample of Registered Nurses: Brief Summary of Results* [Washington, DC: HRSA, 2019]. https://data.hrsa.gov/DataDownload/NSSRN/GeneralPUF18/2018_NSSRN_Summary_Report-508.pdf.)

authority, (2) reduced practice authority, and (3) restricted practice authority. These are defined below[27]:

*Full practice:* State practice and licensure laws permit all NPs to evaluate patients; diagnose, order, and interpret diagnostic tests; and initiate and manage treatments, including prescribing medications and controlled substances, under the exclusive licensure authority of the state board of nursing. Depending on the state, NPs may need to complete an agreement that verifies a consultative relationship with a physician, although no direct supervision is needed.

*Reduced practice:* State practice and licensure laws reduce the ability of NPs to engage in at least one element of NP practice. State law requires a regulated collaborative agreement with another health provider in order for the NP to provide patient care, or it limits the setting of one or more elements of NP practice. This may include written proof of collaboration including plans for coordinating care. This may entail limits on the number and/or types of drugs that can be prescribed (eg, those with little potential for abuse). For controlled substances, the NP and physician may need to practice in the same facility.

*Restricted practice:* State practice and licensure laws restrict the ability of NPs to engage

in at least one element of NP practice. State law requires supervision, delegation, or team management by another health provider in order for the NP to provide patient care. This may include a supervising physician who develops practicing and prescribing guidelines that describe methods the NPs should follow in managing care, as well as plans for quality assurance.

Scope of practice has become an active and growing area of debate in healthcare workforce discussions (see the Critical Thinking Exercise later in this chapter). States have debated the issue of NPs and scope of practice since the profession was founded in the 1960s. Prior to COVID-19, expanded scope was often targeted at reducing care delivery variations across states and promoting transformation from volume to value; since COVID-19, expanded scope is now targeted at meeting increased patient demand in community (nonhospital) settings. Calls to expand scope of practice are often justified by research findings of comparable quality of care at lower cost rendered by PCPs, NPs, and PAs for managing certain types of conditions (eg, diabetes).[28]

Another barrier to use of NPs and PAs, as noted at the end of Chapter 9, is the negative attitude of many physicians regarding the ability of other, nonphysician practitioners to help them improve quality of care. Such attitudes seem to diminish once physicians employ these practitioners in their offices. Another barrier is that many (primarily older) consumers prefer to see a physician as their primary care provider, although there is some receptivity to seeing NPs and PAs.[29] Indeed, those with prior experience seeing an NP or PA are much more willing to see them than those lacking such exposure. Data also show that many consumers are willing to forego seeing the PCP tomorrow for a worsening condition if they can get into the office and see an NP or PA today. Recent data suggest that Millennials are less likely to have a PCP and thus may be more receptive to nonphysician providers.

In 2008, the National Council of State Boards of Nursing (NCSBN) adopted the Consensus Model for APRN Regulation, Licensure, Accreditation, Certification, and Education. The Model addressed the issue that state-level licensing boards are the final arbiters of who is recognized to practice within a given state. Currently, there is no uniform model of regulation of APRNs across states. Each state independently determines the APRN legal scope of practice, the roles that are recognized, the criteria for entry into advanced practice, and the certification examinations accepted for entry-level competence assessment. This has created a significant barrier for APRNs to easily move from state to state, limited their opportunity to enjoy full practice and prescribing authority, and potentially decreased access to care for patients. Supportive APRN legislation has been introduced in many state legislatures; however, not all states have embraced this model, partly due to physician lobbying and resistance.

---

**Critical Thinking Exercise: Proposed Legislation in California to Broaden Scope of Practice**

As of 2019, California was 1 of 22 states that restricted the scope of work of APRNs by requiring that they practice and prescribe with physician oversight. Broadening the scope of practice by APRNs has merit under certain conditions, including the alleviation of shortages of healthcare personnel in rural areas and medically underserved urban areas. The United States has faced a chronic shortage of physicians, both primary care and specialist providers, which is projected to continue. Supplementing the supply of physicians with APRNs can help to mitigate issues of poor access to care. Moreover, during the current COVID-19 pandemic, APRNs may assist the healthcare delivery system by improving patient screening and triage and reducing provider burnout.

However, efforts to address these specific needs perhaps should be cautious about overgeneralizing the roles that APRNs can play. Proposed legislation in California, *AB-890 Nurse Practitioners: Scope of Practice*, and specifically its *Article 8.5 and Section 2837.103*, would allow NPs to "order, perform, and interpret diagnostic procedures" (including x-rays, mammography, and ultrasounds), as well as "prescribe, administer, dispense, and furnish pharmacological agents, including over-the-counter, legend, and controlled substances." Should we have any concerns about allowing APRNs, most of whom have master's degree training, to read mammograms and prescribe opioids? What do you think?

---

## Trends in Nursing Demographics

In complete contrast with the medical profession, the nursing profession has historically been female. There is now a noticeable trend toward greater male representation among RNs and LPNs (9% and 8%, respectively, in 2017). Like the medical profession, the nursing profession has historically been mainly White, but with growing diversity in its racial and ethnic mix. By 2017, there was 19% minority representation among RNs and 29% among LPNs/LVNs. The composition of the RN population is presented in Figure 10-5. Roughly three-quarters of RNs are White, reflecting the racial mix prominent in nursing schools before 1990. However, Figure 10-6 shows increasing racial diversity as newer cohorts of students graduate from nursing school. Moreover, with more nursing graduates in recent years (Figure 10-7), there is a more even distribution in the age mix of the RN workforce (Figure 10-8).

## Supply and Demand Issues Facing the Nursing Workforce

Nursing is the largest professional group in the US healthcare ecosystem. RNs and LPNs/LVNs

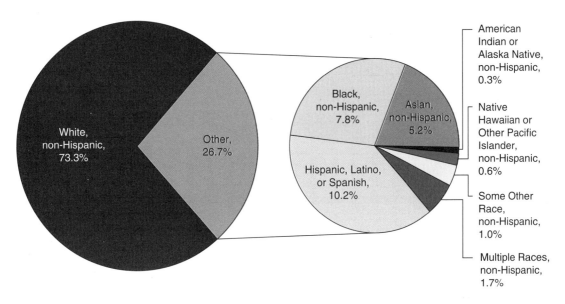

**Figure 10-5** • Distribution of Registered Nurses by Race and Ethnicity. (Source: Health Resources and Services Administration. *2018 National Survey Sample of Registered Nurses: Brief Summary of Results* [Washington, DC: HRSA, 2019]. https://data.hrsa.gov/DataDownload/NSSRN/GeneralPUF18/2018_NSSRN_Summary_Report-508.pdf.)

compose the 2 largest nursing categories. The growth in their numbers between 2000 and 2016 is presented in Figure 10-9.

Like the medical profession, the nursing profession faces personnel issues going forward. And, like the medical profession, the historical relationship between nurse supply and demand has been cyclical, with periodic shortages of nurses (demand exceeds available supply)

followed by periods of nursing surpluses (supply exceeds demand). Part of the problem is the complexity of forecasting demand. Demand drivers include not only the aging of the population, but also the increase in chronic illness, the demand for post-acute care, the supply of PCPs, the alternative employment opportunities available to nurses that might prompt them to leave the nursing labor force, the supply of alternative

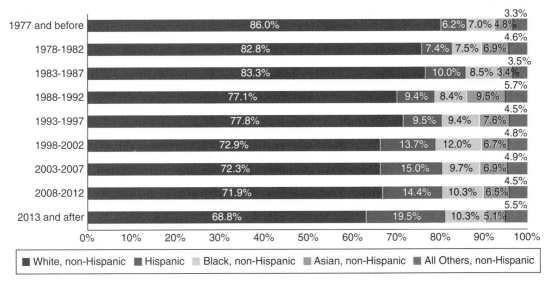

**Figure 10-6** • Distribution of Race and Ethnicity by Initial Nursing Program Graduation Year. (Source: Health Resources and Services Administration. *2018 National Survey Sample of Registered Nurses: Brief Summary of Results* [Washington, DC: HRSA, 2019]. https://data.hrsa.gov/DataDownload/NSSRN/GeneralPUF18/2018_NSSRN_Summary_Report-508.pdf.)

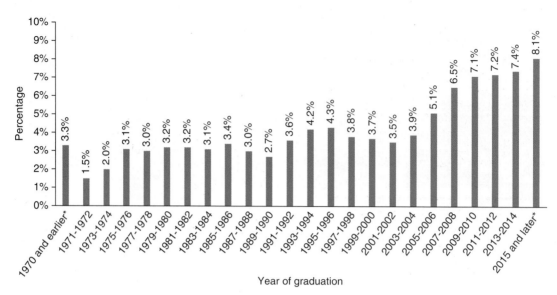

*Data for this time period reflects more than a 2-year interval. As the survey sample was selected from a list of licensed nurses constructed from different sources during year 2017, the count of new graduates in the most recent year(s) may not be fully reflected in the "2015 and later" estimate.

**Figure 10-7 •** Distribution of Registered Nurses by Graduation Year. (Source: Health Resources and Services Administration. *2018 National Survey Sample of Registered Nurses: Brief Summary of Results* [Washington, DC: HRSA, 2019]. https://data.hrsa.gov/DataDownload/NSSRN/GeneralPUF18/2018_NSSRN_Summary_Report-508.pdf.)

models of healthcare delivery such as accountable care organizations, and the possible rise of alternative payment models and risk-based contracting, which prompt greater substitution of nonhospital (ambulatory) and noninstitutional (eg, home healthcare) settings.

A December 2014 report by the federal government's Health Resources and Services Administration (HRSA; see Chapter 25) suggested that 34 states would face a cumulative deficit of 808,000 nurses by 2025.[30] Three years later, everything changed: Only 7 states faced

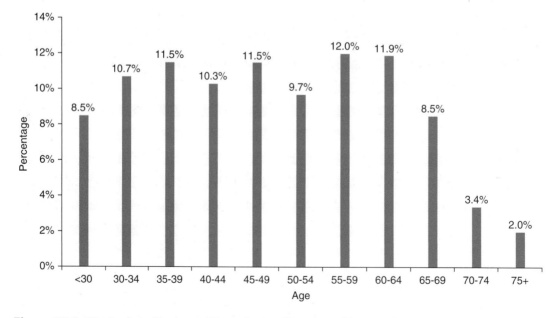

**Figure 10-8 •** Distribution of Registered Nurses by Age. (Source: Health Resources and Services Administration. *2018 National Survey Sample of Registered Nurses: Brief Summary of Results* [Washington, DC: HRSA, 2019]. https://data.hrsa.gov/DataDownload/NSSRN/GeneralPUF18/2018_NSSRN_Summary_Report-508.pdf.)

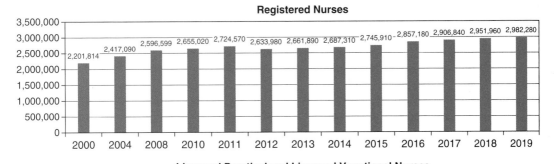

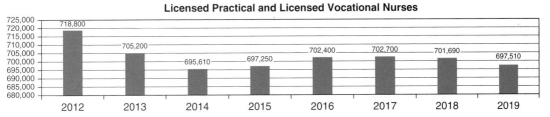

**Figure 10-9** • Number of Employed Registered Nurses and Licensed Practical Nurses/Licensed Vocational Nurses in the United States, 2000 to 2019. (Source: US Bureau of Labor Statistics, Occupational Employment Statistics, www.bls.org; Health Resources and Services Administration. *2018 National Survey Sample of Registered Nurses: Brief Summary of Results* [Washington, DC: HRSA, 2019]. https://data.hrsa.gov/DataDownload/NSSRN/GeneralPUF18/2018_NSSRN_Summary_Report-508.pdf)

a shortage. At the national level, the projected growth in RN supply (39% growth) is expected to exceed growth in RN demand (28% growth), resulting in a projected excess of about 293,800 RNs in 2030 (measured as full-time equivalent positions).[31] So what happened? Forecasters overestimated the percentage of nurses who would retire and failed to account for nurse migration across state lines; they also failed to account for actions by nursing schools and government to recruit new nursing students. HRSA data released in January 2020 showed that roughly 83% of the 3.957 million licensed RNs held nursing-related jobs in 2017.

By contrast, the demand for LPNs is projected to start growing faster than supply starting in about 2022. By 2030, a projected national shortage of about 151,500 LPNs (13% of 2030 demand) could develop, according to HRSA. This shortage reflects the growing need for LPN/LVN personnel in post-acute care settings to care for an aging population. Nearly half (45%) of these personnel work in long-term services and supports (LTSS; a term used in Medicaid, see Chapter 19) settings, contrasted with only 15% of RNs who work in these settings.

HRSA projects state-level disparities in matching supply and demand for both RNs and LPNs by 2030. Some states will experience RN shortages anywhere from 10,000 (South

Carolina) to 44,500 (California); conversely, some states will enjoy RN surpluses ranging from 18,200 (New York) to 53,700 (Florida). Thirty-three states will face an LPN/LVN shortage by 2030.[32] As of 2017, the number of employed RNs per capita varied widely, from fewer than 700 RNs per 100,000 population in Nevada to over 1,500 RNs per 100,000 in the District of Columbia; the ratio of employed LPNs/LVNs varied between 65 and 70 per 100,000 people in Alaska, Oregon, and Utah and over 400 per 100,000 in Arkansas and Louisiana.[33]

There are *some opportunities* here, given the trends noted earlier in the physician workforce. First, the maldistribution of physician personnel (both PCPs and specialists) between urban versus rural areas might be redressed using any excess supply in RNs who can be connected with physicians using telemedicine. Second, research shows that NPs and PAs are more likely than physicians to practice in rural areas (16% vs 11%); NPs and PAs who focus on primary care are much more likely to be rural practitioners (28% and 25%, respectively).[34]

There are also *some problems* here. The number of RNs from the Baby Boomer generation peaked at 1.26 million in 2008. Although the 2008-2009 recession offered a brief respite, Baby Boomer RNs began retiring in large numbers. Between 2012 and 2020, roughly 60,000 RNs are predicted to exit the workforce annually. In 2020, the number of Baby Boomer RNs will be 660,000, roughly half their 2008 peak. Researchers estimate that, by 2015, the nursing workforce lost 1.7 million "experience-years" (the number of retiring RNs multiplied by the years of experience for each RN), double the number in 2005. This trend will continue to accelerate as the largest groups of Baby Boomer RNs reach their middle to late 60s. The anticipated retirement of 1 million RNs between 2015 and 2030 means that patient care settings and other organizations that depend on RNs will face a significant loss of nursing knowledge and expertise.[35]

## Role for NPs, PAs, and Community Health Workers

In 2017, there were 129,961 NPs, with roughly half (52%) practicing primary care, and 83,224 PAs, with less than half (43%) in primary care.[36] Their numbers have been growing since the 1960s, with more expanded roles since the 1980s. The growth rates for these personnel are outstripping the growth rates among PCPs. For example, just between 2001 and 2012, the number of newly certified PAs rose more than 50% (from 4,235 to 6,479).[37]

As new healthcare models move care into the community setting, and as the need for providers in rural and health shortage areas increases, some RN and LPN responsibilities may be provided by nonnursing personnel such as community health workers (CHWs). As of May 2016, 51,900 CHWs were working in the United States, with the highest levels of employment in individual and family services, local government, outpatient care centers, general medical and surgical hospitals, and physician offices. CHWs differ from home healthcare aides, who may assist with ADLs, and from CNAs, who may assist in carrying out a nursing plan of care. CHWs are often part of the patient's community and usually share the language, ethnicity, and life experiences of their patients. This commonality helps them be uniquely valued by both the patient and the healthcare team. Job responsibilities for CHWs often include home visits, follow-up after acute care discharge, monitoring chronic diseases, and educating patients on how to manage their conditions. They also act as specialists who educate the community on best practices for specific conditions, provide outreach to homebound patients on behalf of hospitals and other providers who may be at financial risk for such patients, and convene disparate stakeholders to coordinate a targeted outreach effort.[38]

## Nursing Incomes

As in many other occupations, RNs with graduate degrees earn substantially higher incomes than those without graduate degrees ($95,804 vs $69,663). Among the APRNs, CRNAs earned the highest incomes (Figure 10-10). There is also evidence that male nurses earn higher incomes than female nurses ($79,928 vs $71,960). Nevertheless, NPs and PAs earn much lower incomes compared to PCPs. In 2013, the median income across PCP specialties ranged from $195,000 to $215,000; NPs and PAs earned $91,000 to $92,000.

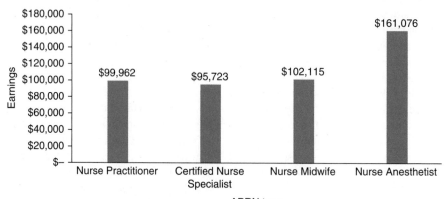

**Figure 10-10** • Median Full-Time Earnings by Advanced Practice Type. APRN, Advanced Practice Registered Nurse. (Source: Health Resources and Services Administration. *2018 National Survey Sample of Registered Nurses: Brief Summary of Results* [Washington, DC: HRSA, 2019]. https://data.hrsa.gov/DataDownload/NSSRN/GeneralPUF18/2018_NSSRN_Summary_Report-508.pdf.)

## Nursing Stress and Burnout

Nurses echo many of the complaints voiced by physicians regarding their work environment. These complaints include understaffing issues (eg, to deal with a more severely ill patient population), workload issues (eg, long shifts), and inadequate involvement in decision making. In a survey of bedside nurses in the Commonwealth of Pennsylvania[39]:

- 94% reported their facility lacks sufficient nurses
- 87% reported staffing levels affecting patient care getting worse
- 84% reported problems with high nursing turnover rates
- 74% reported spending more time on paperwork
- 69% reported decreased time spent on bedside patient care over the past 5 years
- 51% reported decreased input on how things are done at work over the past 5 years
- 46% reported their input was undervalued

In a 2019 survey released by The Joint Commission, 15% of all nurses reported being "burned out"—variously defined as a physical/mental/emotional state of exhaustion, a disconnect from patients, or a lack of confidence to overcome work challenges. The rate was even higher (41%) among nurses who were "not engaged" (eg, not part of a team, those with lower morale).

A host of solutions have been proposed to alleviate the problem. They include increasing nurse staffing ratios and nursing autonomy, decreasing nonnursing tasks they have to perform, involving them more in scheduling and staffing decisions, involving them in policy discussions (eg, patient quality), and improving nursing support services. Such solutions resemble those to address the comparable problems afflicting physicians (see end of Chapter 9).

## PHARMACISTS

The third and final set of professionals considered here, and the third largest professional occupation in healthcare, are pharmacists. To quote the late comedian, Rodney Dangerfield, pharmacists "don't get no respect." Early academic researchers did not consider pharmacy as a "profession," since they did not live up to the standards laid out by sociologists, such as Everett Hughes and (later) Eliot Freidson.[40] Pharmacists advertised their services, failed to control the content of their work, and failed to accumulate a specialized body of knowledge that could only be learned via socialization in their own institutions and training sites. As a result, it has often been treated as much as an occupation or, at most, a quasi-profession.[41]

Pharmacists have been treated more kindly in recent years as an "egalitarian profession" and a "family-friendly occupation."[42] But this is because of (1) the narrowing gender gap in earnings between male and female pharmacists, as well as between racial and ethnic groups, and (2) the decline in independently owned pharmacies, the growth in their employment and part-time employment, and the growing substitutability among pharmacists (allowing easier patient handoffs). These characteristics are not widely shared with other professions, particularly their growing substitutability and the decline in self-employment. This latter trend appears to be associated with a flattening of the age-earnings profile among pharmacists, which is about two-thirds as steep as the typical college graduate.

Pharmacists have witnessed a set of manifold changes in their roles in the US healthcare ecosystem. From dispensing drugs (often as owner-operators) from behind the counter of the freestanding, community pharmacy, they have evolved into salaried employees of large-scale pharmacy chains, (2) valued members of multidisciplinary care teams in hospitals, (3) providers of personalized healthcare at "healthcare hubs" (see Chapter 13), or (4) alternatives to PCPs, among others. The following sections explore these roles.

## Pharmacist Training

Until the 1990s, pharmacists needed a minimum 4-year training in a Bachelor of Science (BS) degree program from an accredited school of pharmacy. The BS degree was considered sufficient preparation for the licensing exam. At that time, only 17 of the country's 72 schools offered a Doctor of Pharmacy (PharmD) degree. During the 1990s, the pharmacy profession moved to raise the entry barrier to the PharmD degree, which was finalized in 2000 when the Accreditation Council for Pharmacy Education announced it would only accredit PharmD programs.[43] The number of programs mushroomed thereafter. Schools of pharmacy grew from 72 to 142 between 1987 and 2018.

Matching the rise in pharmacist programs has been a mushrooming of private and for-profit pharmacy technician training programs, and thus a rise in the number of these personnel. Between 2005 and 2015, the number of technicians grew by 130,640 (a 49% rise). However, their training is highly variable and often limited. For this reason, pharmacists were reluctant to delegate tasks to them and expressed concern that their training might contribute to problems in medication dispensing.[44]

## Supply and Demand

According to the US Bureau of Labor Statistics (BLS), there were 314,300 pharmacists in 2018. However, the BLS forecasted zero growth in the profession over the ensuing 10-year period (2018-2028). This is a remarkable projection, given that the number of pharmacy schools roughly doubled between 1987 and 2018 and that much of this growth occurred after 2000. Why was this so?

In a report to Congress in December 2000, HRSA stated that the current supply was adequate to keep pace with population growth. Between 1991 and 2000, the number of active US pharmacists increased by roughly 14% (from 172,000 to 196,000), whereas the population grew by only 9%. Moreover, the number of active pharmacists per 100,000 population increased

by 5% (from slightly under 68 to 71) over the same period. *However*, the report sounded a warning about an imminent rise in demand that would outstrip current supply. Such demand would be driven by growing efficacy and thus popularity of new drugs for chronic conditions, a resulting rise in prescription volumes (during the era of blockbuster drugs and rising insurance coverage for drugs), rising vacancy for pharmacists in expanding retail chains, changes in the pharmacist workforce that included more females rising from 13% in 1970 to 46% by 2000 (and thus the possibility of part-time employment), advent of direct-to-consumer marketing of drugs (authorized in 1997), limited use at the time of automation and information technology and pharmacist technicians, and recognition that pharmacists could play a larger role in improving quality of care. The Pharmacy Workforce Center also cited the imminent retirement of Baby Boomer pharmacists.

Indeed, between 1992 and 1999, the number of retail prescriptions dispensed rose 44% from 1.9 billion to 2.8 billion; by 2010, volume had grown to roughly 3.7 billion.[45] The huge increase in outpatient prescriptions, driven by new blockbuster drugs in the 1990s and expanded insurance coverage (1990s and 2000s), is depicted in Figure 10-11. The growing intensity of drugs prescribed per capita, driven by direct-to-consumer advertising, is shown in Figure 10-12.

The growth in drug launches and prescriptions dispensed in the 1990s spawned growth in

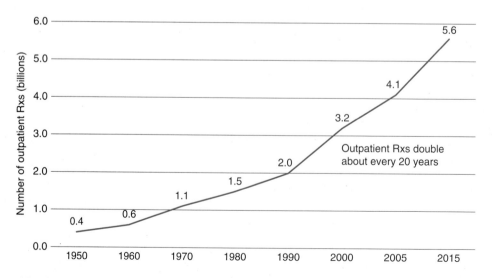

**Figure 10-11** • US Outpatient Prescriptions (Rxs) from 1950 to 2015. (Adapted from Stephen Schondelmeyer, "Recent Economic Trends in American Pharmacy." *Pharm Hist.* 51 (3) (2009): 103-126.)

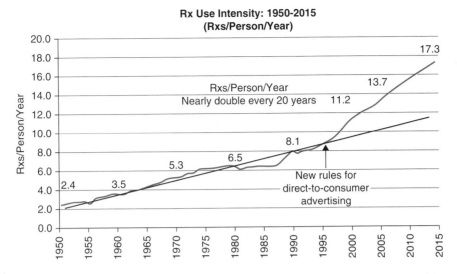

**Figure 10-12** • Prescription (Rx) Use Intensity: 1950 to 2015 (Rx Per Person Per Year). (Adapted from Stephen Schondelmeyer, "Recent Economic Trends in American Pharmacy." *Pharm Hist.* 51 (3) (2009): 103-126.)

the number of retail pharmacies (particularly by supermarkets and mass merchandisers). In 1998, the total number of retail outlets ($n$ = 51,975) included independents (20,644), chain (19,110), supermarkets (6,963), and mass merchandisers (5,258).[46] The number of retail pharmacies increased to 56,000 stores in 2004, to 59,583 in 2010, and then to 62,145 in 2019.[47] Part of this growth may have been spurred by the enactment of Medicare Part D coverage for prescription drugs, part of the Medicare Modernization Act of 2003, which took effect in 2006.[48]

The response to the 2000 HRSA report was a massive expansion of pharmacy schools.[49] The number of schools was roughly flat between 1980 ($n$ = 72) and 2000 ($n$ = 81), and then nearly doubled over the next 2 decades. Existing programs increased their class sizes. Acceptance rates into PharmD programs also skyrocketed from 32% to 82%.[50] By 2011, the United States had 272,320 working pharmacists, along with roughly 343,000 pharmacy technicians. This represented a huge increase from the number of active pharmacists in 2000 (196,000). The ratio of pharmacists to 100,000 population rose from 71 to 87 between 2000 and 2011.

More schools meant more students and more graduates (PharmDs). In 2000, the number of pharmacy graduates was 7,195. During 2014 to 2015, 14,000 to 15,000 students were graduating every year. It is not clear that 5% of the current pharmacist labor force is retiring to offset the new entrants. The oversupply will likely pressure pharmacist salaries, which are now estimated at

$105,000 for entry-level positions. The oversupply is also now showing up in layoffs from the supermarket chains and reduced work hours at pharmacy chains; it may also lead to lower starting salaries and less attractive work conditions going forward. Indeed, the 2 largest pharmacy chains—Walgreens and CVS—have closed or are closing more than 300 underperforming stores as of early 2020 (Figure 10-13); supermarkets are also closing their pharmacies, for different reasons (competition from the chains, as well as the growth of mail-order pharmacies). Both trends are further spurring layoffs.[51] Part of this may be due to trends in automation, which increase productivity per pharmacist and reduce the need for staffing. All of this means fewer stores and reduced geographic access to pharmacy services.

## Work Settings

Pharmacists work in 2 major settings: retail and institutional. In 2000, nearly two-thirds (63%) of pharmacists worked in retail settings; another quarter (25%) worked in hospitals, long-term care facilities, and home health agencies.[52] Only 3% of pharmacists were self-employed.[53]

Retail pharmacy work has morphed over the past decades beyond the independent drugstore and the chain drugstores (CVS, Walgreens, Rite-Aid). It now includes discount stores such as Walmart and Target, as well as supermarkets with pharmacies (Figure 10-14). These sites differ in the percentage of their revenues

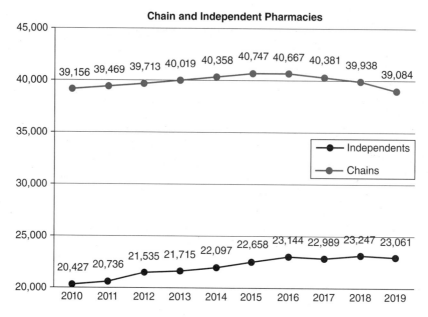

**Figure 10-13** • Numbers of Chain and Independent Pharmacies. (Source: Adam Fein, Drug Channels.)

that come from dispensing prescriptions: independent pharmacies (90%+), chain drugstores (67%+), and supermarkets and mass merchandisers (5%-10%).[54] Prescription activity likewise differs across these settings. In rank order, the number of annual prescriptions filled ranges from chain drugstores (95,000) to supermarkets

and mass merchandisers (55,000-57,000) to independent pharmacies (34,000).[55]

The hospital/institutional track may offer some hopeful alternative to working in retail settings. Pharmacists are seeking and obtaining positions at hospitals (often as residents), which offer full-time employment. Hospitals

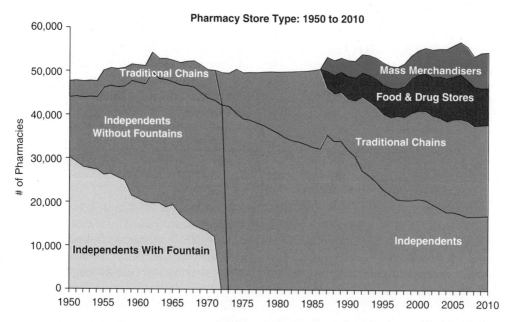

**Figure 10-14** • Pharmacy Ownership Type, 1950 to 2010. (Source: Compiled by Stephen W. Schondelmeyer, PRIME Institute, College of Pharmacy, University of Minnesota; based on annual data reported by American Druggist, Drug Topics, and the National Council of Prescription Drug Programs and reported in the National Association of Chain Drug Stores Industry Profile, the National Community Pharmacists Association Digest, and IMS Health annual reports.)

may account for more than 60% of the employment growth going forward.[56] Hospitals are recognizing the importance of having clinical pharmacy specialists making patient rounds with physicians, recommending drug therapies, monitoring patients' responses to medications, helping reduce medication errors, and helping their institutions deal with value-based payments. Hospitals can also serve as qualifying employers to get Public Service Loan Forgiveness (PSLF), which can help new PharmDs pay back their student loans. That said, however, hospital settings can be stressful places to work due to higher-acuity patients.

## Pharmacist Burnout

Like physicians and nurses, there are growing reports of burnout among pharmacists. According to a recent study, 53% of pharmacists reported a high degree of burnout caused by increasing stresses and demands. Two other studies, one in community pharmacy and the other in institutional practice, found that more than 50% of pharmacists were dissatisfied with their current occupation, to the point of considering quitting their jobs.[57]

The issue of burnout seems especially acute among pharmacists working in retail chains, mass merchandisers, and hospitals, compared to those working in independent pharmacies and supermarkets.[58] Pharmacist Workforce Surveys (PWS) show higher workloads, as measured by prescriptions filled per day or per week at these locations (eg, metrics-driven productivity), although workloads at the independent pharmacies are 15% to 40% higher than at the chains. The growing substitutability among pharmacists—attributable to uniform training, standardization of products handled, and extensive use of information technology (personal computers, point-of-sale computer systems to track inventory, bar coding, and online product ordering using the Internet)—has reduced the premium of owning an independent pharmacy and thus the rise of bureaucratic employment.

What has been the impact of employment by chain pharmacies? According to newspaper reports, chains can impose "sweatshop-style conditions" by virtue of understaffing, lower pharmacist time with patients, and pressure to overprescribe medications (ie, "Did you fill it?").[59] Physicians complain that pharmacies bombard them with refill requests that patients have not asked for and should not receive. Pharmacists are also expected to contact dozens of patients daily using a computer-generated list and then are evaluated based on whether patients do what the pharmacists ask. Other factors contributing to burnout include maintenance of license and certification, increased rules and regulations, heavy workload, high employee turnover, and drug shortages.

## SUMMARY

Chapters 9 and 10 make repeated reference to emerging patterns of burnout among US healthcare professionals. One cannot conclude these chapters without reference to Max Weber, a German historian and social theorist writing at the turn of the 20th century. Weber has become widely known for his views of modernization based on "rationalization," particularly increasing control in social and material life. Weber envisioned a future of rationalization partly in terms of "mechanized petrification," more popularly known as the growth of administrative bureaucracy or the bureaucratic "iron cage." Weber's bureaucracy involved a hierarchy of offices (each under the control of the one above), along with a division of labor based on specialized training and expertise that specified areas of action for which individuals were competent, and the performance of duties based on written rules. This cluster of characteristics afforded the ability to specialize based on expertise, the ability to coordinate roles and functions, and the mechanisms to control the performance of these roles. Although Weber noted the importance of discipline, he emphasized the critical importance of expertise. For him, bureaucracy was rational because it allowed for the exercise of control based on technical knowledge. This may be on the wane.

Chapters 9 and 10 suggest that, at least in healthcare organizations, the bureaucratic emphasis on discipline and control may finally be winning out over the professional emphasis on expertise and exercise of autonomy. The sociology literature of the 1960s discussed the relationship of professionals working in bureaucracies but did not declare the organization supreme. That same literature revisited the issue in the 1980s and concluded a number of relationships were possible by describing 3 forms of professional work in organizations (heteronomous/

independent, conjoint/shared, and custodial/controlled).[60] More recently, organization theorists have suggested the scale is tipping in favor of control.[61]

However, it is important to note that the pressures to which healthcare professionals are subjected are not just the bureaucracies in which they work. They are also bureaucratically imposed by government agencies that (1) control the reimbursement of physicians and (2) mistakenly forecast the future supply and demand needs for these healthcare professionals. They are further imposed by demanding patients who are now "customers" and co-decision makers in healthcare episodes.

---

### QUESTIONS TO PONDER

1. The first part of this chapter presents evidence that primary care can help solve the iron triangle and promote the triple aim. The chapter also presents some counter evidence calling this assertion into question. What do you conclude?
2. Is the trend observed among Millennials of not using a PCP a good thing or a bad thing? Are there other explanations for this trend?
3. Are new models of primary care delivery, such as CareMore, One Medical, and Iora Health, a "path out of the wilderness"?
4. What are the prospects for getting PCPs and NPs to work together in collaborative models of healthcare delivery? Is this the future of healthcare?
5. What do you conclude about the observed burnout reported among physicians, nurses, and pharmacists?

---

## REFERENCES

1. World Health Organization. *The World Health Report 2008—Primary Health Care (Now More Than Ever)* (Geneva, Switzerland: WHO, 2008). Available online: http://www.who.int/whr/2008/en/. Accessed on March 8, 2020.
2. Ann O'Malley, Eugene Rich, Alyssa Maccarone, et al. "Disentangling the Linkage of Primary Care Features to Patient Outcomes: A Review of Current Literature, Data Sources, and Measurement Needs," *J Gen Intern Med.* 30 (Suppl 3) (2015): S576-S585.
3. Barbara Starfield, Leiyu Shi, and James Macinko. "Contribution of Primary Care to Health Systems and Health," *Milbank Q.* 83 (3) (2005): 457-502.
4. Stephen Petterson, Robert McNellis, Kathleen Klink, et al. *The State of Primary Care in the United States* (Washington, DC: Robert Graham Center, January 2018).
5. Sanjay Basu, Seth Berkowitz, Robert Phillips, et al. "Association of Primary Care Physician Supply With Population Mortality in the United States, 2005-2015," *JAMA Intern Med.* 179 (4) (2019): 506-514.
6. David Levine, Bruce Landon, and Jeffrey Linder. "Quality and Experience of Outpatient Care in the United States for Adults With or Without Primary Care," *JAMA Intern Med.* 179 (3) (2019): 363-372.
7. Sara Martin, Robert Phillips, Stephen Petterson, et al. "Primary Care Spending in the United States, 2002-2016," *JAMA.* 180 (7) (2020). 1019-1020.
8. Ishani Ganguli, Zhuo Shi, John Orav, et al. "Declining Use of Primary Care Among Commercially Insured Adults in the United States, 2008-2016," *Ann Intern Med.* 172 (4) (2020): 240-247.
9. Itzik Fadlon and Jessica Van Parys. "Primary Care Physician Practice Styles and Patient Care: Evidence from Physician Exits in Medicare," *J Health Econ.* 71 (2020): 102304.
10. Mark Friedberg, Peter Hussey, and Eric Schneider. "Primary Care: A Critical Review of the Evidence on Quality and Costs of Health Care," *Health Aff.* 29 (5) (2010): 766-772.
11. John Fortney, Diane Steffick, James Burgess, et al. "Are Primary Care Services a Substitute or Complement for Specialty and Inpatient Services?" *Health Serv Res.* 40 (5) (2005): 1422-1442.
12. Deborah Peikes, Erin Taylor, Ann O'Malley, et al. "The Changing Landscape of Primary Care: Effects of the ACA and Other Efforts Over the Past Decade," *Health Aff.* 39 (3) (2020): 421-428.
13. Zirui Song and Suhas Gondi. "Will Increasing Primary Care Spending Alone Save Money?" *JAMA.* 322 (14) (2019): 1349-1350.
14. Timothy Hoff. *Practice Under Pressure: Primary Care Physicians and Their Medicine in the Twenty-First Century* (New Brunswick, NJ: Rutgers University Press, 2010).
15. Sanjay Basu, Seth Berkowitz, Robert Phillips, et al. "Association of Primary Care Physician Supply With Population Mortality in the United States, 2005-2015," *JAMA Intern Med.* 179 (4) (2019): 506-514.
16. Shantanu Nundy, Joseph Kvedar, and Gina Cella. "From One-to-One to One-to Many: Rethinking the Health Care Relationships in the Digital Age," *Health Affairs Blog* (April 6, 2020). Available online: https://www.healthaffairs

.org/do/10.1377/hblog20200320.600000/full/. Accessed on November 5, 2020.

17. Melia Robinson. "After Trying One Medical, I Could Never Use a Regular Doctor Again," *BusinessInsider.com* (January 28, 2016). Available online: https://www.businessinsider.com/what-its-like-to-use-one-medical-group-2016-1. Accessed on November 5, 2020.

18. Eli Adashi, Ryan Clodfelter, and Paul George. "Direct Primary Care: One Step Forward, Two Steps Back," *JAMA.* 320 (7) (2018): 637-638.

19. Niran Al-Agba. "Is the Direct Primary Care Model Dead?" *The Health Care Blog* (June 6, 2017). Available online: https://thehealthcareblog.com/blog/2017/06/06/is-the-direct-primary-care-model-dead/. Accessed on November 5, 2020.

20. Ron Shinkman. "Oak Street Health Moves Forward with National Expansion," *Healthcare Dive* (February 14, 2020). Available online: https://www.healthcaredive.com/news/oak-street-health-moves-forward-with-national-expansion/572330/. Accessed on August 5, 2020.

21. Griffin Myers, Geoffrey Price, and Mike Pykosz. *A Report From the COVID Front Lines of Value-Based Primary Care.* NEJM Catalyst–Innovations in Care Delivery (May 1, 2020).

22. Robert L. Kane, Tatyana A. Shamliyan, Christine Mueller, et al. "The Association of Registered Nurse Staffing Levels and Patient Outcomes: Systematic Review and Meta-Analysis," *Med Care.* 45 (2007): 1195-1204. Koen Van den Heede, Emmanuel Lesaffre, Luwis Diya, et al. "The Relationship Between Inpatient Cardiac Surgery Mortality and Nurse Numbers and Educational Level: Analysis of Administrative Data," *Int J Nurs Stud.* 46 (2009): 796-803. Jack Needleman, Peter Buerhaus, Shane Pankratz, et al. "Nurse Staffing and Inpatient Hospital Mortality," *N Engl J Med.* 364 (2011): 1037-1045.

23. Center for Health Workforce Studies. *Health Care Employment Projections, 2014-2024: An Analysis of Bureau of Labor Statistics Projections by Setting and by Occupation* (Albany, NY: School of Public Health, SUNY, April 2016).

24. Norma E. Anderson. "The Historical Development of American Nursing Education," *J Nurs Educ.* 20 (1) (1981): 18-36.

25. Health Resources and Services Administration. *2018 National Survey Sample of Registered Nurses: Brief Summary of Results* (Washington, DC: HRSA, 2019).

26. National Council of State Boards of Nursing. "National Nursing Workforce Study." Available online: https://www.ncsbn.org/workforce.htm. Accessed on March 8, 2020.

27. American Association of Nurse Practitioners. "State Practice Environment." Updated December 20, 2019. Available online: https://www.aanp.org/advocacy/state/state-practice-environment.

Accessed on March 6, 2020. See also, Catherine Dower, Jean Moore, and Margaret Langelier. "It Is Time to Restructure Health Professions Scope-of-Practice Regulations to Remove Barriers to Care," *Health Aff.* 32 (11) (2013): 1971-1976.

28. Valerie Smith, Perri Morgan, David Edelman, et al. "Utilization and Costs by Primary Care Provider Type: Are There Differences Among Diabetic Patients of Physicians, Nurse Practitioners, and Physician Assistants?" *Med Care.* 58 (8) (2020): 681-688. George Jackson, Valerie Smith, David Edelman, et al. "Intermediate Diabetic Outcomes in Patients Managed by Physicians, Nurse Practitioners, or Physician Assistants," *Ann Intern Med.* 169 (2018): 825-835.

29. Michael Dill, Stacie Pankow, Clese Erikson, et al. "Survey Shows Consumers Open to a Greater Role for Physician Assistants and Nurse Practitioners," *Health Aff.* 32 (6) (2013): 1135-1142.

30. Health Resources and Services Administration. *The Future of the Nursing Workforce: National- and State-Level Projections, 2012-2025* (December 2014). Available online: https://bhw.hrsa.gov/sites/default/files/bhw/nchwa/projections/nursingprojections.pdf. Accessed on March 8, 2020.

31. Health Resources and Services Administration. *Supply and Demand Projections of the Nursing Workforce: 2014-2030* (July 2017). Available online: https://bhw.hrsa.gov/sites/default/files/bhw/nchwa/projections/NCHWA_HRSA_Nursing_Report.pdf. Accessed on March 8, 2020.

32. Health Resources and Services Administration. *Supply and Demand Projections of the Nursing Workforce: 2014-2030* (July 2017). Available online: https://bhw.hrsa.gov/sites/default/files/bhw/nchwa/projections/NCHWA_HRSA_Nursing_Report.pdf. Accessed on March 8, 2020.

33. US Department of Labor 2017 Occupational Employment Statistics. https://www.bls.gov/data/; US Census Bureau, Population. 2017. https://www.census.gov/topics/population.html

34. Personal communication from Julie Sochalski, PhD.

35. Peter Buerhaus, Lucy Skinner, David Auerbach, et al. "Four Challenges Facing the Nursing Workforce in the United States," *J Nurs Regul.* 8 (2) (2017): 40-46.

36. Stephen Petterson, Robert McNellis, Kathleen Klink, et al. *The State of Primary Care in the United States* (Washington, DC: Robert Graham Center, January 2018).

37. National Commission on Certification of Physician Assistants (NCCPA). "Certified Physician Assistant Population Trends," 2012 data from NCCPA.

38. National Council of State Boards of Nursing. "Progress and Precision: The NCSBN 2018 Environmental Scan," *J Nurs Regul.* 8 (4) (2018, Suppl): S1-S48.

39. Nurses of Pennsylvania. *Breaking Point: Pennsylvania's Patient Care Crisis* (September 2017). Available online: https://nursesofpa.org/wp-content/uploads/2017/09/Nurses-of-Pa-Patient-Care-Crisis-Report.pdf. Accessed on July 28, 2020.

40. Everett Hughes. "Professions," *Daedalus* 92 (4) (1965). Eliot Freidson. *The Profession of Medicine* (Chicago, IL: University of Chicago Press, 1970).

41. Norman Denzin and Curtis Mettlin. "Incomplete Professionalization: The Case of Pharmacy," *Social Forces* 46 (3) (1968): 375-381.

42. Claudia Goldin and Lawrence Katz. "A Most Egalitarian Profession: Pharmacy and the Evolution of a Family-Friendly Occupation," *J Labor Econ.* 34 (3) (2016): 705-746.

43. University of California. *An Era of Growth and Change: A Closer Look at Pharmacy Education and Practice* (February 2014). Available online: https://www.ucop.edu/health-sciences-services/_files/pharmacy-an-era-of-growth-and-change.pdf. Accessed on November 5, 2020.

44. Judith Cooksey, Katherine Knapp, Surrey Walton, et al. "Challenges to the Pharmacist Profession From Escalating Pharmaceutical Demand," *Health Aff.* 21 (5) (2002): 182-188.

45. University of California. *An Era of Growth and Change: A Closer Look at Pharmacy Education and Practice* (February 2014). Available online: https://www.ucop.edu/health-sciences-services/_files/pharmacy-an-era-of-growth-and-change.pdf. Accessed on November 5, 2020.

46. Reference for Business. "SIC 5912 Drug Stores and Proprietary Stores." Available online: https://www.referenceforbusiness.com/industries/Retail-Trade/Drug-Stores-Proprietary-Stores.html. Accessed on March 8, 2020.

47. Pete Hatemi and Christopher Zorn. *Independent Pharmacies in the U.S. Are More on the Rise Than on the Decline* (PCMA, March 2020). Available online: https://www.pcmanet.org/wp-content/uploads/2020/03/FINAL_Independent-Pharmacies-in-the-U.S.-are-More-on-the-Rise-than-on-the-Decline.pdf. Accessed on March 8, 2020.

48. Donald Klepser, Liyan Xu, Fred Ullrich, et al. "Trends in Community Pharmacy Counts and Closures Before and After Implementation of Medicare Part D," *J Rural Health.* 27 (2011): 168-175.

49. John Grabenstein. "Trends in the Numbers of US Colleges of Pharmacies and Their Graduates, 1900 to 2014," *Am J Pharm Educ.* 80 (2) (2016): 1-10.

50. Rob Bertman. "Pharmacist Job Outlook: It's Worse Than You Thought," *Student Loan Planner* (September 18, 2019).

51. Sharon Terlep and Jaewon Kang. "The Pharmacist Is Out: Supermarkets Close Pharmacy Counters," *Wall Street Journal* (January 27, 2020).

52. University of California. *An Era of Growth and Change: A Closer Look at Pharmacy Education and Practice* (February 2014). Available online: https://www.ucop.edu/health-sciences-services/_files/pharmacy-an-era-of-growth-and-change.pdf. Accessed on November 5, 2020.

53. Judith Cooksey, Katherine Knapp, Surrey Walton, et al. "Challenges to the Pharmacist Profession From Escalating Pharmaceutical Demand," *Health Aff.* 21 (5) (2002): 182-188.

54. Stephen Schondelmeyer. "Recent Economic Trends in American Pharmacy," *Pharm Hist.* 51 (3) (2009): 103-126.

55. Adam Fein. *The 2018 Economic Report on U.S. Pharmacies and Pharmacy Benefit Managers* (Philadelphia, PA: Drug Channels Institute, February 2018).

56. Alex Barker. "Understanding Pharmacy Job Trends and What They Mean For Your Career," *The Happy PharmD* (November 29, 2018).

57. Mary E. Dunham, Paul W. Bush, and Amanda M. Ball. "Evidence of Burnout in Health-System Pharmacists," *Am J Health Syst Pharm.* 75 (4) (2018): S93-S100. Mark A. Munger, Eliot Gordon, John Hartman, et al. "Community Pharmacists' Occupational Satisfaction and Stress: A Profession in Jeopardy?" *J Am Pharm Assoc.* 53 (3) (2013): 30-44.

58. Claudia Goldin and Lawrence Katz. "A Most Egalitarian Profession: Pharmacy and the Evolution of a Family-Friendly Occupation," *J Labor Econ.* 34 (3) (2016): 705-746.

59. Ellen Gabler. "How Chaos at Chain Pharmacies Is Putting Patients at Risk," *New York Times* (January 31, 2020).

60. W. Richard Scott. "Managing Professional Work: Three Models of Control for Health Organizations," *Health Serv Res.* 17 (3) (1982): 213-240.

61. Robert E. Grant. "The State of U.S. Healthcare: An Iron Cage of Bureaucracy," *The Doctor Weighs In* (July 18, 2018). Available online: https://thedoctorweighsin.com/state-of-u-s-healthcare-iron-cage-of-bureaucracy/. Accessed on March 11, 2020.

# 11

# Hospitals

## OVERVIEW AND TYPES OF HOSPITALS

The United States had 6,146 hospitals as of January 2020 (Figure 11-1). Hospitals are typically classified by the types of services they render, their average length of stay, ownership, and teaching affiliation. With regard to *service*, 5,198 of the 6,146 facilities are considered "community hospitals." These provide either (1) general medical-surgical services that span lots of specialties or (2) specialty services for specific diseases and conditions (eg, rehabilitation, orthopedic, obstetrics/gynecology, ear/nose/throat, long-term acute care). Most of the beds set up and staffed in hospitals are for general medical-surgical patients; only a fraction are set up for intensive care units (ICUs) and other specialized purposes (eg, burn units). There are also more than 400 psychiatric hospitals in the private sector that treat patients with mental health illnesses (severe depression, substance abuse) requiring acute hospital care. Noncommunity ("other" in Figure 11-1) hospitals include prison hospitals and school infirmaries.

With regard to *length of stay*, general medical-surgical hospitals are considered "short term" if they admit patients for less than 30-day stays. By contrast, long-term care hospitals (LTCHs), also known as long-term acute care (LTAC) hospitals, admit patients for stays lasting 30 or more days.

Hospitals can also be classified based on their *ownership*. Roughly 60% of the community hospitals (2,937) are nonprofit institutions owned by their local community; another 25% (1,296) are for-profit hospitals owned by publicly traded companies (hence the label "investor-owned");

the remaining 15% (965) are owned by state and local governments. A small number (200) and percentage of hospitals are owned and operated by the federal government for former or active military personnel (eg, Veterans Administration, Department of Defense).

Community hospitals can be further classified by their *teaching status*. Teaching hospitals train future physicians and other healthcare professionals, conduct research projects and clinical trials on new drugs and therapies, and care for patients with rare or complex conditions. There are various methods used to delineate gradations in the teaching status of a hospital. Some researchers define *major* teaching hospitals as (1) belonging to the Council of Teaching Hospitals (COTH) of the Association of American Medical Colleges; (2) offering a specified ratio of interns and residents to beds, ranging from more than 0.10 to more than 0.27; or (3) being designated as a flagship hospital or major affiliate of a medical school (ie, academic medical center [AMC]). By contrast, *minor* teaching status is alternatively defined as the presence of a residency program, a minor affiliation with a medical school, or simply as those not meeting the criteria for major teaching status outlined earlier. Nonteaching hospitals have professionally trained medical staff that focus on providing essential care for patients in a community rather than conducting medical training and research.

These gradations in teaching status are nearly synonymous with an earlier classification introduced in Chapter 3 about "levels of care" (primary, secondary, tertiary, quaternary). Secondary care is provided by general medical-surgical community hospitals that offer the services of specialist physicians but usually lack teaching functions

| Total Number of All US Hospitals | 6,146 |
|---|---|
| Number of US **Community** Hospitals | 5,198 |
| Number of Nongovernment Not-for-Profit Community Hospitals | 2,937 |
| Number of Investor-Owned (For-Profit) Community Hospitals | 1,296 |
| Number of State and Local Government Community Hospitals | 965 |
| Number of Federal Government Hospitals | 209 |
| Number of Nonfederal Psychiatric Hospitals | 616 |
| **Other** Hospitals | 123 |

| Total Staffed Beds in All US Hospitals | 924,107 |
|---|---|
| Staffed Beds in Community Hospitals | 792,417 |
| **Intensive Care Beds** in Community Hospitals | |
| **Medical-Surgical Intensive Care** Beds in Community Hospitals | 46,825 |
| **Cardiac Intensive Care** Beds in Community Hospitals | 14,439 |
| **Neonatal Intensive Care** Beds in Community Hospitals | 22,860 |
| **Pediatric Intensive Care** Beds in Community Hospitals | 5,131 |
| **Burn Care** Beds in Community Hospitals | 1,198 |
| **Other Intensive Care** Beds in Community Hospitals | 7,323 |
| Total Admissions in All US Hospitals | 36,353,946 |
| Admissions in Community Hospitals | 34,251,159 |

**Figure 11-1** • Characteristics of US Hospitals. (Source: American Hospital Association.)

(eg, residency programs). Tertiary and quaternary care is provided by AMCs and other teaching hospitals; both involve specialized equipment and personnel, with quaternary care being much more unusual and much less prevalent in supply.

AMCs are the most complex type of hospital and feature a dizzying array of organizational arrangements between their constituents—the medical school, the hospital, the physicians, and the host university.[1] Figure 11-2 illustrates the

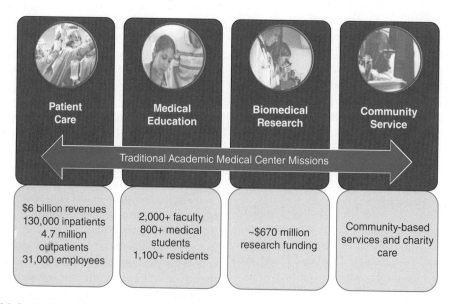

| Patient Care | Medical Education | Biomedical Research | Community Service |
|---|---|---|---|
| | *Traditional Academic Medical Center Missions* | | |
| $6 billion revenues 130,000 inpatients 4.7 million outpatients 31,000 employees | 2,000+ faculty 800+ medical students 1,100+ residents | ~$670 million research funding | Community-based services and charity care |

**Figure 11-2** • Scale and Scope of Academic Medical Center Mission.

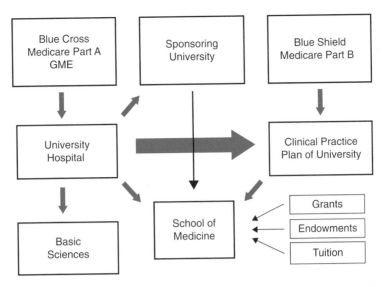

**Figure 11-3** • Following the Money in the Academic Medical Center. GME, Graduate Medical Education.

scale and scope of their multiple missions, using information from the University of Pennsylvania Health System. Figure 11-3 illustrates the complex "flow of funds" that financially support these diverse missions. Inpatient care is reimbursed by private insurers (eg, Blue Cross) and Medicare Part A, as well as supported by graduate medical education (GME) payments from Medicare to defray some of the costs of care rendered by residents. The monies received by the hospital are then disbursed in various directions—some to the sponsoring (parent) university, some to fund the departments of basic sciences, some to fund the school of medicine, and some to fund the clinical practices of physicians that compose the faculty practice plan.

## DISTINGUISHING NONPROFIT AND FOR-PROFIT HOSPITALS

The majority of community hospitals (both in the United States and worldwide) are organized and operated as nonprofit corporations. Nonprofit corporation statutes require that the corporation exist for a limited number of purposes: charitable, scientific, educational, benevolent, religious, etc. The Internal Revenue Service (IRS) Code, Section 501(c)(3), grants tax-exempt status to nonprofit firms provided they are organized and operated for charitable purposes.

Beginning in 1956, the IRS required hospitals to provide charity care (care at free or discounted prices) to be eligible for *federal tax*

exemption. In 1969, the IRS no longer specifically required charitable activity as long as the hospital provided "community benefits" (eg, promotion of health, operation of an emergency room open to all members of the community regardless of ability to pay). That is, healthcare itself was considered a sufficient charitable purpose for exemption, regardless of the level of charity care provided.[2] The 1969 ruling identified other factors that might warrant tax exemption including a governing board composed of community members and using surplus revenues to improve facilities, patient care, medical training, education, and research.[3]

Nonprofit hospitals can also receive exemption from *state and local taxes* by meeting standards that vary by state. In most states, the group of nonprofits eligible for a charitable property tax exemption largely overlaps with those designated as 501(c)(3) charitable nonprofits at the federal level, with the further stipulation that property must be both owned by such a nonprofit and used to serve its exempt purpose. Tax exemption allows nonprofit hospitals to devote their income to internal operations and service expansions that supply these public goods. To retain their tax exemption, hospitals cannot allow their surplus revenues or assets to "inure" to the benefit of (ie, be appropriated by) any private individuals. Nonprofit hospitals are "owned" by a variety of groups, such as local citizens, churches, other philanthropic organizations, and local government. These groups, along with the hospital's managers and physicians, serve as the "residual claimants" in the absence of public shareholders.

The restraint against private inurement represents the major difference between nonprofit and for-profit hospitals. Such restraint leads nonprofit hospitals to engage in different strategies, such as research and education, investments in unprofitable and/or specialty services, and support of nonprofitable services and activities. Indeed, nonprofits hold their assets in the form of a trust, dedicate themselves to serving purposes that states deem charitable, and are less likely to make misleading claims and exploit vulnerable clients.[4]

By contrast, for-profit firms are not exempt from taxes. They are free to distribute their operating surplus to shareholders as partial return on their invested capital. They are not bound by many of the legal and legislative limitations related to exempt status. They may also selectively offer profitable clinical services (eg, open-heart surgery, cardiac catheterization laboratory) while not offering unprofitable services

(eg, psychiatric emergency services, AIDS services, trauma center).[5]

## THE IMPORTANCE AND CENTRALITY OF HOSPITALS

Hospitals are also commonly distinguished in terms of their "bed size" (number of patient beds). The American Hospital Association (AHA) classifies hospitals into 8 bed size categories; the majority (including most rural hospitals) have less than 200 beds, whereas only a few (often AMCs in large metro areas) have 500+ beds. The historical distribution of hospitals by bed size is presented in Figure 11-4.

Make no mistake: Despite their small average size, hospitals are important. Hospitals account for the single largest share (~33%) of national health expenditures in the United States. Their inpatient and outpatient services also account for 2 of the largest expense categories of health

[Data are based on reporting by a census of hospitals]

| Type of ownership and size of hospital | 1975 | 1980 | 1990 | 2000 | 2005 | 2010 | 2013 | 2014 | 2015 |
|---|---|---|---|---|---|---|---|---|---|
| Hospitals | | | | | Number | | | | |
| All hospitals | 7,156 | 6,965 | 6,649 | 5,810 | 5,756 | 5,754 | 5,686 | 5,627 | 5,564 |
| Federal | 382 | 359 | 337 | 245 | 226 | 213 | 213 | 213 | 212 |
| Nonfederal | 6,774 | 6,606 | 6,312 | 5,565 | 5,530 | 5,541 | 5,473 | 5,414 | 5,352 |
| Community | 5,875 | 5,830 | 5,384 | 4,915 | 4,936 | 4,985 | 4,974 | 4,926 | 4,862 |
| Nonprofit | 3,339 | 3,322 | 3,191 | 3,003 | 2,958 | 2,904 | 2,904 | 2,870 | 2,845 |
| For-profit | 775 | 730 | 749 | 749 | 868 | 1,013 | 1,060 | 1,053 | 1,034 |
| State-local government | 1,761 | 1,778 | 1,444 | 1,163 | 1,110 | 1,068 | 1,010 | 1,003 | 983 |
| 6-24 beds | 299 | 259 | 226 | 288 | 370 | 424 | 469 | 486 | 499 |
| 25-49 beds | 1,155 | 1,029 | 935 | 910 | 1,032 | 1,167 | 1,186 | 1,168 | 1,146 |
| 50-99 beds | 1,481 | 1,462 | 1,263 | 1,055 | 1,001 | 970 | 959 | 934 | 916 |
| 100-199 beds | 1,363 | 1,370 | 1,306 | 1,236 | 1,129 | 1,029 | 995 | 1,013 | 983 |
| 200-299 beds | 678 | 715 | 739 | 656 | 619 | 585 | 571 | 536 | 535 |
| 300-399 beds | 378 | 412 | 408 | 341 | 368 | 352 | 334 | 328 | 322 |
| 400-499 beds | 230 | 266 | 222 | 182 | 173 | 185 | 183 | 188 | 177 |
| 500 beds or more | 291 | 317 | 285 | 247 | 244 | 273 | 277 | 273 | 284 |
| Beds | | | | | | | | | |
| All hospitals | 1,465,828 | 1,364,516 | 1,213,327 | 983,628 | 946,997 | 941,995 | 914,513 | 902,202 | 897,961 |
| Federal | 131,946 | 117,328 | 98,255 | 53,067 | 45,837 | 44,940 | 38,747 | 38,893 | 38,863 |
| Nonfederal | 1,333,882 | 1,247,188 | 1,115,072 | 930,561 | 901,160 | 897,055 | 875,766 | 863,309 | 859,098 |
| Community | 941,844 | 988,387 | 927,360 | 823,560 | 802,311 | 804,943 | 795,603 | 786,874 | 782,188 |
| Nonprofit | 658,195 | 692,459 | 656,755 | 582,988 | 561,106 | 555,768 | 543,929 | 534,554 | 530,579 |
| For-profit | 73,495 | 87,033 | 101,377 | 109,883 | 113,510 | 124,652 | 134,643 | 135,909 | 134,569 |
| State-local government | 210,154 | 208,895 | 169,228 | 130,689 | 127,695 | 124,523 | 117,031 | 116,411 | 117,040 |
| 6-24 beds | 5,615 | 4,932 | 4,427 | 5,156 | 6,316 | 7,261 | 7,763 | 7,985 | 8,237 |
| 25-49 beds | 41,783 | 37,478 | 35,420 | 33,333 | 33,726 | 37,446 | 38,039 | 37,559 | 37,020 |
| 50-99 beds | 106,776 | 105,278 | 90,394 | 75,865 | 71,737 | 69,470 | 67,892 | 66,092 | 65,208 |
| 100-199 beds | 192,438 | 192,892 | 183,867 | 175,778 | 161,593 | 148,090 | 143,760 | 147,188 | 142,471 |
| 200-299 beds | 164,405 | 172,390 | 179,670 | 159,807 | 151,290 | 142,616 | 140,113 | 131,526 | 131,287 |
| 300-399 beds | 127,728 | 139,434 | 138,938 | 117,220 | 126,899 | 121,749 | 115,511 | 112,909 | 111,139 |
| 400-499 beds | 101,278 | 117,724 | 98,833 | 80,763 | 76,894 | 82,071 | 81,148 | 83,285 | 78,276 |
| 500 beds or more | 201,821 | 218,259 | 195,811 | 175,638 | 173,856 | 196,240 | 201,377 | 200,330 | 208,550 |

**Figure 11-4** • Trends in Hospitals. (Source: Centers for Disease Control and Prevention.)

insurers: inpatient care (25%) and outpatient care (10%). Some of the most expensive encounters in our healthcare system involve the hospital: an inpatient admission and a visit to the emergency department. Hospitals are a major cause of rising healthcare costs, not only because of the expensive services they render but also because of the high prices they charge insurers for them.

Hospitals are important for other reasons. The history of the US healthcare system dating back to the late 19th century is inextricably tied to the rise of the modern hospital and the shift from primary care provided by a community practitioner to advanced care rendered by a hospital-based specialist. The hospital setting is where most physicians and nurses are trained; 62.4% of registered nurses are employed in hospitals (as of 2016). In the United States as well as in other countries (India, China), the hospital is also the center of the country's healthcare delivery system.

## FUNCTIONS THAT HOSPITALS PERFORM

Hospitals perform a host of important functions as well. First and foremost, they provide secondary and tertiary patient care on both an inpatient and outpatient basis; they may also sponsor the provision of primary care clinics and multispecialty groups in the community. Second, they provide professional education to physicians (eg, residency programs), medical and nursing students, and other trainees. Third, a subset of hospitals (the AMCs) conducts biomedical research, largely funded by the National Institutes of Health (NIH; see Chapter 25). Fourth, hospitals are often the major employer in their local community, serve as a big source of jobs, and exert a major impact on the local economy. Figure 11-5 indicates they are the second largest sector of employment; however, hospital employment levels have been stable over the past few years (Figure 11-6). Fifth, hospitals serve as the "physician's workshop" for community-based practitioners with admitting privileges who send their patients to the facility for treatment. Sixth, hospitals provide educational and health promotion services for community residents (eg, health fairs), as well as important public health functions (eg, quarantine patients with infectious diseases), custodial functions (eg, contain patients with severe psychiatric disorders), and charitable functions (free care for the indigent). Seventh, publicly held (for-profit) hospitals earn financial returns

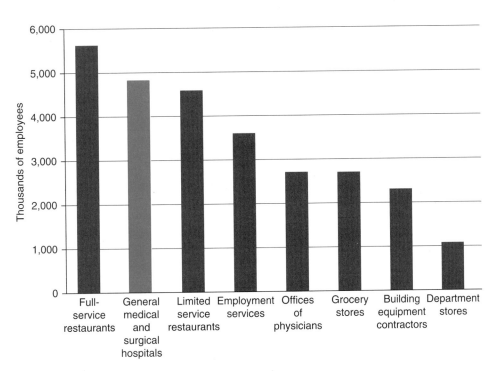

**Figure 11-5** • Hospital Employment Versus Employment in Other Industries, 2020. (Source: Bureau of Labor Statistics.)

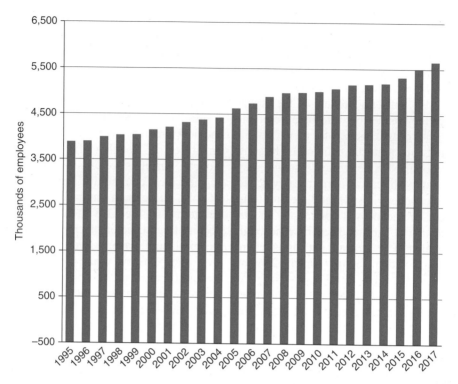

**Figure 11-6** • Number of Full-Time and Part-Time Hospital Employees, 1995 to 2017. (Source: American Hospital Association.)

for investors. Eighth, and finally, hospitals serve as the locus for the major rites of passage in human life: birth, healing, and death—or, as the English say, "hatch 'em, patch 'em, and dispatch 'em."

## THE COMPLEX HOSPITAL STRUCTURE

Hospitals are among the most complex bureaucracies on the face of the earth. This partly reflects the multiple functions they perform (patient care, teaching, research, community service). Their complexity also stems heavily from the multiple occupational groups they house (covered previously in Chapters 9 and 10). But in particular, their real complexity rests elsewhere—on 3 groups of leaders and the presence of a "dual hierarchy" of administrators and physicians (Figure 11-7).

In most organizations, there is a governing body (eg, board of directors) and a body of senior managers composed of the chief executive officer, the chief operating officer, the chief financial officer, and so on (ie, the C-suite; also jokingly referred to as "the O-zone"). But

hospitals feature a third leadership group that creates a dual hierarchy in the institution. On the one hand, there is the *administrative hierarchy*, headed by the C-suite, that oversees a sprawling array of professional departments (eg, nursing, pharmacy, radiology), nonprofessional departments (eg, materials management, central sterile supply), and administrative functions (eg, human resources, finance, planning). On the other hand, there is also the *medical staff hierarchy*, which is not under the supervision of the administrative hierarchy but is separate, parallel, autonomous, and self-governing. This is not found in any other organization. How did we get here?

Since the early part of the 20th century, medical care has become more technologically complex, with a growing reliance on sophisticated equipment, services, and personnel to operate them. The hospital thus became a component of more sophisticated care for the physician's seriously-ill patients. The hospital and physician became more dependent on each other. For their part, hospitals needed physicians to admit their patients to fill the facility's beds, to utilize the facility's ancillary services (eg, laboratory, x-ray), and to refer to the hospital's specialists. For their

**Medical Hierarchy**

**Administrative Hierarchy**

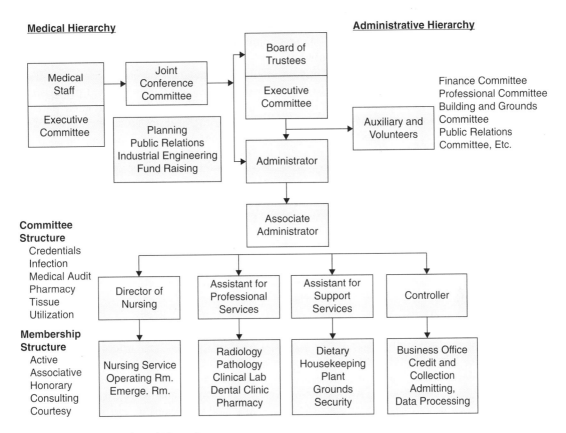

**Figure 11-7** • Hospital Dual Hierarchy.

part, physicians' office practices became more reliant on expensive hospital facilities and services to render quality care to their patients, as well as on the hospital's residents (house staff) to care for their patients when hospitalized. Physicians increasingly sought and obtained privileges at local community hospitals where they could admit and/or treat their patients and enjoy these benefits.

Why is this important? As noted in a prior chapter, physicians are collectively responsible for 85% to 90% of all healthcare spending. Physicians who are members of the hospital's medical staff hierarchy can direct those in the hospital's administrative hierarchy to conduct patient care activities that expend clinical resources (eg, administer drugs, order diagnostic tests, utilize operating rooms) and increase healthcare costs. And yet, these same physicians are not (usually) employees of the hospital or even under the direct supervision of the administrative hierarchy. Instead, they collectively govern their own affairs but are individually responsible for the patients they admit. How did we get here?

The American College of Surgeons (ACS; discussed in Chapter 7) was founded in 1913 to develop standards for surgeons as well as minimum standards for hospitals, in tandem with the standardization of medical education (as part of the Flexner reforms). Its initial standard was issued in 1918; by 1926, it had published a manual to guide hospital standardization. The ACS was reconstituted in 1951 as The Joint Commission on Accreditation of Healthcare Organizations (JCAHO), later renamed The Joint Commission.

The Joint Commission performs the national accreditation function for US hospitals, which is a prerequisite for hospital participation in and reimbursement under the federal Medicare and Medicaid programs. Hospitals need to demonstrate compliance with the Joint Commission standards to receive this accreditation and be certified by the federal government. According to the Joint Commission, its accreditation process and standards (published in a manual) form the basis for an objective evaluation to help healthcare organizations measure, assess, and improve their performance. The standards focus on important patient, individual or resident care, and organization functions that are essential to providing safe, high-quality care.

As the national accrediting body for US hospitals, the Joint Commission issues standards for how hospital medical staffs should be structured. The primary purpose of the "organized medical staff structure," according to the Joint Commission, is to approve the medical staff's bylaws and provide oversight for quality, treatment, and services "provided by practitioners with privileges." These practitioners are medical staff members with independent privileges. While accountable to the hospital's board of trustees for quality of care, the medical staff is self-governing with explicitly recognized oversight regarding quality of care rendered by physician members. That oversight is exercised through 3 mechanisms: organized medical staff activities (eg, establish the criteria for becoming a medical staff member, establish the criteria for credentialing and delineating privileges), delegation to individual practitioners, and development of medical staff bylaws (rules for self-governance). The hospital's board approves these medical staff bylaws, but the medical staff enforces them; the 2 groups are to work collaboratively, but each has clearly recognized roles and responsibilities.

Paradoxically, what is contained herein is a nonhierarchical medical staff hierarchy. The organized medical staff designates member licensed independent practitioners to provide oversight of care rendered by practitioners with privileges. Licensed independent practitioner members of the medical staff are (1) designated to perform the oversight activities of the organized medical staff and (2) responsible for the oversight responsibilities of the organized medical staff. Thus, oversight rests on a collection of individuals rather than a hierarchy of authority within the medical staff; there is no chain of command. The management and coordination of each patient's care are the responsibility of a licensed practitioner with the appropriate clinical privileges. The organized medical staff determines the circumstances under which consultation or management by a physician is required; the hospital administrative hierarchy plays no role here. Thus, "oversight" by the organized medical staff is delegated to individual physician members and exercised through the medical staff membership process such that individual members meet professional criteria.

To the degree that it occurs, physicians supervise the activities of other physicians in the hospital via a process of peer review, as outlined in the hospital medical staff bylaws. In most community hospitals, the vast majority of the physicians included within the medical hierarchy are independent practitioners, have office-based practices, have been granted privileges to admit their patients to and treat their patients at the hospital, and are collectively referred to as the "voluntary" medical staff of the hospital.

These physicians are not salaried employees of the hospital and come and go from the hospital as they please. They view and utilize the hospital as an extension of their office practice; thus, scholars have labeled the hospital as "the physicians' workshop."[6] A State of New Jersey commission report concluded that the physician workshop model accurately describes the state's nonprofit hospital sector.[7] As self-employed professionals, physicians utilize the hospitals where they have privileges

> as free workshops whose resources they can enlist in the treatment of their patients more or less as these physicians see fit. Remarkably, in that arrangement, affiliated physicians do not usually render formal accountability for their use of hospital resources in the treatment of their patients. Because affiliated physicians are the major source of revenue for hospitals, hospital managers have little economic leverage over affiliated physicians in efforts to control the physicians' use of hospital resources.[8]

In an era of bed surpluses and lower than optimal occupancy rates, as is the case in New Jersey, hospitals have even less leverage over, and are even more dependent upon, their physicians.

The persistence of this dual hierarchy has been reinforced by separate payment/reimbursement schemes for the hospital and the physician. Beginning in the early 1930s, hospitals received reimbursement through Blue Cross insurance plans; starting in the late 1930s, physicians received reimbursement through Blue Shield insurance plans. Blue Cross was organized by the AHA; Blue Shield was organized by the American Medical Association. The 2 associations and their insurance schemes were kept separate to prevent either party from exerting any control over the other's income stream. The separation was further institutionalized in the 1965 Social Security Act Amendment XVIII that established the Medicare program: Hospitals were reimbursed under Part A of Medicare (with Blue Cross as the main fiscal intermediary), whereas physicians were reimbursed under Part B (with Blue Shield as the main fiscal intermediary). This separation of payment, in both commercial and public insurance schemes, has largely remained in place.

Dr. Paul Schyve, former senior vice president of the Joint Commission, has complained about the Joint Commission standards. The unique role of independent practitioners on the medical staff has 2 implications for the hospital's ability to achieve its goals, let alone help with the triple aim and iron triangle:

First, the licensed independent practitioners (for example, physicians) cannot be *clinically* supervised by someone who is not a licensed independent practitioner. If an unlicensed individual were to *clinically* supervise a physician or other licensed independent practitioner, that individual would be "practicing without a license," and, therefore, acting illegally. (Note that a licensed independent practitioner may be *administratively* supervised by a non-licensed independent practitioner [for example,

as an employee]; it is *clinical* supervision that can only be provided by someone who is also licensed to practice.)

The second implication for the healthcare organization is that the clinical decisions licensed independent practitioners make about their patients drive much of the rest of the organization's use of resources—from nursing care to diagnostic imaging to laboratory testing to medication use—and affect the organization's ability to achieve its goal of providing high-quality, safe care.[9]

The result, depicted in Figure 11-8, is the "real hierarchy" in the hospital: the individual physician who directs and spends just about everything.

In practice, according to Schyve, this leaves the hospital with multiple leadership silos: the board, the C-suite, the medical staff, and (even) the nursing staff. The hospital organization requires systems thinking and collaboration across these silos, but allows the medical staff to govern itself. Although the medical staff has a medical executive committee and a structure comprised of various leadership roles (eg, president, chief medical officer), departments (eg, surgery, internal medicine), and committees (eg, credentials, infection

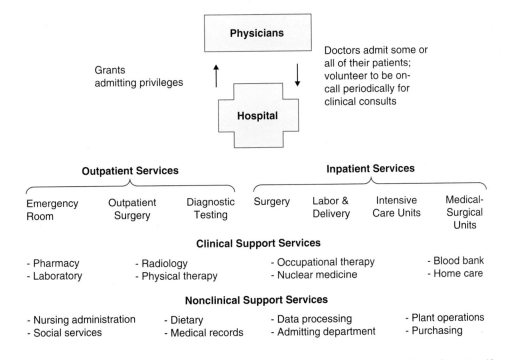

**Figure 11-8** • The Hospital's "Real Hierarchy": Services That Largely Serve the Admitting Physician. (Source: Sean Nicholson, Cornell University.)

| | | | |
|---|---|---|---|
| ☐ Internal Medicine | ☐ Cardiology | ☐ Pulmonary Medicine | ☐ Gastroenterology |
| ☐ Nephrology | ☐ Endocrinology | ☐ Hematology and Oncology | ☐ Radiation Oncology |
| ☐ Rheumatology | ☐ Infectious Disease | ☐ Cardiothoracic Intensive Care | ☐ Family Medicine |
| ☐ General Surgery | ☐ Thoracic Surgery | ☐ Gastrointestinal Surgery | ☐ Colorectal Surgery |
| ☐ Pediatric Surgery | ☐ Resuscitative Intensive Care | ☐ Pediatrics | ☐ Pediatric Oncology |
| ☐ Pediatric Endocrinology | ☐ Pediatric Nephrology | ☐ Pediatric Infectious Diseases | ☐ Pediatric Neurology |
| ☐ Neonatology | ☐ Pediatric Cardiology | ☐ Pediatric Emergency and Clinical Care Medicine | ☐ Obstetrics and Gynecology |
| ☐ Gynecologic Oncology | ☐ Orthopedics | ☐ Joint Reconstruction | ☐ Urology |
| ☐ ENT (Otolaryngology) | ☐ Opthalmology | ☐ Dermatology | ☐ Neurology |
| ☐ Psychiatry | ☐ Rehabilitation | ☐ Anesthesiology (Anesthesia) | ☐ Diagnostic Radiology |
| ☐ Radiotherapy | ☐ Clinical Pathology | ☐ Anatomical Pathology | ☐ Plastic Surgery |
| ☐ Emergency Medicine | ☐ Dentistry (Dental) | ☐ Oral Surgery | ☐ Home Care |

**Figure 11-9** • Medical Staff Fragmentation by Clinical Department. ENT, Ear, Nose, and Throat.

control, pharmacy and therapeutics), these constitute "liaisons" and communication channels more than any formal chain of command. Moreover, there can be lots of clinical departments, which some liken to the pre–World War I Balkan states (Figure 11-9).

But the medical staff is even more complex than this! The medical staff structure is really a "matrix" composed of vertical departments (with their own department chairs) and a horizontal overlay of committees (composed of physicians from different departments). Thus, the hospital has a matrixed medical staff within a dual hierarchy—2 very cumbersome administrative mechanisms that challenge running the organization smoothly.

## HOSPITAL-PHYSICIAN RELATIONSHIPS

The prior section summarized the collective organization of physicians that compose the medical staff. It is also important to describe the relationship of an individual physician with the hospital. As noted earlier, most US physicians were historically autonomous practitioners with private offices in the community. For those patients who needed hospital treatment, office physicians had 2 choices: They could refer their patient to a specialist already on the medical staff at the hospital, or they could themselves obtain privileges to admit and treat their patients at the hospital. To do so, the physician would first apply for membership on the medical staff, wait for a medical staff committee to evaluate and approve his or her credentials (eg, medical school training, medical licensure), and then be granted admitting privileges (at first on a probationary basis).

Physicians thus split their practice time between (1) seeing patients in their community offices and (2) seeing patients in a hospital where they had privileges. To reduce travel time, most physicians located their offices near the hospital they used. Many physicians obtained privileges at multiple hospitals, also located closer (rather than farther away) from their offices, in order

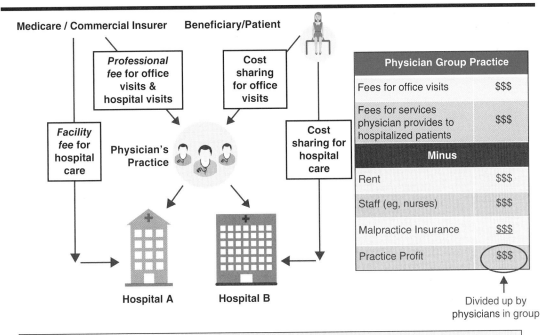

**Figure 11-10** • Historic Relationship Between Physicians and Hospitals: Admitting Privileges and the Voluntary Medical Staff Model. (Source: Sean Nicholson, Cornell University.)

to (1) access a broader range of specialists, services, and facilities; (2) maintain some options in case one hospital's beds and services were too busy; and/or (3) reduce overdependence on one hospital. The relationship between the community physician and the hospital(s) used is depicted in Figure 11-10.

Currently, roughly 40% of physicians practice medicine as solo practitioners or in small partnerships with another physician. Much of the remaining physician population practices in medical groups, defined as groups with 3 or more doctors. Roughly 80% of physicians in group practice are practicing in small groups (ie, groups with <10 doctors). Only 5% of group practices are large in size (50 or more doctors).[10]

The economic model for the office-based physician has historically been driven by *professional fees* for seeing patients in the office and in the hospital. For its part, the hospital's economic model has historically rested on *institutional fees* (also known as facility fees) generated when the patient is admitted to the hospital; these fees cover the hospital's expenditures on staff (eg, nurses, technicians, housekeepers) as well as equipment and supplies used in patient care.

Over time, this traditional model of physician-hospital relationships has diversified to include 2 additional models (Figure 11-11). *First,* there are a handful of physicians who specialize in using diagnostic and therapeutic services typically found only in a hospital, such as radiology, anesthesiology, pathology, and emergency medicine. It is not possible to operate a modern hospital without them. These physicians do not usually see patients in community offices but rather see patients in the hospital based on referrals from colleagues; they are referred to as hospital-based practitioners (HBPs). For example, radiologists are consulted when other doctors require imaging tests to confirm or disconfirm a diagnosis; anesthesiologists accompany the patients of surgeons who are about to enter the operating room; and pathologists typically examine the tissues and specimens of patients seen by other physicians, again to confirm or disconfirm diagnoses. Due to their consultative practices, they have to locate their practices near large groups of physicians or, more typically, by hospitals that contain large numbers of physicians on their medical staffs. Over time, hospitals have come to contract out the management of these areas to physician groups in each of the

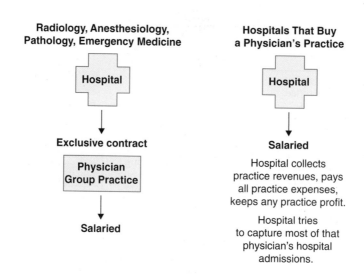

**Figure 11-11** • Two Other Physician-Hospital Practice Relationships. (Source: Sean Nicholson, Cornell University.)

relevant specialties, as well as others like oncology. These practitioners are often organized in local communities as large, single-specialty group practices that contract with one or more hospitals on an exclusive basis and are paid by the hospital for their professional services; in turn, the group practices pay their physician members based on salary.

*Second*, since the 1990s, a growing number of hospitals have employed physicians in certain specialties to treat their patients; these specialties can be community-based primary care physicians, community-based oncologists, hospital-based specialists such as cardiologists, and hospitalists. The percentage of US physicians who are salaried employees of hospitals is approximately 30%; however, half of these are residents who are completing their medical training. If one strips away the residents, the actual (and accurate) percentage of physicians employed by hospitals is 15% but may be rising.[11]

## THE CHALLENGE OF MANAGING A PROFESSIONAL ORGANIZATION

The preceding sections describe the challenge facing the management of healthcare. The single most expensive organizational setting (the hospital) is home to 3 leadership bases (board, executive, medical) and an independent profession, organized as an autonomous medical staff, that controls most of the decisions and the spending. This medical staff is organized, in

turn, as a matrix of lots of clinical departments and an overlay of committees in which most of the collective medical decision making occurs.

The medical staff also consists of physicians who use 1 of 3 different models to contract with the hospital for their services: community-based physician with privileges, hospital-based physicians on contract, and employed physicians who work either on salary or (more commonly) a productivity model. AHA data from 2014 suggest that the percent distribution of the medical staff across these 3 models of contracting is 42%, 38%, and 20%, respectively. Managing the medical staff and relationships with hundreds of autonomous, powerful physicians who control the hospital's fate and who are scattered across lots of specialty silos is thus akin to "herding emperors."

As noted in Chapter 9, physicians have a monopoly over the decision to admit patients, whether from their community offices or from the hospital's emergency room. To stay afloat financially, hospitals must attract physicians (and their patients) in order to generate revenues (facility fees) paid by health insurers. Certain physician specialties contribute significantly to the hospital's revenues and bottom line (Figure 11-12). Due to the presence of physician privileges at multiple hospitals (especially prevalent among active surgeons), hospitals must compete with one another for physicians' loyalty by offering expensive medical technologies that physicians and patients want, availability of beds and operating rooms, excellent nursing care for the physicians' patients, and timely completion of tests and procedures to serve the physician. At the same time, hospitals

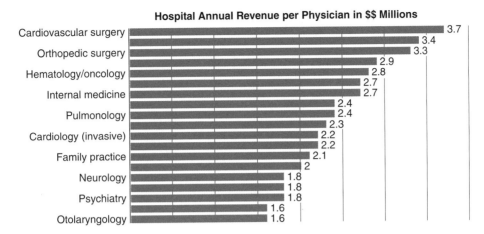

**Figure 11-12** • Specialist Physicians Contribute Substantially to Hospital Profits. (Source: Merritt Hawkins. 2019 Physician Inpatient/Outpatient Revenue Survey. https://www.merritthawkins.com/uploadedFiles/MerrittHawkins_RevenueSurvey_2019.pdf.)

must also try to attract patients from health insurers by cutting costs, accepting lower prices, and gaining inclusion in the insurer's provider network. Most insurers, starting with Medicare and its diagnosis-related groups (DRGs) payment system in the 1980s, have created incentives for hospitals to reduce costs, reduce lengths of stay, and discharge patients from the hospital faster. More recently, the Patient Protection and Affordable Care Act has ushered in new alternative payment methods (ie, not fee-for-service) that encourage physicians and hospitals to work together in an effort to simultaneously reduce costs and improve quality.

## TRENDS IN HOSPITAL CAPACITY AND UTILIZATION

Hospital utilization can be measured by a number of metrics that are used in common parlance. These metrics and their definitions are as follows:

- *Capacity*: The number of hospitals that are operating, as well as the number of beds that hospitals have staffed and made available.
- *Admissions*: The number of people admitted as inpatients to a hospital floor (ward) as inpatients for medically necessary, appropriate care and treatment of an illness or injury.
- *Inpatient days* (IPDs): The total number of patient days of care spent as

inpatients by all those admitted to (or discharged by) the hospital.
- *Average length of stay* (ALOS): The average number of days spent in the hospital by those admitted as inpatients. It is calculated by dividing the total inpatient days by the total number of admissions.
- *Average daily census* (ADC): The total number of patients admitted to a hospital for a given period (eg, by midnight). This can be calculated by adding the daily census for a month and then dividing by the number of days in the month.
- *Occupancy*: The percentage of the hospital's available beds that are occupied by inpatients. This can be calculated by dividing the average daily census by the hospital's bed count.
- *Discharges*: An alternate measure of hospital volume based on the number of patients discharged from the hospital to nonhospital settings.

Over time, the capacity (number) of US community hospitals has fallen slightly. The decline has been bigger among rural than urban hospitals (Figure 11-13). Why has this decline occurred?

The rising cost of healthcare following passage of Medicare and Medicaid in 1965 was heavily concentrated in hospital settings and specialist physicians (many of them hospital based). To combat this problem, public and private insurers encouraged the substitution of outpatient for inpatient care during the 1980s and

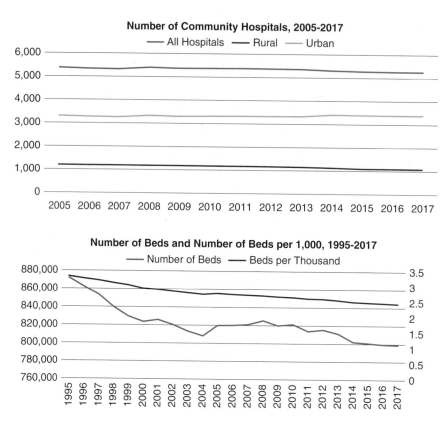

**Figure 11-13** • Number of Community Hospitals and Number of Beds. (Source: American Hospital Association, AHA Chartbook 2019, 2017 Data.)

altered the basis for paying hospitals for their inpatient care. DRGs were one weapon in the arsenal of new payment methods used; another was managed care using new insurance vehicles (eg, health maintenance organizations [HMOs]) to help promote ambulatory care (eg, ambulatory surgery centers) and hospital outpatient care over inpatient care. After 1980, outpatient care began to grow quickly, while inpatient care utilization began to stagnate. Figure 11-14 shows that hospital admissions and inpatient days per 1,000 people have been flat-liners (at best) since 1995; inpatient care is *not* a growth business.

Despite the leveling off of utilization of expensive hospitals, the trajectory of healthcare spending did not really change. As noted in Chapter 2, squeezing the balloon on the inpatient spending was largely offset by expanded spending on outpatient and physician care. Outpatient visits have become the growth market for hospitals (Figure 11-15), thereby explaining why many hospitals are constructing, modernizing, and expanding their outpatient pavilions (hint: look for cranes on the horizon). Outpatient surgeries are garnering a growing share of the hospital's

surgical volume (Figure 11-16), just as outpatient revenues are garnering a growing share of the hospital's revenue base (Figure 11-17). Outpatient care also generates higher margins than does inpatient care (Figure 11-18).

Of course, any discussion of hospital utilization needs to consider the impact of COVID-19. During the 4-month period from March to June 2020, the AHA estimated that hospitals lost $202.6 billion, or an average of $50 billion a month.[12] This largely resulted from the cancellation of elective surgeries and nonessential medical, surgical, and dental procedures. Losses also resulted from the costs of purchasing personal protective equipment (PPE) and providing support to frontline healthcare workers in COVID-19 hotspots. The US Congress moved to offset some of these losses by passing the Coronavirus Aid, Relief, and Economic Security (CARES) Act, which allocated $100 billion for provider relief. Nevertheless, top-flight hospital systems such as the Mayo Clinic and Johns Hopkins estimate a loss of nearly $300 million going into next year; other academic health systems may reportedly lose much more money.[13] Such losses

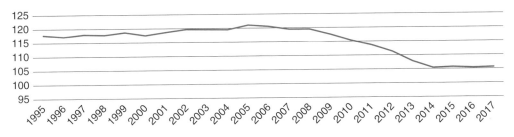

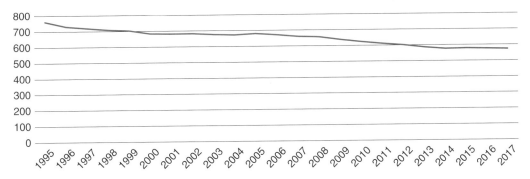

**Figure 11-14** • Trends in Hospital Inpatient Utilization. (Source: American Hospital Association, AHA Chartbook 2019, 2017 Data.)

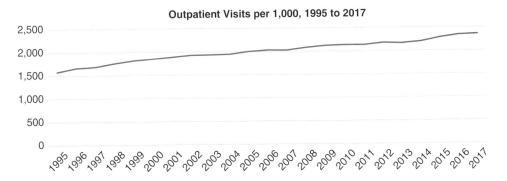

**Figure 11-15** • Hospital Outpatient Visits per 1,000 Persons, 1995 to 2017. (Source: American Hospital Association, AHA Chartbook 2019, 2017 Data.)

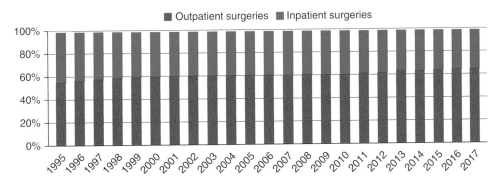

**Figure 11-16** • Percentage Share of Inpatient Versus Outpatient Surgeries, 1995 to 2017. (Source: American Hospital Association, AHA Chartbook 2019, 2017 Data.)

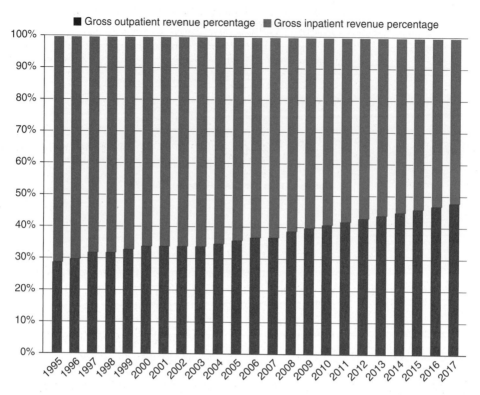

**Figure 11-17** • Distribution of Outpatient Versus Inpatient Revenues, 1995 to 2017. (Source: American Hospital Association, AHA Chartbook 2019, 2017 Data.)

led some analysts to question whether hospitals were indeed "recession proof."[14] Some also suggested that hospitals will develop "hospital-at-home" programs to treat patients where they feel most safe. Eligible patients would include those who are acutely ill, do not require intensive, 24/7 care, and can be monitored via command centers supplemented by daily home visits.[15]

## HOSPITAL FINANCES

Hospitals have 3 main sources of patient revenues: the federal Medicare program, which pays for the elderly and the disabled; the federal-state Medicaid program, which pays for the poor; and private health insurers. Between 1980 and 2017, hospitals have experienced a growth in

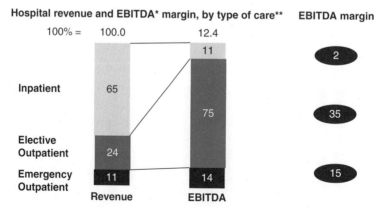

*Earnings before interest, taxes, depreciation, and amortization.
**Represents average margins across a variety of hospital types and settings and may not be representative of margins for any individual hospital.

**Figure 11-18** • Inpatient Care Generates Lower Margins for Hospitals Than Does Outpatient Care. (Source: Hospital Annual Reports; Hospital Cost Data; McKinsey Global Institute Analysis.)

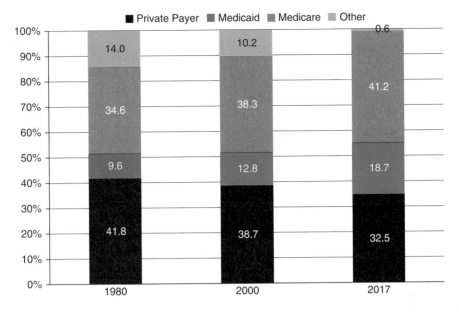

**Figure 11-19** • Distribution of Hospital Cost by Payer Type, 1980, 2000, and 2017. (Source: American Hospital Association, AHA Chartbook 2019, 2017 Data.)

the percentage of revenues coming from Medicare (from 34.6% to 41.2%) and Medicaid (from 9.6% to 18.7%) and a contraction in revenues from private insurers (from 41.8% to 32.5%) (Figure 11-19). This is significant because, in contrast to private insurers, hospitals have no bargaining power over the level of Medicare reimbursements and little to no bargaining power with state governments over the level of Medicaid reimbursements. Hospitals are thus dependent on what these public payers are willing to pay.

Moreover, as Figure 11-20 demonstrates, these public payers typically reimburse hospitals for less than 100% of what the hospitals spend to provide care to their enrollees—referred to as the payment-to-cost (PCR) ratio. Medicaid's PCR can be much lower than Medicare's. For hospital inpatient care in New Jersey, Medicaid pays far less than the full cost of services, estimated to be

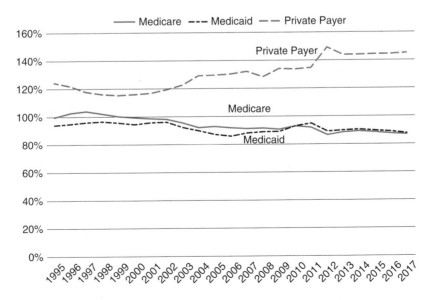

**Figure 11-20** • Aggregate Hospital Payment-to-Cost Ratios for Private Payers, Medicare, and Medicaid, 1995 to 2017. (Source: American Hospital Association, AHA Chartbook 2019, 2017 Data.)

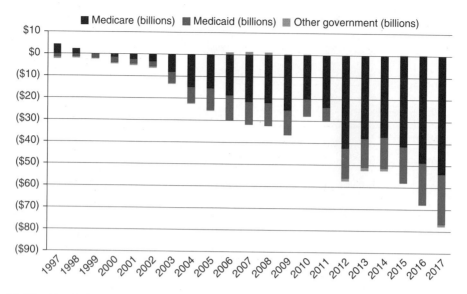

**Figure 11-21** • Hospital Payment Shortfall Relative to Costs for Medicare, Medicaid, and Other Government, 1997 to 2017. (Source: American Hospital Association, AHA Chartbook 2019, 2017 Data.)

as low as 70 to 73 cents for every dollar of costs.[16] Hospitals earn surpluses on the care provided to privately insured patients but suffer shortfalls in caring for publicly insured patients—shortfalls that have accumulated over time (Figure 11-21). Figure 11-22 shows the different methods these payers use to reimburse the hospital for treating their enrollees.

Hospitals are required to earn positive margins of revenues over expenses in order to replace plant and equipment, keep their facilities modern to attract patients and physicians, and to keep up with the rising prices of inputs

(labor and supplies). Healthcare finance scholars suggest hospitals need at least a 5% margin to cover these needs.[17]

Earning such margins has become a more difficult task over time for several reasons noted earlier. First, public payers (eg, Medicare and Medicaid) account for a growing proportion of hospital revenues (see Figure 11-19). Second, public payers reimburse hospitals using "administered" (ie, imposed top-down) prices. Third, the payments from public payers typically do not cover the hospital's costs (see Figure 11-20). Fourth, total Medicare margins for teaching

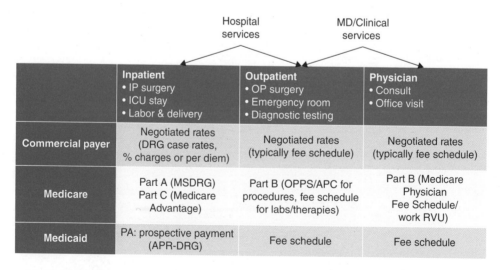

**Figure 11-22** • Methods of Hospital and Physician Payment. APC, Ambulatory Payment Classification; APR, All Patient Refined; DRG, Diagnosis-Related Group; IP, Inpatient; MSDRG, Medicare Severity–Diagnosis-Related Group; OP, Outpatient; OPPS, Outpatient Prospective Payment System; PA, Pennsylvania; RVU, Relative Value Unit.

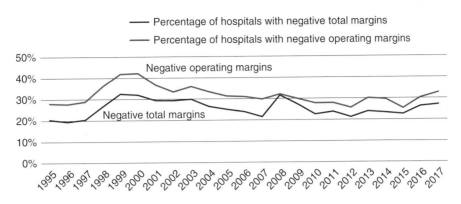

**Figure 11-23** • Percentage of Hospitals with Negative Total and Operating Margins, 1995 to 2017. (Source: American Hospital Association, AHA Chartbook 2019, 2017 Data.)

hospitals have fallen over time; among non-major teaching hospitals, these margins turned negative as early as 2003. Figure 11-23 shows the percentage of US hospitals that historically operate with negative margins; Figure 11-24 shows the aggregate total and operating margins for hospitals over time.

Fifth, hospital finances are heavily driven by "payer mix" (ie, the mix of Medicare, Medicaid, and privately insured patients). Hospitals with more privately insured patients and fewer Medicaid patients typically have healthier operating margins. Hospitals can raise total margins by increasing nonoperating revenues (eg, investments, charitable endowments), but these amounts as a percentage of total net revenues are low (2% or less) and have fallen since the late 1990s. Hospitals can also raise margins by increasing bargaining power over commercial insurers through consolidation. Hospitals that have formed or joined multihospital systems sometimes have greater leverage to negotiate

higher reimbursement rates, since there are fewer available hospitals to staff the insurer's network of providers (see Chapter 12).

However, payers in the private sector have also consolidated and adopted a more aggressive stance in rate negotiations with hospitals. The Federal Trade Commission and the Department of Justice have been more forgiving of health plan mergers and market consolidation on the payer side than they have been of hospital mergers and market consolidation on the provider side.

Hospital finances are also driven by their mix of inpatient and outpatient care services. Within each set of services, there are some services that generate much higher revenues and profit margins (eg, oncology, surgery, interventional cardiology) than others (eg, psychiatric, pediatric, obstetric, pulmonary, neurology, nephrology). The former are used to cross-subsidize the latter. Revenues can also be enhanced by expanding outpatient care (as noted earlier) and

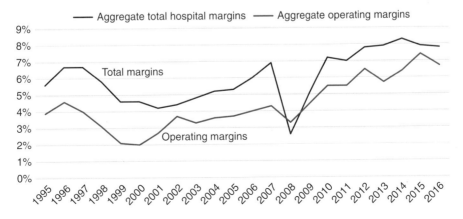

**Figure 11-24** • Aggregate Total Hospital Margins and Operating Margins, 1995 to 2016. (Source: American Hospital Association, AHA Chartbook 2019, 2017 Data.)

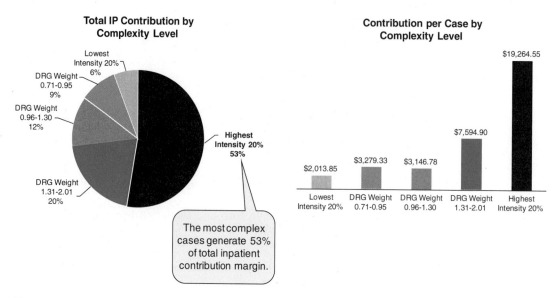

**Figure 11-25** • Inpatient Margins Vary by Complexity of Care: Inpatient Contribution by Level of Complexity, Fiscal Year 10. (Each Complexity Grouping Represents ~16,400 Cases.) DRG, Diagnosis-Related Group; IP, Inpatient.

by adding unique services and therapies that other (especially community) hospitals cannot provide. Such services, including advanced oncology care and transplantation, are often the bailiwick of AMCs. There is evidence that hospitals offering complex services that patients are willing to travel longer distances to utilize command higher reimbursements and enjoy higher contribution margins (Figure 11-25).

## HOSPITAL EFFORTS TO DELIVER VALUE

As intimated earlier, hospitals face enormous reimbursement pressures from public and private insurers to control their costs if they wish to remain profitable. At the same time, hospitals are also being pressured to document the value of the care they render that justifies payer reimbursement. In 2004, Michael Porter popularized the phrase "value," defined as quality divided by cost.[18] Hospitals are being pressured to deliver on both the numerator and the denominator, even though (as described in Chapter 2) they may not be highly correlated. This challenges hospitals to "multitask."

What are hospitals doing here to manage these challenges? Some efforts include the following:

- Improve efficiency by lowering costs and length of stay across all services

- Promote the coordination/integration of patient services across all care settings (eg, hospital, outpatient, home care, rehabilitation; covered in Chapters 13 and 14)
- Manage patient populations at a lower cost (manage the actual costs of care incurred, rather than manage care to match insurance payments)
- Manage the costs and quality of care for patients with high medical complexity and severity of illness across settings
- Build partnerships and create linkages with other providers, hospitals, and community affiliates to manage care across settings (also covered in Chapter 9)
- Improve the coordination of community-based primary care services with community health agencies to improve patient management in select populations
- Leverage a common electronic medical record (EMR) across all settings of care (covered in Chapter 24)
- Expand experimentation with alternative payment models (eg, bundled payments)

At the same time, hospitals need to focus on managing their cost structure, which is depicted in Figure 11-26. Figure 11-26 shows that wages and benefits of personnel are by far the biggest source of hospital costs (50%+). Of these, nursing costs represent the largest component of labor. Cutting nurse labor costs is difficult,

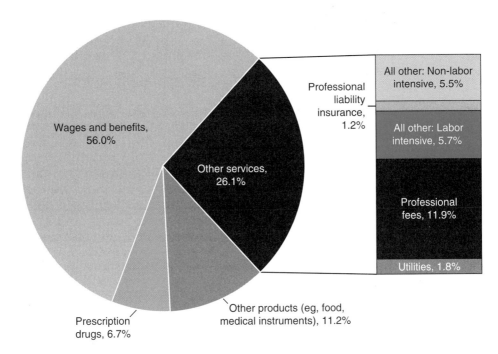

**Figure 11-26** • Percentage of Hospital Costs by Type of Expense, 2015. (Source: American Hospital Association, Centers for Medicare and Medicaid Services.)

because (as noted in Chapter 10) nurse staffing levels are associated with the quality of hospital care. If you try to cut nurse staffing costs, you may hurt quality of care (the iron triangle problem).

Another source of cost savings, and the second largest opportunity after labor, is supplies (20%-30%). This area is now known as supply chain management, which includes not only the costs of the supply items but also the management of supply procurement, storage, and transportation inside the hospital. The challenge here is the sheer number of hospital departments that are involved (Figure 11-27).

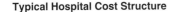

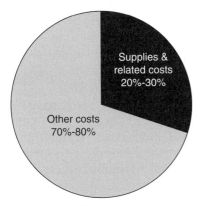

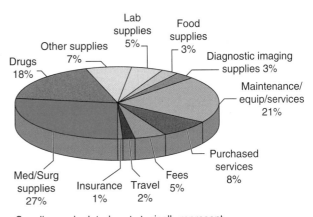

**The Opportunities**
- Complex, manual processes
- Waste and obsolescence
- Vendor/supply proliferation
- Utilization
- Excess inventory/equipment
- Expensive replenishment processes

Supplies and related costs typically represent 20%-30% of a provider cost structure ($100-$150 million in expenses for a $500 million IDN)

**Figure 11-27** • Large Saving Opportunities in Supply Chain Costs. IDN, Integrated Delivery Network.

Like the hospital's medical staff, the hospital's supply areas are fragmented. Over time, the percentage of hospital costs due to nonpayroll expenses has steadily climbed. This growth reflects the rising costs of supplies and services purchased from outside vendors, who steadily raised the prices for their products during the past decade.

---

**Critical Thinking Exercise: ThedaCare Case**

ThedaCare was a 4-hospital system in Northeast Wisconsin (near Appleton) popularized by a Harvard Business School case written by Michael Porter.[19] ThedaCare's strategy was to improve quality of care; its mission was to improve the health status of its community. ThedaCare pursued this by undertaking an impressive array of activities. Among these were the following:

- Employed primary care physicians (PCPs)
- Employer occupational health clinics
- Senior care living facilities
- Home healthcare and home medical equipment
- Ambulance service
- EMR
- Patient-focused care
- Idealized design of clinical office practices
- Lean management via the Toyota Production System (TPS)
- Wisconsin Collaborative for Healthcare Quality
- Wisconsin Health Information Organization

In addition to this array, ThedaCare also pursued quality improvement, oriented itself to patient outcomes and the delivery of "value" to payers and employers, practiced transparency by reporting its quality measures, attempted to promote the sharing of quality data among Wisconsin hospitals, sought to rationalize its service lines to achieve "system-ness," and redesigned patient care by setting up treatment improvement teams. The system was helped here by a good payer mix and the long tenure of its chief executive officer, Dr. John Toussaint.

ThedaCare's self-reported results were impressive. It improved productivity by 12% between 2006 and 2009, achieved savings to its bottom line of $25 million in 2009 (due to TPS), raised its prices to payers by only half of what competitors did, and served as the lowest-cost provider in Wisconsin. And, yet, one rarely hears about ThedaCare's accomplishments. There is little mention of "value healthcare" taking off in that part of the state. It is not clear if employers and/or insurers embraced Michael Porter's "value" approach; it is also unclear if hospitals in the state wanted to collaborate on quality or share their data. It didn't help that no peer-reviewed publications are available to document ThedaCare's results. What might explain its success? What might have limited its impact?

---

## THE HOSPITAL'S REGULATORY ENVIRONMENT

Healthcare is one of the most regulated sectors in the US economy, perhaps lagging behind only nuclear energy. Nearly every aspect of the healthcare industry is subject to governmental oversight, with regulations exerted at both federal and state levels, as well as by private institutions.[20]

Hospitals, in particular, are subject to federal regulations imposed by the Department of Health and Human Services (DHHS) and its constituent bodies, including the Centers for Medicare and Medicaid Services (CMS), the Health Resources and Services Administration (HRSA), and the Office of the Inspector General (OIG). Other federal regulatory bodies include the Environmental Protection Agency (EPA), the Centers for Disease Control and Prevention (CDC), the Federal Trade Commission (FTC), the Office of Occupational and Safety Administration (OSHA), the Drug Enforcement Agency (DEA), and the Departments of Justice (DOJ), Labor (DOL), and Transportation (DOT).

These agencies and departments are profiled in Chapter 25.

Outside of the federal government, hospitals are also subject to scrutiny by state agencies, such as boards of medicine and departments of health, welfare, licensure, and insurance, as well as by local governments and private accrediting bodies (eg, The Joint Commission, National Committee on Quality Assurance). This regulatory scrutiny requires hospitals to hire administrative staff to monitor legislative and regulatory developments and respond to requests for information.

Hospitals are also subject to Certificate of Need (CON) programs, still active in many states, which oversee and restrict capital investments. CON programs place the hospitals at a competitive disadvantage relative to freestanding facilities that are (often) operated by community physicians: The latter are not subject to CON and are often not subject to state licensure. Moreover, the latter are not mandated to provide care to all patients regardless of their ability to pay.

---

## QUESTIONS TO PONDER

1. Decades of research suggest that the distinction between nonprofit and for-profit ownership does not impact the 3 goals of the iron triangle (quality, access, and cost). Why might this be true, given the historical attention and concern paid to for-profit hospitals?
2. Why is the hospital so central to the healthcare delivery system in both the United States and other countries?
3. Can you think of any other organization as bureaucratically complex as the American hospital? What problems does this complexity pose to hospital managers?
4. Some hospital executives say their job is "half political." What do you think they mean by this?
5. What problems do hospitals face in trying to deliver "value"?

---

## SUMMARY

Hospital executives face the daunting task of satisfying stakeholders on every front. They must satisfy regulators (eg, the federal government, The Joint Commission) that their complex organizations are meeting a host of legal and accreditation standards. They must satisfy public and private insurers that their healthcare services are of high quality and reasonable cost to demonstrate "value." They must satisfy the physicians on their medical staffs that they are providing the services, equipment, and specialized personnel needed to deliver quality of care and meet the demands and needs of their patients. They must meet the expectations of their communities that they are seeking to improve the population health of their community, including the containment of pandemics and other contagious diseases. They must also satisfy local and state governments that they are providing charitable services that justify their tax-exempt status.

---

## REFERENCES

1. Bryan J. Weiner, Richard Culbertson, Robert F. Jones, et al. "Organizational Models for Medical School – Clinical Enterprise Relationships," *Acad Med.* 76 (2) (2001): 113-124.
2. Mark Schlesinger and Bradford Gray. "How Nonprofits Matter in American Medicine, and What to Do About It," *Health Affairs Web Exclusive* (June 20, 2006): w287-w303.
3. Government Accountability Office. *Nonprofit, For-Profit, and Government Hospitals: Uncompensated Care and Other Community Benefits* (Washington, DC: GAO, 2005).
4. Mark Schlesinger and Bradford Gray. "How Nonprofits Matter in American Medicine, and What to Do About It," *Health Affairs Web Exclusive* (June 20, 2006): w287-w303.
5. Jill Horwitz. "Making Profits and Providing Care: Comparing Non-Profit, For-Profit, and Government Hospitals," *Health Aff.* 24 (3) (2005): 790-801.
6. Mark Pauly and Michael Redisch. "The Not-for-Profit Hospital as a Physicians' Cooperative," *Am Econ Rev.* 63 (1973): 87-99.
7. State of New Jersey. *New Jersey Commission on Rationalizing Health Care Resources: Final Report* (January 24, 2008).

8. State of New Jersey. *New Jersey Commission on Rationalizing Health Care Resources: Final Report* (January 24, 2008): 3-4.

9. Paul M. Schyve. *Leadership in Healthcare Organizations: A Guide to Joint Commission Leadership Standards*, 2nd ed (Lincoln, NE: The Governance Institute, 2017): 2.

10. Lawton R. Burns, Jeff Goldsmith, and Aditi Sen. "Horizontal and Vertical Integration of Physicians: A Tale of Two Tails." In *Annual Review of Health Care Management: Revisiting the Evolution of Health Systems Organization Advances in Health Care Management*, Volume 15 (Bingley, United Kingdom: Emerald Group Publishing, 2013): 39-117.

11. Lawton R. Burns, Jeff Goldsmith, and Aditi Sen. "Horizontal and Vertical Integration of Physicians: A Tale of Two Tails." In *Annual Review of Health Care Management: Revisiting the Evolution of Health Systems Organization Advances in Health Care Management*, Volume 15 (Bingley, United Kingdom: Emerald Group Publishing, 2013): 39-117.

12. American Hospital Association. *Hospitals and Health Systems Face Unprecedented Financial Pressures Due to COVID-19* (Chicago, IL: AHA, May 2020).

13. Sarah Kliff. "Hospitals Knew How to Make Money. Then Coronavirus Happened," *The New York Times* (May 15, 2020).

14. Ben Teasdale and Kevin Schulman. "Are U.S. Hospitals Still 'Recession-Proof'?" *N Engl J Med.* 383 (2020): e82.

15. Linda Johnson. "Pandemic Pushes Expansion of 'Hospital-at-Home' Treatment," *Modern Healthcare* (August 20, 2020).

16. For outpatient care, Medicaid in New Jersey reimbursed at cost minus 5.8% for a majority of services. Combining both inpatient and outpatient services, Medicaid paid hospitals 75% to 80% of their costs. *State of New Jersey. New Jersey Commission on Rationalizing Health Care Resources: Final Report* (January 24, 2008).

17. Thomas Prince. *Strategic Management for Health Care Entities: Creative Frameworks for Financial and Operational Analysis* (San Francisco, CA: Jossey-Bass, 1988).

18. The term value has been in use since the mid-1990s as a response to employers and provider report cards.

19. Michael Porter and Sachin Jain. *ThedaCare: System Strategy.* Harvard Business School Case 708-424, November 2007. (Revised January 2010.)

20. Robert Field. *Health Care Regulation in America: Complexity, Confrontation, and Compromise* (New York, NY: Oxford University Press, 2007).

# Hospital Diversification, Restructuring, and Integration

# 12

## INTRODUCTION

Chapter 11 described the loose, but nevertheless complex relationship between the hospital and the physicians on its medical staff. Healthcare delivery by hospitals and physicians has grown more intertwined over the past 4 decades. Much of this has been spurred by federal government efforts to control rising healthcare costs, which relied on regulatory approaches in the 1970s (eg, certificate of need legislation), budgetary remedies (eg, diagnosis-related groups [DRGs] and the Inpatient Prospective Payment System [IPPS]) in the 1980s, and an increasingly diverse and complex reimbursement environment for Medicare and Medicaid patients. Federal efforts were supplemented by private sector efforts in the form of "managed care." Most of these efforts were directed at the largest destination of healthcare spending—the hospital (40% of national health expenditures in 1980).

These public and private sector forces jointly motivated a series of organizational responses by hospitals that encompassed (in order) diversification, corporate restructuring to protect some of the newly diversified services, horizontal integration, vertical integration, and payer-provider integration. They are discussed in the following sections.

## DIVERSIFICATION OF SERVICES

Starting in the early 1900s, hospitals began to diversify beyond their core function of inpatient services. The new services included hospital outpatient care, emergency care, ambulatory care, and post-acute care. Outpatient and emergency care have been offered for over a century; their use mushroomed, however, in the 1960s after the passage of Medicare and Medicaid. By contrast, ambulatory care and post-acute care are more recent offerings, dating to the 1980s.

### Outpatient Care

Outpatient care began as a charitable function. Freestanding "dispensaries" began in the late 18th century to serve the urban poor who did not need to be hospitalized. They dispensed medications, performed minor surgery, and extracted teeth. Dispensaries reached roughly 100 in number by 1900 and gradually ceded their role over to the hospitals and their newly opened outpatient departments.

The US hospital sector witnessed rapid growth in the early 20th century, and so did the number of outpatient clinics. In 1914, 250 outpatient clinics were associated with hospitals; by 1926, the number had reached 1,790.[1] Outpatient clinics were used for teaching and training younger physicians, who staffed the clinics in return for hospital admitting privileges, and who could be exposed to diseases in their early stages (before hospitalization was required). They nevertheless remained a "stepchild" of the core inpatient hospital. Medical social workers conducted "means tests" on patients to ensure they were poor enough to qualify for charitable care; the poor patients were routed to the clinics where they were given low priority. The staff at these clinics were almost exclusively young professionals in training, reinforcing this inferiority.

Over time, with the growth of the US hospital, more hospitals opened outpatient departments, and more patients were seen in such settings. Between the late 1920s and the early 1960s, hospital outpatient visits (as a percentage of total nonhospitalized physician visits) increased 50%, rising from 10% to 16% of physician visits.[2] Demand was still limited by the relatively low availability of public and private insurance coverage for outpatient care.

Hospital outpatient departments became more critical (1) in the mid-1960s with the passage of Medicare and Medicaid, which both covered outpatient care, and (2) in the mid-1970s, when the growth in hospital inpatient days plateaued. Between 1965 and 1977, the ratio of outpatient visits to inpatient admissions rose from 4.37 to 7.12. Between 1968 and 1978, Blue Cross enrollees used 18.6% fewer inpatient days and 137.6% more outpatient visits.[3] This shift was driven not only by insurance coverage but also by the rise of ambulatory care, managed care, and post-acute care—all profiled later in this chapter. Still, only a minority of hospitals (30% in 1977) had outpatient departments, and only 5% of the US population reported the outpatient clinic as their usual source of ambulatory care in 1974.

## Emergency Care

Emergency services are considered one type of outpatient care and grew in tandem with outpatient care but became more prevalent across hospitals (79% in 1977). During the first half of the 20th century, emergency medicine was not a defined academic specialty. Hospitals, like the hospital outpatients of old, staffed their emergency services with medical trainees (interns, residents) and other hospital staff physicians or rotated physicians who were "on call." There was no coordination with inpatient hospital care. Often, the emergency service was just a single room (hence, "emergency room"). Ambulance services were often run by morticians or funeral directors who had vehicles that could transport people horizontally, often using untrained staff.

The hospital emergency department (ED) began in the early 1960s, often through the efforts of pioneering physicians.[4] Their efforts were buttressed by a 1966 National Academy of Sciences report titled "Accidental Death and Disability, the Neglected Disease of Modern Society," which described the poor state of emergency care in the United States. This led to the 1966 Federal Highway Safety Act, which for the first time set standards for ambulances and training in the United States. Two years later, the American

College of Emergency Medicine was founded as a new specialty society, later recognized in 1972 by the American Medical Association. During the 1970s, emergency residency programs were also established to train physicians in this specialty.

Hospital EDs serve as an important source of hospital overall volumes. Figure 12-1 shows the rising number of total ED visits and ED visits per 1,000 patients since the 1990s. The EDs also provide an increasing percentage of the hospital's inpatient volume. Between 2003 and 2009, inpatient admissions grew more slowly than the population; however, most of the admissions growth resulted from a 17% increase in unscheduled inpatient admissions from hospital EDs. Moreover, the growth in ED-based admissions more than offset a 10% decline in admissions from doctors' offices and other outpatient settings.[5]

This pattern suggests that physicians directed some of the patients they previously admitted to the hospital to the ED. In addition to serving as an increasingly important portal of hospital admissions, EDs support primary care practices by performing complex diagnostic workups and handling overflow, after-hours, and weekend demand for care. Primary care and specialist physicians alike report that they increasingly rely on EDs to evaluate complex patients with potentially serious problems, rather than managing these patients themselves. As a consequence of these shifts in practice, emergency physicians are increasingly serving as major decision makers for approximately half of all hospital admissions in the United States.

## Ambulatory Care

Hospitals began to diversify into ambulatory care in earnest following the 1983 enactment of the Inpatient Prospective Payment System (IPPS). IPPS eliminated fee-for-service reimbursement for hospitalized Medicare patients and replaced it with a fixed, budgeted reimbursement amount (ie, a budget cap) based on the patient's admitting diagnosis (DRGs). However, IPPS changed reimbursement only on the inpatient side and left Medicare's fee-for-service reimbursement of outpatient and ambulatory care untouched. This began a pattern of "squeezing the balloon" (see Chapter 2): Hospitals could escape the budget constraint on the inpatient side by seeing some Medicare patients on the outpatient side. Cost pressures from managed care were also less intense on the ambulatory care side. Hospitals

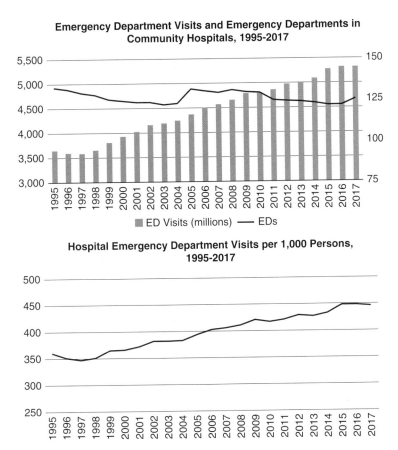

**Figure 12-1** • Emergency Department (ED) Visits and EDs in Community Hospitals and Hospital Emergency Department Visits per 1,000 Persons, 1995 to 2017. (Source: American Hospital Association, AHA Chartbook 2019.)

immediately began to develop outpatient cardiac care rehabilitation programs and outpatient diagnostic centers—all known at the time as "alternative delivery systems." Such ventures capitalized on the growing use of less invasive surgical and diagnostic technologies, which gained momentum during the 1980s.

Other currents already underway by the time IPPS was enacted propelled ambulatory care. Physician entrepreneurs were busy in various markets setting up freestanding emergency centers (FECs), urgent care centers (UCCs or "urgi-centers"), ambulatory surgery centers (ASCs or "surgi-centers"), and chains of physician office clinics ("doc in a box"). The federal government even encouraged the growth of the ASCs, since they were much less expensive than surgeries conducted in hospital operating rooms. The 2 sides—doctors and hospitals—each recognized the opportunity to get into the ambulatory care market. This brought their separate worlds more into contact with one another, much like the Venn diagram in Figure 12-2, and increased their potential rivalry.

## Post-Acute Care

In prior decades, hospitals discharged the patients they admitted back to their homes. Over time, however, several developments complicated the discharge issue.

First, the Medicare IPPS incentivized hospitals to discharge patients sooner given the budget constraint. However, in order to minimize their mortality rates and/or stabilize those who were more seriously ill, hospitals transferred more patients to skilled nursing facilities (SNFs), which, at that time, were not covered by IPPS.

Second, the DRG payments applied to short-term hospitals; the remaining handful of hospitals that treated patients staying more than 30 days were exempt from IPPS and still paid on a fee-for-service basis. These are now known as long-term care hospitals (LTCHs) or long-term acute care (LTAC) hospitals.

Third, another set of facilities exempt from IPPS and DRGs were rehabilitation hospitals, as well as rehabilitation units inside

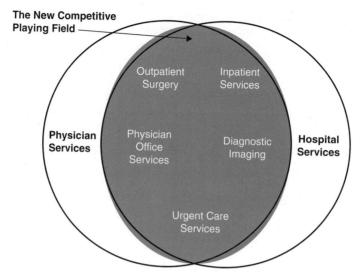

**Figure 12-2** • Venn Diagram of Hospital Services and Physician Services. (Source: Veterans Health Administration's 2003 Research Series, *The Doctor Is Out: Physician Competitors in the Marketplace*.)

community hospitals. The continuance of fee-for-service payment prompted the expansion of these hospitals and units, now known as intermediate rehabilitation facilities (IRFs). As with SNFs, IRFs received a lot more patients from community hospitals that discharged their patients "quicker and sicker." In the decade following IPPS, the number of rehabilitation beds in hospital units and IRFs doubled.[6]

Fourth, over time, patients have developed more chronic conditions that limit the degree to which they can be safely discharged back home to be tended by family members. During the late 1980s and early 1990s, the US Congress was pressured to provide reimbursement to providers who could handle the post-acute care (PAC) needs of discharged patients. This marked the flowering of the PAC segment of the healthcare industry, which now included not only SNFs, but also home health agencies, LTCHs, IRFs, and hospices.

The close interdependence between hospital discharges and use of PAC sites has led many hospitals to develop their own in-house settings for PAC care. Figure 12-3 charts the spread of these hospital-sponsored settings.

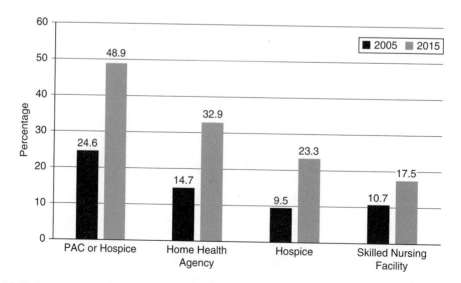

**Figure 12-3** • Percentage of Acute Care Hospitals with Common Investor Linkage to the Post-Acute Care (PAC) and Hospice Sectors, 2005 Versus 2015. (Source: *Health Affairs*.)

## CORPORATE RESTRUCTURING

During the 1980s, hospitals began to develop new organizational structures, whereby the hospital became a subsidiary of a nonhealthcare organization or foundation that had no direct responsibility for healthcare delivery. Such a structure would serve to segregate and insulate the more regulated lines of healthcare business (eg, the inpatient hospital enterprise) from other potentially more profitable lines of growth in outpatient and ambulatory care. The latter could include new ventures with physicians and revenue-generating activities. Without the new corporate structures, the new income streams could be considered as either taxable or as offsets against the hospital's inpatient Medicare and Medicaid reimbursement. Protection of these income streams became an important strategy to deal with growing financial problems faced by hospitals that included access to capital and preservation of the hospital's capital base. The corporate form also served as a vehicle for hospitals to make the acquisition of these new lines of business.

Some analysts suggest that such hospital efforts to (1) redefine their business lines to include ambulatory care, joint ventures with their physicians, and diversified services outside the core hospital and (2) house them as for-profit businesses underneath these corporate structures were needed to survive. Hospitals that did not do so were threatened with extinction.[7]

These structures also served as a vehicle to try to partner with community physicians who were developing their own outpatient businesses and, in some instances, taking the hospital's revenues with them. Hospitals calculated that sharing half of the revenues with physicians was better than sharing in none of them. Some hospitals developed these businesses proactively (rather than reactively) as a means to keep physicians from leaving the hospital.

Finally, these for-profit businesses served the core hospital business by developing new components and venues of patient care delivery outside of the hospital's walls. These could include home health services, imaging services, specialty medical services, and ambulance services. Nevertheless, even though they were organized as for-profit businesses, many new lines of service lost money. Moreover, the revenues generated by these for-profit entities

were miniscule compared to the hospital's core inpatient revenues. The hospital maintained these money-losing operations to partner with its community physicians, to provide needed community services (eg, home health care), to provide affordable care to community residents, and to maintain the community's access to physician care.

## THE 1990s PUSH FOR INTEGRATION

The 1980s and 1990s fomented a 2-fold trend toward new methods of paying providers and new models of provider organization to manage such payment changes. Payers and providers would again embrace dual trends in new payment and organization 2 decades later, much as singer Shirley Bassey noted ("Just a little bit of history repeating.").

### Pressures From Public Insurers and Private Health Plans in the 1980s to 1990s

The impetus for provider integration originated with the 1983 passage of the Medicare IPPS. IPPS replaced traditional fee-for-service payment with fixed budget (DRG) payments. However, IPPS affected only Medicare Part A payments (facility fees) to the hospital and left Medicare Part B's professional fees (based on fee-for-service payments) to physicians unchanged. Faced with a budget constraint and the need to control costs for the first time, hospitals approached the physicians on their medical staffs for their help. Given that the medical staff was composed almost entirely of independent community physicians (ie, no employment), hospitals sought ways to "align" and "partner" with physicians to try to increase ambulatory revenues and control inpatient costs. Hospital partnerships with scattered physicians to develop ambulatory ventures addressed the first need; more inclusive approaches were needed to address the second.

The budgetary pressures exerted by Medicare DRG reimbursement soon intensified due to the efforts of private insurers (health plans) to control utilization and costs for enrollees in employer-based health insurance. The health plans pivoted from merely "reimbursing" their care to "managing" their care and shifting it to outpatient settings. Such efforts led the health plans to be renamed as "managed care organizations" (MCOs). The MCOs began a national trend toward health plan consolidation that increased their bargaining power over providers. The MCOs used this power in calling on hospitals and/or their physicians to shift from fee-for-service to (1) large percentage discounts off their fee-for-service payments (ie, "discounted fees"), and/or (2) new models of payment, such as capitation (fixed reimbursement per month for each enrollee) or percentage of premium (a fixed percentage of the enrollee's premium, much less than 100%). Capitation and percentage of premium constituted "risk-based payment": Providers' profit or loss was tied to their ability to constrain utilization.

The payment pressures observed during the 1980s accelerated during the 1990s due to several environmental forces. The managed care movement reached its zenith in the mid-1990s, when health maintenance organizations (HMOs) penetrated one-third of the large commercially insured market. Such MCO models combined capitated payments with group and staff model clinics (eg, the much-lauded Kaiser model), as well as risk-sharing arrangements with physician-based independent practice associations (IPAs; ie, networks of independent doctors that sought to collectively negotiate with MCOs in risk contracts). Capitated plans now included global capitation, in which providers assumed risk for inpatient, outpatient, and (sometimes) pharmaceutical risk.

The proposed Health Security Act of 1993 (also known as the Clinton Health Plan) intensified these pressures. The plan, based largely on Stanford University economist Alain Enthoven's model of "managed competition," called for "regional health alliances" (insurers typically organized at the state level) that would purchase healthcare services from "accountable health plans" of providers in local markets. The plan envisioned only 3 to 4 provider networks in a local market, which would contract with the state-level insurers on more of a capitated basis.

## Horizontal Integration of Hospitals Into Systems in 1990s

The new constraints posed by public and private sector payers encouraged hospitals to begin another wave of hospital system formation, which had initially begun in the late 1960s and early 1970s following the passage of Medicare (1965). In that earlier era, hospitals formed systems to take advantage of the new (and generous) level of federal government reimbursement for inpatient care. This time around, however, hospitals formed horizontally integrated systems to match the consolidation of insurance plans and thereby hopefully develop some countervailing bargaining power.

Hospitals also consolidated to address the perceived, existential threat of Columbia Healthcare, a large for-profit chain that was gobbling up community hospitals in selected markets. Columbia threatened to physically combine the hospitals it acquired, thereby reducing excess bed capacity and lowering inpatient costs. By doing so, it could charge MCOs lower rates and thereby take business away from community hospitals. In the early 1990s, Columbia was commonly referred to as "the 800-pound gorilla" in healthcare.

The dual impact of MCOs and Columbia spurred a massive consolidation of hospitals into systems. After a decade of only 16 hospital mergers per year, hospital merger activity skyrocketed in the wake of the Clinton Health Plan's announcement and then plateaued (Figure 12-4).

The shape of the curve in Figure 12-4 should look familiar to anyone who has studied

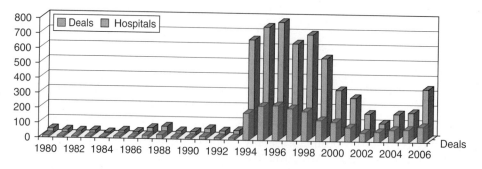

**Figure 12-4** • Hospital Consolidation.

the diffusion of innovations: It is the S-shaped (or logistic) curve. There is a very slow ramp-up, followed by a steep rate of adoption, and then a quick leveling off. Such curves are also known as "contagion curves," reminiscent of the spread of a contagious virus (like the Coronavirus in spring 2020). Contagions work when one infected person comes into contact with others, leading to an exponential increase in the disease. Such is the case here with managerial innovations like hospital mergers: One hospital "gets the bug" to do a merger, which leads to neighboring hospitals feeling pressured or threatened or unsure about what to do, so they follow suit. Such contagions (or "managerial bandwagons") are facilitated not only by others nearby getting the bug but also by consultants and academic researchers who tout the advantages of the newly-merged organizations.

As with many bandwagon movements, the reasons for adopting the innovation are more normative than rational (ie, others are doing it, so you should be doing it too). This was clearly the case in the 1990s. The research evidence from the 1990s showed that, with few exceptions, these newly merged systems failed to improve the quality of care or to reduce the cost of care.[8] They would come to have other benefits in the new millennium, however, that had nothing to do with higher-quality, lower-cost healthcare (covered later).

## Vertical Integration With Physicians Into Integrated Delivery Networks in the 1990s

Legal rulings during the decade of the 1980s (eg, *Arizona v Maricopa County Medical Society*) froze any movement toward a similar consolidation of physicians and blocked independent physicians from collectively negotiating higher reimbursement rates from MCOs. The result was an increasingly uneven playing field between national chains of MCOs, national and regional chains of hospitals, and independent, fragmented physicians.

The rise of MCOs (HMOs, in particular) and the threat of the Clinton Health Plan induced hospitals and physicians to form a variety of integrated delivery networks (IDNs) to overcome the fragmentation between hospitals and physicians (and other providers). The IDNs included a wide array of arrangements (see Figure 12-5 for brief definitions). These included not only the IPAs already established, but new models including (1) physician-hospital organizations (PHOs; ie, alliances of doctors and hospitals that form to engage in risk contracting with MCOs); (2) management services organizations (MSOs), which provided back-office support functions to physician practices; (3) equity models that took an ownership interest in the physician's practice; (4) foundation models, which were owned by hospitals and employed the physicians (rather than the hospital) to comply with state laws dealing with the corporate practice of medicine; and (5) integrated salary models (ISMs; ie, hospital acquisition and/or employment of physicians). The IPAs and PHOs were loosely linked "alliance models" involving no common asset base or ownership; the ISM and foundation models were tightly linked "employment models" that did involve a common asset base and ownership.

The IDNs represented a collaborative effort by hospitals and physicians to confront the threat of managed care and develop contracting vehicles for joint hospital-physician bargaining with MCOs and thereby level the playing field with health plans. Hospital consolidation and physician employment were often explicitly pursued to offset the bargaining power of health plans. IDNs were initially compelling to physicians because they believed capitated payments under health reform would be made only to large institutions, not individual physicians who were constrained by antitrust laws from organizing into larger economic units. Physicians, especially primary care physicians (PCPs), were now more attractive to IDNs due to the shift to ambulatory care and managed care. Hospital systems sought to become sole-source contractors for MCOs by offering broad, accessible, and proprietary physician networks. Hospitals also formed IDNs in an effort to try to further "align incentives" between themselves and their physicians to work within the budgetary constraints imposed by IPPS and the MCOs. Finally, IDNs expressed a commitment to "developing a seamless continuum of care" that (1) spanned inpatient, outpatient, and community health settings as part of an effort to develop "integrated care," and (2) provided the capability to manage the risk of global capitation. They also espoused the commitment to improving the health status of their local population that would keep their capitated patients out of the hospital.

**Physician-Hospital Models of Organization**

| Type of organization | How organized |
|---|---|
| Hospital medical staff | Collectivity of independent physicians with admitting privileges at the hospital |
| Independent practice association (IPA) | A loosely linked IDN that includes independent physicians and medical groups that come together to contract jointly with health plans through the IPA. The physicians work through the IPA to control the cost and increase the quality of healthcare. |
| Closed physician-hospital organization (closed PHO) | A loosely linked IDN that can be structured in various ways. It is typically created as a joint venture with joint ownership by physicians and a hospital. They are usually formed to jointly contract with health plans. Closed PHOs exclude some medical staff members. |
| Open physician-hospital organization (open PHO) | A loosely linked IDN that can be structured in various ways. It is typically created as a joint venture with joint ownership by physicians and a hospital. They are usually formed to jointly contract with health plans. Open PHOs include most medical staff members. |
| Equity model | A moderately linked IDN that allows physicians to become shareholders in a professional corporation in exchange for the tangible and intangible assets of their practices. |
| Foundation model | A tightly linked IDN organized as a hospital subsidiary or affiliate. The foundation purchases the tangible and intangible assets of one or more medical groups. The foundation employs all non-medical staff. Physicians remain in a separate corporate entity but sign a professional services agreement with the foundation. |
| Integrated salary model (ISM): hospital-employed physicians | The most tightly linked IDN. The hospital directly employs physicians by purchasing physician practices and/or by hiring physicians (new physicians and physicians moving from other communities) |
| Accountable care organization (ACO) | A voluntary association of providers that come together to accept responsibility and accountability for the cost and quality of the patients attributed to them. The providers can include physicians only, hospitals only, or (more commonly) physicians and hospitals together. They can also include other types of providers such as nursing homes and home healthcare entities. |
| Clinically integrated network (CIN) | An alliance of physicians and hospitals in regional markets who wish to pursue clinical integration and jointly engage in risk-based or value-based contracts with health plans. It functions as a PHO on a wider geographic scale. |

**Figure 12-5 •** Physician-Hospital Models of Organization. IDN, Integrated Delivery Network.

Much of this effort was in vain. The Clinton Health Plan was "dead on arrival" in Congress in spring of 1994 due to Clinton's failure to rally enough support from his own party. Employers and their employees resisted the push to capitation and HMOs due to the narrow network of providers they offered and the utilization controls they imposed. The failure of capitation to spread as a new payment model scuttled efforts to both develop a full continuum of care and improve health status since payers were not paying for it. By the late 1990s, broadly based and open-panel provider networks, such as preferred provider organizations (PPOs), triumphed over closed-panel HMOs and marked a return to largely fee-for-service payments. For their part, MCOs initiated disease management programs to manage subsets of their enrollees who had chronic conditions (eg, asthma, congestive heart failure) that placed them at higher risk for emergency room visits, hospitalization, and thus high cost.

Figure 12-6 reveals that the IDN vehicles had a rapid takeoff in the early 1990s, peaked in 1996, and then fell off in prevalence (like the hospital mergers in Figure 12-4). The only model that endured (and subsequently grew) is the ISM, the physician employment model.

Hospitals used these vertically integrated IDNs, particularly the PHOs and IPAs, to try to leverage commercial insurers for higher reimbursement rates to be paid to their physician partners. The Department of Justice (DOJ) and Federal Trade Commission (FTC) developed guidelines for such hospital-physician combinations to be considered procompetitive rather than antitrust. These guidelines outlined the types of "financial integration" and "clinical integration" that must be present for provider groups to engage in collective contracting with MCOs.

Financial integration encompassed provider efforts to jointly engage in risk-based contracting and share in risk-based payments, such as bonuses (withholds) for meeting (missing) cost and utilization targets. Clinical integration encompassed the joint efforts of providers to coordinate patient care services across caregivers and care sites in an attempt to improve the quality of patient care. Such efforts could include care guidelines, care coordination, disease management, clinical information systems (eg, electronic medical records), and disease registries. Clinical integration also encompassed efforts to monitor and control utilization of care (see the end of Chapter 7).

Such efforts marked an important step beyond developing structures like the physician-hospital IDN vehicles discussed earlier because these represented nascent efforts at changing clinician

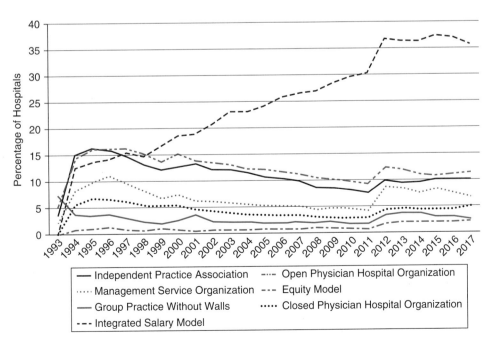

**Figure 12-6** • Physician-Hospital Contracting Vehicles, 1993 to 2017. (Source: American Hospital Association Database.)

processes and behaviors. Unfortunately, during the 1990s at least, they were relatively underdeveloped. The FTC succeeded in bringing several antitrust cases against these IDNs in the early 2000s and enjoined them from this joint bargaining in the absence of true financial and clinical integration. This contributed to the decline in these IDN types in the early 2000s (see Figure 12-6).[9]

The failure of hospital efforts to support networks of PCPs left a bad taste in physicians'

mouths and increased their cynicism and suspicion of the corporate practice of medicine. Despite the rhetoric about "aligned incentives," these efforts failed to improve relationships between the 2 parties. Many of the IDNs dissolved during the late 1990s and early 2000s; many hospitals divested themselves of the PHOs they had developed and the physicians they had acquired. As a result of the failed 1990s experiment with global capitation, few providers wanted to assume risk.

---

### Critical Thinking Exercise: Allina Case

One of the first major IDNs to form during the 1990s was Allina Health System in the Twin Cities (Minneapolis). Allina was constructed by merging several hospitals and several health plans into one organization and then developing an employed medical group. A timeline of its formation is depicted below. It developed in anticipation of the 1994 passage of the Health Security Act (also known as the Clinton Health Plan) as well as in response to similar, enabling legislation at the state level in 1992. Providers also believed that employers and purchasers wanted to contract with IDNs. For example, the Business Health Care Action Group (BHCAG) issued a "request for proposals" in 1992 for a cost-effective integrated delivery system to meet the needs of multiple employer purchasers.

Multiple assumptions underlay the formation of the Allina IDN. These included the following:

- Integrated care is cheaper, better, and more accessible.
- Payers and employers want it and will pay for it.
- Patients want integrated healthcare.
- The "California/Kaiser" model is coming eastward.
- Hospital systems can enjoy scale economies.
- IDNs can enjoy synergies among their hospital, physician, and insurer businesses.
- The continuum of care is the delivery model of the future.
- Hospitals can partner with physicians.

These were a lot of assumptions. What was the evidence base to support them all? If you are going to base your corporate strategy on such a list, what should you do as you roll out the strategy?

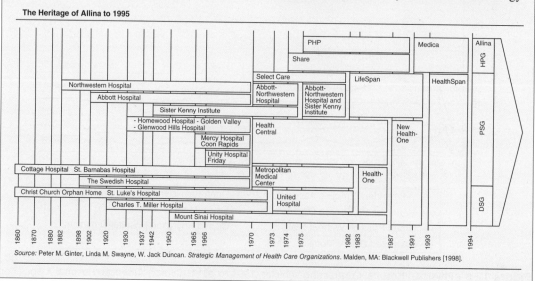

The Heritage of Allina to 1995

Source: Peter M. Ginter, Linda M. Swayne, W. Jack Duncan. *Strategic Management of Health Care Organizations*. Malden, MA: Blackwell Publishers [1998].

## Vertical Integration by Hospitals Into Insurance Plans in the 1990s

Hospitals and some physician groups also pursued integration into the insurance sector by establishing their own health plans. Many IDNs wanted to emulate Kaiser and thus felt they either had to offer a health insurance plan or assume full capitated risk. Kaiser had worked on these issues for decades; IDNs were in a hurry. They developed their own health plans as neophytes, experiencing widespread failures with insurance products as a result of (1) low capitalization, (2) conflicting capital needs between the core hospital and the new health plan, (3) lack of expertise in actuarial science and marketing, and (4) competition from larger and savvier insurers.[10] Moreover, empirical research showed that hospital diversification into health plans (and other lines of business) was associated with lower operating margins and higher debt-to-capitalization ratios.[11] By the end of the 1990s, hospital systems began shedding their insurance products (Figure 12-7), much as they began to shed their IDN vehicles with physicians (see Figure 12-6).

### RENEWED PUSH FOR INTEGRATION IN THE NEW MILLENNIUM

Figures 12-4, 12-6, and 12-7 illustrate "the rise and fall" of integration efforts in the last decade of the past century. But, like everything else in healthcare, "history repeats" (see Chapter 2), and it did not take long to do so. The 2009 American Recovery and Reinvestment Act (ARRA), the 2010 Patient Protection and Affordable Care Act (PPACA), and the subsequent use of value-based purchasing (VBP) programs by the Centers for Medicare and Medicaid Services (CMS) set in motion an ongoing stream of changes in how providers were paid that incented them to once again integrate both horizontally and vertically.

ARRA included incentives and subsidies to physicians to encourage them to move away from paper-based medical records and both adopt and use electronic medical records (EMRs) in their offices. Many physicians could not afford the EMR investment and turned to hospitals (and, sometimes, hospital employment) as a

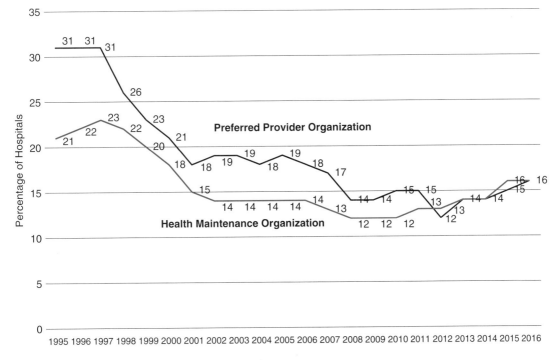

**Figure 12-7** • Percentage of Community Hospitals With Insurance Products (Preferred Provider Organizations and Health Maintenance Organizations), 1995 to 2016. (Source: American Hospital Association.)

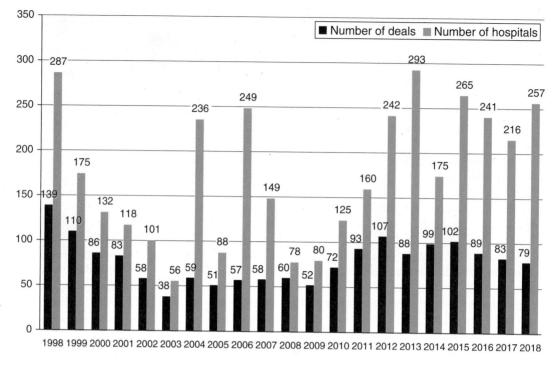

**Figure 12-8** • Hospital Mergers and Acquisitions, 1998 to 2018. (Source: Irving Levin Associates.)

funding source. PPACA posed new opportunities and uncertainty for hospitals. Hospitals responded as they had to Medicare's passage in 1965 and the Clinton Health Plan in 1993: They engaged in mergers and acquisitions (M&A). Finally, VBP programs tied payment to performance on a host of quality metrics. These programs have largely been targeted at hospitals, including the End-Stage Renal Disease Quality Incentive Program, the Hospital Value-Based Purchasing Program, the Hospital Readmission Reduction Program, the Value Modifier Program (also called the Physician Value-Based Modifier [PVBM]), and the Hospital-Acquired Conditions Reduction Program. Just as physicians had turned to hospitals, hospitals now turned to their physicians for help with quality improvement.

## Hospital Systems Redux

Hospital M&A served as a hedge against the uncertain future posed by the PPACA. It also served other purposes, including a strategy to bolster the hospital's existing market position and services relative to local rivals, a strategy of regional expansion into new geographies and ancillary areas, a means to improve access to capital (by virtue of being bigger and more

credit worthy), an avenue to gain bargaining leverage over MCOs, and (hopefully) a means to achieve cost efficiencies. Figure 12-8 shows the growing trend toward system formation following 2010.

What did hospitals achieve through their M&A efforts? It depended on how they executed the mergers. The (handful of) hospitals that physically merged facilities lowered their costs, sometimes increased their volumes, achieved scale economies (up to a bed size of 300), but did not necessarily improve quality. The (majority of) hospitals that did not merge facilities but rather just combined them under one administrative roof did not lower costs, sometimes saw their costs increase (especially true in larger and more geographically dispersed systems), made greater capital investments in quality improvement that might not necessarily improve quality, and did not increase their level of charity care.

In tandem with the shift to (more and bigger) systems, PPACA offered incentives to hospitals to form accountable care organizations (ACOs) that would share in any savings they generated for the Medicare program if they (1) hit their quality metrics and (2) reduced costs 2% or more below historical benchmarks. An example of the ACO model is presented in Figure 12-9. ACOs combined under one organizational roof the

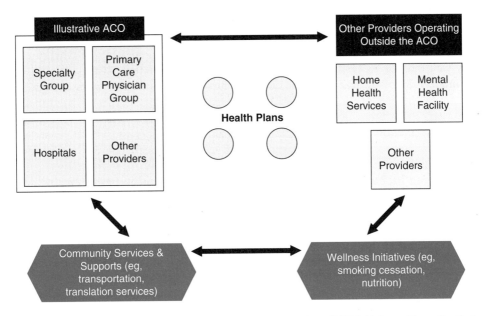

**Figure 12-9** • Integrating Care Through Accountable Care Organizations (ACOs). (Adapted from the Dartmouth Institute for Health Policy and Clinical Practice.)

practitioners and sites of care needed to manage a population of patients (eg, PCPs, specialty physician groups, multiple hospitals, and post-acute care providers), as well as network alliances with community-based services.

Figure 12-10 shows the rapid formation of ACOs across the United States following the passage of PPACA. The total number of ACOs rose over time from 58 (quarter [Q] 1 2011) to 1,011 (Q1 2018), whereas the number of ACO enrollees grew to 32.7 million. This growth has been driven primarily by growth in Medicare ACOs. Medicare ACOs account for 37% of all ACO-covered lives and 46% of all ACO contracts.[12] The most populous form of ACOs are known as Medicare shared savings plans (MSSPs), which serve Medicare FFS beneficiaries. Two other ACO models were the Pioneer

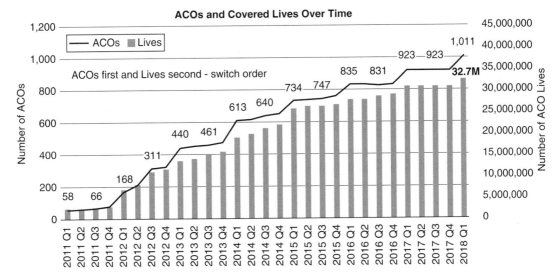

**Figure 12-10** • Recent ACOs and Covered Lives Over Time. (Reproduced from David Muhlestein, Robert Saunders, Robert Richards, and Mark McClellan. "Recent Progress in the Value Journey: Growth of ACOs and Value-Based Payment Models in 2018," Health Affairs Blog, August 14, 2018. https://www.healthaffairs.org/do/10.1377/hblog20180810.481968/full/.)

ACOs, which were more advanced and took on more risk, and the Next Generation ACOs, which succeeded them.

How well did the ACOs fare? Among the Pioneer models, 23 of 32 had dropped out of the program by the time of its "sunset" in 2016. Program year 2015 data showed an average savings of $2.7 million among the remaining 12 participants; however, of the $34 million earned, one ACO accounted for 72% of the savings.[13] Between 2012 and 2014, many showed improvement on the 30+ quality metrics, but less than 30% sufficiently reduced costs to earn shared savings. Research suggests that medical group participation in Medicare ACOs failed to change use of either high-value or low-value specialty care.[14] Additional research suggests little or no impact on hospital readmission rates.[15]

Roughly half of the ACOs reduced spending. The percentage of ACOs achieving savings was correlated with earlier start years and higher benchmark spending levels per beneficiary. ACOs led by physicians achieved a higher savings rate compared to hospital-led ACOs; smaller ACOs (with a mean number of beneficiaries <10,000) achieved greater net savings per beneficiary than larger ACOs. The relatively small size of ACOs and thus the relatively low percentage of providers' patients who have been attributed to the ACO provide only weak incentives to pursue hospital-wide strategies to reduce costs that might have spillovers to non-ACO patients.

In August 2016, ACO analysts engaged in an interesting exchange on the savings potential of ACOs. CMS pronounced it had reaped $1.29 billion in total savings from Pioneer and MSSP models since 2012, with $429 million savings in 2015. That same month, Harvard researchers replied that half of the ACOs made money while half lost money in 2015. After paying providers their bonuses, CMS lost a net of $216 million, which did not include CMS program costs.[16] In September 2016, Leavitt Partners reported lots of variation in ACO cost and quality, and that quality was unrelated to both spending and savings. The savings rate was tied to the benchmark rate.

In October 2016, other Harvard researchers reported savings of $287 million in 2014.[17] Savings totaled $685 million after taking account of estimated spillover effects to non-ACO patients and reduced Medicare Advantage cost due to lower benchmarks; as noted earlier, spillovers in smaller ACOs may be questionable. According to the Department of Health and Human Services (DHHS), ACO savings totaled nearly $1 billion, or roughly 0.15% of Medicare spending. CMS reported that ACOs achieved gross savings of $1.6 billion between 2013 and 2016. In December 2018, another study estimated savings of $2.66 billion.[18] After accounting for bonuses paid to providers, the MSSP generated net savings to the federal government of $542 million during 2013 to 2015. Based on $2,124 billion in Medicare expenditures over this time period, this translated into a whopping 0.02% saving in total Medicare spending.[19] The Medical Payment Advisory Commission (MedPAC) called the MSSP savings "incredibly unsatisfying."

Among those ACOs that reduced costs, the biggest reductions were in inpatient care and post-acute care (hospice, SNFs), largely driven by declines in volumes rather than cost per admission.[20] Recent research suggests that ACOs achieve savings in nonhospital, nonphysician care. In one study, hospitals affiliated with ACOs achieved lower readmissions from SNFs than non–ACO-affiliated hospitals.[21] In another study, ACOs reduced admissions and stays to post-acute sites without harming quality.[22] There were no changes in hospital readmissions or mortality. These results suggest the ACOs' incentives rest on reducing services used outside rather than inside the hospital. Overall, however, ACOs do not appear to have substantially or significantly reduced spending on end-of-life care.[23]

## Reprise of the Physician Integration Strategy in the 2000s

During the new millennium, hospitals returned to employment models as vehicles to partner with physicians, this time employing specialists as well as PCPs. With the impending retirement of the Baby Boom generation of physicians and stagnating physician incomes, hospital employment offered physicians a buffer from market competition and a revenue "float" until retirement. Hospitals began to employ specialists, collectively referred to as hospitalists, to cover a variety of inpatient and outpatient services such as the intensive care unit (intensivists) and the delivery room (laborists). Hospitals also began to employ certain types of specialists such as (1) cardiologists and radiologists, both of whom had suffered fee decreases from the Deficit Reduction Act of 2005, and (2) oncologists and PCPs, both of whom could now bill for higher reimbursement by virtue of calling themselves extensions of the hospital outpatient department. As noted later, hospital efforts to employ physicians were also spurred by enactment of the PPACA in 2010, which is evident from the spike in the ISM model in Figure 12-6.

An increasing percentage of physicians became reliant on the hospitals for a portion of their incomes. As Baby Boom PCPs retired, their practices were increasingly absorbed into the hospital, and new PCPs became hospital employees. Hospital employment did not entail guaranteed salaries, however. Instead, hospitals used productivity systems to reward employed physicians for their inpatient work, including physicians' production of relative value units (RVUs) in their clinical practice. Community-based physician groups grew more reliant on hospitals to help them recruit and finance new members. Hospitals witnessed rising levels of admissions from the ED (upward of 40% in many institutions)—admissions that were not directed by any community practice but were now instead managed by hospitalists.

Consolidation of physicians into hospital systems increased substantially between 2016 and 2018. According to one data source, the percentage of PCPs affiliated with vertically integrated systems rose from 38% to 49%; the share of all affiliated physicians rose from 40% to 51%. The median number of physicians per system rose from 285 to 369. By contrast, the percentage of hospitals that were horizontally integrated with other hospitals rose only 2% (from 70% to 72%).[24]

What was the impact of physician-hospital integration this time around? Vertical integration of physicians and hospitals does not lead to lower volume or utilization. Instead, it can (but does not always) lead to higher resource use in hospitals (eg, higher procedure rates), higher levels of ambulatory care–sensitive admissions and rates of ED use, and thus higher hospital spending and costs.[25] For example, salaried models lead to higher resource use, whereas capitated models reduce it.[26] Some reports also indicate higher spending in outpatient testing, outpatient procedures, and post-acute areas.[27] There is some evidence that patients of employed physicians are treated at higher-cost, lower-quality (ie, low-value) hospitals and receive a higher use of low-value services.[28]

Hospital employment of physicians not only leads to higher spending but also to higher prices for physician services charged to insurers.[29] Researchers recently estimated that the increase in hospital-employed physicians translated into a 12% increase in premiums for patients covered under the PPACA, a 9% rise in specialist prices, and a 5% hike in primary care prices during 2013 to 2016.[30] Consistent with the evidence cited earlier, the price effects are more pronounced for outpatient prices and volumes than for inpatient prices and volumes, perhaps due to the growing trend to employ specialists in outpatient clinics and the higher compensation they are offered compared to community-based specialists.[31] Higher prices resulted from the increased bargaining power over insurers that hospitals had when integrating with doctors. There do not appear to be any care coordination efficiencies flowing from physician employment. Moreover, there is some evidence that physician productivity declines after employment.[32]

Findings regarding quality are mixed. On the one hand, vertical integration is associated with higher levels of several process quality measures, such as use of care management practices, health promotion activities, health screenings, outcome improvements for ambulatory care–sensitive conditions, EMR adoption and clinical information technology capabilities, use of chronic disease registries, and use of reminders for both patients and physicians.[33] On the other hand, vertical integration is associated with lower levels of several other quality measures, such as Healthcare Effectiveness Data and Information Set (HEDIS) scores, avoidable hospitalizations, and inappropriate ED visits.[34] There is no consistent impact on mortality rates and patient safety; some studies find lower mortality rates in hospital-owned practices.[35]

## Reprise of the Health Plan Strategy

Providers went further than developing hospital systems and ACOs. They reprised the in-house health plan strategy they had pursued earlier in the 1990s. This time, rather than responding to the Clinton Health Plan or the Balanced Budget Act or trying to emulate Kaiser, hospitals sought to position themselves to manage risk-based contracts, position themselves to become ACOs, position themselves for population health management, gain some leverage over payers, disintermediate the MCOs, and/or manage the care continuum and triple aim.

The results were the same, however. Hospitals that got into risk contracts and/or developed their own health plans did not improve their quality of care or patient satisfaction. Moreover, rather than lowering costs, their average costs of care and the costs of care for patients in the last 2 years of life were higher than their competitors. There was also no relationship between the amount of "revenue at risk" and either their profitability or cost of care.[36]

Another study similarly suggested that nearly half of provider plans suffered negative margins in some or all of the period from 2011 to 2014, partly due to losses in most lines of business (except large employer groups).[37] Such expenses can hurt the underlying hospital system's cash flow margin, operating margin, and reserves, and delay the time to plan profitability. McKinsey concluded there is no guarantee for value creation by payer-provider integration, particularly in the commercial market, since the costs incurred may outweigh the cost savings.[38]

## Recent, Ongoing Changes in Provider Payment and Organization

The US healthcare ecosystem is currently attempting a massive "transformation from volume to value." This had been brewing since roughly 2005, with the advent of pay-for-performance (P4P) programs in Medicare reimbursement advocated by CMS. In 2015, DHHS secretary Sylvia Burwell announced that Medicare payments would transition from fee-for-service (FFS) to value-based payments between 2016 and 2018.[39]

What did these governmental initiatives portend? First, they served as a signal to MCOs to accelerate their move to alternative payment models (APMs) and place providers under risk-based contracts. The federal government would take the lead with the enactment of new legislation, the Medicare Access and CHIP Reauthorization Act (MACRA) of 2015. MACRA called for new payment models to physicians in Part B of Medicare, including the Merit-based Incentive Payment System (MIPS). Second, they served as a signal to the provider sector to integrate, both horizontally and vertically, in order to manage cost and quality under new payment schemes. Both signals meant that providers would be increasingly accountable to payers (public and private) for both the quality and cost of care they provided.

Transformation in payment encompasses a gradual shift away from FFS to a host of new APMs (Figure 12-11). Transformation in organization encompasses a gradual shift away from solo physician practice to group practice, IPA and PHO models, ACOs and IDNs, and physician employment by hospitals (see Figure 12-5). The goal of every combination of payment method and provider organization is to deliver the best possible quality of care in the most efficient (ie, lowest cost) way possible and improve patient outcomes (health status).

Perhaps the most prevalent type of APM has been (and still is) "bundled payment." In bundled payment, the total allowable acute and/or post-acute expenditures (target price) for an episode of care are predetermined. Participant providers share in any losses or savings that result from the difference between this target price and actual costs incurred in delivering care to beneficiaries. Similar to episode payments, bundled payment requires participating providers to assume risk, as they must cover costs that go above the target price for an episode of care, including those that arise from complications and hospital readmissions. Providers share in the savings (upside risk) if they keep costs below the target price while maintaining quality standards.[40]

Bundled payment was initially floated as a demonstration program by CMS in the early 1990s for treatment of patients undergoing coronary artery bypass with graft (CABG) procedures. The program was followed by a second demonstration in 2009, the Acute Care Episode (ACE) program, for both orthopedic and cardiac surgery patients. CMS's pursuit of bundled payment as an APM widened in more recent years to include the following:

- 2013 Medicare Bundled Payment for Care Improvement (BPCI) initiative
- 2015 Oncology Care Model
- 2016 Comprehensive Care for Joint Replacement (CCJR) model
- 2018 BPCI Advanced model

This chronicle suggests that bundled payments have become a permanent fixture in healthcare and will continue to dominate the APM landscape going forward. Research suggests that bundled payments could account for as much as 17% of all payments by 2021.

On the organization side, ACOs call for hospitals and community physicians in a wide

| Type of payment | Description |
| --- | --- |
| Fee-for-service (FFS) | Physicians are paid for every service and test that they provide based on the usual, customary, and reasonable (UCR) charges of physicians in the local area. These fees are usually "discounted" by health plans using a fee schedule or predetermined discount of the UCRs. |
| Pay-for-performance (P4P) | Hospitals and/or physicians receive payment rewards (penalties) for meeting (missing) performance benchmarks. |
| Shared savings | Providers can share in the cost savings achieved for managing the care of a population over a specific period of time, contingent on their meeting quality metrics and cost benchmarks. |
| Episode of care | Payment is based on episodes of care, which can be defined in multiple ways. Usually, the episode is tied to a set of diagnoses and services provided over a specified time frame. For example, an episode of care could include an inpatient hospital stay plus all services provided during a window surrounding the inpatient stay. |
| Bundled payment | A single payment is made to cover all costs of care associated with a single episode of care for a particular condition. In contrast to episode payments, bundled payment covers multiple providers in different care settings. The payment is for a specific condition or procedure rather than the total care delivered over a specified time period. |
| Professional capitation | Physicians are paid a fixed amount per enrollee, not per service, on a monthly basis. |
| Global capitation | All stipulated providers (usually physicians and hospitals) are paid a fixed amount per enrollee on a monthly basis. |
| Global budget/payment | A single payment is made for all services rendered on a per member per month basis (like capitation). However, payment adjustments are made for performance and risk. |
| Salary | Physicians are paid an annual amount that is not tied to the number of enrollees treated. The payment can be fixed up front or can be tied to the number of relative value units (RVU productivity). Either way, it can be adjusted based on other parameters such as quality of care and patient satisfaction. |

**Figure 12-11 •** Alternative Payment Models (APMs).

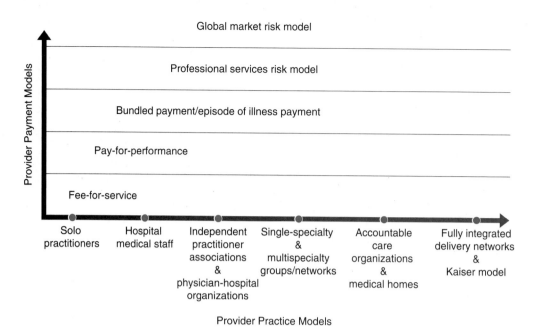

**Figure 12-12** • Simultaneous Change in Payment and Provider Organization.

geographic catchment area to coordinate patient care under shadow capitated arrangements called "shared savings." Calls for clinical integration have fostered a return of some of the IDN models from the 1990s, such as IPAs and PHOs, which can serve as the chassis for an ACO. Newer versions have also been developed, such as "clinically integrated networks," which are super-PHOs that span multiple hospital and physician providers across a wide geographic area (see Figure 12-5). All of these arrangements are now called upon to develop care coordination and clinical integration that manage the cost and quality of care.

This 2-fold transformation of the US healthcare ecosystem is depicted in Figure 12-12. The chart suggests that the country should achieve progress on both cost containment as well as quality improvement as we move along both axes (ie, as payment models migrate away from FFS, and as provider organizations migrate away from solo practice and the traditional hospital medical staff). A 2018 literature review suggests that progress has been slow on all fronts. FFS payment still dominates how hospitals and physicians are paid; small physician practices still dominate how doctors are organized;

and the demonstrable impact of both axes on cost containment and quality improvement remains elusive.[41]

## SUMMARY

The end result of all of this diversification and integration conducted since the 1960s can be described by contrasting Figure 12-13 (the 1960s) with Figure 12-14 (the situation since the 1990s). On top of the complexity of a single hospital and its relationships with the medical staff, diversification and integration have overlaid a superstructure of even greater complexity. Over time, the US hospital has migrated outward from its core focus on inpatient specialty care to embrace outpatient care, post-acute care, and a host of future possibilities (Figure 12-15).

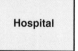

**Figure 12-13** • The Old Days (1960s): Freestanding Community Hospital.

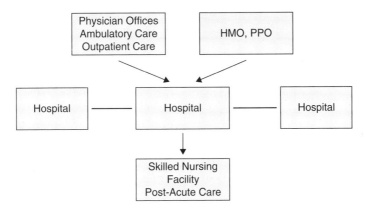

**Figure 12-14** • Hospital Diversification and Integration. HMO, Health Maintenance Organization; PPO, Preferred Provider Organization.

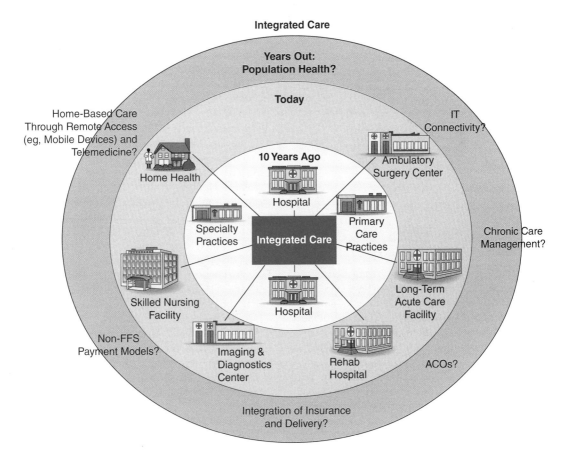

**Figure 12-15** • Integrated Care. ACO, Accountable Care Organization; FFS, Fee for Service; IT, Information Technology.

| | |
|---|---|

**QUESTIONS TO PONDER**

1. This chapter chronicles hospital efforts to mimic corporate America and adopt the same strategies and structures deployed in other industries. How successful have hospitals been?
2. The growth avenue for the hospital is no longer in its core inpatient business, but rather in new areas such as outpatient care and (perhaps) post-acute care. Are hospitals well-positioned and capable of success here? Should they own these new lines of business or partner with others who may know more about them?
3. Hospitals have sought to develop horizontally integrated multihospital chains on a local, regional, and national basis. Is any one geographic strategy better than the others? Is the formation of such chains a good thing for the hospital? For society at large?
4. Hospitals have also sought to develop vertically integrated continua of care (eg, the IDN, the ACO). Is the formation of such continua a good thing for the hospital? For society at large?
5. Does it make sense for hospitals to get into the insurance business?

## REFERENCES

1. Milton Roemer. *Ambulatory Health Services in America: Past, Present, Future* (Rockville, MD: Aspen Publishers, 1981).
2. Jerry Solon. "An Overview of Outpatient Services," *Inquiry* 2 (3) (1965): 3-15.
3. Jeff C. Goldsmith. *Can Hospitals Survive* (Homewood, IL: Dow Jones-Irwin, 1981).
4. Arthur Kellerman, Renee Hsia, Charlotte Yeh, et al. "Emergency Care: Then, Now, and Next," *Health Aff.* 32 (12) (2013): 2069-2074. Robert Suter. "Emergency Medicine in the United States: A Systemic Review," *World J Emerg Med.* 3 (1) (2012): 5-10.
5. Kristy Morganti, Sebastian Bauhoff, Janice Blanchard, et al. *The Evolving Role of Emergency Departments in the United States* (Santa Monica, CA: Rand Corporation, 2013).
6. Randall Braddom. "Medicare Funding for Inpatient Rehabilitation: How Did We Get to This Point and What Do We Do Now?" *Arch Phys Med Rehabil.* 86 (2005): 1287-1292.
7. Jeff C. Goldsmith. *Can Hospitals Survive* (Homewood, IL: Dow Jones-Irwin, 1981).
8. Lawton R. Burns and Mark V. Pauly. "Integrated Delivery Networks (IDNs): A Detour on the Road to Integrated Healthcare?" *Health Aff.* 21 (4) (2000): 128-143.
9. Lawrence Casalino. "The Federal Trade Commission, Clinical Integration, and the Organization of Physician Practice," *J Health Polit Policy Law.* 31 (3) (2006): 569-585.
10. Lawton R. Burns and Darrell P. Thorpe. "Why Provider-Sponsored Health Plans Don't Work," *Healthcare Financial Management: 2001 Resource Guide* (2001): 12-16.
11. Lawton R. Burns, Gilbert Gimm, and Sean Nicholson. "The Financial Performance of Integrated Health Organizations (IHOs)." *J Healthc Manag.* 50 (3) (2005): 191-213.
12. David Muhlestein, Robert Saunders, Robert Richards, and Mark McClellan. "Recent Progress in the Value Journey: Growth of ACOs and Value-Based Payment Models In 2018," *Health Affairs Blog* (August 14, 2018). Available online: https://www.healthaffairs.org/do/10.1377/hblog20180810.481968/full/. Accessed on January 17, 2019.
13. David Muhlestein, Robert Saunders, and Mark McClellan. "Growth of ACOs and Alternative Payment Models in 2017," *Health Affairs Blog* (June 28, 2017). Available online: https://www.healthaffairs.org/do/10.1377/hblog20170628.060719/full. Accessed on November 27, 2017.
14. John M. Hollingsworth, Brahmajee K. Nallmothu, Phyllis Yan, et al. "Medicare Accountable Care Organizations Are Not Associated with Reductions in the Use of Low-Value Coronary Revascularization," *Circ Cardiovasc Qual Outcomes.* 11 (6) (2018): e004492.
15. Ryan Duggal, Yongkang Zhang, and Mark L. Diana. "The Association Between Hospital ACO Participation and Readmission Rates," *J Healthc Manag.* 63 (5) (2018): e100-e114.
16. Ashish K. Jha. "ACO Winners and Losers: A Quick Take," *An Ounce of Evidence* blog (August 30, 2016). Available online: https://blogs.sph.harvard.edu/ashish-jha/2016/08/30/aco-winners-and-losers-a-quick-take. Accessed on November 27, 2017.
17. J. Michael McWilliams. "Changes in Medicare Shared Savings Program Savings from 2013 to 2014: Research Letter," *JAMA.* 316 (16) (2016): 1711-1713.
18. Allen Dobson, Sarmistha Pal, Alex Hartzman, et al. *2016 Updates: MSSP Savings Estimates: Program Financial Performance 2013-2016* (Vienna, VA: Dobson DaVanzo & Associates, December 7, 2018).

19. K. John McConnell, Stephanie Renfro, Benjamin K.S. Chan, et al. "Early Performance in Medicaid Accountable Care Organizations: A Comparison of Oregon and Colorado," *JAMA Intern Med.* 177 (4) (2017): 538-545.

20. John Schulz, Matthew DeCamp, and Scott A. Berkowitz. "Spending Patterns Among Medicare ACOs That Have Reduced Costs," *J Healthc Manag.* 63 (6) (2018): 374-381.

21. Ulrika Winblad, Vincent Mor, John P. McHugh, et al. "ACO-Affiliated Hospitals Reduced Rehospitalizations From Skilled Nursing Facilities Faster Than Other Hospitals," *Health Aff.* 36 (1) (2017): 67-73.

22. J. Michael McWilliams, Lauren G. Gilstrap, David G. Stevenson, et al. "Changes in Postacute Care in the Medicare Shared Savings Program," *JAMA Intern Med.* 177 (4) (2017): 518-526.

23. Lauren G. Gilstrap, Haiden A. Huskamp, David G. Stevenson, et al. "Changes in End-of-Life Care in the Medicare Shared Savings Program," *Health Aff.* 37 (10) (2018): 1693-1700.

24. Michael Furukawa, Laura Kimmey, David Jones, et al. "Consolidation of Providers Into Health Systems Increased Substantially, 2016-2018," *Health Aff.* 39 (8) (2020): 1321-1325.

25. Kristin Madison. "Hospital–Physician Affiliations and Patient Treatments, Expenditures, and Outcomes," *Health Serv Res.* 39 (2) (2004): 257-278. John E. Kralewski, Eugene C. Rich, Roger Feldman, et al. "Effects of Medical Group Practice and Physician Payment Methods on Costs of Care," *Health Serv Res.* 35 (3) (2000): 591-613. John E. Kralewski, Bryan E. Dowd, Yi "Wendy" Xu, et al. "The Organizational Characteristics of Best Medical Group Practices," unpublished manuscript (February 2011). Michael F. Pesko, Andrew M. Ryan, Stephen M. Shortell, et al. "Spending per Medicare Beneficiary Is Higher in Hospital-Owned Small- and Medium-Sized Physician Practices," *Health Serv Res.* 53 (4) (August 2018): 2133-2146. Rachel Mosher Henke, Zeynal Karaca, Brian Moore, et al. "Impact of Health System Affiliation on Hospital Resource Use Intensity and Quality of Care," *Health Serv Res.* 53 (1) (February 2018): 63-86.

26. John E. Kralewski, Terence D. Wingert, David J. Knutson, et al. "The Effects of Medical Group Practice Organizational Factors on Physicians' Use of Resources," *J Healthc Manag.* 44 (3) (1999): 167-182. John E. Kralewski, Eugene C. Rich, Roger Feldman, et al. "Effects of Medical Group Practice and Physician Payment Methods on Costs of Care," *Health Serv Res.* 35 (3) (2000): 591-613.

27. Michael F. Pesko, Andrew M. Ryan, Stephen M. Shortell, et al. "Spending per Medicare Beneficiary Is Higher in Hospital-Owned Small- and Medium-Sized Physician Practices," *Health Serv Res.* 53 (4) (August 2018): 2133-2146.

28. Tara F. Bishop, Stephen M. Shortell, Patricia P. Ramsay, et al. "Trends in Hospital-Ownership of Physician Practices and the Effect on Processes to Improve Quality," *Am J Manag Care.* 22 (3) (2016): 172-176. John N. Mafi, Christina C. Wee, Roger B. Davis, et al. "Association of Primary Care Practice Location and Ownership with the Provision of Low-Value Care in the United States," *JAMA Intern Med.* 177 (6) (2017): 838-845.

29. Caroline S. Carlin, Roger Feldman, and Bryan Dowd. "The Impact of Provider Consolidation on Physician Prices," *Health Econ.* 26 (12) (December 2017): 1789-1806.

30. Richard M. Scheffler, Daniel R. Arnold, and Christopher M. Whaley. "Consolidation Trends in California's Health Care System: Impacts on ACA Premiums and Outpatient Visit Prices," *Health Aff.* 37 (9) (September 2018): 1409-1416.

31. Vance M. Chunn, Bisakha Sen, Stephen J. O'Connor, et al. "Integration of Cardiologists with Hospitals: Effects on Physician Compensation and Productivity," *Health Care Manag Rev.* (October 5, 2018). Available online: https://journals.lww.com/hcmrjournal/Abstract/9000/Integration_of_cardiologists_with_hospitals_.99693.aspx. Accessed July 29, 2020.

32. Vance M. Chunn, Bisakha Sen, Stephen J. O'Connor, et al. "Integration of Cardiologists with Hospitals: Effects on Physician Compensation and Productivity," *Health Care Manag Rev.* (October 5, 2018). Available online: https://journals.lww.com/hcmrjournal/Abstract/9000/Integration_of_cardiologists_with_hospitals_.99693.aspx. Accessed on July 29, 2020.

33. Stephen M. Shortell, Julie Schmittdiel, Margaret C. Wang, et al. "An Empirical Assessment of High Performing Physician Organizations: Results from a National Study," *Med Care Res Rev.* 62 (4) (August 2005): 407-434. Diane R. Rittenhouse, Stephen M. Shortell, Robin R. Gillies, et al. "Improving Chronic Illness Care: Findings from a National Study of Care Management Processes in Large Physician Practices," *Med Care Res Rev.* 67 (3) (June 2010): 301-320. James C. Robinson, Lawrence P. Casalino, Robin R. Gillies, et al. "Financial Incentives, Quality Improvement Programs, and the Adoption of Clinical Information Technology," *Med Care.* 47 (4) (April 2009): 411-417. Stephen M. Shortell, Robin R. Gillies, Juned Siddique, et al. "Improving Chronic Illness Care: A Longitudinal Cohort Analysis of Large Physician Organizations," *Med Care.* 47 (9) (September 2009): 932-939. Diane R. Rittenhouse, Lawrence P. Casalino, and Stephen M. Shortell. "Small and Medium-Size Physician Practices Use Few Patient-Centered Medical Home Processes," *Health Aff.* 30 (8) (August 2011): 1575-1584.

34. John E. Kralewski, Bryan E. Dowd, Yi "Wendy" Xu, et al. "The Organizational Characteristics of Best Medical Group Practices," unpublished manuscript (February 2011).

35. Rachel Mosher Henke, Zeynal Karaca, Brian Moore, et al. "Impact of Health System Affiliation on Hospital Resource Use Intensity and Quality of Care," *Health Serv Res.* 53 (1) (February 2018): 63-86.

36. Jeff Goldsmith, Lawton R. Burns, Aditi Sen, et al. *Integrated Delivery Networks: In Search of Benefits and Market Effects* (Washington, DC: National Academy of Social Insurance, 2015).

37. Gunjan Khanna, Deepali Narula, and Neil Rao. *The Market Evolution of Provider-Led Health Plans* (New York, NY: McKinsey, 2016).

38. Shubham Singhal. "Payors in Care Delivery: When Does Vertical Integration Make Sense?" *Health Affairs Blog* (February 5, 2014). Available online: https://www.healthaffairs.org/do/10.1377/hblog20140205.036950/full/. Accessed on July 23, 2020.

39. Sylvia Burwell. "Setting Value-Based Payment Goals—HHS Efforts to Improve U.S. Health Care," *N Engl J Med.* 372 (2015): 897-899.

40. NEJM Catalyst. "What Are Bundled Payments?" *NEJM Catalyst* (February 28, 2018).

41. Lawton R. Burns and Mark V. Pauly. "Transformation of the Healthcare Industry: Curb Your Enthusiasm?" *Milbank Q.* 96 (1) (2018): 57-109.

# 13

# Organized Ambulatory Care

## INTRODUCTION

Ambulatory care accounts for approximately one-quarter to one-third of healthcare spending in the United States.[1] Ambulatory care includes physician offices, hospital outpatient departments, hospital emergency departments (EDs), and other sites. According to the Centers for Disease Control and Prevention (CDC), the number of ambulatory visits has been growing steadily in the new millennium, rising from 1 billion to 1.25 billion between 2000 and 2011. The volume of such visits going to physician offices may be declining, however. CDC data suggest that physician office visits declined from 1 billion (2009-2010) to 884 million (2016). During the same period, visits to hospital EDs remained relatively stable, rising slightly from 133 million (2009-2010) to 145 million (2016). The remainder of the increase occurred in hospital outpatient departments (see Chapter 11) and a wide array of newer, "organized ambulatory care" settings.[2] These settings are profiled in the following sections.

## CONSUMER- AND INDUSTRY-SPONSORED GROUP PRACTICES

One of the earliest examples of organized ambulatory care were the consumer-sponsored group practices and "medical cooperatives"— forerunners of the health maintenance organizations (HMOs). Early developers sought a system of family-oriented care in which the interests of the patient and the physician were parallel and directed to the goals of good care, health maintenance, and prevention and that was supported by monthly (capitated) payments by enrollees. Care was to be "comprehensive," combining the primary care physician (PCP), the specialist, and any consultants needed. This meant the provision of care in groups of physicians and other needed practitioners. A number of such cooperatives were established in the late 1920s (Elk City, Oklahoma), 1930s (Group Health Association, Washington, DC), and 1940s (Health Insurance Plan of Greater New York; Group Health Cooperative of Puget Sound).

The movement received a huge lift with the Kaiser Foundation Medical Care Program. During the 1930s and 1940s, Kaiser was engaged in the construction of a rural aqueduct in the southern California desert, the Boulder Dam, the Grand Coulee Dam in the state of Washington, and then ship construction in San Francisco and Portland. Kaiser partnered with Dr. Sidney Garfield in establishing the first Kaiser prepaid plans and clinics for its workers on these projects. Kaiser Foundation Plans were later opened to the public following World War II. The "Kaiser model" came to include an organized group practice of physicians (Kaiser Permanente Medical Group), prepayment of care using an in-house health plan (Kaiser Foundation Health Plan), integration with Kaiser Foundation Hospitals, and an emphasis on prevention.

With a handful of exceptions (eg, Mayo Clinic, Cleveland Clinic), physician group practices were quite rare before 1930. The Committee on the Costs of Medical Care recommended in its 1933 report that medicine be practiced in groups rather than in solo practice. The committee's recommendations were not warmly received by the American Medical Association (AMA), which viewed group practice, salaried medical practice, and prepayment as "unethical" (and even "communist"). Local medical societies opposed the consumer- and industry-sponsored group plans; they were enjoined during the 1940s by several major decisions rendered by the US Supreme Court. The AMA did not officially relax its opposition to medical groups until 1959. As Chapter 9 shows, physician group practice took off in subsequent decades (see Figure 9-5).

## COMMUNITY HEALTH CENTERS AND FEDERALLY QUALIFIED HEALTH CENTERS

Organized ambulatory care came to the disadvantaged beginning in 1965. The first community health centers (CHCs) were launched under the auspices of President Johnson's Office of Economic Opportunity (OEO) as part of the War on Poverty. Although Medicaid and Medicare were also created in 1965, these health insurance programs were not integrated with the CHCs until later.

Presidents Nixon and Ford subsequently dismantled the OEO and transferred the CHCs to the Department of Health, Education, and Welfare (DHEW). In 1975, Congress passed a special Community Health Center program, authorized under Section 330 of the Public Health Service Act, which provided grants to what were now called federally qualified health centers (FQHCs). This program highlighted the main focus of CHCs on underserved patients, thereby serving as "safety-net providers." In addition, these facilities were defined as sites for comprehensive primary care. The centers were supposed to involve the local community and deliver high-quality primary care with the help of qualified professional staff. Additionally, these centers were given an opportunity to establish connections and partnerships with the private and public sector and had a governing board that included individuals served by the CHC.[3]

Over time, congressional authorizations added migrant health centers and primary care programs for the homeless and residents of public housing. The Health Centers Consolidation Act (1996) combined these separate authorities (community, migrant, homeless, and public housing) under Section 330 of the Public Health Service Act (PHSA), thereby creating the consolidated health centers program.

CHC grantees are thus alternatively called "330 grantees" or Community, Migrant, Homeless, and Public Housing Health Centers (sorry, no easy acronym for this).

In 1990, Congress established the FQHC benefit under Medicare and Medicaid in response to concerns that CHCs were using 330 grant funds to subsidize low reimbursement for Medicaid patients rather than their intended purpose of paying for the uninsured. The benefit paid CHCs a cost-based reimbursement rather than any rate negotiated with the government. Three types of centers were now eligible to become FQHCs: the 330 grantees, clinics that looked like the grantees but did not receive the grants, and certain outpatient clinics run by the Indian Health Service. As of 2011, 1,131 centers received grants under Section 330, and 106 received grants as look-alikes. CHCs composed 80% of all FQHCs. The 2000 Benefits Improvement and Protection Act established a prospective payment system (PPS) for Medicaid reimbursement to FQHCs; the 2010 Patient Protection and Affordable Care Act (PPACA) followed suit by instituting a PPS for Medicare reimbursement starting in 2014.

CHCs must be located in federally designated medically underserved areas (MUAs) or serve federally designated medically underserved populations (MUPs). The criteria for "medically underserved" are designed to capture community need along several dimensions, including existing primary care capacity, health status, economic vulnerability, and demand for care. These dimensions of need are quantified in the Index of Medical Underservice (IMU), which is calculated from 4 data variables: ratio of primary medical care physicians per 1,000 population, infant mortality rate, percent population with incomes below the poverty level, and percent population age 65 or older. In addition, CHCs have several other defining characteristics:

- They are governed by community boards, at least 51% of whose members are health center patients.
- They provide comprehensive primary healthcare services as well as supportive and enabling services (eg, education, translation, transportation) that promote access to healthcare.
- They are open to all, regardless of insurance status or ability to pay, and offer fees adjusted based on ability to pay.

CHCs serve a low-income, predominantly female, and relatively young population. In 2017, 92% of grantee FQHC patients lived below 200% of the federal poverty level. Health center patients are less likely than the general population to be covered by insurance and, when insured, rely heavily on public insurance programs like Medicaid. In 2015, 44% of FQHC revenues came from Medicaid; in 2016, 49% of FQHC patients were on Medicaid. The population is also racially, ethnically, and linguistically diverse; almost two-thirds of health center patients are members of racial or ethnic minority groups, primarily Hispanic/Latino (35% in 2017) and African American (23%).[4]

This demographic profile influences the types of services that CHCs offer. The combination of a young and largely female patient population creates demand for obstetric/gynecologic, family practice, and pediatric services. The combination of low incomes, linguistic barriers, and poor health status requires CHCs to offer comprehensive primary care as well as such enabling services as case management, translation, transportation, outreach, eligibility assistance, and health education.

Today, roughly 1,400 federally funded FQHC grantees deliver comprehensive primary care to roughly 29 million Americans, providing a safety net to people who would otherwise be unable to access or afford care, including those living in poverty, rural residents, children, and veterans. Over the past decade, health centers have undergone significant changes, in large part because of the PPACA. First, the PPACA's insurance expansions, including the option for states to expand Medicaid eligibility, contributed to an increase in the share of insured patients and a decrease in the share of uninsured patients that health centers see. This shift boosted health centers' revenue from Medicaid while increasing patient access to care and the affordability of care. The overall number of patients served by health centers also rose following the PPACA's coverage expansions, from 21.7 million in 2013 to 27.2 million in 2017. Second, the PPACA's Community Health Center Fund (CHCF) doubled federal funding and improved the financial stability of health centers. The fund was authorized for 5 years (2011-2015) and has been renewed incrementally ever since (but is set to expire in November of 2020). CHCF funds compose most of the federal subsidies of FQHCs, which account for 20% of

their revenues. Third, PPACA incentives, such as training opportunities and tuition reimbursement, have encouraged providers to practice in health centers.

The current COVID-19 crisis is now jeopardizing FQHCs. The centers have been hit by staffing furloughs, reduced hours of operation, reduced services, and reduced visits, which have hurt patient revenues and led to temporary facility closures (as many as 1,900 [or 15%] by May 2020). More than 40% of FQHCs had negative operating margins in 2018. At the same time, the disproportionate impact of COVID-19 on minority populations makes FQHCs a main line of defense in tackling the virus.[5] In recognition of this role, the administration authorized $100 million in supplemental funding in March 2020 to deal with the crisis. However, the administration has also placed heavy emphasis on telemedicine visits to manage care delivery in the midst of COVID-19. The Coronavirus Aid, Relief, and Economic Security (CARES) Act of 2020 injected $1.32 billion for virus response efforts, which helps to pay for telemedicine visits. Unfortunately, 56% of FQHCs did not have any telehealth use in 2018 and are underresourced to participate in this virtual care solution, including inadequate funding for equipment and staff training, as well as a historical lack of reimbursement needed to invest here.[6]

## RURAL HEALTH CLINICS

Congress designated the rural health clinic (RHC) in 1977 to facilitate payment to support primary care delivery in rural areas to Medicare and Medicaid beneficiaries who lacked access. The RHCs were organized clinics staffed by both physicians and non-physicians. RHCs must have at least one physician and at least one nurse practitioner, physician assistant, or certified nurse midwife at least 50% of the time the clinic is open to see patients.

In 2010, there were 3,820 RHCs in 45 states, both provider-based and freestanding, under different ownership auspices (for-profit, nonprofit, state/local government). There are currently about 4,500 RHCs in operation.

RHCs and FQHCs are both found in rural areas and thus need to be distinguished. RHCs can be for-profit, can be part of a Medicare participating hospital or skilled nursing facility or home health agency, cannot be both an RHC and an FQHC, and are *not* mandated to provide care to everyone regardless of their ability to pay. RHCs do serve some Medicaid and uninsured patients, but the majority of their patients are covered by Medicare or private insurance. Medicare reimburses RHCs using an all-inclusive payment that entails per-visit payment limits ($78.07 in 2011), compared to FQHC limits of $109.24 and $126.22 for rural and urban centers, respectively. The 2000 Benefits Improvement and Protection Act established a PPS for Medicaid reimbursement to RHCs as well as FQHCs.[7]

## COMMUNITY MENTAL HEALTH CENTERS

In 1963, President Kennedy signed into law the Community Mental Health Act (CMHA), also known as the Mental Retardation and Community Mental Health Centers Construction Act. The CMHA provided grants to states for the establishment of community mental health centers (CMHCs), under the overview of the National Institute of Mental Health, to offer a community-based care alternative to institutionalization in state mental hospitals. Such hospitals had come under severe criticism following the publication of several popular books, including *One Flew Over the Cuckoo's Nest* and *Asylums*.

The act provided grants to states for the construction of CMHCs, facilities specially designed for the delivery of mental health prevention, diagnosis, and treatment services to individuals residing in the community. CMHC patients could be treated at the centers while working and living at home. Each center was required, at a minimum, to provide 5 essential services: consultation and education on mental health, inpatient services, outpatient services, emergency response, and partial hospitalization.

The CMHA marked a major transformation of the public mental health system by shifting resources away from large institutions toward community-based mental health treatment programs. Starting in the 1960s, states emptied out the patient populations in their mental hospitals—a process known then as "deinstitutionalization." States did this for 3 reasons: Mental hospitals were believed to "warehouse" the mentally ill, new psychotropic medications and psychotherapies were introduced that allowed (many thought) patients to

be managed in community settings, and state hospitals were expensive to run. A growing body of evidence at the time also suggested that mental illness could be treated more effectively and in a more cost-effective manner in community settings than in traditional psychiatric hospitals.

The CMHA grants were intended to fund 1,500 to 2,500 new CMHCs nationwide to serve roughly 40 million people. Only half of the proposed centers were ever built; none were fully funded; and the act failed to provide long-term funding for their operations. Between 1963 and 1980, the federal government funded only 789 CMHCs to the tune of $2.7 billion. During those same years, the number of patients in state mental hospitals fell by three-quarters from 504,604 to 132,164; 90% of beds were closed down. In 2000, approximately 55,000 patients remained in these institutions, representing less than 10% of those institutionalized just 50 years prior.

What happened? Some states took the opportunity to close expensive state facilities without redirecting some of their hospital funding to community-based care. Some observers suggest the states did not treat the most seriously ill patients. Under President Reagan, the Omnibus Budget Reconciliation Act (OBRA) of 1981 converted the remaining funding for the act into a mental health block grant to the states. The CMHC program had failed—not because of President Reagan, but because it did not provide care for the sickest patients. President Reagan did not kill the CMHA program; he was merely disposing of the corpse.[8]

Public mental health systems largely failed to develop sufficient resources and staffing adequate to treat and support individuals in home- and community-based settings. Part of the problem is that there has historically been no standard definition for CMHCs in federal law.[9] Moreover, the service array in many communities was, and often continues to be, insufficiently comprehensive and intensive to meet the needs of young people and adults returning from or at risk of institutional care. Many public mental health systems were, and remain, critically underfunded and understaffed. From 2014 to 2017, the number of CMHCs decreased by 14% nationally (from 3,406 to 2,920)[10]; as of 2018, there were 2,553 CMHCs in the United States.

What about the patients? Approximately half of the mentally-ill individuals discharged from state mental hospitals, many of whom had family support, sought outpatient treatment and have done well. The other half, many of whom lack family support and suffer from the most severe illnesses such as schizophrenia and bipolar disorder, have done poorly.

According to multiple studies summarized by the Treatment Advocacy Center, the untreated mentally-ill are responsible for 10% of all homicides (and a higher percentage of the mass killings), constitute 20% of jail and prison inmates, and compose at least 30% of the homeless. Severely mentally-ill individuals now inundate hospital emergency rooms and have colonized libraries, parks, train stations, and other public spaces. The quality of their lives mocks the lofty intentions of the founders of the CMHC program.

Another remarkable aspect of this federal experiment has been its inordinate cost. In 2009, 4.7 million Americans received Supplemental Security Income or Social Security Disability Insurance (SSI or SSDI; see Chapter 19) because of mental illnesses, not including intellectual disability. This represented a 10-fold increase since 1977. The total Medicaid and Medicare costs for mentally ill individuals in 2005 were more than $60 billion.

In 2013, an estimated 10 million adults in the United States (4.2% of the country's adult population) had experienced serious mental illness (SMI) in the past year. The Substance Abuse and Mental Health Services Administration (SAMHSA) defines SMI—such as schizophrenia, bipolar disorder, and major depression—as "mental, behavioral, or emotional disorders that substantially interfere(s) with or limit(s) one or more major life activities." For the roughly 60% of adults with SMI who receive mental health treatment, the most common treatment settings are outpatient settings, such as CMHCs. CMHCs provide counseling and medication management; some may also provide short-term residential services, substance abuse treatment, and support linking consumers to needed community services.

Over the past decade, experts have called for the integration of physical and behavioral healthcare services to improve quality of care and overall health outcomes for adults with SMI. Integrated care involves systematic collaboration between behavioral health providers and general medical providers. Early integrated care initiatives focused on bringing behavioral health services into medical settings, such as primary care clinics. More recent initiatives that specifically target adults with SMI (eg, SAMHSA's Primary and Behavioral Health Care Integration program [PBHCI]) focus on bringing physical healthcare into community behavioral health settings, such as CMHCs. CMHCs may partner with other organizations, such as FQHCs, to provide physical healthcare services for their integrated care consumers. Among the first 3 cohorts of PBHCI grantees, most ($n$ = 45, 82%) had partnered with other healthcare and community organizations (eg, hospitals, CHCs, FQHCs). FQHCs and FQHC look-alikes are becoming increasingly involved in integrated care.

## URGENT CARE CENTERS

The first urgent care centers (UCCs) opened in the United States in the late 1970s to a big splash. Labeled at the time as "urgi-centers" or "emergency offi-centers," they were often founded by entrepreneurial physicians (eg, Dr. Bruce Flashner in Chicago). Such physicians felt they could (1) offer more convenient care via walk-in (no appointment basis) clinics without sacrificing the qualifications of doctors, (2) offer more expanded access (eg, 16 hours per day) than a physician's office, (3) reduce the unnecessary utilization of EDs for nonemergent care, and (4) strip away some of the business from the hospital ED and thus potential admissions through the ED. As a result, and serving as a source of their "buzz," urgi-centers were viewed as an early form of disruptive innovation that could render hospital EDs "vulnerable to replacement" due to their lower-cost structure, focus on a narrow range of services, and increased consumer convenience.[11]

Like other so-called disruptive innovations, this scenario did not materialize. Hospitals played aggressive defense and called on state regulators to subject the urgi-centers to the same regulatory standards they were held to, including their trained personnel and expensive, life-saving equipment. Some states heard the call; others did not.[12] But the urgi-centers got the message and backed off of the use of "emergency" in their marketing and promotion.

The disruption strategy failed for another reason: Incumbents commandeered the disrupters. Physician ownership of UCCs has fallen over time (from 54% to 40% between 2008 and

2014), while hospital ownership has risen from 25% to 37%. Some insurers such as United's Optum division have also gotten into the UCC business via its recent acquisition of DaVita Medical Group and its 35 UCCs and its 2015 acquisition of MedExpress Urgent Care.

Over time, the urgi-centers have become known as *urgent care centers* (UCCs). Unlike some of the organized ambulatory care models chronicled earlier, UCCs operate almost exclusively on a walk-in basis and are frequently found in convenient locations in areas of high foot or vehicle traffic. Many also provide transparent pricing, with the menu and price of services often listed online or onsite. The modal staffing model is a mix of physicians, advanced practice registered nurses, nurse practitioners, and physician assistants. Almost all UCCs are staffed by primary care and/or emergency physicians, and approximately half employ physician assistants and nurse practitioners as additional providers.[13]

The estimated number of UCCs ranges widely. The Urgent Care Association (UCA) puts the total number at 9,616 centers (as of 2019, up from 6,400 in 2014; Figure 13-1). Part of the reason for the discrepancy is that there is no single nationally accepted definition of what a UCC is or what the scope of services should be. According to the UCA, the UCC is "a medical clinic with expanded hours that is specially equipped to diagnose and treat a broad spectrum of non-life or limb-threatening illnesses and injuries. . . . Care is rendered under the medical direction of an allopathic or osteopathic physician. UCCs accept unscheduled, walk-in patients seeking medical attention during all posted hours of operation."[14]

The scope of UCC services and acuity of conditions treated fall between those of a PCP and an ED. However, the lines between these facilities are often blurred, due in part to the overlapping scope of services delivered across the sites of care. More than half of UCCs render treatments and services considered to be primary care, and nearly two-thirds offer routine immunizations.[15] Unlike EDs, UCCs are generally not equipped to deal with trauma, resuscitation, or other life-threatening conditions and are not open 24/7.[16] Nevertheless, one study reported an overlap of 60% in the top 20 diagnoses treated by EDs and UCCs in Texas, although the ED cost of treatment for the same diagnoses was 10 times higher.[17] Others put the cost differential more at 3:1 ($500 vs $160).[18]

In terms of utilization, UCA data indicate a median number of 32 patients treated per day, or 89 million patient visits annually (2017 data). This compares with 922 million physician office visits, 53% of which are PCP visits (2013 data). Thus, UCCs provide roughly 18% of primary care visits and nearly 10% of all outpatient visits in the United States.[19] There is some dispute as to whether the presence of UCCs helps to reduce visits to hospital EDs, however, despite the overlap in many of the services they render.[20]

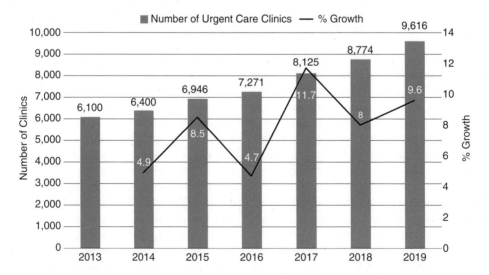

**Figure 13-1** • US Urgent Care Clinic Growth, 2013 to 2019. (Source: Urgent Care Association 2019 Benchmarking Report.)

| **Critical Thinking Exercise: Urgent Care Centers—Cost-Saving or Costly?** |
| --- |

UCCs offer patients an alternative to using the hospital ED, which is expensive. They are open for extended hours, although not 24/7 (the way EDs work), and thus serve the "access" angle of the iron triangle. They are clearly less costly and may also not interfere with a patient's existing relationships with their own PCP. But are there any downsides to the growth of UCCs? Critics suggest they do little to address the fragmentation of care and may actually add to the problem. They may also not be linked to the patient's PCP, which poses an issue of care coordination. Finally, there is some evidence that UCCs locate in more affluent areas with insured patients and may not reduce unnecessary use of the ED. So, overall, are UCCs cost-saving or costly?

## STAND-ALONE EMERGENCY DEPARTMENTS

UCCs need to be distinguished from stand-alone EDs (ie, facilities devoted primarily to ED services but located apart from hospitals). The majority of stand-alone EDs have opened since 2010, either reflecting or causing the growth in ED volumes noted in Chapter 12. Between 2010 and 2015, the number of hospital outpatient ED visits per capita increased by more than 7%, more than triple the number of physician office visits per capita (<2%). In 2016, there were 566 freestanding EDs—some hospital-affiliated ($n = 363$) and some independent ($n = 203$). Such growth has been partly driven by Medicare reimbursement that rewards treating lower-severity cases in the higher-paying ED settings, competition among hospitals for market share, and an exemption in the Bipartisan Budget Act (2015) that allows stand-alone EDs to receive higher hospital outpatient payments for non-ED services.[21]

The regulation of stand-alone EDs occurs primarily at the state level, and states take varying approaches in their standards and regulations regarding staffing and clinical capabilities. Most hospital-affiliated stand-alone EDs must be within 35 miles of the main campus to capture hospital-based billing under Medicare; this results in most being located in metropolitan (rather than rural) areas.

Stand-alone EDs vie to treat patients with lower-severity conditions with a host of competitors: the 200,000+ community-based PCPs (see Chapter 10), the 9,000+ UCCs discussed earlier, and the 1,800 or so retail clinics covered later in this chapter. They offer overlapping services and overlapping access, but at a higher cost. This is because the competitors bill Medicare under the outpatient prospective payment system (OPPS) and the physician fee schedule (PFS); by contrast, stand-alone EDs can also bill for the ED's facility services. Medicare's total ED payment combines a facility fee, an OPPS fee for any outpatient services (eg, lab, imaging), and a professional fee.

Stand-alone EDs also compete for paying patients. They are concentrated in zip codes with above-average incomes and higher shares of patients with private insurance coverage. Research suggests that use of ED services, both in the Medicare and commercially insured populations, grew more rapidly in recent years in a few large metro areas with higher rates of stand-alone EDs per capita.

## AMBULATORY SURGERY CENTERS

Ambulatory surgery centers (ASCs), originally labeled "surgi-centers," preceded the establishment of urgi-centers, with the first one founded in 1970. The concept caught on slowly: By the end of the decade, there were only 100 ASCs. And like the "urgi-centers," they were often founded by entrepreneurial physicians who followed up after patient office visits with procedures conducted in their own surgical centers.[22] This act of entrepreneurism led to the development of a new organizational form for conducting non–hospital-based outpatient surgery.

Such procedures were performed by the same surgeons who practiced in hospital-based operating rooms, with the same quality of care, but at a much lower cost. A Government

Accountability Office study found that the costs of care in freestanding ASCs are much lower than the costs of care provided in hospital-based ASCs.[23] A subsequent review concluded that ASCs save considerable monies for both the Medicare program and Medicare beneficiaries.[24] A review of the literature on ASCs conducted by the Medicare Payment Advisory Commission (MedPAC), the congressional watchdog over provider payments made by the Medicare program, suggests further benefits provided by freestanding ASCs.[25] These benefits included more convenient locations for patients, shorter waiting times for patients, easier scheduling of surgery for patients, greater operating efficiency, availability of more specialized staff, lower Medicare reimbursement rates, and greater physician control over the work environment. There are also quality-enhancing benefits when physicians concentrate their practice schedules at one site of care. These benefits derive from the physician's familiarity with the operating room staff and the teamwork that develops from performing multiple procedures together. It is also important to point out that there are no data that physician ownership of ASCs either increases costs or decreases the quality of care provided to patients.

In this manner, ASCs outcompeted hospital-based surgery centers and gradually dominated them in terms of numbers and patient volume. Their cost advantage led the federal government to approve Medicare reimbursement to ASCs for 200 procedures in 1982; commercial insurers began supporting ASC utilization as a mechanism to reduce utilization of more expensive hospital-based facilities. The number of ASCs grew from 293 in 1982 to 1,000 by 1988, followed by rapid growth after 2000 (Figure 13-2).

| | |
|---|---|
| • 2000 | 3,028 |
| • 2010 | 5,135 |
| • 2011 | 5,217 |
| • 2012 | 5,287 |
| • 2013 | 5,363 |
| • 2014 | 5,437 |
| • 2015 | 5,475 |
| • 2016 | 5,519 |
| • 2017 | 5,602 |
| • 2018 | 5,700 |
| • 2019 | 5,788 |

**Figure 13-2** • Number of Medicare-Certified Ambulatory Surgery Centers by Year. (Source: VMG Health. "ASCs in 2019: A Year in Review." https://vmghealth.com/blog/ascs-in-2019-a-year-in-review.)

There has been enormous growth in ambulatory surgeries, with a tripling of outpatient procedures between 1990 and 2010 (Figure 13-3). Much of that increase has taken place in ASCs. Studies show that ASCs lead to lower levels of hospitalization, lower costs for the same procedure, increased consumer convenience (shorter travel distance, faster throughput), and no difference in quality of care (eg, patient mortality).[26] This suggests that ASCs contribute to both iron triangle and triple aim goals.

Surgeons established ASCs for several reasons, including delays in scheduling patient surgeries at the hospitals where they held privileges, limited operating room capacity at those hospitals, and challenges in obtaining new equipment due to constrained hospital finances. Sometimes, surgeons who wished to develop joint ventures with their hospitals in developing ASCs were rebuffed by their hospitals who (1) wanted to maintain 100% control, (2) limited the hours during which physicians could operate, and/or (3) wanted physicians to assume partial debt for the facility. In such cases, the surgeons sought and obtained outside financing partners (management services organizations) who put up the money to construct the facility, hired the administrative staff for the ASC, and retained minority ownership.

There were some definite financial advantages to the surgeons to do so. Not only did they collect their professional fees for performing the surgery but, as owners of the ASC, they could collect a portion of the facility fees that commercial insurers paid; this is not allowed under Medicare, however. Most freestanding ASCs are owned, at least in part, by the surgeons and anesthesiologists who practice there. This can create a potential conflict of interest because ownership may come with financial incentives to maximize throughput and increase utilization. The potential for physician-induced demand, wherein thresholds for intervention are lowered, is made possible by the discretionary nature of outpatient surgery. Some state-level studies, although limited in clinical scope, showed a relationship between physician ownership of an ASC and the volume of outpatient surgeries performed and that the rates of some procedures increased dramatically after a facility opened.[27]

However, prior research has uncovered only limited evidence of a *causal* relationship between physician ownership and surgical volume. Instead, the relationship could be spurious

| Year | Inpatient Surgeries | Outpatient Surgeries | Total Surgeries | Outpatient Surgeries as a % of Total | Inpatient Surgery Growth | Outpatient Surgery Growth |
|---|---|---|---|---|---|---|
| 1993 | 10,181,703 | 12,624,292 | 22,805,995 | 55.4% | NA | NA |
| 1994 | 9,833,938 | 13,154,838 | 22,988,776 | 57.2% | −3.4% | 4.2% |
| 1995 | 9,700,613 | 13,462,304 | 23,162,917 | 58.1% | −1.4% | 2.3% |
| 1996 | 9,545,612 | 14,023,651 | 23,569,263 | 59.5% | −1.6% | 4.2% |
| 1997 | 9,509,081 | 14,678,290 | 24,187,371 | 60.7% | −0.4% | 4.7% |
| 1998 | 9,735,705 | 15,593,614 | 25,329,319 | 61.6% | 2.4% | 6.2% |
| 1999 | 9,539,593 | 15,845,492 | 25,385,085 | 62.4% | −2.0% | 1.6% |
| 2000 | 9,729,336 | 16,383,374 | 26,112,710 | 62.7% | 2.0% | 3.4% |
| 2001 | 9,779,583 | 16,684,726 | 26,464,309 | 63.0% | 0.5% | 1.8% |
| 2002 | 10,105,010 | 17,361,176 | 27,466,186 | 63.2% | 3.3% | 4.1% |
| 2003 | 9,940,922 | 17,165,616 | 27,106,538 | 63.3% | −1.6% | −1.1% |
| 2004 | 10,050,346 | 17,351,490 | 27,401,836 | 63.3% | 1.1% | 1.1% |
| 2005 | 10,097,271 | 17,445,587 | 27,542,858 | 63.3% | 0.5% | 0.5% |
| 2006 | 10,095,683 | 17,235,141 | 27,330,824 | 63.1% | 0.0% | −1.2% |
| 2007 | 10,189,630 | 17,146,334 | 27,335,964 | 62.7% | 0.9% | −0.5% |
| 2008 | 10,105,156 | 17,354,282 | 27,459,438 | 63.2% | −0.8% | 1.2% |
| 2009 | 10,100,980 | 17,357,534 | 27,458,514 | 63.2% | 0.0% | 0.0% |
| 2010 | 9,954,821 | 17,357,177 | 27,311,998 | 63.6% | −1.4% | 0.0% |
| 2011 | 9,368,467 | 17,269,245 | 26,637,712 | 64.8% | −5.9% | −0.5% |
| 2012 | 9,513,598 | 17,297,663 | 26,811,261 | 64.5% | 1.5% | 0.2% |
| 2013 | 9,147,264 | 17,418,773 | 25,566,037 | 65.6% | −3.9% | 0.7% |
| 2014 | 9,015,000 | 17,386,000 | 26,401,000 | 65.9% | −1.5% | −0.2% |
| 2015 | 8,920,775 | 17,588,335 | 26,509,110 | 66.3% | −1.05% | 0.01% |
| 2016 | 8,982,309 | 18,224,816 | 27,207,125 | 67.0% | 0.7% | 3.6% |
| 2017 | 9,146,015 | 19,075,759 | 28,221,774 | 67.6% | 1.8% | 4.7% |

**Figure 13-3** • Hospital Inpatient and Outpatient Surgeries, 1993 to 2017. NA, Not Applicable. (Source: American Hospital Association.)

or driven by other factors. For example, research has shown that ASCs attract high-volume and entrepreneurial surgeons.[28] Such physicians do not become high-level users of the ASC because they have an ownership interest; instead, they acquire an ownership interest because they are already high-volume surgeons. These physicians see many of their patients in the ASC because it is more convenient to them and their patients to do so. This maximizes their surgical productivity and patient access, both of which increase public welfare. Other reasons for the association include meeting previously unmet patient demand.

The federal government issued "Safe Harbor" guidelines for physician-owned ASCs such that they are not subject to antikickback statutes and are exempt from the Stark II laws (Section 1877 of the Social Security Act) as long as physicians conduct at least one-third of their cases there. According to the Office of the Inspector General, the ASC is an "extension of the physician's office practice."[29] This has lessened some (but not all) of the concerns over conflict of interest.

MedPAC is now concerned that freestanding ASCs may be an endangered species.[30] This is because Medicare pays hospital-based ASCs 81% higher rates than what is paid freestanding ASCs. Due to the payment differential, physician owners of ASCs are selling their facilities to hospitals and often entering employment arrangements with those hospitals. Both trends increase healthcare costs. They also reduce patient access to community physicians and sites of care. Hospital sites of surgery are not only higher cost but also less efficient and less productive than freestanding ASCs. According to MedPAC officials, "we believe it is desirable to maintain beneficiaries' access to ASCs because services provided there are less costly [than hospital outpatient departments]." The disappearance of the freestanding ASCs may harm adequate access of Medicare beneficiaries to ASC services.

ASCs currently appear to be enjoying several favorable tailwinds.[31] First, the CMS 2019 final payment rule stated that CMS would use the hospital market basket to update ASC payments from 2019 to 2023, an effective update of 2.1% on average over all covered procedures for 2019. CMS also lowered the device-intensive procedure threshold, resulting in more than 140 new device-intensive procedures for which ASCs can receive Medicare reimbursement. Second, patients continue to migrate away from hospital-based sites to ASCs, partly due to advanced technology and anesthetics (and increased safety in performing higher-acuity procedures), physician comfort with minimally invasive approaches, consumer and payor demand for lower-cost care, and tightening reimbursement. Third, a 2018 national survey showed the huge interest of health systems in owning or affiliating with a freestanding ASC.[32] Fourth, the health systems face stiffening competition here from ASC management companies (eg, AMSURG, Surgical Care Affiliates [SCA], United Surgical Partners International, Surgery Partners) that continue to seek new partnership opportunities with surgeons and build ASCs. The 2017 acquisition of SCA by Optum, a division of UnitedHealth Group, suggests that payers are interested in adding surgery centers to their portfolio. Finally, consumers may desire "one-stop shopping" for ASCs that offer such ancillary services as imaging, pathology, and physical therapy. Such investments can make an ASC more attractive to patients, physicians, and potential business partners.

Figure 13-4 shows the growth in outpatient surgeries captured by the ASCs.[33] Figure 13-5 shows the mix in ASC ownership structures and the growth in for-profit management companies involved in the ASC sector. The majority of ASCs (90%+) have some degree of physician ownership.[34] Nearly all of these ASCs (97%) are investor-owned and for-profit. Nearly one-quarter (22%) are owned or managed by ASC management and development companies.[35]

## RETAIL CLINICS

Retail clinics (RCs) are healthcare clinics located in retail settings, such as supermarkets and pharmacies, that treat simple medical conditions and provide basic preventive care. They are also labeled "convenient care clinics" or "store-based health clinics" and are usually open extended weekday hours and weekends. The average cost of services offered by RCs ranges from $30 to $110.

RCs offer healthcare almost exclusively through nurse practitioners or physician assistants, providing a limited scope of care under physician supervision.[36] They do not treat medical emergencies and are not intended for people with recurring illnesses. A typical RC treats about 30 minor illnesses, performs health screenings, and administers vaccines. Ten acute conditions and preventive care account for the vast majority (90.3%) of RC visits: upper respiratory infections, sinusitis, bronchitis, pharyngitis, immunizations, otitis media (middle ear infection), otitis externa (outer ear infection, also known as "swimmer's ear"), conjunctivitis, urinary tract infections, and screening lab test or blood pressure check. The most frequently provided service is strep throat testing.

Although almost all RCs offer basic exams, vaccines, and preventive care, some clinics are adding risk assessment and management services. These services create more opportunities to serve patients, generate revenue, and increase volume through lab testing and other screening. With the 2018 merger of CVS Health and Aetna, RCs appear to be expanding their range of offered preventive and proactive services to help patients to better manage their health, rather than just providing treatment for illnesses.

### Types of RCs

Three types of retail stores typically host RCs: (1) pharmacies who see RCs as a way to increase prescription spending (65%); (2) discounters or mass merchandisers who see RCs as a venue for consumer services (20%); and (3) grocers who see RCs as a way to increase store visits and "basket" size (15%). RCs are commonly structured as 1 of 3 models. In the retailer leasing model, the retailer leases space to an independent retail medical clinic operator that employs clinicians. Both profits and losses flow to the RC operator. Under the retailer ownership model, the retailer owns the RC and employs clinicians. Profits and losses flow to the retailer in this model. In the retailer practice management model, the retailer leases space and nonclinical items (equipment, furniture, health information technology, administrative staff) to the independent clinic operator, who employs physicians and/or mid-level practitioners. Profits and losses flow to the RC operator, but the retailer shares risk in the form of a practice management fee.

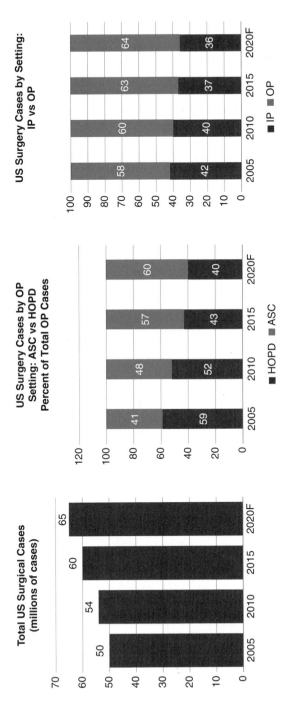

**Figure 13-4** • Surgical Volumes, by Setting. ASC, Ambulatory Surgery Center; HOPD, Hospital Outpatient Department; IP, Inpatient; OP, Outpatient. (Source: L.E.K.)

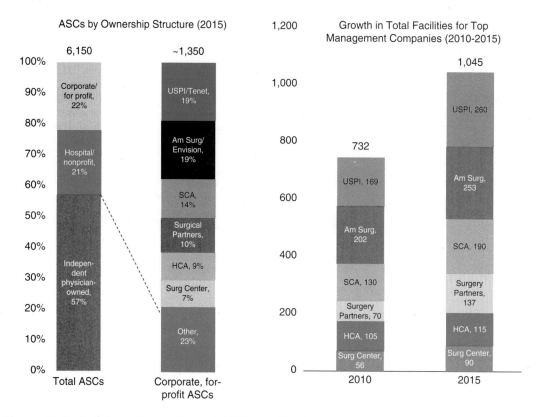

**Figure 13-5** • Ambulatory Surgery Center (ASC) Ownership. (Source: L.E.K.)

RCs can also take on 1 of 2 types of partnerships with mainstream providers.[37] In an integrated model, the RC is owned and operated by larger providers such as hospital chains or physician groups, and is linked to one of the provider's PCP practices via a shared electronic medical record. In a hybrid model, the RC collaborates with the larger provider via co-branding and (in some cases) a shared electronic medical record.

## History of RCs

The first retail medical clinic was established in St. Paul, Minnesota, in 2000 after founder Rick Krieger waited over 2 hours in a UCC for his son to get a strep throat test. According to Krieger[38]:

We started talking about why there was not a way to just get a simple question answered or a simple test, like strep throat, done. Why was there not some way to just slip in and be seen quickly? Wasn't there some way to get care in a timely manner for a relatively simple illness? A quick convenient way to diagnose without waiting in the ER or clinic for two hours? We are not talking about diabetes, cancer, or heart disease! We are talking about colds and throat and ear infections.

Krieger created QuickMedx and partnered with Cub Foods to offer medical services in a retail setting. Centers offered treatment for 7 common medical conditions: strep throat, mono, flu, pregnancy testing, and bladder, ear, and sinus infections. Centers offered a more affordable alternative to EDs and UCCs and were cash pay only. The demand for walk-in convenience led to quick growth, with several large employers asking their health plans to include QuickMedx in their networks. With the advent of insurance coverage, QuickMedx became MinuteClinic in December 2003 and added clinics in more stores (and more cities like Baltimore). By 2005, MinuteClinic launched its relationship with CVS Corporation (now CVS Health) and opened its first walk-in medical clinics based in CVS Pharmacy stores in Minneapolis-St. Paul and Baltimore. This led to national expansion in CVS Pharmacy locations and, in 2006, acquisition by CVS for an estimated $170 million. RCs took off that same year: 220 new clinics opened, and 130 more opened before April 2007. Year-over-year growth rates in the number of RCs were an astounding 422% (2005), 170% (2006), and 157% (2007).[39]

There followed some sector consolidation, some RC closures, and slowing growth from 2008 to 2015. Several explanations for the slowdown include low RC patient volumes for many services other than flu shots (which are seasonal), the uncertainty posed by PPACA and reimbursement, an unproven business model, and the lack of partnerships with other mainstream providers (some of whom saw the RCs as a competitive threat). There were also concerns that RCs constituted yet more fragmentation in a fragmented delivery ecosystem and undermined efforts by mainstream providers to develop patient-centered medical homes (PCMHs). Analysts nevertheless touted the "disruptive innovation" that RCs entailed and forecasted aggressive growth over the next 2 decades, rising to perhaps 2,800 by 2015.[40]

## RCs' Failure to Disrupt

The anticipated rapid expansion of RCs failed to materialize, however. Trend data over the past 3 years indicate that growth in the total number of RCs stalled between 2015 and 2018 (Figure 13-6). RCs reached a plateau below 2,000 sites by 2015 with a slight decline by 2018, perhaps due to the expansion of UCCs.[41] The trend holds for both CVS Health, which operates roughly half of all such clinics, and

Walgreens, which operates roughly one-fifth. Indeed, Walgreens has shifted its strategy away from in-house clinics to partnerships with local health systems that own and operate the clinics inside Walgreens, effectively moving away from a vertically integrated model to a strategic alliance model. Other RC chains have also stopped their expansion. RCs are thus not a booming industry. The stall in RC capacity suggests that the upward trend in RC visits may have likewise plateaued since 2015. At present, RCs may supply as little as 1% to 2% of all primary care in the United States, much less than the 5% estimated a few years ago.[42]

Contrary to Clay Christensen's theory, RCs were not disruptive.[43] Even one of Christensen's colleagues and early advocate of RCs has admitted this.[44] The RCs "cherry-picked" patients instead of targeting those market segments that have been neglected (eg, the poor, the rural, the uninsured, those in poor health—even those covered by the PPACA) with a more affordable if less complex (fewer "bells and whistles") product offering (as suggested by the "theory" of disruption). This was deliberate. The clinics were disproportionately located in urban areas and, within those areas, in higher-income neighborhoods. RCs targeted more affluent people who could pay cash for the clinic's services or who had insurance (that later covered these services). Not only did they target wealthier neighborhoods, but they also attracted patients who were disproportionately younger adults, females, and those without any chronic conditions.[45] This was not "the low end of the market" who were "less-demanding customers."[46] For their patients (many of whom are Millennials), convenience

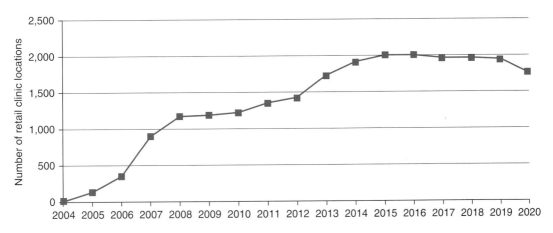

**Figure 13-6 •** Number of US Retail Clinics, 2004 to 2020. (Source: Adam Fein. *The 2020 Economic Report on U.S. Pharmacies and Pharmacy Benefit Managers*. Drug Channels Institute, 2020.)

served as the strongest predictor of RC use. The clinics also did not target the poor or those without a physician—ironically, those who used a hospital ED as their primary source of care. This is perhaps why the entrance of an RC has failed to reduce ED utilization for low-acuity conditions.[47]

A related explanation for the failure of RCs to disrupt was their reluctance to accept Medicaid patients. Research suggests that only 60% of RCs accept Medicaid.[48] This is consistent with the disproportionate location of these clinics in more affluent neighborhoods and is similar to the proportion of physicians who accept Medicaid. As a result, any long-term impact on RC volume via expanded health insurance coverage through the PPACA (half through Medicaid, half through narrow network exchange plans) may have been blunted.

## Impact of RCs

Academic evidence on RCs suggests their ability to impact the iron triangle (access, quality, cost) is limited and difficult to summarize.[49] With regard to *access*, RCs treat patients who are not necessarily treated by other providers. The vast majority of RC patients (60%+) have no PCP, partly reflecting the fact they are also much younger in age than other patients. RCs are almost exclusively located in urban areas; 13% are located in underserved areas (health professional shortage areas) where 21% of the US population resides. Moreover, despite the claims for convenience, RCs do not uniformly enjoy customer praise. An analysis of social media reveals that Walmart's RCs achieve higher positive evaluations than do CVS's MinuteClinics. Forty-one percent of users posted negative comments on MinuteClinics; 38% reported long wait times, suggesting the stores be relabeled as "HourClinic." Customers of both complained about the level of medical expertise, with some claiming they had been misdiagnosed.[50]

With regard to *quality*, RCs perform the same or better on several process measures (Healthcare Effectiveness Data and Information Set [HEDIS] measures, care coordination) compared with other sites of care. However, contrary to Christensen, the disruptive effect of RCs is not always positive.[51] When asked if RCs were helping or hurting primary care, only 22% of physicians responded favorably; by contrast, 36% felt RCs were hurting primary care.

Overall, 79% of respondents said that market disruption fragmented the physician-patient relationship, 47% stated it fostered inaccurate medical information, 47% said it resulted in less coordinated care, and 33% felt it increased the overall cost of care. In another recent survey of healthcare executives, clinical leaders, and clinicians, two-thirds of respondents said that convenient care sites (like RCs) offer care of lower quality compared to PCPs.[52]

Analyses of PCPs suggest that the shift to RCs and other convenient care sites harms the physician-patient relationship and the benefits of such encounters (eg, trust, empathy, information exchange, compliance, emotional bonding, reassurance, and anxiety reduction).[53] One recently completed study shows that the loss of continuity in seeing one's PCP—as often happens when patients seek care from an RC and do not return—leads to higher utilization of specialists and higher healthcare spending.[54] Folding RCs (whose purpose is convenient treatment for episodic complaints) into a continuum of care has so far proven elusive. Patients with symptoms want relief or reassurance, not a personal relationship.

With regard to *cost*, a recent literature review suggests that RCs exhibit lower costs, but often due to lower spending for lower-acuity conditions and for the "evaluation and management" service components of a physician office or ED visit, components that patients may actually value (particularly those with chronic conditions who need or wish to discuss them with their doctor). However, because RC patients typically lack a PCP, there is no explicit substitution of RCs for other types of utilization. Instead, RCs can add to patient demand rather than substitute for other types of utilization, and thereby add to total healthcare utilization and spending.[55] Much of RC utilization (estimated at 58%) would not otherwise occur.[56] The patient who goes to an RC may well follow up with a visit to a PCP to confirm the diagnosis and get advice.

## Profitability of RCs

RCs may have failed to spread because they are often unprofitable, losing $41,000 annually on average.[57] RCs are reportedly unprofitable until they reach a critical volume, after which they earn a small margin. The low profitability of clinics may result from an inability to "cross-sell."

Analysts suggest that MinuteClinic generates less than 1% of CVS retail pharmacy dispensing revenues.[58] Thus, there is little evidence that such cross-selling is working.

RCs hope that they can drive business around customer health and wellness, in addition to filling prescriptions and buying consumer products. Despite the promise, senior pharmacy chain executives acknowledge limits on their ability to cross-sell the front-end and back-end of the store: "health and beauty aids" (HABA) and minor acute care services in the RC. Most customers visit pharmacies for one side of the business but not the other (at least on the same visit). This threatens the business model of RCs, which must compete on the metric of "revenue per square foot" against the higher-margin HABA products.

The clinics are also a high fixed-cost business using labor, space, and some technology. They can cost $50,000 to $250,000 to build out, can typically see 10 to 30 patients per day, and may generate revenues upward of $500,000 per year. Profits of $200,000+ reported for "best-in-class" clinics rest on an ambitious volume of 30 visits per day.

### Critical Thinking Exercise: Aetna Case

In a recent Harvard Business School case, Aetna's chief executive officer Mark Bertolini laid out part of the strategy behind the merger of CVS and Aetna (pharmacy chain and insurer).[59] His strategic intent encompassed the following:

- Pioneer a new model of healthcare.
- Put consumers at the center of their own care.
- Have consumers see Aetna as a "trusted guide" rather than an antagonist.
- Help its members lead healthier lives.
- Organize disparate digital platform investments under "Aetna Digital."
- Support digital interactions to address the majority of members' health needs.

- Be a single front door to guide the member seamlessly through their health journey.
- Use big data and analytics to predict those likely to use EDs unnecessarily.
- Use behavioral economics to figure out customers' preferences and motivate them.
- Have "boots on the ground" in local communities to coordinate care.
- Develop a "community care program"—an individualized approach to deliver services—that identifies what each member's health goals are and help them to achieve them.

What do you make of this strategy? Is this doable with the assets of the two parties?

## RETAIL PHARMACIES

Chapter 10 discussed pharmacists; the previous section discussed RCs, three-quarters of which are owned and operated by community pharmacy chains (CVS, Walgreens, and Rite-Aid). This is depicted in Figure 13-7. The role of pharmacies in ambulatory care is discussed here.

### Overview

There is no federal definition of what a pharmacy is, since the board of pharmacy in each state possesses the authority to license and regulate pharmacies. The National Association of Boards of Pharmacy defines the practice of pharmacy as "the interpretation, evaluation, dispensing, and/or implementation of medical orders, and the initiation and provision of pharmacist care services . . . also includes continually optimizing patient safety and quality of services through effective use of emerging technologies competency-based training."

### Types of Pharmacies

Drugs are dispensed through 3 main formats. *Retail community pharmacies* are retail locations that dispense drugs to the public and include independents, chain drugstores, supermarkets, and mass merchandisers. These outlets differ in the percentage of their store revenues that derive from the sale of drugs (independent is the highest at 90%, followed by chain at 69%, and then supermarket and mass merchandisers at 5%-10%). In terms of annual prescription volume per location, chain stores rank ahead of

| Clinic Location | Clinic Operator(s) | Number of Retail Clinics, Jan. 2020 | Share of Retail Clinics | Change in Number of Retail Clinics vs Jan. 2019 |
|---|---|---|---|---|
| CVS retail pharmacy | MinuteClinic[1] | 1,009 | 57% | −12 |
| Walgreens | Various[2] | 215 | 12% | −187 |
| Kroger[3] | The Little Clinic | 215 | 12% | −10 |
| Target[4] | MinuteClinic; Kaiser Permanente | 102 | 6% | +8 |
| Hy-Vee | Various[5] | 71 | 4% | n.a. |
| Walmart[6] | Care Clinic; Clinic at Walmart | 41 | 2% | −13 |
| Rite Aid | RediClinic | 30 | 2% | −1 |
| HEB | RediClinic | 36 | 2% | 0 |
| All others | | 38 | 2% | |
| **Total** | | 1,757 | 100% | |

Totals may not sum due to rounding.
1. Includes two locations inside Navarro Discount Pharmacy locations in Florida. CVS acquired Navarro in 2014.
2. Clinics are operated by health systems within Walgreens retail locations. In 2019, Walgreens shut down its 184 Walgreens Healthcare Clinic locations.
3. Includes all banners (Kroger; Fry's; Dillons; King Sooper, JayC).
4. Includes 77 locations operated by MinuteClinic and 25 locations operated by Kaiser Permanente.
5. Clinics are operated by hospitals and health systems with Hy-Vee retail locations.
6. Includes 20 Walmart Care Clinics and 22 independently owned and operated Clinic at Walmart locations. Excludes Walmart Health location in Georgia.

**Figure 13-7** • Number of Retail Clinics, by Chain Location, 2020. (Source: Adam Fein. *The 2020 Economic Report on U.S. Pharmacies and Pharmacy Benefit Managers*. Drug Channels Institute, 2020.)

everyone (94,000), followed by the supermarkets and mass merchandisers (57,000-59,000), with independents having the lowest volume (37,000). The vast majority of pharmacists engaged in retail-based, outpatient dispensing are employed by independents and chains; fewer are employed by supermarkets and mass merchandisers.

*Mail pharmacies* are automated facilities that fulfill a patient's prescription at a central location and then deliver via the mail. They focus on 90-day refills of maintenance drugs for chronic conditions and are now the leading dispenser of patient-administered specialty drugs. *Long-term care pharmacies* serve the post-acute care market such as nursing homes and residential care facilities, as well as mental health facilities. Figure 13-8 shows the distribution of drug sales and pharmacy outlets across these settings.

As noted in Chapter 10, pharmacist employment has been shifting from retail to (certain) nonretail settings over time. Employment at retail, mail, long-term care, and specialty pharmacies fell from 65.2% to 59.4% between 2010 and 2018; hospital employment rose from 23.2% to 25.8% of all pharmacists. Hospitals operate their own pharmacies and employ 87% of all pharmacists engaged in nonretail dispensing.

## Types of Drugs Dispensed

Pharmacies dispense and administer 2 types of prescription drugs: brand and generic. Brand drugs have exclusive marketing rights conferred on their manufacturers by the US Food and Drug Administration (FDA). Brands constituted 9% of all outpatient prescriptions in 2019. Generic drugs are drugs that have lost patent and marketing exclusivity but have the same dosage, strength, route of administration, quality, performance characteristics, and intended use as the branded drug; they accounted for 91% of all outpatient prescriptions in 2019, up from a "generic dispensing rate" of 54% in 2002.

Drugs differ in their method of administration. "Patient-administered drugs" include oral medications (eg, pills) and self-injected medications (eg, insulin). They are typically covered under the patient's "pharmacy benefit" and reimbursed by insurers and are dispensed through retail, mail, and specialty pharmacies. "Provider-administered drugs," by contrast, are received via infusions or injections by a clinician in their offices or in hospital outpatient departments. Such drugs are usually covered by

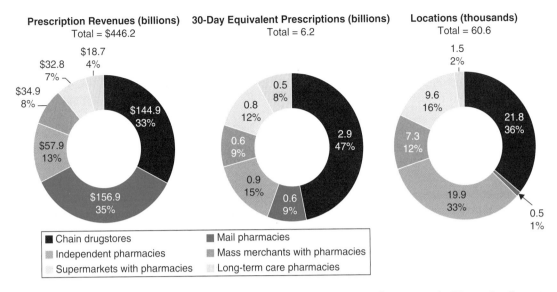

**Figure 13-8** • Total US Pharmacy Prescription Revenues, Prescriptions, and Locations, by Dispensing Format, 2019. (Source: Adam Fein. *The 2020 Economic Report on U.S. Pharmacies and Pharmacy Benefit Managers*. Drug Channels Institute, 2020.)

the patient's medical benefit and are usually dispensed through specialty pharmacies.

## Pharmacy Trends

The US prescription market witnessed significant prescription growth between 2000 and 2016, with a growing share of generics. Since 2016, there has been no growth in prescription drug volumes. Growth in pharmacy prescription revenues began to flatten out starting in 2015 (see Figure 13-9), rising anywhere from 0% to 4% annually between 2016 and 2019. The slowdown has been driven by higher generic

dispensing rates, the deflation in generic drug prices (due to more competitors and competitors' products), lower inflation in the prices for branded drugs, lower prescribing of opioids (43% drop 2011-2018), reduced spending on hepatitis C drugs due to more competitors, and stagnation in the individual insurance market.

## Stalled Growth of Retail Pharmacy and RCs: Trouble in River City

Given the slowdown in retail pharmacy prescriptions and revenues, it is not surprising to find a slowdown in retail pharmacies (and

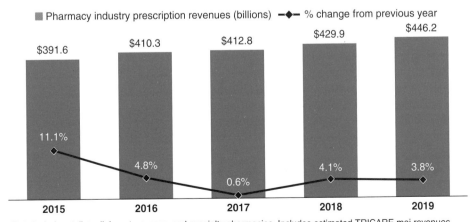

Data include retail, mail, long-term care, and specialty pharmacies. Includes estimated TRICARE mai revenues.

**Figure 13-9** • Pharmacy Industry Prescription Revenues, Annual Total and Growth, 2015 to 2019. (Source: Adam Fein. *The 2020 Economic Report on U.S. Pharmacies and Pharmacy Benefit Managers*. Drug Channels Institute, 2020.)

their RCs). Drug volumes and general margins in retail pharmacies (including the market leader, CVS Health) remain stagnant at best.[60] The retail pharmacy market suffers from excess capacity; retrenchment may be likely, due to falling drug reimbursement rates, mandatory mail-order plans, the growth of generic drugs, and the growth of narrow networks. Retail pharmacy is a mature industry with low annual revenue growth and more players vying for these revenues. Retail pharmacies face mounting competition from mass merchandisers (eg, discount stores, supercenters, and warehouse clubs), mail-order prescription providers, online pharmacies, convenience stores, wholesalers (eg, Costco), and other health clinics (eg, UCCs). If that were not enough, in May 2017, Amazon announced it would enter the pharmacy distribution business, a move threatening both retail pharmacy and mail-order pharmacy businesses.

Over the past 3 years, growth in Minute-Clinics (like all RCs) has stalled because growth in CVS Health pharmacies has stalled.[61] CVS undertook 2 mergers during 2015—with Omnicare and Target—that focused its attention on internal integration issues. Compounding (or exacerbating) the stagnation in CVS stores has been CVS's financial losses. CVS suffered a near 20% drop in its stock price in 2016 and a 17% drop in net income (year-over-year) in the first quarter of 2017. CVS has been hampered by falling revenues from its retail pharmacy business as a percentage of total revenues from 2010 to 2017. Most of the decline is traced to competitive actions taken by Walgreens to win over 2 contracts (Prime Therapeutics in August 2016 and TriCare in September 2016) that steered enrollees away from CVS pharmacies. In 2014, Walgreens Boots Alliance formed a strategic alliance with Prime Therapeutics, the pharmacy benefit manager (see Chapter 16) serving Blue Cross-Blue Shield (BCBS) plans in several states. As a result of this alliance, BCBS members were steered away from other pharmacies (including CVS) to Walgreens as their national preferred pharmacy network.

As a further sign of weakness in both the retail pharmacy and RC markets, Walgreens (the number 2 player in the chain pharmacy segment) announced in October 2019 that it would shutter 150 RCs (40% of its capacity, all of them owned) but continue to operate 200 in-store RCs operated by third parties (an initiative begun in 2015)

due to the losses sustained over several years of operation. During 2019, Walgreens closed down 187 RCs, leaving it with a much smaller footprint of 215 stores. Walgreens was not alone. During 2019, Walmart closed down 13 of its RCs, as did CVS (12 stores) and Kroger (10 stores).

In December 2017, as perhaps a defensive move to all of the above, CVS Health and Aetna announced their intention to merge. The newly merged organization will combine a pharmacy, RC provider, pharmacy benefit manager, and an insurer—"integrating more closely the work of doctors, pharmacists, and other health care professionals and health benefits companies to create a platform that is easier to use and less expensive for consumers."[62] This community-based platform, built around CVS's pharmacies and RCs, will serve as a community-based "healthcare hub" and "America's front door to quality health care."

Much of the supposed benefit of the proposed merger rests on CVS Health's network of RCs. CVS Health operates roughly 1,000+ MinuteClinics in some of its pharmacies. Company executives and analysts assert that as much as 70% of the US population lives within 10 to 15 minutes of a pharmacy (or within 3 miles of a CVS pharmacy).[63] Following the merger, these RCs will become mini-health centers or health hubs that expand access to lower-cost healthcare services and improve care convenience. These pharmacy-based sites would become the new point of entry for patients with symptoms seeking relief or information and for asymptomatic consumers looking to reduce the chance of illness. They would thus replace both emergency care settings (either hospital based or freestanding) and PCP practices (general practice, pediatrics). Some liken them to new CHCs.

One problem the merger will encounter is the mismatch in capacity between CVS Health's chain of pharmacies ($n = 9{,}847$) and its chain of RCs ($n = 1{,}111$ as of March 2018). This means that as few as 11% of CVS pharmacies have such a clinic inside the store. Although 70% of the US population may reportedly live within 3 miles of a CVS pharmacy (according to Leerink), they may not live anywhere near a MinuteClinic. Thus, to deliver on the promised merger benefits outlined earlier, CVS would need to embark on a massive expansion of its RCs and trust that they would be utilized.

Such demand may not be present, given the stalled growth in the total number of RCs. This capacity mismatch in the components of CVS Health (pharmacies and RCs) will hamper the vertical integration effort.

There may also be a mismatch in the geographical location of the merged entities' operations. Only a fraction of CVS Health pharmacies has an RC, and these tend to be disproportionately located in wealthier neighborhoods. It is not clear whether these clinic locations overlap with the geographic location of Aetna's enrollees, who are expected to be directed to CVS pharmacies and hopefully use its pharmacists and MinuteClinics. A preliminary analysis of available data indicates that Aetna has high enrollment in some states (eg, Alaska, Arizona, West Virginia) where CVS has no RCs; in other high-enrollment states, CVS has very few such clinics. To the degree that the geographic overlap is low, there is little synergy likely between these businesses (at least in the short term until the mismatch in capacity issue is addressed).

## Revamping the RC: Doctors' Offices in Pharmacies

Pharmacy RCs are staffed by nurse practitioners. Some pharmacy chains are now pursuing a parallel strategy with doctors' offices attached to the drug store, perhaps as a remodeled version of retail healthcare provider. In summer 2020, Walgreens announced a partnership with VillageMD, a Chicago-based primary startup with a network of 1,000 clinics and 2,800 physicians in 9 states. Walgreens plans to open 500 to 700 clinics at its stores in 30+ markets across the United States over the next 5 years using VillageMD providers. Walgreens reportedly agreed to pay VillageMD $1 billion in equity and debt in exchange for a 30% ownership stake in VillageMD. It should be noted that both parties experienced downturns in their business volume during the COVID-19 crisis and thus may have viewed the partnership as a growth vehicle.

Walgreens will reportedly develop its own version of a neighborhood health hub, called "Neighborhood Health Destinations," to compete with CVS Health. Walgreens will offer many solutions under one roof, including chronic care, pharmacy care, home care, and virtual around-the-clock care. It also hopes to cross-sell prescription drugs and other retail products to patients who visit the VillageMD clinics.

## SUMMARY

There is no shortage of vehicles that offer organized ambulatory care services. This chapter has profiled a number of them, and this does not even begin to exhaust the list of possibilities (eg, school clinics, industrial clinics, insurer-sponsored primary care clinics). Health insurers are resurrecting the primary care clinic strategy they pursued in the late 1980s, led by Optum (a division of UnitedHealthcare) and more recently by several Blue Cross plans.[64] The plethora of care sites has undoubtedly increased access to primary care and healthcare in general for the US population. It is not clear that it has reduced the cost of healthcare (eg, by substituting for more expensive sites like hospitals). Particular ambulatory settings like ASCs and RCs also failed to disrupt the more expensive sites. What all of these settings have achieved is growing complexity and fragmentation of care (as noted in Chapter 1).

## QUESTIONS TO PONDER

1. Multispecialty group practices have been around for nearly a century and a half, stemming back to the Mayo Clinic in the late 19th century and the Cleveland Clinic in the 1920s. Why don't more physicians form multispecialty group practices? Why has the number of such medical groups been relatively flat?
2. Why has the United States lagged in developing community-based primary care sites such as CHCs, FQHCs, and CMHCs?
3. One concern with physician ownership of ASCs is the potential threat of doctors referring their patients to their own ASCs rather than to a hospital-based ASC. Where is the danger in this potential conflict of interest? Might doctors refer patients who do not need surgery? Or is it that doctors do not inform patients they are getting surgery at a site the physician owns?
4. Does it make sense to turn your local community pharmacy into a "healthcare hub"? Why or why not?
5. Do you think the growth of UCCs is a positive development? Why or why not?

## REFERENCES

1. See Kaiser Family Foundation. *Distribution of Health Care Expenditures by Service by State of Residence (in millions)*. Available online: https://www.kff.org/other/state-indicator/distribution-of-health-care-expenditures-by-service-by-state-of-residence-in-millions/?currentTimeframe=0&sortModel=%7B%22colId%22:%22Location%22,%22sort%22:%22asc%22%7D. Accessed on August 6, 2020. Also see: Jeffrey M. Gonzalez. "AHRQ Medical Expenditure Panel Study: National Health Care Expenses in the U.S. Civilian Noninstitutionalized Population, 2011." Available online: https://meps.ahrq.gov/data_files/publications/st425/stat425.shtml. Accessed on July 25, 2020.

2. Ji Eun Chang. *The Urgent Care Connection*. Dissertation Proposal. New York University, 2015.

3. Alice Sardell. *The U.S. Experiment in Social Medicine: The Community Health Center Program, 1965-1986* (Pittsburgh, PA: University of Pittsburgh Press, 1988). Jessamy Taylor. *The Fundamentals of Community Health Centers* (Washington, DC: George Washington University–National Health Policy Forum, August 31, 2004).

4. Medical Payment Advisory Commission. "Federally Qualified Health Centers," in *Report to the Congress: Medicare and the Health Care Delivery System* (Washington, DC: MedPAC, June 2011): 144-160. Medicaid and CHIP Payment and Access Commission. *Medicaid Payment Policy for Federally Qualified Health Centers* (Washington, DC: MACPAC, December 2017).

5. Sanjay Kishore and Margaret Hayden. "Community Health Centers and Covid-19—Time for Congress to Act," *N Engl J Med.* 383 (August 20, 2020): e54(1)-e54(3).

6. June-Ho Kim, Eesha Desai, and Megan Cole. "How the Rapid Shift to Telehealth Leaves Many Community Health Centers Behind During the Covid-19 Pandemic," *Health Affairs Blog* (June 2, 2020). Available online: https://www.healthaffairs.org/do/10.1377/hblog20200529.449762/full/. Accessed on November 11, 2020.

7. Corinne Lewis, Yaphet Getachew, Melinda K. Abrams, et al. *Changes at Community Health Centers, and How Patients Are Benefitting* (New York, NY: Commonwealth Fund, August 20, 2019).

8. E. Fuller Torrey. "Fifty Years of Failing America's Mentally Ill," *Wall Street Journal* (February 5, 2013): A13. Available online: https://www.treatmentadvocacycenter.org/storage/documents/2_5_13_wsj_oped.pdf. Accessed on March 28, 2020.

9. The Centers for Medicare and Medicaid Services (CMS) requires a core set of services to be provided by Medicare-certified CMHCs (eg, outpatient mental health services for any area residents discharged from inpatient mental health facilities and 24-hour-a-day emergency care services). Nicole Hackbarth. *Financing Integrated Care for Adults With Serious Mental Illness in Community Mental Health Centers: An Overview of Program Components, Funding Environments, and Financing Barriers* (Santa Monica, CA: RAND Health, 2015).

10. Peiyin Hung, Susan Busch, Yi-Wen Shih, et al. "Changes in Community Mental Health Services Availability and Suicide Mortality in the US: A Retrospective Study," *BMC Psychiatry*. Available online: https://www.researchsquare.com/article/rs-15835/v1. Accessed on March 28, 2020.

11. Jeff Goldsmith. *Can Hospitals Survive?* (Homewood, IL: Dow Jones-Irwin, 1981).

12. Currently, many states do not have any UCC-specific regulations. Applicable rules are those that apply to opening a medical office (eg, medical licenses, business licenses, and registration of lab and x-ray equipment). Some states have developed UCC-specific regulations that require licensure, registration, or accreditation and may define "urgent care" in regulation. Other states have limited the scope of UCCs; for example, Illinois restricts the use of the term *emergency* to EDs. Some state regulations mention acceptance of, requirement for, or other reference to the use of accreditation standards (eg, The Joint Commission, Urgent Care Association, American Academy of Urgent Care Medicine). Arizona is the only state that has a licensure program that requires a specific license for UCCs; other states such as Florida put UCCs under a more general licensure category, calling them licensed clinics. American College of Emergency Physicians. *Freestanding Emergency Departments and Urgent Care Centers: An Information Paper*. (2015). Available online: https://www.acep.org/globalassets/uploads/uploaded-files/acep/clinical-and-practice-management/resources/administration/fsed-and-ucs_info-paper_final_110215.pdf. Accessed on March 28, 2020. Ramy Yakobi. "Impact of Urgent Care Centers on Emergency Department Visits," *Health Care Curr Rev.* 5 (3) (2017): 1-5.

13. Robin M. Weinick, Steffanie J. Bristol, and Catherine M. DesRoches. "Urgent Care Centers in the U.S.: Findings from a National Survey," *BMC Health Serv Res.* 9 (2009): 79. Robin M. Weinick, Steffanie J. Bristol, and Catherine M. DesRoches. "The Quality of Care at Urgent Care Centers," *J Urgent Care Med.* (2009): 27-32.

14. Laurel Stoimenoff and Nate Newman. *The Essential Role of the Urgent Care Center in Population Health: Urgent Care Industry White Paper* (Warrenville, IL: Urgent Care Association, 2018): 3.

15. Robin M. Weinick, Steffanie J. Bristol, and Catherine M DesRoches. "Urgent Care Centers in the U.S.: Findings from a National Survey," *BMC Health Serv Res.* 9 (2009): 79.

16. Tracy Yee, Amanda E. Lechner, and Ellyn R. Boukus. *The Surge in Urgent Care Centers: Emergency Department Alternative or Costly Convenience?* Center for Studying Health System Change, Research Brief 26 (July 2013).

17. Vivian Ho, Leanne Metcalfe, Cedric Dark, et al. "Comparing Utilization and Costs of Care in Freestanding Emergency Departments, Hospital Emergency Departments, and Urgent Care Centers," *Ann Emerg Med.* 70 (6) (2017): 846-857.

18. Ramy Yakobi. "Impact of Urgent Care Centers on Emergency Department Visits," *Health Care Curr Rev.* 5 (3) (2017): 1-5.

19. Laurel Stoimenoff and Nate Newman. *The Essential Role of the Urgent Care Center in Population Health: Urgent Care Industry White Paper* (Warrenville, IL: Urgent Care Association, 2018).

20. Ramy Yakobi. "Impact of Urgent Care Centers on Emergency Department Visits," *Health Care Curr Rev.* 5 (3) (2017): 1-5.

21. Medical Payment Advisory Commission. "Standalone Emergency Departments," in *Report to the Congress: Medicare and the Health Care Delivery System* (Washington, DC: MedPAC, June 2017): 243-262.

22. Lawrence Casalino. *Physician Self-Referral and Physician-Owned Specialty Facilities.* Research Synthesis Report No. 15. (Princeton, NJ: Robert Wood Johnson Foundation, June 2008).

23. Government Accountability Office. *Medicare: Payment for Ambulatory Surgical Centers Should be Based on the Hospital Outpatient Payment System* (Washington, DC: GAO, 2006).

24. Brent Fulton and Sue Kim. *Medicare Cost Savings Tied to Ambulatory Surgery Centers* (Berkeley, CA: University of California, 2013).

25. Medicare Payment Advisory Commission. *Medicare Payment Policy* (Washington, DC: MedPAC, March 2014).

26. Brent Hollenbeck, Rodney Dunn, Anne Suskind, et al. "Ambulatory Surgery Centers and Their Intended Effects on Outpatient Surgery," *Health Serv Res.* 50 (5) (2015): 1491-1507.

27. Brent Hollenbeck, Rodney Dunn, Anne Suskind, et al. "Ambulatory Surgery Centers and Outpatient Procedure Use Among Medicare Beneficiaries," *Med Care.* 52 (10) (2014): 926-931.

28. Christine Yee. *Why Surgeon Owners of Ambulatory Surgery Centers Do More Surgery Than Non-Owners* (Cambridge, MA: Workers Compensation Research Institute, 2012).

29. 58 Federal Register (September 21, 1993), and OIG Advisory Opinion No. 98-12.

30. Medicare Payment Advisory Commission. *Medicare Payment Policy* (Washington, DC: MedPAC, March 2014).

31. Hilsman Knight. "7 Trends Transforming the Ambulatory Surgery Center Industry," *Salient Value* 6 (7) (2019). Available online: https://salientvalue.com/7-trends-transforming-the-ambulatory-surgery-center-industry/. Accessed on March 28, 2020.

32. Avanza Healthcare Strategies. *Positioning Ambulatory Surgery Center for Success.* (2018). Available online: https://avanzastrategies.com/wp-content/uploads/2018/11/Positioning-ASCs-for-Success-112518.pdf. Accessed on March 28, 2020.

33. Bill Frack, Kevin Grabenstatter, and Jeff Williamson. "Ambulatory Surgery Centers: Becoming Big Business," *LEK Executive Insights* XIX(25) (2017). Available online: https://www.lek.com/sites/default/files/insights/pdf-attachments/1925_Ambulatory_Surgery_Centers_Executive_Insights_v2.pdf. Accessed on March 28, 2020.

34. Medical Payment Advisory Commission. *MedPac Report to Congress: Medicare Payment Policy* (Washington, DC: MedPac, March 2012): 119.

35. *VMG Health's 2011 Intellimaker ASC Benchmarking Study.* Available online: http://www.vmghealth.com/. Accessed on November 11, 2020.

36. Kristin Schleiter. "Retail Medical Clinics: Increasing Access to Low Cost Medical Care Amongst a Developing Legal Environment," *Ann Health Law.* 19 (3) (2010): 527-575.

37. Craig Pollack, Courtney Gidengil, and Ateev Mehrotra. "The Growth of Retail Clinics and the Medical Home: Two Trends in Concert or in Conflict?" *Health Aff.* 29 (5) (2010): 998-1003.

38. JUCM. "The Emergence of Retail Clinics." https://www.jucm.com/emergence-retail-clinics/. Accessed on August 6, 2020.

39. Allen Nalle and Drew Boston. *Retail Clinic Counts Will Double Between 2012 and 2015 and Save $800 Million Dollars per Year* (Accenture, 2014). Available online: https://www.accenture.com/_acnmedia/accenture/conversion-assets/dotcom/documents/global/pdf/dualpub_21/accenture-retail-medical-clinics-from-foe-to-friend.pdf. Accessed on March 29, 2020.

40. Kalorama Information. *Retail Clinics 2017* (New York, NY: Kalorama, May 2017). Allen Nalle and Drew Boston. *Retail Clinic Counts Will Double Between 2012 and 2015 and Save $800 Million Dollars per Year* (Accenture, 2014). Available online: https://www.accenture.com/_acnmedia/accenture/conversion-assets/dotcom/documents/global/pdf/dualpub_21/accenture-retail-medical-clinics-from-foe-to-friend.pdf. Accessed on March 29, 2020.

41. Adam Fein. "As CVS-Aetna Looms, Retail Pharmacy Clinic Growth Stalls," *DrugChannels* (March 6, 2018). Available online: http://www.drugchannels.net/2018/03/as-cvs-aetna-looms-retail-pharmacy.html. Accessed on July 30, 2020.

42. Blue Cross and Blue Shield. *Retail Clinic Visits Increase Despite Use Lagging Among Individually Insured Americans* (Blue Cross and Blue Shield, 2017). Available online: https://www.bcbs.com/sites/default/files/file-attachments/health-of-america-report/BCBS.HealthOfAmericaReport.Retail.pdf. Accessed on July 30, 2020. Rand Corporation. *The Evolving Role of Retail Clinics* (Santa Monica, CA: Rand Corporation, 2016). Available online: https://www.rand.org/pubs/research_briefs/RB9491-2.html. Accessed on June 10, 2018.

43. Clayton M. Christensen, Richard M.J. Bohmer, and John Kenagy. "Will Disruptive Innovations Cure Health Care?" *Harvard Business Review* (September-October 2000). Available online: https://hbr.org/2000/09/will-disruptive-innovations-cure-health-care. Accessed on July 30, 2020.

44. Jason Hwang and Ateev Mehrotra. "Why Retail Clinics Failed to Transform Health Care," *Harvard Business Review* (December 25, 2013). Available online: https://hbr.org/2013/12/why-retail-clinics-failed-to-transform-health-care. Accessed on June 10, 2018.

45. J. Scott Ashwood, Rachel Reid, Claude Setodji, et al. "Trends in Retail Clinic Use Among the Commercially Insured," *Am J Manag Care.* 17 (11) (2011): e443-e448.

46. Clayton M. Christensen, Richard M.J. Bohmer, and John Kenagy. "Will Disruptive Innovations Cure Health Care?" *Harvard Business Review* (September-October 2000). Available online: https://hbr.org/2000/09/will-disruptive-innovations-cure-health-care. Accessed on July 30, 2020.

47. Grant Martsolf, Kathryn Fingar, Rosanna Coffey, et al. "Association Between the Opening of Retail Clinics and Low-Acuity Emergency Department Visits," *Ann Emerg Med.* 69 (4) (2017): 397-403.

48. Grant Martsolf, Kathryn Fingar, Rosanna Coffey, et al. "Association Between the Opening of Retail Clinics and Low-Acuity Emergency Department Visits," *Ann Emerg Med.* 69 (4) (2017): 397-403.

49. Timothy Hoff and Kathryn Prout. "Comparing Retail Clinics With Other Sites of Care: A Systematic Review of Cost, Quality, and Patient Satisfaction," *Med Care.* 57 (9) (2019): 734-741.

50. Stace Aversa. "Comparing Social Sentiment on Convenient Care Clinics: How Convenient Are They?" *Crimson Hexagon* (September 9, 2013).

51. Amy Compton-Phillips. "Care Redesign Survey: In the Push for Convenient Care, Protect the Patient-Doctor Relationship," *NEJM Catalyst* (July 14, 2016). Available online: https://catalyst.nejm.org/care-redesign-report-push-convenient-care-protect-patient-doctor-relationship/. Accessed on November 11, 2020.

52. Ateev Mehrotra and Edward Prewitt. *Convenient Care: Opportunity, Threat, or Both? NEJM Catalyst*, Insights Report (July 2019).

53. Timothy Hoff. *Next in Line: Lowered Care Expectations in the Age of Retail- and Value-Based Health* (Oxford, United Kingdom: Oxford University Press, 2018).

54. Stephen Schwab. *The Effects of Disruptions to the Patient-Physician Relationship.* Doctoral Dissertation. Department of Health Care Management, The Wharton School (2018).

55. Ateev Mehrotra. *Impact of Retail Clinics on Quality and Costs.* Available online: https://static1.squarespace.com/static/573a188740261dc86d93cf71/t/5888be7bebbd1af0a2f9ba63/1485356671639/Ateev+Mehrotra.pdf. Accessed on July 30, 2020.

56. J. Scott Ashwood, Martin Gaynor, Claude Setodji, et al. "Retail Clinic Visits for Low-Acuity Conditions Increase Utilization and Spending," *Health Aff.* 35 (3) (2016): 449-455.

57. Jordan Stone. *Profit From Convenient Primary Care.* Health Care Advisory Board (2013-2014). Available online: https://www.advisory.com/-/media/Advisory-com/Research/HCAB/Events/Webconference/2014/Profit-from-Convenient-Primary-Care-052914.pdf. Accessed on July 30, 2020.

58. Adam Fein. "Retail Clinic Check Up: CVS Retrenches, Walgreens Outsources, Kroger Expands," *Drug Channels* (February 16, 2017). Available online: http://www.drugchannels.net/2017/02/retail-clinic-check-up-cvs-retrenches.html. Accessed on July 30, 2020.

59. Rebecca Henderson, Russell Eisenstat, and Matthew Preble. *Aetna and the Transformation of Health Care.* HBS Case # 9-318-048 (revised February 1, 2018). (Boston, MA: Harvard Business School, 2018).

60. David Larsen and Matt Dellelo. *HCIT and Distribution* (Boston, MA: Leerink, December 18, 2017).

61. Statista. "CVS Health's Number of Stores From 2005 to 2019." Available online: https://www.statista.com/statistics/241544/cvs-caremark—number-of-stores-since-2005/. Accessed on August 6, 2020.

62. CVS Health. "CVS Health to Acquire Aetna," *CVS Health Press Release* (December 3, 2017).

63. David Larsen. Leerink Partners. As quoted in Zachary Tracer. "CVS's $68 Billion Bid to Bring One-Stop Shopping to Health Care," *Bloomberg* (December 7, 2017). Available online: https://www.bloomberg.com/news/articles/2017-12-07/cvs-s-68-billion-bid-to-bring-one-stop-shopping-to-health-care. Accessed on July 30, 2020.

64. Anna Matthews. "Physicians, Hospitals Meet Their New Competitor: Insurer-Owned Clinics," *Wall Street Journal* (February 23, 2020).

# Post-Acute Care

# 14

## THE CONTINUUM OF POST-ACUTE CARE (PAC)

The post-acute care (PAC) sector is a continuum of businesses that serve patients discharged from acute care hospitals for follow-up care in less-intensive, more-appropriate, and lower-cost settings (Figure 14-1). PAC settings include: home healthcare agencies (HHAs), intermediate rehabilitation facilities (IRFs), skilled nursing facilities (SNFs), and long-term care hospitals (LTCHs); some classifications also include hospices.

Figure 14-2 shows the cost advantage of using PAC settings over acute care hospitals, and using noninstitutional over institutional PAC settings.[1] For example, home healthcare represents roughly 5% of the cost of a hospitalization and roughly 20% of the cost of an SNF. Due to the growing costs of healthcare (particularly for seniors), the US federal government has exerted considerable effort over time to (1) promote PAC as a cheaper alternative to hospitalization and (2) apply prospective payment systems (PPSs) to generate even greater efficiencies within PAC.

The majority of patients using PAC sites and services are Medicare enrollees.[2] Medicare is a major payer of PAC services; Medicare spending is an important driver of PAC utilization and PAC profitability; and PAC providers are heavily reliant on this public funding—all of which bring federal scrutiny. Any analysis of PAC must consider the role played by the Centers for Medicare and Medicaid Services (CMS), which serves as the major federal agency paying for PAC care. Any analysis must also consider the role played by the Medicare Payment and Advisory

Commission (MedPAC), which serves as a congressional watchdog over the Medicare program and makes proposals regarding PAC payment.

Following is a brief history of these initial federal efforts. This is followed by a thumbnail description of the 5 major PAC sectors (HHA, IRF, LTCH, SNF, and hospice).[3]

## EARLY FEDERAL EFFORTS TO PROMOTE AND (THEN) CURB PAC SPENDING

Traditionally, the Medicare program paid for skilled care, therapy, and other services provided by HHAs, SNFs, IRFs, LTCHs, and hospice on a fee-for-service (FFS) basis. Each PAC provider was paid its average costs, subject to limits, for treating Medicare beneficiaries. As with the case of inpatient acute care, the FFS model for PAC provided no incentives for efficiency but instead incentives to spend more.

There was plenty of supply and demand to fuel this spending. When Medicare was first enacted in 1965, it was primarily an acute care program covering hospital and physician care. During the 1980s, several court challenges forced the Health Care Financing Administration (now known as CMS) to cover services provided by SNFs (1988) and HHAs (1989)—in the latter case, more frequent visits for more people.[4] This encouraged the growing supply of PAC providers. Over time, as more of the population aged into Medicare and as their chronic disease burden increased, Medicare spending tilted more toward PAC.

Reliance on PAC nevertheless fit with the government's desire to substitute outpatient for

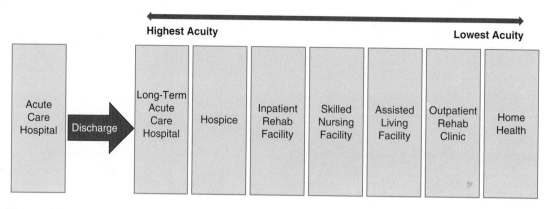

**Figure 14-1** • Continuum of Post-Acute Care.

inpatient care that began with the 1983 inaugura-tion of the inpatient prospective payment system (IPPS; 1983)[5] and the need of acute care hospitals to discharge patients sooner in the presence of capped, diagnosis-related group (DRG) pay-ments. However, gradual spending increases on PAC care in the 1980s mushroomed into rapid spending increases during the 1990s. PAC ser-vices soon represented the most rapidly growing component of Medicare spending. From 1990 to 1995, Medicare's spending on PAC grew by a 30% average annual rate; total PAC spending grew from about $8 billion to $30 billion. Med-icare spending on home health exhibited a simi-lar pattern, rising 29% from 1990 to 1995, due to more people using the benefit and users consum-ing more HHA visits per year. Between 1990 and 1996, home health's share of Medicare spending jumped from 3.6% to 9.2%.[6]

To deal with this issue, Medicare applied a PPS to each type of PAC provider near the turn of the millennium. The Balanced Budget Act (BBA; 1997) mandated prospective payment for

HHAs, SNFs, and IRFs. The Balanced Budget Refinement Act of 1999 and the Medicare and Medicaid Benefits Improvement and Protection Act of 2000 mandated PPS for LTCHs. These PPS models, implemented between 1998 and 2002, set rates on the basis of historical national average costs for each provider type.

## HOME HEALTH AGENCIES

Beneficiaries who are generally restricted to their homes and need skilled care on a part-time or intermittent basis are eligible to receive certain medical services at home. These include skilled nursing care; physical, occupational, and speech therapy; medical social work; and home health aide services.

Home healthcare has been a popular benefit. The number of HHAs grew from roughly 7,500 in 2000 to over 12,300 by 2012. There has been a significant shift in the preference of individu-als for receiving care in the comfort of their own

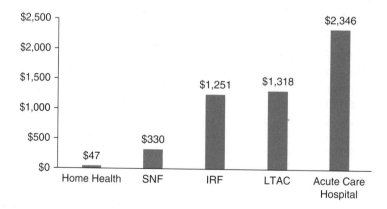

**Figure 14-2** • Medicare Cost by Care Setting. IRF, Inpatient Rehabilitation Facilities; LTAC, Long-Term Acute Care; SNF, Skilled Nursing Facility. (Source: Medicare Payment Advisory Commission, LHC Group.)

homes in comparison to SNFs. A 2010 AARP survey found that nearly 75% of those aged 45+ strongly agreed with the statement, "What I'd really like to do is stay in my current residence for as long as possible."[7] Dartmouth Atlas researchers found that over 80% of patients say that they "wish to avoid hospitalization and intensive care during the terminal phase of life."[8] More recent data indicate that 90% of seniors want to age in their own homes and communities.

Home healthcare is still a fragmented market. The 5 largest companies represent only approximately 17.5% of the broader HHA market; for Medicare home health, the top 4 public providers represent approximately 20% of the market.[9] Currently, Medicare spends $18.1 billion on HHA; the broader HHA sector is estimated to be a $54 billion market.[10]

In October 2000, CMS adopted a PPS that pays HHAs a predetermined rate for each 60-day home healthcare episode. The payment rates are based on patients' conditions and service use and are adjusted to reflect input prices (eg, wages) in local markets. The base payment rate for an episode in 2017 was $2,989.97. To capture differences in expected resource use, patients receiving 5 or more visits are assigned to 1 of 153 home health resource groups (HHRGs) based on clinical and functional status and service use as measured by the Outcome and Assessment Information Set (OASIS).[11]

The home health PPS has 2 programs intended to improve quality. The first is a pay-for-reporting program under which HHAs must report quality-of-care data using standardized measures (eg, in the OASIS) to avoid a 2 percentage point reduction in their annual rate update. In 2018, Medicare began implementing a home health value-based purchasing (VBP) program in 9 states that will adjust Medicare payments (upward or downward) to HHAs based on their performance on a set of quality measures relative to their peers.[12]

## SKILLED NURSING FACILITIES

Beneficiaries who need short-term skilled care (nursing or rehabilitation services) on an inpatient basis following a hospital stay of 3 or more days are eligible to receive covered services in SNFs. Medicare covers up to 100 days of SNF care per spell of illness. SNFs are the most commonly used PAC setting: In 2016, Medicare spent $31.1 billion for SNF care. The number of SNFs grew slightly between 2012 and 2017 to roughly 15,200.

SNFs can be hospital-based units or free-standing facilities. In 2015, 95% of stays were in freestanding facilities. With approval from CMS, certain Medicare-certified hospitals (typically small, rural hospitals and critical access hospitals) may also provide skilled nursing services in the hospital beds used to provide acute care services. These are called swing-bed hospitals.

The Medicare SNF benefit covers skilled nursing care, rehabilitation services, and other goods and services. Prior to PPS, SNFs were paid on the basis of their costs, subject to limits on their per-diem routine costs (room, board, and routine nursing care); no limits were applied for ancillary services (eg, drugs and therapy). Medicare's PPS for SNF services began paying facilities a predetermined daily "base rate" for each day of care starting July 1998. PPS rates are expected to cover all operating and capital costs that efficient facilities were expected to incur in furnishing most SNF services.

The BBA of 1997 exerted serious, downside pressures on SNFs. As part of PPS, BBA 1997 mandated the use of resource utilization groups (RUGs) to pay nursing homes. This effectively capped payments for rehabilitation therapy and ancillary services, which had been growing. Between 1998 and 1999, Medicare payments to nursing homes fell roughly $8 billion, leading to nearly 2,000 nursing home bankruptcy filings (roughly 11% of total homes). The Congressional Budget Office forecasted cuts twice that size over the first 5 years of the BBA's impact. By 2000, 5 of the 7 largest nursing home operators were in bankruptcy protection.

Daily payments to SNFs are determined by adjusting the base payment for case mix using a system known as RUGs.[13] Each RUG has associated nursing and therapy weights that are applied to the base payment rates. A patient's day of care is assigned to 1 of 66 RUGs based on patient characteristics and service use that are expected to require similar resources. The base rates are computed separately for urban and rural areas and are updated annually based on increases in local market input prices (eg, wages). In 2018, for SNFs located in urban areas, the nursing component base rate for urban SNFs was $177.26, whereas the therapy component base rate was $133.52; for rural SNFs, the 2 rates were $169.34 and $153.96, respectively.

## INPATIENT REHABILITATION FACILITIES

Following an illness, injury, or surgery, some patients need intensive inpatient rehabilitation services such as physical, occupational, or speech therapy. Such services are frequently provided in SNFs but are sometimes provided in IRFs. Comparatively few Medicare beneficiaries use IRFs, in part because nationwide there are fewer IRFs than SNFs but also because, to be eligible for treatment in an IRF, the patient generally must be able to tolerate and benefit from 3 hours of therapy per day. According to MedPAC, the number of IRFs has remained stable over the past 5 years (roughly 1,170), while patient volumes and Medicare spending on IRF services have increased.[14]

IRFs may be freestanding facilities or specialized units within acute care hospitals. To qualify as an IRF, a facility must meet Medicare's conditions of participation for acute care hospitals. In addition, the facility must meet a "compliance threshold" whereby no less than 60% of an IRF's patient population (Medicare and other) have as a primary diagnosis or comorbidity at least 1 of 13 conditions that typically require intensive rehabilitation therapy.[15] The intent of the compliance threshold is to distinguish IRFs from acute care hospitals.[16]

Since January 2002, Medicare has paid IRFs predetermined, per-discharge base rates based primarily on the patient's condition (diagnoses, functional and cognitive statuses, and age) and local market input prices. In fiscal year (FY) 2018, the IRF base payment rate was $15,838. Medicare patients are assigned to case-mix groups (CMGs) based on the primary reason for intensive rehabilitation care (eg, a stroke or hip fracture), age, and level of motor and cognitive function. Within each of these CMGs, patients are further categorized into 1 of 4 tiers based on the presence of specific comorbidities that increase the cost of care. Payment rates are also adjusted to account for certain facility characteristics. Rural facilities' payment rates are increased by 14.9% because they tend to have fewer cases, longer lengths of stay, and higher average costs per case.[17]

IRFs have benefited from the unfortunate increase in the number of brain, neurologic, and spinal trauma injuries. Every year, more than 3.3 million people suffer traumatic brain injury, which results in over $77 billion in direct and indirect medical costs.[18] Brain and spinal trauma accounts for an exceedingly large portion of annual incidents by disease, outnumbering prostate and breast cancer (combined) by more than 8 times. Because of this, there is growing awareness of brain trauma and the long-term care needs of those that it afflicts. Combined with the increasing life spans of those affected by these traumas, this should significantly increase the number of patients who seek brain trauma rehabilitation.

## LONG-TERM CARE HOSPITALS

Some patients need hospital-level care for relatively extended periods. These include patients with chronic critical illness (ie, those who exhibit metabolic, endocrine, physiologic, and immunologic abnormalities that result in profound debilitation and often ongoing respiratory failure). Nationwide, most chronic, critically-ill patients are treated in acute care hospitals, but some are admitted to LTCHs. These facilities can be freestanding or co-located with other hospitals as hospitals-within-hospitals or satellites. To qualify as an LTCH for Medicare payment, a facility must meet Medicare's conditions of participation for acute care hospitals and have an average length of stay greater than 25 days for certain Medicare patients.

Under the LTCH PPS, Medicare set per-discharge payment rates for different CMGs called Medicare severity long-term care DRGs (MS-LTC-DRGs) based on the expected relative costliness of treatment for patients in the group. Patients are assigned to these groups based on their principal diagnosis, secondary diagnoses, procedures performed, age, sex, and discharge status. The MS-LTC-DRGs are the same groups used in the acute IPPS but have relative weights specific to LTCH patients, reflecting the average relative costliness of these cases.

Beginning in FY 2016, LTCH cases that immediately follow an acute care hospital stay that included 3 or more days in an intensive care unit (ICU), or LTCH cases for which the LTCH stay includes mechanical ventilation services for at least 96 hours, are paid under the LTCH PPS. For patients not meeting these criteria, including any discharges assigned to psychiatric or rehabilitation MS-LTC-DRGs (regardless of intensive care use), Medicare pays "site-neutral" rates (ie, based on what Medicare pays for similar cases in acute care hospitals).[19]

The LTCH PPS payment (base rate) for a typical discharge in FY 2018 was $41,430.56.[20] The base rate is adjusted to account for differences in local market prices. Payments to LTCHs that fail to provide data on specified quality indicators are reduced by 2%.

In FY 2005, CMS established "the 25% rule," which was intended to help ensure that (1) LTCHs do not function as units of acute care hospitals and (2) decisions about admission, treatment, and discharge in both acute care hospitals and LTCHs are made for clinical rather than financial reasons. The rule set a limit on the share of an LTCH's cases that can be admitted from certain referring acute care hospitals. Subsequent legislation substantially changed the implementation of the 25% rule; in the 21st Century Cures Act, Congress delayed implementation of the 25% rule until FY 2018, whereas CMS further delayed implementation until FY 2019.[21]

## HOSPICES

Hospice became a Medicare benefit in 1983 pursuant to the Tax Equity and Fiscal Responsibility Act (TEFRA) of 1982. The hospice benefit covers palliative services for beneficiaries who have a life expectancy of 6 months or less, as determined by their physician. The benefit is designed to provide pain relief, comfort, and emotional and spiritual support to patients with a terminal diagnosis. To provide this type of care, the benefit covers an array of services, such as skilled nursing services; drugs and biologicals for pain control and symptom management; physical, occupational, and speech therapy; counseling (dietary, spiritual, family bereavement, and other counseling services); home health aide and homemaker services; short-term inpatient care; inpatient respite care; and other services necessary for the palliation and management of the terminal illness.

Beneficiaries who elect the Medicare hospice benefit agree to forgo curative treatment for their terminal condition; for conditions unrelated to their terminal illness, Medicare continues to cover items and services outside of hospice. Typically, hospice care is provided in patients' homes, but hospice services may also be provided in nursing facilities and other inpatient settings. Hospice providers can include freestanding entities, hospital-based entities, SNFs, or HHAs. In 2016, nearly 50% of Medicare patients who died that year used the benefit. Hospice is not an allowed benefit under Medicare Advantage, however.

Medicare pays hospice agencies a daily rate for each day a beneficiary is enrolled in the hospice benefit, adjusted for local market prices, regardless of the amount of services provided on a given day and on days when no services are provided. Payments are made according to a fee schedule that has 4 different levels of care: routine home care (RHC), continuous home care (CHC), inpatient respite care (IRC), and general inpatient care (GIC). The 4 levels of care are distinguished by the location and intensity of the services provided. RHC is the most common level of hospice care, accounting for more than 95% of all hospice days. Other levels of care (GIC, CHC, and IRC) are available to manage needs in certain situations.[22]

Prior to January 2016, Medicare had a single base rate for each RHC day in an episode. Beginning January 1, 2016, there were 2 RHC base payment rates: a higher rate for days 1 to 60 and a lower rate for days 61 and beyond. These were the first changes to the hospice payment system since its inception in 1983. The new RHC payment structure was intended to better align payments with the costs of providing hospice care throughout an episode. Hospices tend to provide more services at the beginning and end of an episode and less in the middle.

Two caps limit the amount and cost of care that any individual hospice agency provides in a single year. One cap limits the number of days of inpatient care an agency may provide to not more than 20% of its total patient care days. The other cap is an absolute dollar limit on the average annual payment per beneficiary a hospice can receive.

Like home healthcare, hospice has become a popular benefit. End-of-life care has shifted from a sole focus on curative medicine to include quality of life. This shift is evident in the change in share of decedents using hospice, growing from 22.9% in 2000 to 48.6% in 2015. It is also evident from the growth in Medicare beneficiaries using hospices from 0.5 million to 1.4 million, the rise in Medicare payments to hospices from $2.9 billion to $16.8 billion (2016), and the 86% increase in number of hospice agencies from 2000 to 2015.[23] By 2017, there were more than

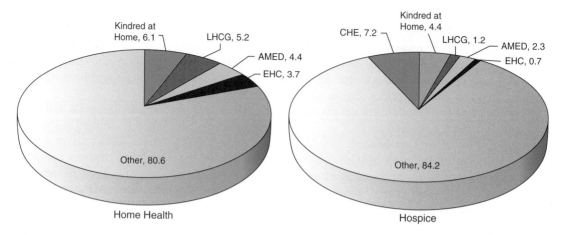

**Figure 14-3** • Home Health and Hospice Market Shares by Company as a Percentage of Medicare Home Healthcare Agency Spend. CHE, Chemed Corp; AMED, Amedisys; LHCG, LHC Group; EHC, Encompass Health Corp.

4,400 hospices. The 5 largest operators account for only 16.5% of the market, and over 90% of businesses are sole proprietorships, indicative of substantial fragmentation within this sector.[24] The fragmentation of the HHA and hospice sectors is depicted in Figure 14-3. Medicaid pays hospice services in 40+ states with similar coverage to Medicare but accounts for a much smaller share of hospice revenues.

## PAC GROWTH UNDER PROSPECTIVE PAYMENT

Despite the implementation of PPS around 2000, PAC spending continued to grow for (at least) the next decade, and sometimes longer. Between 2003 and 2013, overall PAC spending increased by 74%. Spending doubled for LTCHs and SNFs; spending for HHAs and IRFs increased by 77% and 10%, respectively.

The advent of PPS for PAC did succeed in reducing PAC spending as a proportion of total Medicare spending between 1997 and 2015 (from 16% to 10%), driven primarily by reduced spending on SNFs. However, total PAC spending increased from roughly $33.6 billion to $60.5 billion.[25] Home healthcare led the PAC spending increase with 41% growth in spending and 47% growth in count of providers. HHA spending growth was driven by an increase in the number of agencies, the number of users, and the number of episodes per user, as well as a shift in the mix of services used away from home health aide visits toward more costly skilled nursing and therapy visits. SNF spending growth was not driven by more users or more days of care, but mostly by an increase in the intensity of services (primarily therapy). In contrast to SNFs, spending on other PAC services as a percentage of Medicare spend has been more steady and predictable over time (HHAs account for 4%-5% of Medicare spend, IRFs account for 1%-2%).

Not only is the percentage of Medicare spending allocated to these PAC sectors fairly stable, but their profitability is also stable. According to MedPAC, Medicare payments exceed provider costs in HHAs, IRFs, and SNFs. PAC providers enjoy high payment-to-cost ratios (PCRs), largely due to flaws in the PPS systems designed for PAC. Overall, PAC PCRs have averaged 111% under PPS. The enduring profitability of PAC rests on PPS payments that have consistently and substantially exceeded costs, the ability of PAC providers to reduce per-episode costs, and efforts to keep cost growth below annual payment updates.[26] In summary, many PAC sectors have enjoyed strong underlying demand, as evidenced by significant growth in patient volumes and spending, and high margins. To wit, according to MedPAC data:

- **HHAs:** Between 2000 and 2015, the number of HHAs grew 64%, HHA users grew 38%, HHA visits grew 27%, and HHA spending grew 113%.[27] HHA capacity and spending have remained stable since then.[28] On the Medicare side, freestanding HHAs enjoyed high margins that averaged 16.4% between 2001 and 2015 and a rise in the percentage of HHA episodes not preceded by hospitalization.

- **Hospices:** Between 2000 and 2014, hospice users grew 6.7% annually, hospice days rose 9.5% annually, and hospice spending rose 12.4% annually. Spending rose 5% to 6% annually between 2014 and 2016 due to more users, higher Medicare base payments, and longer lengths of stay. In total, Medicare hospice expenditures rose from $2.8 billion in FY 2000 to an estimated $18.7 billion in FY 2018, up from $16.8 billion 2 years earlier. The number of Medicare beneficiaries receiving hospice services grew from 513,000 in FY 2000 to over 1.5 million in FY 2018. Hospice margins increased from 8.2% in 2014 to 10.0% in 2015 and then to 10.9% in 2016. Freestanding hospices had even higher margins (13.8% in 2015).

- **IRFs:** The IRF market has witnessed steady volume growth since 2008, averaging 1% annually, with case volume rising faster during 2015 to 2016 (2.4%). Overall, Medicare program spending on IRFs has grown steadily since 2008 at roughly 3% annually.[29] The market has also enjoyed 2% to 3% annual growth in Medicare spend per case since 2008.[30] Medicare margins have risen since 2010, reaching 13% in 2016; among freestanding IRFs, the margins were much higher (25.5%). IRFs experienced steady growth in provider supply during 2013 to 2016 (0.8% annual change) but are currently decreasing in number as state-run rehabilitation centers close due to declines in inpatient census combined with rising operating costs.[31] Diminishing supply, though, is being met by increasing demand, as aging Baby Boomer caregivers who can no longer care for their adult children or their aging parents turn to IRFs to meet their needs.

- **LTCHs:** LTCHs suffered slight declines in patient volumes after going through 2 federally imposed moratoriums on new construction, but nevertheless maintained stable occupancy rates with little change in profitability among those facilities meeting patient criteria requirements. Over the period from 2012 to 2016, the number of LTCHs slightly declined (–1.1%), as did patient volumes (–2.3%, 2012-2015) and total Medicare spending (–1.3%, 2012-2015) on LTCH services.[32]

- **SNFs:** Between 2010 and 2017, SNFs experienced an 11.5% decline in covered admissions per 1,000 beneficiaries, a 17.7% decline in covered days per 1,000 beneficiaries, and a 7.4% drop in covered days per admission. The number of facilities has been stable since 2014, and Medicare program spending on SNFs has increased over time. The profitability of SNFs has remained stable at roughly 10%.

## PAC GROWTH DRIVERS

PAC used to be called "long-term care." The topic, like the title, sounded boring. Today, PAC is a "hot topic." PAC services have been isolated as the area with greatest geographic variations in care provision, which may indicate overuse of care. Figure 12-3 in Chapter 12 illustrates the growing popularity of PAC services provided by hospitals. Figure 14-4 shows their enduring profitability. At least 2 sets of trends, covered in the following sections, explain why PAC is so hot.

### Favorable Patient Demographic Trends

The aging of the US population has meant stronger demand for healthcare in general and PAC in particular. PAC providers will continue to experience robust demand for their services due to an increasing number of seniors and the growing complexity of their disease states. By 2050, the population aged 65 and older is projected to be 83.7 million, nearly double the estimated population of 43.1 million in 2012. The number of people aged 65 and older is expected to increase at an annualized rate of 3.2% through 2022, significantly faster than the overall population's growth of 0.8% during the same period. Although life expectancies are longer and smoking rates have declined among the current population, Medicare-eligible patients have higher rates of obesity and diabetes compared with previous generations. According to the Medicare Chronic Conditions Dashboard, 17% of Medicare patients live with more than 6 chronic conditions, accounting for half of all spending on beneficiaries with chronic disease (averaging $30,000 per patient each year).

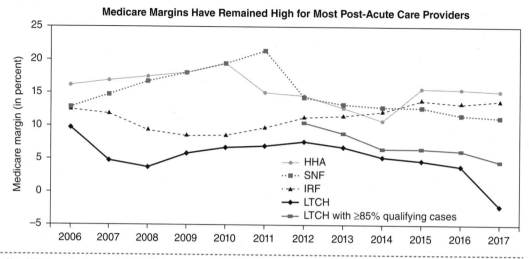

**Figure 14-4** • Post-Acute Care Margins. (Source: MedPac.)

## Favorable Economic Trends

The rising cost of healthcare, an ongoing trend for decades, has increased providers' and regulators' interest in lower-cost, noninstitutional sites of care (eg, HHA and hospice). Figure 14-2 (presented earlier) shows the cost advantage of using certain PAC sites of care.

Moreover, most PAC providers are paid on an FFS basis, even under PPSs, with little entrance of managed care or capitated care into these segments. PAC businesses have enjoyed a stable and perhaps rising share of Medicare discharges from acute care hospitals between 2012 and 2017 (roughly 36%-40%). There is also the possibility that one PAC segment can substitute for another PAC segment as Medicare changes its payment system, particularly given some overlap in the types of patients they treat, helping diversified PAC providers weather threats to any particular PAC segment.

## RECENT FEDERAL EFFORTS TO CONTAIN PAC SPENDING

The federal government has repeatedly tried to address PAC spending over the past decade. As a consequence, most PAC sectors have experienced more stable spending and capacity; hospices are the only outlier here, having risen considerably since 2012 (Figures 14-5 and 14-6). These changes are briefly detailed in the following sections.

**Medicare Spending for PAC Remained Stable but Increased for Hospice Services Since 2012**

|  | 2012 | 2013 | 2014 | 2015 | 2016 | 2017 |
|---|---|---|---|---|---|---|
| All PAC | $58.4 | $58.9 | $59.3 | $60.5 | $59.8 | $59.6 |
| SNF | 28.2 | 28.7 | 29.1 | 29.7 | 29.1 | 28.8 |
| HHA | 18.2 | 18.1 | 18.0 | 18.4 | 18.3 | 18.4 |
| IRF | 6.7 | 6.9 | 7.2 | 7.4 | 7.7 | 7.9 |
| LTCH | 5.3 | 5.2 | 5.0 | 5.0 | 4.7 | 4.5 |
| Hospice | 15.1 | 15.1 | 15.1 | 15.9 | 16.8 | 17.9 |

Note: PAC (post-acute care), SNF (skilled nursing facility), HHA (home health agency), IRF (inpatient rehabilitation facility), LTCH (long-term care hospital). Data include spending for beneficiaries discharged from an acute care hospital to a post-acute care provider and beneficiaries directly admitted to a post-acute care provider from the community.

**Figure 14-5** • Medicare Spending on Post-Acute Care. (Source: MedPac.)

**Between 2012 and 2017, the Number of PAC and Hospice Providers Remained Stable**

| | Number of providers | | | Share of ACH discharges using PAC services within 7 days of discharge | | |
|---|---|---|---|---|---|---|
| | 2012 | 2016 | 2017 | 2012 | 2016 | 2017 |
| All PAC | 28,768 | 29,078 | 28,710 | 36% | 38% | 36% |
| SNF | 15,139 | 15,263 | 15,277 | 51 | 50 | 52 |
| HHA | 12,026 | 12,204 | 11,844 | 36 | 37 | 35 |
| IRF | 1,166 | 1,188 | 1,178 | 9 | 9 | 10 |
| LTCH | 437 | 423 | 411 | 3 | 3 | 3 |
| Hospice | 3,720 | 4,382 | 4,488 | 3 | 4 | 4 |

Note: PAC (post-acute care), ACH (acute care hospital), SNF (skilled nursing facility), HHA (home health agency), IRF (inpatient rehabilitation facility), LTCH (long-term care hospital). The provider counts include all facilities or providers, including those not paid under the prospective payment system.

**Figure 14-6** • Post-Acute Care Providers. (Source: MedPac.)

## The Patient Protection and Affordable Care Act (PPACA 2010)

As part of the PPACA, CMS initiated several quality reporting programs (QRPs) and VBP programs. In general, the QRPs required PAC providers to submit quality reporting data from several data sets or face a 2% reduction in the applicable annual payment update. VBPs for SNFs and HHAs are to be used to compute bonuses/penalties for quality performance.

In addition, the PPACA called for annual rebasing of HHA payments by 3.5% for the years 2014 to 2017, reductions in annual payment updates that account for inflation for several PAC providers (HHA, IRF, and LTCH) by 1.1% for the years 2014 to 2023, and penalties for LTCHs and IRFs that did not report quality measures to CMS starting in 2014. It also included productivity adjustments to the annual inflation updates in the 4 major PAC settings (HHA, IRF, SNF, and LTCH). PPACA did not impact hospice payments at all. Finally, PPACA created financial incentives for states to shift Medicaid patients out of SNFs into home- and community-based services (HCBS). It did so by providing increases in federal medical assistance percentage (FMAP) rates to states to rebalance spending by October 2015.

## The Budget Control Act/ Sequestration (2011)

Congress enacted the Budget Control Act in 2011 to try to force themselves to reach a bipartisan agreement on how to reduce the US budget deficit. When they could not agree, the cuts went into effect. Known as "sequestration," these budget cuts amount to $1.1 trillion over 10 years, with an equal amount (~$110 billion) taken out every year. The Medicare program was hit by an $11.1 billion (or 2%) reduction in provider payments in FY 2013. The mandated cuts reduced Medicare payments to PAC providers annually by 2% starting in April of 2013. This explains the lower level of spending on PAC (and other healthcare services) for several years after 2012 compared to several years before.[33]

## The Pathway for SGR Reform Act (2013)

The major purpose of the Pathway for SGR Reform Act (2013) was to postpone implementation of reimbursement cuts to physicians as mandated by the sustained growth rate (SGR) provisions of the BBA of 1997. It also extended the sequestration's 2% cut to Medicare payments to 2023. However, one part of the 2013 act contained changes to the regulation and payment of LTCHs.

Why the focus on LTCHs? LTCHs were administratively created in the early 1980s to protect 40 chronic disease hospitals from the new IPPS introduced for acute care hospitals. What began as a regulatory carve-out for a few dozen specialty hospitals subsequently expanded into an industry with over 400 LTCHs and billions in annual Medicare spending. CMS became concerned that the patients treated in LTCHs resembled those treated in cheaper SNFs or HHAs, where they might be more appropriately discharged.

In this light, the Pathway for SGR Reform Act also instituted a moratorium on LTCH construction in 2013, following a similar moratorium enacted in 2007. The new moratorium would run from April 2014 through September 2017. Not surprisingly, these moratoria exerted a dampening effect on the number of LTCH facilities and LTCH bed capacity.

Beginning in FY 2016, LTCH-level payments would be made only for patients whose transfer to the LTCH was preceded by at least a 3-day stay in an acute care hospital's ICU or whose diagnosis at discharge from the LTCH indicated that they received mechanical ventilation services for at least 96 hours. Patients not meeting the 3-day ICU stay or ventilation threshold "criteria" would be paid at a lower rate comparable to that paid to an acute care hospital. This became known as the "dual payment rate" structure.[34]

From 2013 to 2016, aggregate spending decreased 2.1% annually; the cost-per-case increase for LTCHs fell from 2% (2012-2015) to 1.3% (2016) and then to 1.1% (2017). This was likely the result of reducing admits and stays for patients not meeting the criteria. The short-term results were dramatic: The percentage of LTCH cases meeting criteria rose from 65% in 2015 to 95% by 2017.[35] That year, as CMS began phasing in dual payment, LTCHs with more than 85% of their patients meeting the criteria were much more profitable (4.6%) than the industry average. As with IRFs, for-profit LTCHs were able to achieve lower cost growth due to their ability to manage length of stay, input costs, patient mix, and short-stay outliers.

For most of the past decade, LTCHs have remained profitable, holding cost growth below the rate of market basket increases. In 2016, cost growth was only 1%, the slowest growth since 2011. At the same time, the Medicare payment-per-case rose 1.0% annually from 2012 to 2015.[36] Medicare payments grew more slowly than the rate of provider costs, resulting in an aggregate 2016 Medicare margin of 4.1%. For-profit LTCHs enjoyed higher margins (5.7%).[37]

## The Home Health Groupings Model

CMS proposed a Home Health Groupings Model (HHGM) as a new payment methodology for home healthcare services in July 2017. HHGM would have made certain changes to reimbursement, such as basing payment off a 30-day (rather than 60-day) episode of care and comorbidities.[38] Due to HHGM, PAC providers anticipated a $950 million cut (15%-17%) to HHA reimbursement. In November 2017, HHGM was "off the table" as CMS finalized the FY 2018 payment update for home health without finalizing HHGM. The Bipartisan Budget Act of 2018 (see later discussion) required CMS to (1) delay implementation of the HHGM proposal and (2) implement it in a budget-neutral manner.

In July 2018, CMS proposed to replace HHGM with a new case-mix system called the Patient-Driven Groupings Model (PDGM), set to initiate in 2020; 60-day payment episodes were replaced with 30-day periods.[39] Payments are expected to increase for some HHAs but decrease for others, including larger, freestanding, and for-profit providers. This is thus designed to be implemented in a budget-neutral fashion.

## MedPAC's Repeated Recommendations to Cut PAC Payments

Every year, MedPAC prepares 2 lengthy reports for Congress offering advice on the financing and delivery of all healthcare services that Medicare covers (including the major PAC sectors). They are great, recommended reading. Over the past decade, MedPAC has consistently called for cuts to PAC reimbursement; these recommendations have rarely been adopted and implemented by Congress.

MedPAC advised Congress to cut PAC payments to HHAs, IRFs, LTCHs, and hospices for FY 2019.[40] To an uninformed observer, these recommendations represented an imminent threat to the financial stability and success of PAC providers. What observers failed to notice, however, were 2 key facts: (1) MedPAC had been making these recommendations to Congress for years, and (2) these recommendations were rarely implemented. Figure 14-7 lists MedPAC's recommendations for payment rate increases for 5 different PAC sites for FYs 2017, 2018, and 2019; the recommended updates were always zero or negative. Figure 14-7 also lists the actions taken by CMS during those same fiscal years; the actual updates were almost always nonzero and positive. The updates were, nonetheless, low in magnitude, which helped to reduce growth in PAC spending.

**PAC Site Payment Rate Increases FY 2017-2019: MedPAC Recommendations vs. CMS Actions**

| PAC Site | 2017 MedPAC Recommendation | 2017 CMS Action | 2018 MedPAC Recommendation | 2018 CMS Action | 2019 MedPAC Recommendation | 2019 CMS Action |
|---|---|---|---|---|---|---|
| IRF | 0.0% | +1.65% | −5.0% | +1.0%[a] | −5.0% | +1.3% |
| LTCH | 0.0% | +1.75% | 0.0% | +1.0%[b] −2.4%[c] | 0.0% | +1.35%[b] +0.9%[c] |
| HHA | 0.0% | −0.7% | −5.0% | −0.4%[d] | −5.0% | +2.2% |
| SNF | 0.0% | +2.4% | 0.0% | +1.0% | 0.0% | +2.4% |
| Hospice | 0.0% | +2.1% | 0.0% | +1.0% | 0.0% | +1.8% |

[a]+1.0% increase based on MACRA update, with −0.1% decrease based on outlier threshold

[b]+1.0% increase based on MACRA update for facilities meeting criteria

[c]−2.4% decrease for facilities not meeting criteria

[d]+1.0% increase based on MACRA update, −0.97 adjustment, and sunset of rural add-on

**Figure 14-7** • Post-Acute Care (PAC) Site Payment Rate Increases. CMS, Centers for Medicare and Medicaid Services; FY, Fiscal Year; HHA, Home Healthcare Agency; IRF, Inpatient Rehabilitation Facilities; LTCH, Long-Term Care Hospitals; MedPAC, Medicare Payment and Advisory Commission; SNF, Skilled Nursing Facility. (Source: MedPac.)

## STRONG PAC TAILWINDS

In contrast to the series of headwinds posed by the previously discussed regulatory and legislative actions, PAC providers have benefited from a host of real tailwinds driven by broader trends in the healthcare industry.

## PAC Growth Prospects Reflected in Merger Activity

Strong growth prospects are reflected by a significant number of mergers and acquisitions (M&A) that occurred in the PAC sector during 2017 (Figure 14-8).[41] In particular, long-term care had the highest number of deals (297, or

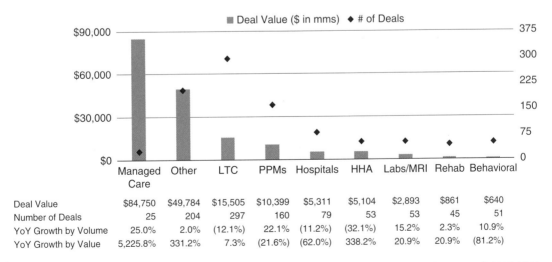

| | Managed Care | Other | LTC | PPMs | Hospitals | HHA | Labs/MRI | Rehab | Behavioral |
|---|---|---|---|---|---|---|---|---|---|
| Deal Value | $84,750 | $49,784 | $15,505 | $10,399 | $5,311 | $5,104 | $2,893 | $861 | $640 |
| Number of Deals | 25 | 204 | 297 | 160 | 79 | 53 | 53 | 45 | 51 |
| YoY Growth by Volume | 25.0% | 2.0% | (12.1%) | 22.1% | (11.2%) | (32.1%) | 15.2% | 2.3% | 10.9% |
| YoY Growth by Value | 5,225.8% | 331.2% | 7.3% | (21.6%) | (62.0%) | 338.2% | 20.9% | 20.9% | (81.2%) |

**Figure 14-8** • US Health Services Deal Volume, Value, and Year-Over-Year (YoY) Growth, Year End 2017. HHA, Home Healthcare Agency; LTC, Long-Term Care; MRI, Magnetic Resonance Imaging; PPMs, Physician Practice Management. (Source: PWC.)

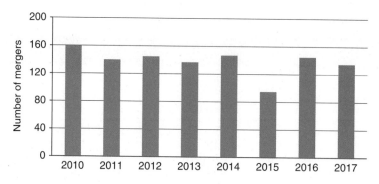

**Figure 14-9** • Home Healthcare Merger Activity, 2010 to 2017.

31% of deals; 9% of deal value); HHA exhibited the highest growth rate (338%) in deal value, compared to 146% overall for all health services. Rehabilitation also exhibited a nearly 21% increase in deal value during the prior year. Figure 14-9 shows the M&A trend for HHA.

## Growth Prospects Reflected in Private Equity Interest

Over the past few years, private investors have latched onto healthcare as a safe haven (ie, an industry with proven resilience to economic turbulence). Long-term growth in healthcare is powered by several immutable trends noted earlier (eg, aging population, chronic illness, and the ongoing need to deliver those services more efficiently in noninstitutionalized settings). Impelled by this logic and helped by low interest rates and readily available capital, private equity funds pushed the total disclosed deal value for

healthcare private equity to $36.4 billion in 2016, the highest level since 2007. The provider sector was the most active sector in healthcare for private equity deals in 2016 (Figure 14-10). Bain & Company research shows a 17% increase in the value of private equity deals between 2016 and 2017.[42] Total disclosed deal value reached $42.6 billion, the highest level since 2007, whereas deal count rose from 206 to 265.

Humana's December 2017 acquisition of Kindred, one of the largest PAC providers, represented the second largest private equity deal in 2017. In April 2018, just 4 months later, Humana announced similar deals with Curo Health Services (chain of hospice sites) and Landmark (home-based care company) as well as a national hospital incentive program to tie hospital compensation to how well hospitals coordinated care across sites. Humana's stated goal was to create a platform of providers to help manage costs and outcomes for the Medicare Advantage (MA)

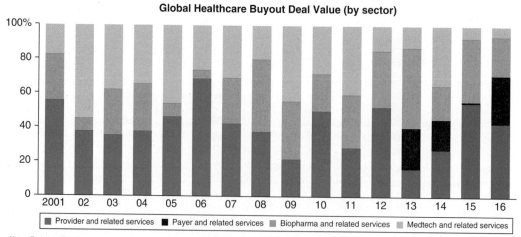

**Global Healthcare Buyout Deal Value (by sector)**

■ Provider and related services  ■ Payer and related services  ■ Biopharma and related services  ■ Medtech and related services

Notes: Excludes spin-offs, add-ons, loan-to-own transactions and acquisitions of bankrupt assets; based on announcement date; includes announced deals that are completed or pending, with data subject to change; deal value does not account for deals with undisclosed values.

**Figure 14-10** • Deal Activity in Healthcare Sectors. (Source: Dealogic; AVCJ; Bain analysis.)

population by treating patients in the most appropriate care setting.

## The Bipartisan Budget Act (2018)[43]

The Bipartisan Budget Act (2018) raised the spending caps imposed by the Budget Control Act of 2011 for 2 years, paving the way for a longer-term spending agreement. The bill made changes to the Medicare home health benefit, in part by reducing the unit of payment for a home health episode from 60 days to 30 days, beginning in 2020, and by eliminating the use of therapy thresholds that CMS uses to make case-mix adjustments to home health payments. It also modified the eligibility determination process for home health services. Beginning in 2019, Medicare will be allowed to base eligibility determinations for home health services on a review of the patient's medical record, including documentation in the home health agency records.

## Growth Prospects Reflected in Federal Medicare Spending Projections

Overall, the Bipartisan Budget Act of 2018 highlighted the government's willingness to spend money on critical healthcare services like home health and outpatient rehabilitation at the risk of increasing federal debt. Indeed, in June 2018, the federal government released its Annual Report of the Boards of Trustees of the Federal Hospital Insurance and Federal Supplementary Medical Insurance Trust Funds. The report contained projections over the next

decade in FFS expenditures on various provider services. The report projected 7.3% annual growth in HHA spending, 7.8% annual growth in hospice spending, and 8.0% annual growth in SNF spending (Figure 14-11). These PAC spending rates exceeded the overall projected growth in national health expenditures of 5.5% (2020-2027). These projections confirmed that federal spending on healthcare would increase and that PAC spending increases would continue to outpace spending on other services—a trend evident as early as the late 1980s. They further suggested that the stable profit margins earned during the 2006 to 2017 period by many PAC businesses (eg, HHAs, IRFs, and those LTCHs meeting the patient criteria) would likely continue into the future.[44]

## Shift to Value-Based Purchasing and Alternative Payment Models

Another strong tailwind behind the PAC sector was the rise of VBP and alternative payment models (APMs) (see Chapter 12). The former heralded the importance of delivering high-quality healthcare in lower-cost sites; the latter heralded the importance of ambulatory-based care sites (as opposed to inpatient sites) that could partner with hospital systems for patients with lower acuity of illness. Large PAC providers offered a solution to both.

APMs like bundled payments are largely directed at spending on hospital and physician services, which account for roughly 53% of every dollar spent on healthcare. Like other APMs, bundled payments seek to incentivize these providers to utilize their services more parsimoniously and, where appropriate, use PAC sites of care (especially HHA and hospice) rather than institutional sites of care. There exists a great savings opportunity in bundled payment for care delivered after discharge from the hospital. Hospital linkages to these PAC sites are needed, suggesting such vertical integration is likely to accelerate (see Chapter 12).

For years, there was often no real incentive for hospitals to direct patients to the highest-quality, most-appropriate PAC facility, coordinate care, or continue to track the patient. Like Ed Murrow, the broadcast journalist, many hospitals would say "good night, and good luck" to their patients as they left the hospital. They had no accountability for what happened to patients afterward. Now, due to

| Calendar Year | Inpatient Hospital | Skilled Nursing Facility | Home Health Agency | Hospice |
|:---:|:---:|:---:|:---:|:---:|
| | | | (see note 4) | |
| 2006 | 0.4 | 7.7 | 2.3 | 16.9 |
| 2007 | 0.6 | 8.3 | 3.9 | 12.3 |
| 2008 | 2.8 | 9.2 | 7.8 | 8.4 |
| 2009 | 1.4 | 5.5 | 4.4 | 7.6 |
| 2010 | 1.5 | 6.2 | 3.3 | 6.9 |
| 2011 | 1.5 | 11.7 | −5 | 6.6 |
| 2012 | 1.7 | −9.5 | −1.4 | 8.4 |
| 2013 | 1.7 | 1.6 | 0 | −0.2 |
| 2014 | 0.1 | 1.4 | −1.1 | 0 |
| 2015 | −0.2 | 1.9 | 4.3 | 5.2 |
| 2016 | 4.2 | −2.2 | −1 | 6.1 |
| 2017 | 0.9 | −1.2 | −0.5 | 6.5 |
| 2018 | 0.8 | −1.6 | −0.6 | 7.2 |
| 2019 | 0.1 | −1.3 | 3.3 | 8.4 |
| 2020 | 2.4 | 2.3 | 7.1 | 9.5 |
| 2021 | 3.8 | 4.9 | 6.1 | 8.1 |
| 2022 | 5.1 | 6.4 | −4.7 | 7.5 |
| 2023 | 5.1 | 6.7 | 16 | 7.3 |
| 2024 | 4.6 | 6.2 | 7 | 7.5 |
| 2025 | 4.7 | 6.2 | 7.1 | 7.6 |
| 2026 | 4.6 | 6.3 | 7 | 7.7 |
| 2027 | 4.6 | 6.4 | 7.1 | 8.1 |
| 2028 | 4.5 | 6.5 | 7.2 | 8.1 |
| 2029 | 4 | 5.9 | 6.5 | 8.6 |
| 2030 | 7.1 | 9.1 | 9.7 | 11.3 |

Notes
1. Percent increase in year indicated over previous year.
2. Includes costs of quality improvement organizations.
3. The ratio of the increase in HI costs to the increase in taxable payroll. This ratio is equivalent to the percent increase in the ratio of HI expenditures to taxable payroll (the cost rate).
4. Includes the declining share of costs drawn from HI for coverage of certain home health services transferred from HI to SMI Part B.

**Figure 14-11** • Federal Projections in Post-Acute Care Spending. HI, Hospital Insurance; SMI, Supplementary Medical Insurance.

VBP and bundled payment, hospitals have a financial reason to care about what happens to their patients after leaving the hospital and pay close attention to PAC.

Recently published research on the Comprehensive Care for Joint Replacement (CCJR) program for bundled payment suggests what the overall impact of this APM might be. Unlike prior bundled payment models, CCJR is a mandatory program implemented in 67 different metropolitan statistical areas; it was implemented in April 2016 and is scheduled to run until December 2020. Study findings published during 2018 to 2019 on the first 2 years of the CCJR program reveal that bundled payment reduces utilization of institutional PAC providers (SNFs) with observed shifts to HHA use.[45] These findings are consistent with prior

research that shows an inverse relationship between SNFs' share of PAC spending and HHAs' share of PAC spending and research that shows an inverse relationship between hospital lengths of stay and PAC (SNF, IRF) lengths of stay. They are also consistent with evidence that the use of PPS for SNFs occasioned a shift of patients to HHAs and that the use of PPS for IRFs occasioned a shift of patients to SNFs.[46] This suggests a substitution of lower-cost PAC sites for higher-cost PAC sites, similar to a shift from inpatient care to outpatient care following the 1983 IPPS (and squeezing the balloon). The same substitution mechanism is built into VBP arrangements that seek to promote the use of PAC over rehospitalization and use of inpatient days. This may help to explain why regulatory and legislative efforts to curb PAC spending and growth have not been successful.

## Rise of Medicare Advantage Plans

Since the early 2000s, Medicare has incentivized the transition of its beneficiaries to managed care plans offered under the MA program, previously known as Medicare Part C. In contrast to FFS Medicare, MA plans are run by private sector insurers, are paid a capitated fee, and develop more narrow provider networks using health maintenance organization (HMO) and preferred provider organization (PPO) models.

MA has enjoyed bipartisan political support and encouragement from the federal government over the past decade. MA is one of the few growth markets in health insurance (other than Medicaid). MA enrollment has been steadily increasing since 2005, penetrating 31% of the Medicare population by 2015, with an anticipated 11.5% increase in enrollment in 2018 that will raise the MA penetration level to 36% by 2019. To manage the capitated payments they receive from CMS, the MA plans have incentives to reduce unnecessary hospitalization, lengths of stay, and unnecessary readmissions. To facilitate this, many have sought to develop proprietary networks of primary care physicians as well as PAC sites (especially HHAs and hospices) to manage postdischarge transitions and avoid hospitalizations.

Moreover, in April 2018, the CMS administrator announced new rules that broadened the definition of "primarily health-related" benefits that MA plans are allowed to include in their policies. Plans could now add adult day care, home aides to help with activities of daily living (ADLs), and home-based palliative care. In 2019, CMS expanded the supplemental benefits (to be covered in 2020) to include nonskilled home health-based support services, adult day care, and home modifications to assist patients with ADLs and instrumental ADLs (IADLs). Such benefits are designed to help improve the functioning of beneficiaries with chronic conditions. According to a survey conducted by Avalere, 40% or more of MA plans intend to offer these benefits in 2019.

This policy change suggests that not only is the government willing to see more Medicare beneficiaries join MA plans but is also willing to pay for more services to the enrollees of these plans. This suggests a strong tailwind to the HHA and hospice segments of PAC, thereby reversing an earlier trend (2007-2013) in which MA plans used less home healthcare than FFS Medicare. It is less clear that the spread of MA plans will provide similar tailwinds to SNFs and IRFs; research suggests that enrollees in MA plans use these PAC sites less than FFS Medicare beneficiaries do.[47]

## Accountable Care Organizations and Vertically Integrated Hospital-PAC Networks

Accountable care organizations (ACOs) and hospital-PAC networks constitute 2 examples of vertical integration efforts identified in Chapter 12. Both seek to assemble a panel of providers operating across the care continuum to take responsibility for the cost and quality of care of a defined population of patients. This is at the heart of care provision under VBPs and APMs. Some ACOs may have the care continuum in house as part of their vertical integration efforts; other ACOs may contract for the continuum of care services needed as part of a virtual integration strategy. All observers agree that home healthcare and hospice care are necessary components of ACOs.[48]

Because Medicare payments to PAC providers doubled between 2001 and 2015, PAC sites represent a growth opportunity for ACOs to generate savings. Moreover, PAC networks can help ACOs to decrease episode costs and increase quality outcomes.[49] ACOs and other vertically integrated providers recognize network development and partnerships with PAC sites of care as a major preparatory task (Figure 14-12).[50]

## SUMMARY

PAC has assumed tremendous importance and stature in the healthcare ecosystem in just a few decades. The hitherto-neglected sectors of HHA, IRF, LTCH, and hospice have joined SNFs as major players in the provider space—not only by themselves, but also in terms of their collaboration with major providers (like hospitals) and payers. PAC providers are now considered key to cost containment and the reduction of fragmentation in healthcare.

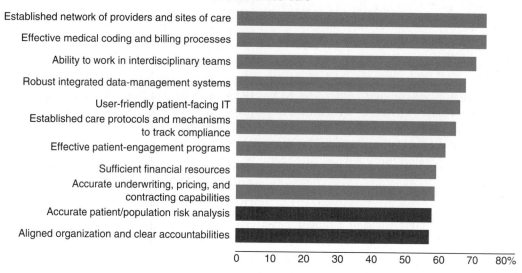

**Figure 14-12** • Network Development as Number 1 Way to Prepare for Value-Based Care. (Source: Tim van Biesen, Josh Weisbrod, Michael Brookshire, et al. (2017), Front Line of Healthcare Report 2017: Why Involving Doctors Can Help Improve US Healthcare. Used with permission from Bain & Company. https://www.bain.com/insights/front-line-of-healthcare-report-2017/.)

## QUESTIONS TO PONDER

1. Like the hospital sector, the PAC sector features a mix of nonprofit and for-profit facilities. Unlike the hospital sector, there is some serious concern about the large presence of for-profit PAC facilities. Why might their presence be of concern?
2. Why is the PAC sector so fragmented? Why didn't it consolidate the way that hospitals did several decades ago?
3. What is the promise of PAC? What are the major problems of PAC?
4. Have federal government efforts to rein in PAC spending succeeded? Why or why not?

## REFERENCES

1. Harris Williams & Co. *Home Health Market Overview* (Richmond, VA: Harris Williams & Co., December 2013): 2. Available online: https://www.harriswilliams.com/system/files/industry_update/2013.12.16_home_health_market_overview.pdf. Accessed on March 20, 2018.
2. Wen Tian. *An All-Payer View of Hospital Discharge to Postacute Care 2013* (Washington, DC: Agency for Healthcare Research and Quality, May 2016).
3. These descriptions are based on primers published by the Medicare Payment and Advisory Commissions (MedPAC), which serves as Congress's watchdog over the Medicare program. MedPAC. *Home Health Care Services Payment System* (October 2017). Available online: http://www.medpac.gov/docs/default-source/payment-basics/medpac_payment_basics_17_hha_final.pdf. Accessed on July 20, 2020. MedPAC. *Inpatient Rehabilitation Facilities Payment System* (October 2017). Available online: http://www.medpac.gov/docs/default-source/payment-basics/medpac_payment_basics_17_irf_final93a311adfa9c665e80adff00009edf9c.pdf?sfvrsn=0. Accessed on July 30, 2020. MedPAC. *Long-Term Care Hospitals Payment System* (October 2017). Available online: http://www.medpac.gov/docs/default-source/payment-basics/medpac_payment_basics_17_ltch_final.pdf. Accessed on July 30, 2020. MedPAC. *Hospice Services Payment System* (October 2017). Available online: http://www.medpac.gov/docs/default-source/payment-basics/medpac_payment_basics_17_hospice_final4ea311adfa9c665e80adff00009edf9c.pdf?sfvrsn=0. Accessed on July 20, 2020.
4. *Duggan v. Bowen*. U.S. District Court for the District of Columbia. Number 87-0383, August 1, 1988.
5. PPS was initially targeted at inpatient stays at acute care hospitals. It is often denoted as IPPS.
6. Harriet Komisar and Judith Feder. *The Balanced Budget Act of 1997: Effects on Medicare's Home Health Benefit and Beneficiaries Who Need Long-Term Care* (New York, NY: The Commonwealth Fund, February 1998).

7. AARP. "Home and Community Preferences of the 45+ Population, 2014." Available online: https://www.aarp.org/content/dam/aarp/research/surveys_statistics/il/2015/home-community-preferences.doi.10.26419%252Fres.00105.001.pdf. Accessed on August 6, 2020.

8. Steven Landers, Elizabeth Madigan, Bruce Leff, et al. "The Future of Home Health Care: A Strategic Framework for Optimizing Value," *Home Health Care Manag Pract.* 28 (4) (October 2016): 262-278.

9. Encompass Health Corporation. *Investor Reference Book* (March 5, 2019): 57.

10. IBISWorld. *Home Care Providers in the US*. Available online: https://www.ibisworld.com/industry-statistics/market-size/home-care-providers-united-states/. Accessed on November 12, 2020.

11. Centers for Medicare and Medicaid Services. *Home Health Payment Refinement* (Washington, DC: CMS, January 18, 2017). Available online: https://www.cms.gov/Outreach-and-Education/Outreach/NPC/Downloads/2017-01-18-HH-Presentation.pdf. Accessed on September 19, 2019. The HHRGs range from groups of relatively uncomplicated patients to those of patients who have severe medical conditions, who have severe functional limitations, and who need extensive therapy. Each HHRG has a national, relative weight reflecting the average relative costliness of patients in that group compared with the average Medicare home health patient. If fewer than 5 visits are delivered during a 60-day episode, the agency is paid per visit by visit type, rather than by the episode payment method.

12. Centers for Medicare and Medicaid Services. *Home Health Value-Based Purchasing Model* (Washington, DC: CMS). Available online: https://innovation.cms.gov/initiatives/home-health-value-based-purchasing-model. Accessed on July 20, 2019. Quality bonus payments are funded through a payment withhold of 5% in 2018, increasing to 8% by 2021. Performance will be evaluated on a set of 24 measures that include outcome measures collected in the OASIS, patient experience survey measures from the Home Health Consumer Assessment of Health Providers and Systems (HH CAHPS), and claims-based quality measures.

13. The 66 RUGs in the classification system include 14 rehabilitation groups; 9 groups for days with rehabilitation and extensive services (eg, ventilator care); 3 groups for extensive services; 16 groups for special care (eg, patients who have chronic obstructive pulmonary disease); and 10 groups for clinically complex care (eg, patients with pneumonia).

14. Medicare Payment Advisory Commission. "Inpatient Rehabilitation Facility Services," Chapter 10 in *Report to the Congress: Medicare Payment Policy* (Washington, DC: CMS, March 2018).

15. Centers for Medicare and Medicaid Services. *Inpatient Rehabilitation Facility Prospective Payment System* (Washington, DC: CMS). Available online: https://www.cms.gov/Outreach-and-Education/Medicare-Learning-Network-MLN/MLNProducts/Downloads/InpatRehabPaymtfctsht09-508.pdf. Accessed on September 18, 2019.

16. Facilities that cannot demonstrate compliance with the 60% rule are paid as acute care hospitals under the inpatient PPS (IPPS). IRFs must meet other requirements such as having a medical director of rehabilitation who provides services in the facility on a full-time basis (or for at least 20 hours per week in hospital-based units).

17. Federal Register. *Medicare Program; Inpatient Rehabilitation Facility (IRF) Prospective Payment System for Federal Fiscal Year 2020 and Updates to the IRF Quality Reporting Program* (August 8, 2019). Available online: https://www.federalregister.gov/documents/2019/08/08/2019-16603/medicare-program-inpatient-rehabilitation-facility-irf-prospective-payment-system-for-federal-fiscal. Accessed on September 16, 2019.

18. Centers for Disease Control and Prevention. "Severe TBI" (March 30, 2017). Available online: https://www.cdc.gov/traumaticbraininjury/severe.html. Accessed on November 12, 2020.

19. Medicare Payment Advisory Commission. "Long-term Care Hospital Services," Chapter 10 in *Report to the Congress: Medicare Payment Policy* (Washington, DC: MedPAC, March 2016). Beginning with cost reporting periods starting in FY 2016 and 2017, cases that do not meet the specified criteria receive a blended rate of one-half the standard LTCH payment and one-half the site-neutral payment. These cases receive 100% of the site-neutral payment rate or 100% of the cost of the case (whichever is lower), beginning with hospital cost reporting periods starting on or after October 1, 2017.

20. ReedSmith. *CMS Finalizes IPPS/LTCH Payment and Policy Changes for FY 2018*. Available online: https://www.healthindustrywashingtonwatch.com/2017/08/articles/department-of-health-and-human-services/cms-finalizes-ippsltch-payment-and-policy-changes-for-fy-2018/. Accessed on September 16, 2019.

21. Stephen H. Cooper, Corbin T. Santo, and Ryann D. Roberts. "Implications of the Medicare and Medicaid Provisions in the 21st Century Cures Act," *National Law Review* 6 (348) (December 13, 2016). Neda Ryan. *Medicare Reimbursement Policy Changes Under the 21st Century Cures Act* (Miramed, July 5, 2017). Available online: https://www.miramedgs.com/blog/medicare-reimbursement-policy-changes-under-the-21st-century-cures-act. Accessed on July 30, 2020.

22. Department of Health and Human Services. "Medicare's Hospice Benefit: Revising the Payment System to Better Reflect Visit Intensity"

(May 28, 2016). Available online: https://aspe
.hhs.gov/basic-report/medicares-hospice-benefit-
revising-payment-system-better-reflect-visit-
intensity. Accessed on September 16, 2019.

23. Amedisys, Inc. *Amedisys Presentation*. J.P. Morgan
Health Care Conference 2018 (January 2018): 3.
Available online: https://seekingalpha.com/article/
4136653-amedisys-and-nbsp-amed-presents-
36th-annual-j-p-morgan-healthcare-conference-
slideshow?page=2. Accessed on March 20, 2018.

24. KaufmanHall. "Home Health and Hospice Services." Available online: https://www.kaufmanhall
.com/sites/default/files/documents/2020-03/ma_
flash_report_09_2018_home_health_and_hospice_
kaufmanhall.pdf. Accessed on August 6, 2020.

25. Total Medicare spending during this period rose
from $210.4 billion to $648.9 billion.

26. MedPAC. *Medicare Payment Policy: Report to
the Congress* (March 2018): 242, 257. Several
problems have plagued the PPS systems aimed
at PAC. These include inaccuracy of payment
(ie, overpayment, a problem that MedPAC has
worked on unsuccessfully since 2008), huge differ-
entials between high-cost and low-cost providers,
imprecise adjustment for differences in patient
needs (known as case-mix adjustment), inadequate quality measurement, uniform payment for
care delivered despite variations in quality, and
insufficient criteria to inform decisions on the
appropriate PAC site for treatment. Moreover,
hospital discharge planners are not allowed by
law to direct patients to specific discharge settings.

27. MedPAC. *A Data Book: Health Care Spending
and the Medicare Program*. June 2018. MedPAC.
*Medicare Payment Policy: Report to the Congress*
(March 2018): Table 9-1.

28. MedPAC. *Medicare Payment Policy: Report to
the Congress* (March 2018): 246. MedPAC. *Medicare Payment Policy: Report to the Congress*
(March 2019). Chapter 9.

29. MedPAC. *Medicare Payment Policy: Report to
the Congress* (March 2018): 283, Figure 10-1.

30. MedPAC. *Medicare Payment Policy: Report to
the Congress* (March 2018): 278, Table 10-5.

31. Ben Schmitt and Natasha Lindstrom. "Children's
Institute of Pittsburgh to Close Rehab Hospital,"
*Trib Total Media* (March 13, 2018).

32. MedPAC. *Medicare Payment Policy: Report to
the Congress* (Spring 2018): Tables 11-1, 11-2.

33. Laura Keohane, Salama Freed, David G.
Stevenson, et al. *Trends in Postacute Care Spending
Growth During the Medicare Spending Slowdown*
(Commonwealth Fund Issue Brief, December 1,
2018): 1-11.

34. The dual-rate payment structure exerted less of
an immediate impact on the LTCH sector than
anticipated for 2 reasons. First, many of the
LTCH closings that occurred after 2015 took
place in markets with lots of LTCH capacity; due

to certificate of need (CON) laws, LTCHs are
located in only 8.5% of US counties. As a result,
with the closings, competitors could thus absorb
the patients, particularly those who met the new
patient criteria, and thereby become more profitable. Despite the closings, LTCH occupancy has
remained stable (~66%) over time (2012-2016). Second, LTCHs also instituted managerial responses
to adapt: (1) admit more cases that meet criteria,
(2) expand their referral regions, (3) educate
physicians and nurse case managers at acute care
hospitals about their LTCH's capabilities, (4) build
affiliations with acute care hospitals, (5) contract
with Medicare Advantage plans, and (6) reduce
their costs per discharge.

35. Kindred's analysis of its own LTCHs classified
them into 3 buckets based on their "Criteria
Performance." The first bucket contained those
"clearly viable under the criteria"; the second
bucket contained those "that will have to supplement their operations with targeted managed
care contracting or ancillary services"; the third
bucket contained those "that would be targets for
a more dramatic transformation (or closure)."
Kindred's classification allocated them into the 3
buckets as follows: 70% to 75%, 10% to 15%, and
10%. The last group was largely concentrated in
specific geographic areas.

36. MedPAC. *Medicare Payment Policy: Report to
the Congress* (Spring 2018): Table 11-2.

37. MedPAC. *Medicare Payment Policy: Report to
the Congress* (Spring 2018): 311.

38. Kindred Healthcare. *10-K* (December 2017): 27.

39. Centers for Medicare and Medicaid Services.
*CMS Takes Action to Modernize Medicare
Home Health* (July 2, 2018). Available online:
https://www.cms.gov/Outreach-and-Education/
Outreach/FFSProvPartProg/Provider-Partnership-
Email-Archive-Items/2018-07-02-eNews-Se.html.
Accessed on September 20, 2019.

40. MedPAC. *Medicare Payment Policy: Report to
the Congress* (Spring 2018): 260, 289, 315, 346.

41. Thaddeus Kresho et al. *US Health Services Deals
Insights: Year-End 2017* (PricewaterhouseCoopers, 2018). Available online: https://www.pwc
.com/us/en/health-industries/publications/health-
services-quarterly-deals-insights.html. Accessed
on March 20, 2018.

42. Bain & Company. *Global Healthcare Private
Equity and Corporate M&A Report 2018* (Bain &
Company, 2018).

43. John B. Larson, February 9, 2018. H.R. 1892–
Bipartisan Budget Act of 2018, 115th Congress
(2017-2018) (US Congress, February 9, 2018).
Available online: https://www.congress.gov/
bill/115th-congress/house-bill/1892. Accessed
on November 13, 2020.

44. Vernon Smith, Kathleen Gifford, Eileen Ellis,
et al. *Implementing Coverage and Payment*

*Initiatives: Results From a 50-State Medicaid Budget Survey for State Fiscal Years 2016 and 2017* (Kaiser Family Foundation Report, October 2016).

45. Amy Finklestein, Yunan Ji, Neale Mahoney, et al. "Mandatory Medicare Bundled Payment Program for Lower Extremity Joint Replacement and Discharge to Institutional Postacute Care: Interim Analysis of the First Year of a 5-Year Randomized Trial," *JAMA.* 320 (9) (2018): 892-900. Michael Barnett, Andrew Wilcock, J. Michael McWilliams, et al. "Two-Year Evaluation of Mandatory Bundled Payments for Joint Replacement," *N Engl J Med.* 380 (2019): 252-262. Derek A. Haas, Xioran Zhang, Robert S. Kaplan, et al. "Evaluation of Economic and Clinical Outcomes Under Centers for Medicare & Medicaid Services Mandatory Bundled Payments for Joint Replacements," *JAMA Int Med.* 179 (7) (2019): 924-931.

46. Melinda Buntin, Carrie Colla, and Jose Escarce. "Effects of Payment Changes on Trends in Post-acute Care," *Health Serv Res.* 44 (4) (2009): 1188-1210.

47. Peter Huckfeldt, Jose Escarce, Brendan Rabideau, et al. "Less Intense Postacute Care, Better Outcomes for Enrollees in Medicare Advantage Than Those in Fee-for-Service," *Health Aff.* 36 (1) (2017): 91-100.

48. Susan Block, Vicki Jackson, and Thomas Lee. "Care Delivery and Coordination in the Accountable Care Environment," *Health Affairs Blog* (February 19, 2014). Amy Kelley and Diane Meier. "The Role of Palliative Care in Accountable Care Organizations," *Am J Managed Care.* 21 (6) (April 2015). Alana Stramowski. "How Home Health Can Win ACO Partners," *Home Health Care News* (October 18, 2016).

49. Leavitt Partners. *Six Characteristics of Successful Post-Acute Care (PAC) Value Networks* (Washington, DC: Leavitt Partners, April 18, 2017).

50. Bain & Company. *Front Line of Healthcare Report 2017: Giving Physicians a Say: Why Involving Doctors Can Help Improve US Healthcare* (Bain, 2017). Available online: https://www.bain.com/insights/front-line-of-healthcare-report-2017/. Accessed on November 13, 2020.

# SECTION III

## Payer Sectors in the Ecosystem

# 15

# Employer-Based Health Insurance

## OVERVIEW OF CHAPTERS 15-19

There are 3 main types of insurance coverage in the United States today (Figure 15-1): private sector insurance sponsored by employers, public sector insurance through the Medicare program (for the elderly), and public sector insurance through the Medicaid program (for the poor). As of 2015, private insurance covered over half (56%) of the population and 62% of the nonelderly population (Figure 15-2).

This chapter reviews the role of employers in the healthcare system, the goals behind employer-based health insurance (EBHI), the tools at their disposal to influence the cost and quality of healthcare, and their degree of success in doing so. Chapter 16 continues the discussion of employers in managing a particularly difficult and little understood subject—pharmacy benefits (drug coverage) and the chain of participants in the drug channel. Chapter 17 analyzes the role of health insurers who work on behalf of the employers and who also contract with the public insurers. Chapters 18 and 19 examine the Medicare and Medicaid programs, respectively.

## HISTORICAL ORIGINS OF PRIVATE HEALTH INSURANCE

As covered in Chapter 13, the first insurance plans were community-based schemes covering local workers in specific industries (eg, teachers, Kaiser construction). Many of these schemes were capitated, prepaid plans that presaged the rise of health maintenance organizations (HMOs). These plans, organized by local hospitals to help finance themselves, were known as "hospital service plans." The hospitals called on their national association, the American Hospital Association (AHA), for guidance, which set up a committee and began approving them. This culminated in the establishment of the AHA Blue Cross Commission in 1946. Similarly, local medical societies established "medical service plans" to finance physician services, which were approved by the American Medical Association (AMA). In contrast to the hospital plans, these were indemnity plans where the insurer paid the patient, who, in turn, paid the physician. In this manner, local nonprofit Blue Cross and Blue Shield plans (covered in Chapter 17) were organized by the AHA and AMA, respectively, starting in the 1930s to help pay for the services rendered by their members.

Three major changes over the next 50 years transformed this landscape. The *first* major change was the rapid development of private sector insurance coverage during World War II. The federal government imposed wage and price controls in 1942 to stem inflation to help the war effort. This prevented private companies from offering higher wages to attract scarce labor, however. To alleviate the problem, the National War Labor Board ruled that health insurance was not to be considered a "wage," thereby encouraging employers to offer healthcare coverage as a fringe benefit. In 1943, the Internal Revenue Service ruled that such benefits were not subject to federal income taxation. This made healthcare insurance tax-free income to both the employer and employee, encouraging the adoption of a tax-free benefit over taxable income. In 1947, the Supreme Court and the Taft-Hartley Act ruled that health insurance

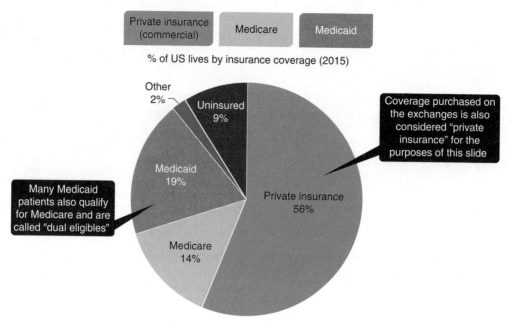

**Figure 15-1** • Three Main Types of Insurance Coverage in the United States.

was also a condition for employment and thus a negotiable item in collective bargaining agreements. Health coverage expanded quickly to organized labor.

Insurers favored the large employers over individuals, who were not part of a natural risk pool and whose benefits were expensive to administer. This led to the dominance of group insurance coverage over individual plans. Employers altered their compensation packages to now pay health insurance premiums on behalf of their workers. By 1950, health insurance coverage had become a standard feature of and closely linked to private sector employment. The enrollments in Blue Cross and Blue Shield plans swelled.

The 1940s and 1950s witnessed the entrance of commercial for-profit insurers. They competed with the nonprofit plans by offering "experience rating"; that is, charging healthier

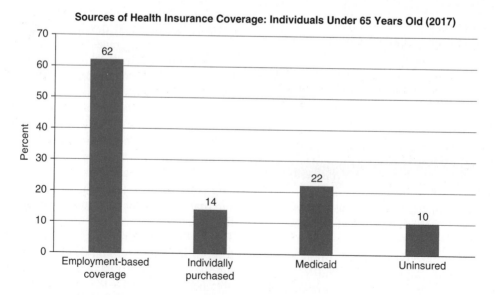

**Figure 15-2** • Insurance Coverage for Non-Medicare Population. (Source: Employee Benefit Research Institute Estimates of the Current Population Survey, March 2018 Supplement.)

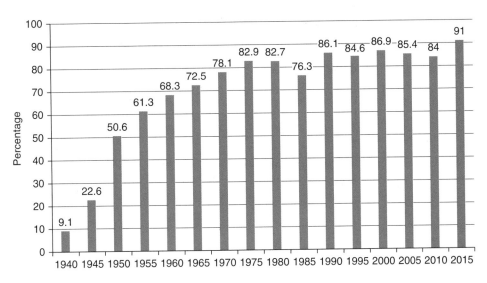

**Figure 15-3** • Percent US Population with Insurance Coverage, 1940 to 2015. (Source: US Census Bureau.)

workers (little "experience" in using services) a lower premium. With the end of World War II, there was an acceleration of enrollment of workers into these plans. Employers now competed for workers not only in terms of offering insurance coverage for health, life, and disability but, now, also offering retiree benefits that included health coverage. Figure 15-3 charts the rapid growth in private sector coverage.

The *second* major change occurred in 1974 with passage of the Employee Retirement and Income Security Act (ERISA). ERISA was designed primarily to protect underfunded pension plans; however, it also contained provisions regarding health insurance plans. ERISA allowed firms to "self-insure" (ie, to assume the financial risk themselves for the expenditures on their employees' healthcare benefits, rather than pass the risk on to insurance companies). By doing so, employers could avoid (1) paying monthly premiums to insurers, (2) paying state taxes (which ranged from 2% to 4%) based on those health insurance premiums, and (3) state-mandated health insurance benefits. Firms now bore their own health claims risk but outsourced the processing of claims to third-party administrators (TPAs), often the health insurers. The insurers responded by establishing new product lines called "administrative services only" (ASO).

The *third* major change was the rise of managed care organizations (MCOs) in the 1980s and (especially) the 1990s. From the 1940s through the early 1980s, employers were generally passive about the amounts they spent on their employees'

health insurance coverage. However, due to the rising cost of care after 1965 (see Chapter 6) and growing competition from other countries (eg, Japan), employers got more engaged in several ways. They organized local and regional business coalitions to study the problem; some pooled their purchasing of healthcare benefits through these coalitions. They saw the results of the Health Insurance Experiment conducted by the Rand Corporation, which showed that cost sharing with enrollees reduced utilization and spending. They also embraced the HMO model, which had been developed decades earlier (Kaiser) and legitimized in the 1973 HMO Act. ERISA had also spawned a second model called "preferred provider organizations" (PPOs) in the 1980s, which (unlike the HMOs) were not always insurers, did not bear underwriting risk, and negotiated contracts with a provider network for use by self-insured employers.

During the early to mid-1980s, employers began requiring more cost sharing from their employees: The percentage using deductibles rose from 30% to 63%, whereas the percentage using copayments rose from 58% to 74% (1982-1984). Shortly thereafter, a handful of large employers got serious about their rising healthcare premium costs and began to push or entice their employees away from indemnity plans to join the new MCO plans (HMOs and PPOs). The growing demand for managed care by employers was quickly met by a growing supply of managed care plans offered by insurers; by 1996, there was a massive switch of employees from indemnity plans to HMOs and PPOs. In 1984, 95% of employees were covered by fee-for-service (FFS) plans compared to only 5% in managed care plans; by 1997, 85% of employees were in managed care plans compared to 15% in FFS.

## UNDERSTANDING EMPLOYER HEALTH COVERAGE TODAY

### Salary and Benefits

To attract more and better-qualified labor, employers offer prospective employees a combination of salary and benefits. Together, salary and benefits are considered the employee's total compensation and the employee's money.[1] Employer payments for health insurance premiums ultimately come out of what would otherwise have been paid to workers as money wages. As of the mid-1990s, consultants estimated that 88% of premiums were offset by money wage reductions.[2] Thus, it is the employee and not the employer who is paying for the health insurance premium.

Employees have the discretion to accept the total compensation package in return for contributing their labor. However, it is financially disadvantageous for employees to forego the health insurance coverage since their wages may not rise, they would forego the savings on their income and payroll taxes, and they would have to spend more on their own to obtain coverage without the group discount.[3] Employees also have discretion in determining the mix of the total compensation going to the various components of the benefit package.

Employer-sponsored benefit plans that provide insurance coverage to employees are known as ERISA-covered health plans; the employers serve as ERISA plan sponsors, while the employees are known as ERISA plan participants. The ERISA plans (employers) pay premiums and/or administrative fees to health insurers who serve as third parties that underwrite and/or administer health insurance plans on behalf of the employers.

The employee's benefit package includes a mix of retirement plan benefits and "health and welfare plan" benefits.[4] The latter center on the provision of group health plans that provide medical care benefits for ERISA plan participants or their dependents.[5] They usually include hospital, medical, and drug insurance coverage; they can also cover life, disability, and long-term care insurance, as well as other types of health benefits (dental, vision).[6] According to data from the Bureau of Labor Statistics, insurance benefits represented 7% to 9% (depending on firm size) of total worker compensation in 2020.[7]

### Employer Offer Rates and Employee Take-Up Rates of Health Insurance

Figure 15-4 shows that slightly more than half (57%) of all firms offer workers health insurance coverage. Coverage is nearly universal in large firms (200+ employees) and quite available in middle-sized firms (10-199 employees), due to risk pooling advantages and purchasing efficiencies (ability to obtain coverage at relatively lower cost). Among those firms that offer health benefits, most offer them to spouses and dependents; few offer them to part-time and temporary workers. However, not all employees who are offered coverage accept the coverage. The "take-up" rate is roughly three-quarters of employees, a figure that has fallen slightly over time (from 85% to 76% between 1999 and 2019). Take-up rates are lower in firms with a higher share of lower-wage, nonunionized, and younger workers.

### Variation in Employer Financing of Health Plan Coverage

Employers may sponsor their health insurance plans in 2 ways: (1) offer a fully insured plan whereby the employer purchases coverage from a health insurer who then bears the risk, or (2) offer a self-insured plan where the employer bears the risk and the insurer serves as a TPA that administers the benefits, processes and pays the claims, and assembles the provider network under ASO contracts. Between 1999 and 2019, a higher percentage of covered workers were employed by firms that self-insured, rising from 44% to 61%; in large firms with 1,000 or more workers, the increase was from 62% to 82%.[8]

### Variation in Health Plan Options Offered by Employers

Employers can offer their employees a range of health insurance coverage options. These

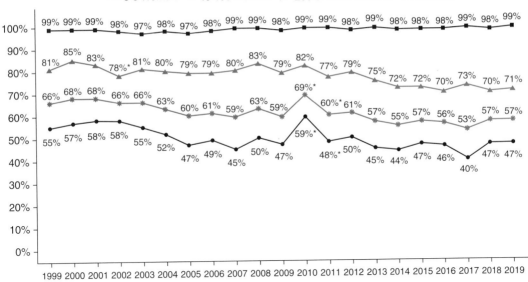

**Percentage of Firms Offering Health Benefits, by Firm Size, 1999-2019**

→ 3-9 Workers → 10-199 Workers → 200 or More Workers → All Firms

*Estimate is statistically different from estimate for the previous year shown (p <.05).

NOTE: As noted in the Survey Design and Methods section, estimates are based on the sample of both firms that completed the entire survey and those that answered just one question about whether they offer health benefits.

**Figure 15-4** • Firms Offering Health Benefits. (Source: KFF Employer Health Benefits Survey, 2018-2019; Kaiser/HRET Survey of Employer-Sponsored Health Benefits, 1999-2017.)

include HMOs, PPOs, point-of-service (POS), and high-deductible health plans (HDHPs) with a savings option (SO).[9] The distribution in the percentage of employees selecting these plans has changed over time to higher enrollment in HDHPs.[10] The largest share of participants are still enrolled in PPOs. This is portrayed in Figure 15-5. These aggregate figures mask a lot of variation that has occurred over time and among different types of firms.

There is also temporal variation in the number of plan options that ERISA plan sponsors offer to their employees. The vast majority (87%) of firms offering healthcare benefits offered only 1 type of plan in 2007, with larger firms more likely to offer more than 1 plan than smaller firms (44% vs 11%). Nevertheless, 49% of all workers in firms were offered more than 1 plan.[11] Consistent with the data presented earlier, only 10% of firms offered an HDHP/SO in 2007, and only 18% of workers were offered such a plan. In 2019, by contrast, fewer (75%) firms offering healthcare benefits offered only 1 type of health insurance plan; large firms (those with 200+ workers) are much more likely to offer more than 1 plan type than smaller firms (61% vs 24%). As a result, the majority (64%)

of covered workers are employed in firms offering more than 1 plan and thus have discretion in their health insurance coverage. Among firms offering only 1 plan, the majority (56%) offer a PPO plan; 27% are offered an HDHP/SO plan. These trend data suggest that, over the period of 2007 to 2019, more firms offered workers a choice of more than 1 plan, more workers were offered more than 1 plan, workers in both large and small firms were offered more than 1 plan (with workers in larger firms having more choice), and more workers were enrolled in an HDHP/SO plan.

## Employee Choices and Trade-Offs Among Health Plans Offered

The choice among these plans entails a fundamental, well-known trade-off that workers consciously make: pay a higher premium with lower out-of-pocket costs *or* a lower premium with higher out-of-pocket costs.[12,13] According to Figure 15-6, the HDHP/SO plan option entails the lowest premiums and the lowest worker contributions in exchange for worker responsibility for higher, up-front costs paid out of pocket before the insurance coverage begins.[14]

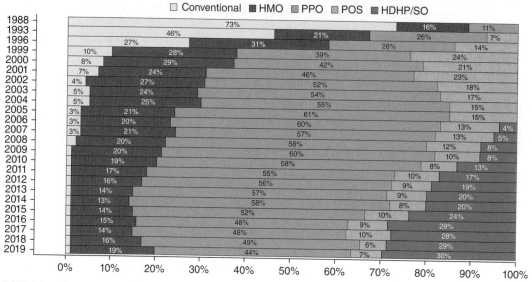

NOTE: Information was not obtained for POS plans in 1988 or for HDHP/SO plans until 2006. A portion of the change in 2005 is likely attributable to incorporating more recent Census Bureau estimates of the number of state and local government workers and removing federal workers from the weights. See the Survey Design and Methods section from the 2005 Kaiser/HRET Survey of Employer-Sponsored Health Benefits.

**Figure 15-5** • Health Plan Enrollment for Covered Workers. (Source: KFF Employer Health Benefits Survey, 2018-2019; Kaiser/HRET Survey of Employer-Sponsored Health Benefits, 1999-2017; KPMG Survey of Employer-sponsored Benefits, 1993 and 1996; The Health insurance Association of America (HIAA), 1988.)

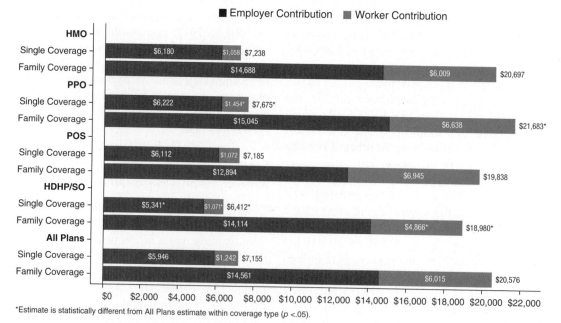

*Estimate is statistically different from All Plans estimate within coverage type ($p$ <.05).

**Figure 15-6** • Annual Worker and Employer Premium Contributions and Premiums. (Source: KFF Employer Health Benefits Survey, Kaiser Family Foundation, 2019.)

Workers select the plan with the trade-off they prefer. This is (purportedly) an exercise in consumerism.[15] According to researchers, HDHPs are designed to make the healthcare system more responsive to consumers and make consumers more responsible for the cost of healthcare by exposing them to larger, up-front out-of-pocket expenses. HDHPs entail 3 types of cost sharing: the annual deductible to be paid before coverage begins, the percentage of cost sharing (coinsurance) once the insurance coverage kicks in, and the annual out-of-pocket maximum.[16] Kaiser trend data indicate that workers have increasingly chosen the plan (the HDHP/SO) with a lower annual premium but higher out-of-pocket cost.[17]

Over the time period from 2007 to 2019, more employers have chosen to offer the HDHP/SO plan to their workers and more workers have elected this plan. Although the Kaiser data do not directly indicate whether the HDHP is an "option" or a "replacement," other data reveal that the vast majority (66%) of enrollees in HDHPs had a choice of plan.[18] Indeed, a higher percentage of HDHP enrollees have greater choice among 2 or 3 plans compared to enrollees in national and traditional health plans. The plans from which they choose can include open-network models such as PPOs or more restricted models such as HMOs and POS plans.

## Degree of "Informed Consumerism" in Employee Choice of HDHPs

Of course, workers may not be fully informed when making their choice among health plans and the types of cost sharing they entail. In one

study, when presented with descriptions of possible provider network features, 50% or fewer of consumers could correctly describe HMO and PPO network characteristics.[19] In another study, only 14% of individuals could correctly identify 4 basic components of traditional insurance design: deductible, copay, coinsurance, and out-of-pocket maximum (defined later).[20] A 2014 survey by the Kaiser Family Foundation reported low consumer literacy regarding health insurance terms and concepts (Figure 15-7).

## Employer Concerns With HDHP Plans

A 2018 survey asked employers what they considered the number 1 challenge with HDHPs.[21] The most frequent response (29%) was medications unaffordable to members before the deductible is met, followed by members not understanding how deductibles work (25%) and lack of member engagement (19%). The increased use of HDHPs has raised other concerns including lack of affordability of needed care before the deductible is met, delaying or forgoing high-value treatment, and an increase in the proportion of household income dedicated to healthcare.

Employer concerns are echoed by self-employed physicians. Physicians likewise report that patients have inadequate knowledge of their insurance coverage: In a recent survey, only 1% of physicians said their patients' understanding was "excellent," and only 14% described it as "good." The same survey reveals that 51% of physicians report that more than half of their patients ask about their responsibility for the

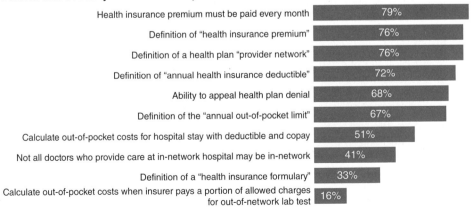

Percent who correctly answered each question:

- Health insurance premium must be paid every month — 79%
- Definition of "health insurance premium" — 76%
- Definition of a health plan "provider network" — 76%
- Definition of "annual health insurance deductible" — 72%
- Ability to appeal health plan denial — 68%
- Definition of the "annual out-of-pocket limit" — 67%
- Calculate out-of-pocket costs for hospital stay with deductible and copay — 51%
- Not all doctors who provide care at in-network hospital may be in-network — 41%
- Definition of a "health insurance formulary" — 33%
- Calculate out-of-pocket costs when insurer pays a portion of allowed charges for out-of-network lab test — 16%

**Figure 15-7** • Knowledge of Health Insurance Terms and Concepts. (Source: Assessing Americans' Familiarity With Health Insurance Terms and Concepts (Conducted October 17-27, 2017), Kaiser Family Foundation.)

cost of their care. Conversely, 40% of physicians report they are only slightly or not at all prepared to have these discussions; three-quarters say they have little or no access to the necessary information (eg, deductibles). Finally, physicians report their patients frequently delay or refuse care due to cost concerns.[22]

## Trends in Employer Cost Sharing for Health Plan Coverage With Employees

To control their health benefits costs, employers have increasingly shifted some of the responsibility for the cost of coverage to their employees. Known as "cost sharing," this shift began with the advent of managed care in the 1980s and increased in earnest during the 1990s. This cost sharing takes many manifestations.

### Cost Sharing: Premium Contributions

Cost sharing starts with the worker's share of the health insurance premium. Figure 15-8 depicts the annual rise in the worker's contribution over time, with the average percentage of premium paid by the worker rising from 25% in 1999 to 30% by 2019.[23]

### Cost Sharing: Deductibles

Beyond the premium contribution, and regardless of the health plan chosen, most employees share additional costs for the health plan coverage they select. According to Kaiser[24]:

> In addition to any required premium contributions, most covered workers must pay a share of the cost for the medical services they use. The most common forms of cost sharing are: deductibles (an amount that must be paid before most services are covered by the plan), copayments (fixed dollar amounts), and coinsurance (a percentage of the charge for services). Sometimes cost sharing forms are mixed, such as assessing coinsurance for a service up to a maximum amount, or assessing coinsurance or copayment for a service, whichever is higher. The type and level of cost sharing often vary by the type of plan in which the worker is enrolled. Cost sharing may also vary by the type of service, such as office visits, hospitalizations, or prescription drugs.

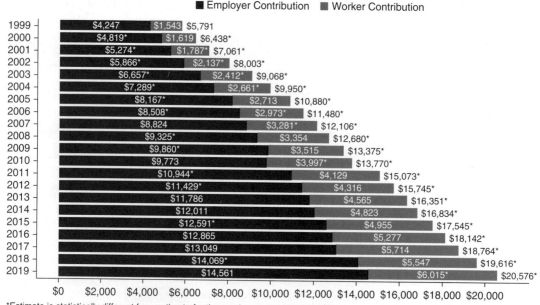

**Average Annual Worker and Employer Contributions to Premiums and Total Premiums for Family Coverage, 1999-2019**

■ Employer Contribution  ■ Worker Contribution

| Year | Employer Contribution | Worker Contribution | Total |
|------|----------------------|---------------------|-------|
| 1999 | $4,247 | $1,543 | $5,791 |
| 2000 | $4,819* | $1,619 | $6,438* |
| 2001 | $5,274* | $1,787* | $7,061* |
| 2002 | $5,866* | $2,137* | $8,003* |
| 2003 | $6,657* | $2,412* | $9,068* |
| 2004 | $7,289* | $2,661* | $9,950* |
| 2005 | $8,167* | $2,713 | $10,880* |
| 2006 | $8,508* | $2,973* | $11,480* |
| 2007 | $8,824 | $3,281* | $12,106* |
| 2008 | $9,325* | $3,354 | $12,680* |
| 2009 | $9,860* | $3,515 | $13,375* |
| 2010 | $9,773 | $3,997* | $13,770* |
| 2011 | $10,944* | $4,129 | $15,073* |
| 2012 | $11,429* | $4,316 | $15,745* |
| 2013 | $11,786 | $4,565 | $16,351* |
| 2014 | $12,011 | $4,823 | $16,834* |
| 2015 | $12,591* | $4,955 | $17,545* |
| 2016 | $12,865 | $5,277 | $18,142* |
| 2017 | $13,049 | $5,714 | $18,764* |
| 2018 | $14,069* | $5,547 | $19,616* |
| 2019 | $14,561 | $6,015* | $20,576* |

$0  $2,000  $4,000  $6,000  $8,000  $10,000  $12,000  $14,000  $16,000  $18,000  $20,000

*Estimate is statistically different from estimate for the previous year shown ($p < .05$).

**Figure 15-8** • Annual Worker and Employer Contributions to Premiums and Total Premiums for Family Coverage. (Source: KFF Employer Health Benefits Survey, 2018-2019; Kaiser/HRET Survey of Employer-Sponsored Health Benefits, 1999-2017, Kaiser Family Foundation.)

. . . Some plans require enrollees to meet a service-specific deductible, such as for prescription drugs or hospital admissions, in lieu or in addition to a general annual deductible.

In 2019, the vast majority of workers were enrolled in a plan with a general annual deductible (82% of workers with both single and family coverage). Kaiser data indicate that the only health plans that sometimes exempt employees from a general annual deductible are the HMOs, which account for only 19% of enrollees in 2019. By contrast, the vast majority of employees enrolled in all other plans (for family coverage) are subject to an annual deductible (Figure 15-9).[25] These deductibles themselves vary in terms of how they are structured: as either a family aggregate amount or a per-person family member amount. The former is more common.

Moreover, there is a clear trend among employers since 2007 to expose their employees to cost sharing using annual deductibles, regardless of the plan they choose.[26] Between 2007 and 2019, the percentage of workers with an annual deductible rose from 59% to 82%. There is also a clear trend in the size of this deductible over time,

for both single and family coverage, across all plan types. However, the size of the deductible varies considerably by plan type, with HMO plans having the lowest deductible ($881 per person in 2019 for family coverage with aggregate structure deductibles, or an average of $2,905 in aggregate) and HDHP/SO plans having the highest ($3,078 per person, or $4,779 in aggregate).[27]

## Cost Sharing: Out-of-Pocket Maximums

Another type of cost sharing is the out-of-pocket maximum that limits the amount workers must pay in a given year. The Patient Protection and Affordable Care Act (PPACA) required nongrandfathered health plans to have a maximum of no more than $7,900 for single coverage and $15,800 for family coverage in 2019. Out-of-pocket limits for HSA-qualified HDHP/SOs are required to be lower. There has been a significant increase over time in the percentage of covered workers with out-of-pocket maximums for single coverage, rising from 81% in 2009 to 99% by 2019. There is also growing variation in the spending limit thresholds between 2009 and 2019 (Figure 15-10).[28] Finally, there is enormous variation in the out-of-pocket maximum by plan type (Figure 15-11).[29]

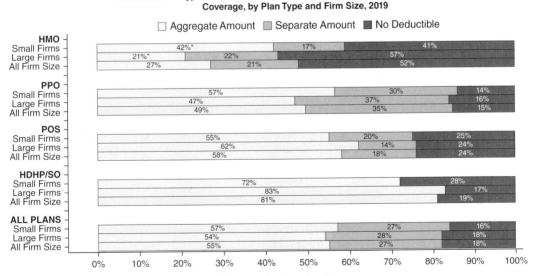

Distribution of Type of General Annual Deductible for Covered Workers With Family Coverage, by Plan Type and Firm Size, 2019

☐ Aggregate Amount ☐ Separate Amount ■ No Deductible

**HMO**
Small Firms: 42%* | 17% | 41%
Large Firms: 21%* | 22% | 57%
All Firm Size: 27% | 21% | 52%

**PPO**
Small Firms: 57% | 30% | 14%
Large Firms: 47% | 37% | 16%
All Firm Size: 49% | 35% | 15%

**POS**
Small Firms: 55% | 20% | 25%
Large Firms: 62% | 14% | 24%
All Firm Size: 58% | 18% | 24%

**HDHP/SO**
Small Firms: 72% | 28%
Large Firms: 83% | 17%
All Firm Size: 81% | 19%

**ALL PLANS**
Small Firms: 57% | 27% | 16%
Large Firms: 54% | 28% | 18%
All Firm Size: 55% | 27% | 18%

0%  10%  20%  30%  40%  50%  60%  70%  80%  90%  100%

*Estimate is statistically different between All Small Firms and All Large Firms estimate (*p* <.05).

NOTE: Small Firms have 3-199 workers and Large Firms have 200 or more workers. HDHP/SOs are defined as having a minimum deductible of $1,000 for single coverage and $2,000 for family coverage and either an HRA or HSA. Among workers with a general annual family deductible, 57% in HMOs, 58% in PPOs, and 77% in POS plans. The survey distinguishes between plans that have an aggregate family deductible and plans that have a separate per-person deductible, typically with a limit on the number of family members required to reach that amount. N/A: Not Applicable.

**Figure 15-9** • Distribution of Type of General Annual Deductible for Covered Workers With Family Coverage. (Source: KFF Employer Health Benefits Survey, Kaiser Family Foundation, 2019.)

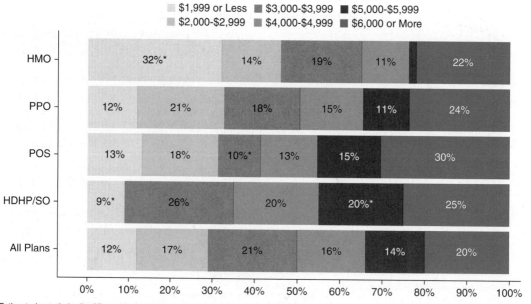

**Percentage of Covered Workers in a Plan with an Out-of-Pocket Maximum Above Certain Thresholds for Single Coverage, 2009-2019**

→ OOP Maximum Above $3,000   → OOP Maximum Above $6,000   → OOP Maximum Above $7,900

*Estimate is statistically different from estimate for the previous year shown ($p$ <.05).

NOTE: OOP is 'out-of-pocket'. OOP maximums are for in-network services. Values include covered workers without an OOP max. Covered workers without an OOP maximum are considered to be exposed to at least the specified threshold. Some of these workers may be enrolled in plans whose cost-sharing structure has other limits that make it impossible to reach the specified threshold.

**Figure 15-10** • Covered Workers in a Plan With an Out-of-Pocket Maximum Above Certain Thresholds for Single Coverage. (Source: KFF Employer Health Benefits Survey, 2018-2019; Kaiser/HRET Survey of Employer-Sponsored Health Benefits, 2009-2017, Kaiser Family Foundation.)

**Among Covered Workers With an Out-of-Pocket Maximum for Single Coverage, Distribution of Out-of-Pocket Maximums, by Plan Type, 2019**

*Estimate is statistically different from All Plans estimate within plan type ($p$ <.05).

**Figure 15-11** • Distribution of Out-of-Pocket Maximums. (Source: KFF Employer Health Benefits Survey, Kaiser Family Foundation, 2019.)

## HDHP/SO Plans

As demonstrated earlier, ERISA plan participants have increasing discretion (choice) among different types of health plans, which entail different levels of premiums, worker contributions, and cost-sharing amounts. The degree of choice and cost sharing extends even further. While HDHP plans are always paired with a health savings account (HSA-qualified HDHPs), employees who select an HDHP plan may have further discretion in choosing to pair it with a health reimbursement account (HRA). In the Kaiser survey, HRAs and HSAs are financial accounts that workers or their family members can use to pay for health care services.[30]

> The survey treats high deductible plans paired with a savings option as a distinct plan type, High-Deductible Health Plan with Savings Option (HDHP/SO), even if the plan would otherwise be considered a PPO, HMO, POS plan, or conventional health plan. Specifically, for the survey, HDHP/SOs are defined as (1) health plans with a deductible of at least $1,000 for single coverage and $2,000 for family coverage offered with an HRA (referred to as HDHP/HRAs); or (2) high deductible health plans that meet the federal legal requirements to permit an enrollee to establish and contribute to an HSA (referred to as HSA-qualified HDHPs).

The Kaiser data reveal that the percentage of firms offering these options has increased markedly over time. In 2007, only 10% of firms offered an HDHP/SO (7% HDHP/SO, 3% HDHP/HRA); in 2019, 28% of firms offered an HDHP/SO (26%) and/or an HDHP/HRA (4%).[31] The increase is particularly evident among larger firms (1,000+ workers). Enrollment in these plans has also increased over time from 5% in 2007 to 30% in 2019; the percentage of workers enrolled in HDHP/SO grew from 3% to 23%, while the percentage enrolled in HDHP/HRA grew from 3% to 7%.

Between 2007 and 2016, the mix of HDHP enrollees has shifted over time from the small group and individual market to the large group market.[32] The majority of the HDHP enrollees (66%) had a PPO product, while 31% had an HMO/POS product. There is considerable variation in HDHP enrollment by state.[33] There is also variation among the insurers offering these plans in their provision of online, consumer decision-support tools to manage their HSA accounts.[34]

It is important to distinguish these 2 types of HDHP plan options since they entail different levels of premiums and employee contributions. For example, premiums for family coverage are lower for the HSA-qualified HDHPs ($18,433) than for HDHP/HRAs ($21,002); as noted earlier, both are much lower than premiums for the HMO, PPO, and POS options. The average annual worker contribution to premiums for family coverage is $4,376 for the HSA-qualified HDHP and $6,729 for the HDHP/HRA. These contributions are also much lower than contributions to HMO, PPO, and POS options. Finally, employer contributions to both the premium and to the HDHP account are much lower for the HSA-qualified HDHP option than for the HDHP/HRA option.[35] There is considerable variation in the amounts that employers contribute to these 2 options.[36]

As a trade-off for the lower premiums, enrollees of HDHP plans with family coverage face much higher deductibles than enrollees in HMO, PPO, and POS plans: $4,673 for HSA-qualified HDHPs and $5,335 for HDHP/HRA plans.[37] Data for workers with single coverage indicates there is (1) wide variation in the range of deductibles paid by employees for these 2 plans, (2) variation in the amounts paid depending on the size of the employer,[38] and (3) variation in the amounts paid depending on whether there are aggregate or per-person deductibles.

There is also variation in the out-of-pocket maximums faced by enrollees in these 2 HDHP options. HSA-qualified HDHPs were legally required to have an annual out-of-pocket maximum of no more than $6,750 for single coverage and $13,500 for family coverage in 2019. Nongrandfathered HDHP/HRA plans were required to have out-of-pocket maximums of no more than $7,900 for single coverage and $15,800 for family coverage in 2019. The average annual out-of-pocket maximum for single coverage is $4,492 for HSA-qualified HDHPs and $4,822 for HDHP/HRAs.

## Overall Variation in HDHP Plans

The foregoing review reveals tremendous variation among HDHP plans, both HSA-qualified

HDHPs and HDHP/HRAs, on a number of dimensions. As summarized by researchers, HDHP products differ with regard to[39]:

- Size of the deductible
- Maximum out-of-pocket expense
- Whether the employer contributes to the HDHP
- Size of the employer contribution
- Size of the provider network (eg, PPO vs HMO/POS)
- Range of covered services (eg, PPO vs HMO/POS)
- Degree of online consumer decision-making support
- Whether the employer offers the HDHP as another choice or as a replacement
- Whether the employer linked the HDHP to either an HRA or HSA
- Whether the employee opens the HSA
- How much the employee chooses to contribute to the HDHP

Researchers also characterize the variables that affect the employee's decision to select the HDHP option. These include employee characteristics such as age, gender, education level, income, number of dependents, perceived health risk, and prior healthcare utilization and costs. Enrollees who are more likely to select an HDHP are younger, female, and more educated; they also have more dependents, face lower health risks, and have incurred lower prior utilization and costs. For those enrollees selecting family coverage, choice of an HDHP is less likely when the family has a sick member. Blacks are less likely to opt into an HDHP, perhaps due to risk aversion. Research also suggests that health insurance choices are "sticky": Individuals rarely switch plans over time.[40]

Research has also documented the differential impact of HDHPs on different types of employees. In general, HDHP enrollees incur lower healthcare costs, largely due to lower outpatient utilization and lower expenditures on higher-cost prescription drugs. However, counterbalancing their lower premiums, some may incur an "excessive financial burden of out-of-pocket costs" (defined as out-of-pocket costs exceeding 3% of their income). Those particularly affected include the lower-income population and those with chronic conditions.[41] The higher out-of-pocket costs may occasion the lower utilization of certain healthcare services.[42]

Under certain conditions, HDHPs can lead to overall savings for employees even if they meet their high annual deductibles. These conditions include (1) the combined lower premium and the tax advantage of the dollars contributed to the HSA account exceed the cost of the deductible; (2) the higher the employee's income level and thus tax rate, the higher the tax subsidy of the HSA; and (3) the degree to which the worker's employer passes on any premium savings to the employee.[43]

## Employer Benefits Management and Health Strategies

Surveys of employers suggest they have a lot on their minds when thinking about their workforce. Five of the top challenges they mention are workforce engagement and motivation, employee retention, healthcare costs, linking pay and performance, and managing a global workforce.[44] When it comes to their overall healthcare strategy, employers state the goals are to improve workforce health and productivity, reduce the trend in healthcare expenditures ("bend the trend"), and create a culture of participant responsibility and accountability. The strategy is to motivate behavioral change through benefits design, financial incentives, and communication.

Benefits management is becoming much more important. In 2004, benefits accounted for roughly 36% of the employee's total compensation from their employer; by 2014, that percentage had crept up to 39%. That 39% was comprised of benefits funded by the employer (27%) and the employee (12%). Healthcare benefits drove nearly one-third (32%) of the benefits amount. By 2024, according to Aon Hewitt, employee benefits may reach 44% of the employee's total compensation, with healthcare driving 35% of that amount. Healthcare benefits cost as a percentage of the worker's total compensation will rise to 15% by 2024, up from 12% in 2014; these costs as a percentage of the worker's contribution will rise from 6% to 8%.

For employers, keeping a budgetary lid on these outlays is universally recognized as a top priority in their health/benefits strategy. Other (somewhat competing) goals include offering competitive benefits to attract workers, promoting the health of their workforce, and increasing "employee engagement" in health and well-being programs. To achieve their goals, employers are offering navigation tools to their employees to select the right insurance plan design (covered earlier) and choose the right total benefits (flex or cafeteria) design and improving consumerism and transparency tools. They are also offering other tools like high-cost claimant care management, high-performance networks, centers of excellence, value-based management, and prescription drug management.

To do so, many employers are segmenting their workforce by age groups and differentiating the benefit packages and approaches taken. According to one classification, the age groups include "traditional employees" (born 1930-1945), "Boomers" (1946-1964), "Gen X'ers" (1965-1979), "Gen Y'ers" or "Millennials" (1980-1994), and "Gen Z'ers" (1995-2012).[45] Shifting demographics are also necessitating this approach. In 2015, the Millennials outnumbered both the Gen X'ers and the Boomers (53.5 million vs 52.7 million and 44.6 million, respectively). For their part, 80% of consumers want benefits customized to their age and circumstance, while 40% want help in achieving financial security via their benefits.[46] Employers are now tailoring their base compensation, pay increases, rewards, benefits, and incentives. Boomers, for example, are more likely to value base compensation and the medical benefit package most highly, whereas Millennials are likely to place relatively greater value on work-life balance, workplace flexibility, and well-being. Employers pursue this differentiated approach in the belief that employee health is "good for business"—lower turnover, higher productivity, and higher job performance.

## EMPLOYER COST AND QUALITY APPROACHES

Employers have expressed great interest in "value-based purchasing," "value-based insurance designs," and "value-based care delivery." These are portrayed in Figure 15-12. As we noted in prior chapters, "value" has been defined as quality divided by cost. Employers have focused their efforts on both the numerator and the denominator.

With regard to the numerator, sources of quality improvement include reductions in defensive medicine, reductions in treatment variations, and reductions in a host of what are called "potentially avoidable complications" (eg, preventable hospital readmissions, poorly managed chronic care conditions, unnecessary

| Value-Based Benefits Design | Value-Based Purchasing | Valued-Based Care Delivery |
|---|---|---|
| • **Plan Design**<br> • Defined contribution<br> • Cost sharing and risk transfer<br> • Absence management<br>• **Financial Incentives**<br> • Copays and deductibles<br> • Chronic condition management<br> • Health improvement and prevention<br> • Steerage (network formulary)<br> • Behavior change and compliance<br> • Vendor alignment<br>• **Communications**<br> • Behavioral economics<br> • Company-specific data<br> • Segmented and targeted messaging<br> • Health competency | • **Product Specification Features**<br> • Evidence-based care<br> • Quick access to care<br> • Rapid return to work and full functionality<br> • Total cost of care reduction<br> • Patient engagement and satisfaction<br> • Data transparency<br> • Utilization<br> • Provider costs<br> • Plan payments<br> • Payment flexibility<br> • Value-added services<br> • Cost-inefficient treatment<br> • Cost-inefficient or inappropriate service | • **Vendor Selection (RFP)**<br> • Commercial ACOs<br> • Integrated delivery network<br> • High performance network<br> • Centers of excellence<br> • Primary care medical home<br> • Chronic care models<br>• **Vendor Performance Metrics**<br> • Efficiency standards<br> • Lean production results<br> • Cost reduction (facility and professional)<br> • Potentially preventable events<br>• **Clinical Value Streams Metrics**<br> • High-cost and high-volume procedures<br> • Chronic condition (cost, quality, productivity, patient experience)<br> • Clinical integration and care coordination<br>• **Vendor Implementation**<br> • Communications<br> • Evaluation and correction |

**Figure 15-12 •** Value-Based Contracting Components. ACO, Accountable Care Organization; RFP, Request for Proposal.

emergency department [ED] visits, medical errors, and hospital-acquired infections). Employers have sought to engage the delivery system on these matters over time through an array of initiatives: the Leapfrog Group (transparency focused), Bridges to Excellence (pay-for-performance focused), Catalyst for Payment Reform (value-based contracting focused), and Prometheus (episode of care payment focused). Some employers have also employed on-site case managers and preventive screenings, as well as vaccine coverage by their health insurers, and membership in regional employer purchasing coalitions to measure insurer and provider quality. With regard to the denominator, employers have focused on cost sharing, increasing workers' share of the insurance premiums, use of financial incentives, tiered networks and centers of excellence with bundled value pricing, and reductions in scope of benefits offered (including retiree health benefits or offering benefits at all) (Figure 15-13).

Employers have a robust toolkit for trying to manage their employees' healthcare benefits costs and the quality of care they receive. Broadly stated, the toolkit encompasses (1) cost sharing, (2) consumer accountability, (3) care management, (4) the delivery system, and (5) worker

health and productivity. One way to view these efforts is that employers are fighting a war on 2 fronts: one dealing with their employees, and the other dealing with the healthcare delivery system that is treating them (Figure 15-14). Moreover, some believe that population health begins with workplace initiatives.

A healthy workplace is one in which the employer and employees collaborate to protect and promote the health and well-being of all workers and the sustainability of the workplace by pursuing the following, based on identified needs:

- Incorporate positive health practices into the physical work environment
- Make health easy to obtain and sustain through a supportive workplace culture
- Provide individual health resources in the workplace and at home
- Identify ways of participating in the community to improve the health of workers, their families, and other members of the community

These efforts are discussed in the following sections; 2 efforts (cost sharing and accountability) have been partly dealt with earlier and are only briefly described.

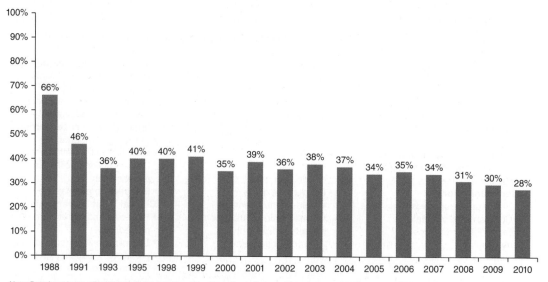

Note: Data have been edited to include the less than 1% of large firms who report "yes, but no retiree" responses in 2010. Historical numbers have been recalculated so that the results are comparable.

**Figure 15-13** • Percentage of Firms Offering Retiree Health Benefits Among all Large Firms (200 or More Workers) Offering Health Benefits to Active Workers, 1988 to 2010. (Source: Kaiser/HRET Survey of Employer-Sponsored Health Benefits, 1999-2010; KPMG Survey of Employer-Sponsored Health Benefits, 1991, 1993, 1995, 1998; The Health Insurance Association of America (HIAA), 1988.)

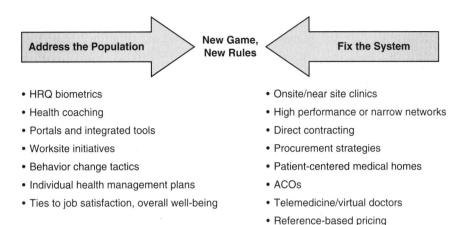

**Figure 15-14** • For Employers: A War on 2 Fronts. ACOs, Accountable Care Organizations; HRQ, Health-Risk Questionnaire.

## Cost Sharing

Cost sharing includes not only deductibles, copayments, and coinsurance. It can also include efforts to migrate employee benefits from "defined benefits" that the employer will cover to "defined contributions" (fixed amount of dollars) that the employer will make. Other approaches include eliminating working spouses from coverage and reducing subsidies for dependents. Research shows that cost sharing does not adversely affect outcomes for the average patient. Cost sharing may increase the expenditures of vulnerable populations and Medicare enrollees, who use more expensive services and/or have more adverse events.[47] Reductions in utilization and costs are less likely to derive from the half of the covered population with low medical expenses to begin with. Most employers encounter the Pareto Rule whereby 20% of their population accounts for 80% of the cost, or even more alarmingly, 5% accounts for 50% of costs.

## Consumer Accountability

Accountability involves workers (and their dependents) taking more personal responsibility for their health and the costs of their health. It includes the use of HDHPs, HRAs, and, for some employers, the full replacement of other plans with HDHPs as the only option. Other avenues to improve consumerism include personal health records, transparency tools (eg, provider cost and quality), value-based medical designs, employee access to web-based portals that supply cost information to support cost-based decisions, employee access to quality and outcomes information, navigation and advocacy services, and web-based programs to support member outreach.

## Care Management

Care management approaches can include prevention, comprehensive health management programs, mandatory condition or case management, integration of medical care and disability management, and disease management (DM) programs. It can also include expanded benefits for mental health and other behavioral health issues. Employers spend quite a bit of time looking at this issue, but rarely interfere with the providers of care management services; the latter typically include insurers, providers, and stand-alone start-ups.

## Delivery System

Delivery system initiatives range from using accountable care organizations, narrow provider networks, tiered provider networks, lab and radiology networks, bundled payment packages for specific procedures (eg, coronary artery bypass graft, hip implants), centers of excellence (requiring higher cost sharing if enrollee goes outside the designated provider network), steerage to preferred providers, selective contracting with providers on "value," retail and on-site clinics, on-site pharmacies, employee assistance programs, and reference-based pricing (which requires patient cost sharing for choosing provider/service above the reference price). More recently, due to the COVID-19 crisis, employers are boosting their virtual care options for acute care, mental healthcare, and emotional well-being services.

One impediment to such initiatives is the low take-up rate by employers. For example, only 16% of employers encourage their employees to receive care at a center of excellence, and only 19% of those cover the cost of travel and lodging. Similarly, a low percentage of employers contract with a local accountable care organization. A second impediment—and perhaps the driver of the first—is employer skepticism that such initiatives can lead to higher quality.[48] A third impediment is employers' reported difficulty in measuring and comparing provider quality and thus the difficulty in designing narrow or tiered networks. A fourth impediment is provider pushback; for example, refusing to treat employees of employers who participate in reference-based pricing. Fifth, there is considerable distrust of providers due to a lack of price transparency and suspicion of overcharging. Sixth, and finally, there is a lack of resources in Human Resources departments. They have been shrinking in recent years just when they need more personnel to monitor and manage all their health programs. It is one of the reasons why direct contracting by employers has been so slow to increase.

### Worker Health and Productivity

Health and productivity initiatives include health risk questionnaires (HRQs) that assess risky behaviors and solicit biometric data, health coaches, behavioral economics, health promotion, promoting a culture of health, sit-to-stand workstations, healthy cafeteria food, stress management sessions, standing/walking meetings, health coaches and advocates to help workers manage chronic conditions, and wellness programs. Employers are also tinkering with ways to gamify healthy behavior and reward it with prizes that further encourage such behavior, creating virtuous cycles. Prizes can include gift cards, raffle drawings, recognition programs, or bonuses. Finally, such initiatives can include predictive modeling, data warehouses, and analytics to study the patterns in worker health and utilization. There has been increasing employer interest in the impact of the "social determinants of health" on their workforce.

## HEALTH PROMOTION EFFORTS

To understand the possible effects of wellness and health promotion programs, it is important to distinguish those that are employer-sponsored from those that are clinically delivered.

### Employer-Sponsored Programs

Many employers believe that their main issue is the poor health habits of their own employees (Figure 15-15). Employers have used incentives

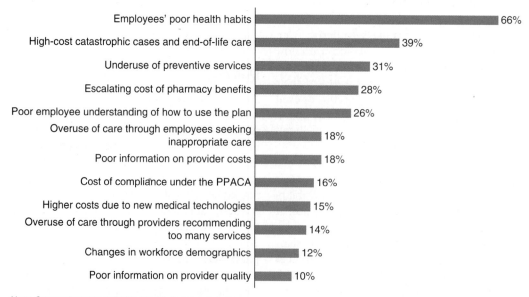

Note: Companies were asked to identify their top 3 challenges.

**Figure 15-15** • Employers: Employees' Poor Health Habits Are Top Challenge to Maintaining Affordable Coverage. PPACA, Patient Protection and Affordable Care Act. (Source: 2012 Towers Watson/National Business Group on Health Employer Survey on Purchasing Value in Health Care.)

for the past decade in an effort to change employee behavior. PPACA increased the amount of money that employers could use to incentivize employee health behaviors by 50%. This was known as the "Safeway amendment," based on a 2009 *Wall Street Journal* opinion piece authored by Safeway CEO Steve Burd, who claimed that his company's "Healthy Measures" incentives program could cut the nation's healthcare costs by 40%. The amendment let companies reimburse employees as much as 20% of their insurance premiums if they take part in wellness programs; this percentage rose to 30% in 2014 and to 50% with special governmental approval. In a similar vein, the National Business Group on Health (which represents large employers including Walmart and Wendy's) stated that roughly two-thirds of its members either offered a discount of several hundred dollars on health insurance premiums to employees who quit smoking or provided other incentives or penalties to make it happen.

And, yet, there are disquieting signs that employees were not so engaged. In a survey published in 2010, 55% of respondents said health and wellness programs are not exciting or relevant to them or they don't know about them.[49] In another survey, employees stated they wanted financial incentives (ie, to be paid) to participate in wellness programs.[50]

To combat this, employers have pursued at least 2 approaches. One approach is the use of "participatory wellness programs" that are voluntary and open to all. These can include gym memberships and weight-loss programs. No health metrics or standards need to be met to earn rewards. A second approach is the use of "health-contingent wellness programs" where the worker must meet health metrics or standards to earn rewards (eg, insurance premium discounts, lower cost sharing, more benefits). In a few cases, such metrics serve as a gatekeeper to receiving any benefits at all.

According to Kaiser, many large firms offer health screening programs, including (1) HRQs asking workers about lifestyle, stress, or physical health, and (2) biometric screening (in-person health examinations conducted by a medical professional). Firms and their insurers can use the biometric data to target wellness offerings or other services to high-risk workers with certain conditions or behaviors. Some companies have incentive programs that reward or penalize workers for different activities, including participating in wellness programs or completing health screenings. Among large firms offering health benefits, 65% offered workers the opportunity to complete an HRQ in 2019, up from 52% in 2010; roughly half of all large firms offered incentives to complete it. In addition, 52% offered workers the opportunity to complete a biometric screening, and 84% offered workers wellness programs (eg, smoking cessation, weight loss, lifestyle and behavioral coaching) in 2019.

There was a smaller increase in the percentage of firms offering biometric screening: from 48% to 52% among large firms and from 14% to 27% among all firms. Two other facts are important to understanding the potential for biometric screening. First, 58% of all large firms offer incentives to complete the screening, but only 14% offer incentives to achieve biometric outcomes. Second, the level of incentives offered varies widely among large firms: In 2019, 17% of firms offered incentives of $150 or less, and another 28% offered incentives of $151 to $500. There has been a slow, upward trend in the distribution of incentives since 2015, however. Finally, some employers (11%) and their insurers are now incorporating information collected from mobile phone applications of wearable devices (eg, Fitbits, Apple Watches) into their health promotion programs.

A large percentage of employers continue to offer wellness and health promotion programs to help workers engage in healthy lifestyles and reduce health risks, including exercise programs, health education classes, health coaching, smoking cessation, weight loss, and stress management counseling. These programs may be offered by the firm, their insurer, or a third-party. Overall, 50% of small firms and 84% of large firms offering health benefits offer at least one of the smoking, weight-loss, or behavioral coaching programs. Forty-one percent of large firms offering one of these programs include an incentive to participate in or complete the programs. The absolute amount of the financial incentive to participate resembles that for biometric screening.

Employers also employ DM programs to improve the health status and reduce the healthcare costs for employees with chronic illness (eg, diabetes, asthma, hypertension, high cholesterol). DM programs educate workers about their disease and suggest treatment options.

Among firms offering health benefits, 28% of small firms and 68% of large firms offer DM programs. Among large firms with a DM program, 13% offer incentives or penalties for workers to participate in or complete the programs. Both the presence of a DM program and the presence of incentives increase with firm size.

The "theory of action" underlying employers' wellness and disease management efforts is that improved health status of workers will positively impact employee productivity, reduce employee absenteeism, increase the affordability of healthcare coverage, and improve the employer's competitiveness and profitability. There are 3 assumptions behind this model, which drive the points at which employers hope to have an influence (Figure 15-16). The first is that health screening will identify those workers at risk; the second is that primary prevention can change behaviors of those at risk with targeted interventions; the third is that secondary prevention via DM programs can address the issues not dealt with by primary prevention.

There may be several problems with this "theory," however. *First*, the assessment of health risks (even including feedback) exerts only a small effect on health behaviors and on physiologic outcomes.[51] Some barriers include concerns over confidentiality of health records, those with important health risks are least likely to participate in HRQs, and HRQ interventions may only attract the "worried well."

Moreover, there is considerable variation in worker motivation in terms of how much they care about health and prevention. Workers who participate in wellness programs already care about their health and do not need incentives. *Second*, there is also variation in how responsive workers are to incentives. Employers may waste incentives on (1) those who will do it anyway and (2) those who will never do it. There is the further issue, found in the literature on behavioral economics, that behavioral change is difficult to sustain over time. Smoking cessation programs reduced smoking levels in one study by only 9%; moreover, there was higher recidivism among those receiving the financial incentives. Once the incentives were withdrawn, people quit the program.[52] Researchers have also noted several potential ethical problems with using incentives: infringement on autonomy, preferential targeting of the poor, privacy concerns, justice of rewarding those who do what others have done for free, extrinsic incentives crowding out intrinsic motivations, and discrimination among heterogeneous populations.[53] Indeed, some research suggests that wellness programs shift costs from the healthy to the unhealthy workers—who happen to be in lower socioeconomic strata—who end up subsidizing their healthy coworkers.[54] *Third*, DM programs have a shaky track record of performance and rarely achieve their stated return on investment.[55]

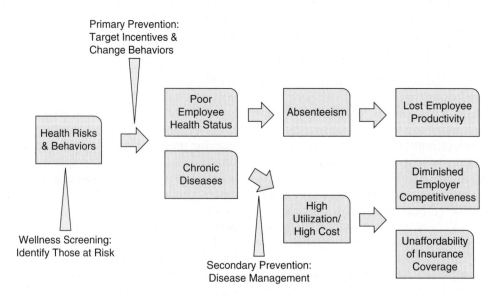

**Figure 15-16** • Goal of Wellness Programs: Interventions and Assumptions.

Employers have also faced a number of logistical issues in conducting employee wellness programs. First, many employers have workforces that are scattered across many states, making it hard to offer on-site resources for all, especially in smaller locations. Second, these programs address the employees only, not their dependents (who may equal the number of employees) or the company's retirees. Third, much of what the employers are battling are the "social determinants of health" (see Chapters 3 and 4)—the personal behaviors of workers, the physical and economic environments in which they reside, and their genetics. Such issues cannot be addressed in worksite clinics.

Overall, the literature on employer-sponsored programs has largely failed to document their impact on overall costs after accounting for the costs of conducting the wellness program.[56] A RAND report showed that most employers do not evaluate whether or not their wellness programs actually work.[57] The RAND researchers found that, over time, participants can reduce their healthcare costs and utilization (eg, 5 years), pointing to the necessity of sustaining these approaches. However, the difference in spending was only $157 annually, an amount that was not statistically significant. Wellness programs can reduce risk factors and increase healthy behaviors and thus can produce clinically meaningful results that are sustainable. Most recently, a randomized clinical trial found that wellness programs exerted no effects on biometric screening outcomes, medical diagnoses, or medical utilization after 12 and 24 months. It did find that the program increased the percentage of employees having a primary care physician and employees' self-reported beliefs regarding their own health.[58]

Such results have led a growing number of employers to show "tough love" to their employees. Rahm Emanuel, the past Mayor of Chicago, enacted a "Shape Up or Pay Up" citywide wellness program for city employees. They could either voluntarily enroll *or* pay higher insurance premiums. The goal was part of an effort to save $500 million in the city's healthcare bills by forcing employees to be "good stewards of their own health." Even tougher efforts have been undertaken by AmeriGas Propane and the Cleveland Clinic (among others): Enroll in these programs or lose your insurance coverage, and choose between being hired or remaining a smoker.

---

## Critical Thinking Exercise: Pitney Bowes Case

Pitney Bowes was a large employer. It had 26,000 employees who made postage stamping equipment at many sites scattered around the country, with many working at the sites of clients. A famous Harvard Business School case written by Michael Porter depicts the efforts of Pitney Bowes to improve the health of its employees while reducing the firm's healthcare expenses.[59] The company also sought to customize healthcare for its employees. The company's strategy, as laid out in the case, was as follows:

- Improve employee loyalty
- Improve employee recruitment and retention
- Manage employees as assets
- "Do the right thing"
- Take a leadership role as a big employer and receive recognition
- Earn a clear return on equity by investing in worker health
- Adopt a long-term, prevention-oriented solution to lower healthcare costs
- Engage employees to take responsibility for their health
- Share the burden of lowering costs and improving health with employees
- Reduce cost of its products to help the company compete

In pursuit of these goals, the chief executive officer switched from fee-for-service to managed care plans, offered HDHPs, increased employee cost sharing, piloted wellness programs at the company's main campus, offered primary care on site as well as prevention screenings, offered voluntary health risk assessments, offered on-site fitness centers, conducted health education, and other initiatives. Nevertheless, the company was not that successful in reducing its healthcare spend or improving its employees' health. What do you think happened?

## Clinically Delivered Programs

An example of a clinically delivered program is the Medicare Health Support (MHS) program, enacted as part of the Medicare Modernization Act (2003). This was a 3-year randomized controlled study of chronic care management in the fee-for-service Medicare population. Two hundred thousand patients with chronic health conditions (eg, diabetes and congestive heart failure) were assigned to companies that specialized in helping the chronically ill to lower their medical costs and keep them from getting sicker. The program also involved nurse contacts to ensure patients followed doctors' instructions to take their medications and reduce their sodium intake. The program failed to reduce acute hospitalizations, readmissions, and ED visits; it also did not lower patients' costs to offset program costs.

The MHS findings are consistent with the broader literature on health prevention and promotion. Much of this evidence was summarized long ago by Louise Russell, who concluded that prevention adds rather than reduces costs.[60] If true, then the question becomes, "When is prevention worth the cost?" or "When is prevention cost-effective?" There is a vast literature on the cost-effectiveness of prevention. An earlier summary of this literature found that less than 20% of preventive interventions, and a similar share of treatment interventions, reduced medical spending.[61] A Congressional Budget Office (CBO) report similarly found that for preventive medical care (eg, cancer screening, cholesterol management, vaccines), an ounce of prevention was true at the individual level, but not so at the population level: Expanded utilization leads to higher medical spending that outweighs savings from averted illness. An estimated 60% of preventive services added costs that were reasonable given the clinical benefits. The impact of "wellness services," such as encouraging healthy habits (eg, eating healthy, exercising), on medical spending showed limited evidence, the effects took years to emerge, and sustained behavioral changes were hard to achieve. For example, the large reduction in smoking took decades, while tackling obesity may take longer (due to multiple contributing factors).

Researchers conclude that prevention is incredibly complicated. Medical science can only identify those at risk of heart disease, a much larger group than those who will someday be candidates for bypass surgery. Prevention must be delivered to all people at risk, often repeatedly over many years, to prevent some from developing disease; these costs mount up. Some develop disease anyway, since prevention is not 100% effective; some do not develop it even without prevention; all receive prevention, but not all experience savings.

There is hope. Some research evidence suggests that a small number of prevention interventions can have a large impact on population health. These include "sin taxes" on tobacco, alcohol, and unhealthy foods (eg, soda tax). Recent research suggests that sugar-sweetened beverage taxes generate substantial health gains (eg, reduced diabetes and cardiovascular disease), increases in quality-adjusted life-years, and huge tax revenues.[62] However, the soda tax is incredibly controversial: When originally proposed in Philadelphia, it was vigorously opposed by the union representing delivery truck drivers. Other helpful interventions include mandatory limits on salt in 3 basic food items (bread, cereal, margarine), intensive "sun-smart" campaigns to limit sun exposure, and gastric banding for severe obesity.[63]

There may also be corporate returns to such investments in the form of higher profitability. Employers are beginning to recognize that engaged and healthy employees (and their dependents) have a big impact on their bottom line and profitability. At the same time, many employers remain risk averse to implementing health interventions that might generate employee noise, and seldom exert their potential marketplace leverage over payers and providers concerning their healthcare expenditures.

## SUMMARY

EBHI has become an important part of the employee's benefits and total compensation package. It has also become an important part of the employer's costs and thus an important target for employers to manage. Although employers potentially have lots of contacts with and opportunities to engage with employees, they have not yet discovered the "silver bullet" solution to motivate or incent workers to take better care of themselves.

## QUESTIONS TO PONDER

1. EBHI began in the United States during the 1940s, took root, and has become the modal way to provide health insurance in the private sector. Why didn't this happen in other Western countries? Why did many of them develop national health insurance schemes instead?

2. Employers typically offer their workers "choice" among different insurance plans. These plans involve trade-offs. What are the major trade-offs that workers make in selecting a given plan? Are they aware of the trade-offs?

3. Is the employer's use of cost sharing with workers a good thing to do? What are the downsides?

4. What are the "plusses" and "minuses" of employers' use of HDHPs?

5. Why are employers a good place to start in efforts to tackle the iron triangle? What problems have employers faced here?

## REFERENCES

1. Mark V. Pauly. *Health Benefits at Work* (Ann Arbor, MI: University of Michigan Press, 1997).
2. Lewin-VHI. *The Financial Impact of the Health Security Act* (Fairfax, VA: Lewin-VHI, 1993).
3. Mark V. Pauly. *Health Benefits at Work* (Ann Arbor, MI: University of Michigan Press, 1997): 9.
4. U.S. Department of Labor, Employee Benefits Security Administration. "Fact Sheet: What Is ERISA." Available online: https://www.dol.gov/agencies/ebsa/about-ebsa/our-activities/resource-center/fact-sheets/what-is-erisa. Accessed on August 1, 2020.
5. US Department of Labor. "Health Plans and Benefits." Available online: https://www.dol.gov/general/topic/health-plans. Accessed on August 1, 2020.
6. Anthem BlueCross BlueShield. *Trends in Health Benefits*. 2018. Available online: https://ga.beerepurves.com/news/carriernews/anthem/bcs2018NationalHealthBenefitsStatisticsTrends-Report.pdf. Accessed on January 26, 2020.
7. US Bureau of Labor Statistics. *Economic News Release* (September 20, 2020).
8. Unless otherwise specified, all "Kaiser Figures" reproduced in Chapter 15 are taken from the following source: Kaiser Family Foundation. *Employer Health Benefits 2019 Annual Survey*. Available online: https://www.kff.org/health-costs/report/2019-employer-health-benefits-survey/. Accessed on January 20, 2020. These data are taken from Kaiser Figure 10.2.
9. The Kaiser survey defines an HMO as a plan that does not cover nonemergency out of network services. The survey defines PPOs as plans that have lower cost sharing for in-network provider services and do not require a primary care gatekeeper to screen for specialist and hospital visits. POS is a point of service plan. The survey defines POS plans as those that have lower cost sharing for in-network provider services but do require a primary care gatekeeper to screen for specialist and hospital visits. The survey defines HDHP/SO as a high-deductible health plan with a savings option such as an HRA or HSA. HDHP/SOs are treated as a distinct plan type even if the plan would otherwise be considered a PPO, HMO, POS plan, or indemnity plan. These plans have a deductible of at least $1,000 for single coverage and $2,000 for family coverage and are offered with an HRA or are HSA-qualified. The survey defines conventional or indemnity plans as those that have no preferred provider networks and the same cost sharing regardless of physician or hospital.
10. Kaiser Family Foundation. *Employer Health Benefits 2019 Annual Survey*. Available online: http://files.kff.org/attachment/Report-Employer-Health-Benefits-Annual-Survey-2019. Data are taken from Kaiser Figure 5.1.
11. Kaiser Family Foundation. *Employer Health Benefits 2007 Annual Survey*. Available online: https://www.kff.org/wp-content/uploads/2013/04/76723.pdf. Accessed on November 13, 2020.
12. Neeraj Sood. *What Do We Know About High Deductible Health Plans* (Los Angeles, CA: Leonard Schaeffer Center for Health Policy & Economics, University of Southern California, October 2017). Available online: https://www.bakerinstitute.org/files/12279/. Accessed on January 20, 2020.
13. The same trade-off characterizes consumer choice among the tiered plans on the public insurance exchanges: The bronze tier has the lowest premium but highest average medical deductible, whereas the platinum tier has the highest premium but the lowest deductible. The same is true for other types of cost sharing on the exchanges, such as coinsurance levels. See data on cost of metal plans on Covered California's insurance exchange for 2019. Data available at: https://apply.coveredca.com/hix/private/planselection?-insuranceType=HEALTH. Accessed on January 28, 2020. Tellingly, the vast majority (roughly 85%)

of exchange enrollees chose the bronze and (especially) the silver plans with the lower premiums but also the higher out-of-pocket costs.

14. Kaiser Family Foundation. *Employer Health Benefits 2019 Annual Survey.* Available online: http://files.kff.org/attachment/Report-Employer-Health-Benefits-Annual-Survey-2019. Accessed on November 13, 2020. Data are taken from Figure 6.6.

15. The evidence on the impact of HDHPs is mixed. There is some evidence that healthcare spending is less for those enrolled in HDHPs and that patients switch to lower-cost providers. The intention that HDHPs will increase consumerism and engagement, however, has been less rosy. A recent study of consumer behaviors found that most Americans who are enrolled in HDHPs do not use information about price or quality of services, talk to providers about costs, or negotiate prices. When prices are compared or conversations occur with providers, however, it is predominantly for prescription drugs. Of those in the study who had compared prices, 61% did so for prescription drugs, while two-thirds of those who had talked to providers about cost discussed prescription drugs.

16. Judith R. Lave, Aiju Men, Brian Day, et al. "Employee Choice of a High-Deductible Health Plan Across Multiple Employers," *Health Serv Res.* 46 (1) (2011): 138-154.

17. The trend data on HDHP/SO enrollment in the Kaiser data are mirrored in data released by the US government. Robin Cohen and Emily Zammitti. *High-Deductible Health Plan Enrollment Among Adults Aged 18-64 With Employment-Based Insurance Coverage* (Hyattsville, MD: National Center for Health Statistics, NCHS Data Brief No. 317, August 2018).

18. *The EBRI/Greenwald & Associates Consumer Engagement in Health Care Survey* (Washington, DC: EBRI and Greenwald & Associates, December 2019). Available online: https://www.ebri.org/docs/default-source/cehcs/2019-cehcs-report.pdf?sfvrsn=b7293d2f_10. Accessed on January 22, 2020.

19. Source: Data extract from AIR's new health insurance literacy measurement tool. See: American Institutes for Research. Available online: https://www.air.org/project/measuring-health-insurance-literacy. Accessed on August 6, 2020.

20. George Loewenstein, Joelle Y. Friedman, Barbara McGill, et al. "Consumers' Misunderstanding of Health Insurance," *J Health Econ.* 32 (2013): 850-862.

21. Pharmacy Benefit Management Institute. *Trends in Drug Benefit Design 2018.* Available online: https://www.pbmi.com/ItemDetail?iProduct Code=BDR_2018&Category=BDR. Accessed on January 19, 2020.

22. National Opinion Research Center. *The Effects of High-Deductible Health Plans (HDHPs) on Patients and Independent Physicians* (Chicago, IL: NORC, June 2020).

23. Kaiser Family Foundation. *Employer Health Benefits 2019 Annual Survey.* Available online: http://files.kff.org/attachment/Report-Employer-Health-Benefits-Annual-Survey-2019. Accessed on November 13, 2020. Data are taken from Kaiser Figure 6.5.

24. Kaiser Family Foundation. *Employer Health Benefits 2019 Annual Survey*: 107.

25. Kaiser Family Foundation. *Employer Health Benefits 2019 Annual Survey.* Data are taken from Kaiser Figure 7.21.

26. Kaiser Family Foundation. *Employer Health Benefits 2019 Annual Survey.* Data are taken from Kaiser Figure 7.2.

27. Kaiser Family Foundation. *Employer Health Benefits 2019 Annual Survey.* Data are taken from Kaiser Figure 7.22.

28. Kaiser Family Foundation. *Employer Health Benefits 2019 Annual Survey.* Data are taken from Kaiser Figure 7.44.

29. Kaiser Family Foundation. *Employer Health Benefits 2019 Annual Survey.* Data are taken from Kaiser Figure 7.45.

30. Kaiser Family Foundation. *Employer Health Benefits 2019 Annual Survey*: 139.

31. Twenty-six percent of firms offered an HDHP/SO, and 4% of firms offered an HDHP/HRA.

32. America's Health Insurance Plans. *2016 Survey of Health Savings Account-High Deductible Health Plans.* (February 2017): Figure 2.

33. America's Health Insurance Plans. *2016 Survey of Health Savings Account-High Deductible Health Plans.* (February 2017): Table 3, Figure 6.

34. America's Health Insurance Plans. *2016 Survey of Health Savings Account-High Deductible Health Plans.* (February 2017): Figure 5.

35. Kaiser Family Foundation. *Employer Health Benefits 2019 Annual Survey.* Available online: http://files.kff.org/attachment/Report-Employer-Health-Benefits-Annual-Survey-2019. Accessed on November 13, 2020. Data are taken from Kaiser Figure 8.10.

36. Kaiser Family Foundation. *Employer Health Benefits 2019 Annual Survey.* Data are taken from Kaiser Figure 8.17.

37. Kaiser Family Foundation. *Employer Health Benefits 2019 Annual Survey.* Data are taken from Kaiser Figure 8.7.

38. Kaiser Family Foundation. *Employer Health Benefits 2019 Annual Survey.* Data are taken from Figure 8.13.

39. Judith R. Lave, Aiju Men, Brian Day, et al. "Employee Choice of a High-Deductible Health Plan Across Multiple Employers," *Health Serv Res.* 46 (1) (2011): 138-154.

40. Judith R. Lave, Aiju Men, Brian Day, et al. "Employee Choice of a High-Deductible Health Plan Across Multiple Employers," *Health Serv Res.* 46 (1) (2011): 138-154.

41. Neeraj Sood. *What Do We Know About High Deductible Health Plans* (Los Angeles, CA: Leonard Schaeffer Center for Health Policy & Economics, University of Southern California, October 2017).

42. Olena Mazurenko, Melinda Buntin, and Nit Menachemi. "High-Deductible Health Plans and Prevention," *Ann Rev Public Health.* 40 (2019): 411-421.

43. Rachel Dody. "High-Deductible Health Insurance Policies With Health Savings Accounts: A Policy Review," *SPNHA Rev.* 10 (1) (2014).

44. Towers Perrin Survey. Presentation by Mike Taylor to the Wharton School (2017).

45. Career Planner. "The Generations." Available online: https://www.careerplanner.com/Career-Articles/Generations.cfm. Accessed on August 6, 2020.

46. Aon. *2016 Consumer Health Mindset Study.* Available online: https://www.aon.com/human-capital-consulting/thought-leadership/commu-nication/2016-consumer-health-mindset.jsp. Accessed on November 13, 2020.

47. *Impact of Cost Sharing* (Princeton, NJ: Robert Wood Johnson Synthesis Project Brief, December 2010).

48. Stephen Parodi, Norman Chenven, and Michael Thompson. *Better Together: Exploring Employer-Physician Collaborations to Deliver Quality Care* (Alexandria, VA: Council of Accountable Physician Practices, July 2020).

49. North American Technographics Healthcare and Communications Online Survey, Q2 2010 (US); Forrester Research, Inc.

50. EBRI and Greenwald & Associates. *The EBRI/Greenwald & Associates 2012 Consumer Engagement in Health Care Survey* (Washington, DC: EBRI and Greenwald & Associates, 2012): Figures 14 and 15.

51. Robin Soler, Kimberly Weeks, Sima Razi, et al. "A Systematic Review of Selected Interventions for Worksite Health Promotion," *Am J Prev Med.* 38 (2S) (2010): S237-S262.

52. Kevin Volpp, Andrea Trorei, Mark Pauly, et al. "A Randomized, Controlled Trial of Incentives for Smoking Cessation," *N Engl J Med.* 360 (February 12, 2009): 699-709.

53. Scott D. Halpern, Kristin M. Madison, and Kevin G. Volpp. "Patients as Mercenaries? The Ethics of Using Financial Incentives in the War on Unhealthy Behaviors," *Circ Cardiovasc Qual Outcomes.* 2 (2009): 514-516.

54. Jill Horwitz, Brenna Kelly, and John DiNardo. "Wellness Incentives in the Workplace: Cost Savings Through Cost-Shifting to Unhealthy Workers," *Health Aff.* 32 (2) (March 2013). Available online: https://www.healthaffairs.org/doi/full/10.1377/hlthaff.2012.0683. Accessed on August 4, 2020.

55. David Bott, et al. "Disease Management for Chronically Ill Beneficiaries in Traditional Medicare," *Health Aff.* 28 (1) (January-February 2009): 86-98. Congressional Budget Office. *Lessons from Medicare's Demonstration Projects on Disease Management, Care Coordination, and Value-Based Payment Issue Brief* (Washington, DC: CBO, January 2012).

56. Gautam Gowrisankaran, Karen Notberg, Steven Kymes, et al. "A Hospital System's Wellness Program Linked to Health Plan Enrollment Cut Hospitalizations but Not Overall Costs," *Health Aff.* 32 (3) (2013): 477-485.

57. RAND Health. *Workplace Wellness Programs Study* (Santa Monica, CA: RAND, 2013).

58. Julian Reif, David Chan, Damon Jones, et al. "Effects of a Workplace Wellness Program on Employee Health, Health Beliefs, and Medical Use: A Randomized Clinical Trial," *JAMA Int Med.* 180 (7) (2020): 952-960.

59. Michael Porter and Jennifer Baron. *Pitney Bowes: Employer Health Strategy HBS Case 9-709-458* (Revised February 24, 2009). (Boston, MA: Harvard Business School, 2009).

60. Louise B. Russell. *Is Prevention Better Than Cure?* (Washington, DC: Brookings, 1986).

61. Joshua T. Cohen, Peter J. Neumann, and Milton C. Weinstein. "Does Preventive Care Save Money? Health Economics and the Presidential Candidates," *N Engl J Med.* 358 (February 14, 2008): 661-663.

62. Yujin Lee, Dariush Mozaffarian, Stephen Sy, et al. "Health Impact and Cost-Effectiveness of Volume, Tiered, and Absolute Sugar Content Sugar-Sweetened Beverage Tax Policies in the United States—A Microsimulation Study," *Circulation.* 142 (2020): 523-534.

63. Theo Vos, Rob Carter, Jan Barendregt, et al. *Assessing Cost-Effectiveness in Prevention (ACE-Prevention): Final Report* (Melbourne, Australia: University of Queensland, Brisbane and Deakin University, 2010).

# Contracting for Prescription Drug Benefits: Role of Employers, Insurers, and Pharmacy Benefit Managers

16

## INTRODUCTION

Until the 1980s, drug coverage was not a distinct benefit in employer-based health insurance. Instead, it was included in major medical plans (when it was included). Such plans were developed by the commercial insurance companies in the late 1950s to compete with Blue Cross and Blue Shield (which covered the services of hospitals and physicians, respectively). Major medical plans served as the start of "catastrophic coverage," reimbursing up to $10,000 in expenses that were not restricted to specific categories of hospital or physician expense (ie, they could include drugs).[1] Coverage was usually subject to an overall deductible for all services and to the same coinsurance amounts (usually 20%) that applied to all medical care.[2] It was thus a limited feature of private insurance plans.[3]

Two factors led to growth in the provision of drug benefits during the 1980s and 1990s: the rise of managed care and the rise of pharmacy benefit managers (PBMs). The 2 factors evolved simultaneously in symbiotic fashion. The growth of the PBMs was further spurred by rising expenditures on pharmaceuticals and the employers' need to control these costs. These events are chronicled in the next 2 sections.

## THE RISE OF MANAGED CARE AND DRUG BENEFITS

The first key event was the rise of managed care organizations (MCOs) such as the health maintenance organization (HMO) and preferred provider organization (PPO) models.

The 1973 HMO Act legitimized HMOs and provided some initial funding for planning. The HMO industry took off in the 1980s, fueled by employer interest in cost containment and controlling health insurance premiums. Total HMO enrollment increased rapidly between 1980 and 2000 (Figure 16-1).

The HMOs offered a distinct drug benefit with minimal deductibles and copayments. The drug benefit could be included as part of the basic benefit package (23% of HMOs in 1989) or in a rider typically purchased with that package (74% of HMOs in 1989).[4] Two-thirds of HMOs provided coverage to 90% or more of their enrollees. The MCOs offered such coverage to reduce (ie, substitute for) more expensive, downstream care in hospitals and emergency departments (EDs), and thereby manage the capitated payments they received.

Third-party insurance coverage for drug benefits expanded rapidly during the 1990s (Figure 16-2). In 1996, 55% of the commercial population and 67% of the non-Medicare population had drug coverage.

## THE RISE OF PHARMACY BENEFIT MANAGERS

The second key event was the rise of PBMs, who worked initially with the HMOs to administer drug benefit coverage. The PBM industry got its start in the late 1960s when one company developed a plastic drug benefit identification card that facilitated the processing and payment of drug claims incurred by employees. Formerly, employees had to pay cash for the

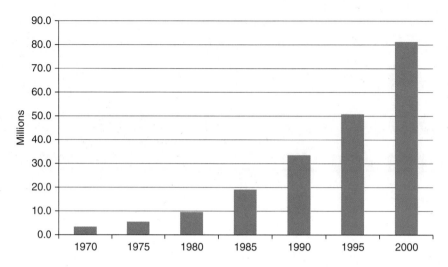

**Figure 16-1** • Growth in US Health Maintenance Organization Enrollment.

prescription at the pharmacy and then wait to get reimbursed; the PBMs made life more convenient for them and the pharmacy using data standardization and electronic linkages to pharmacies in a defined network. Now, an eligible employee armed with an identification card and using a network pharmacy paid only a small copayment. The pharmacy electronically submitted a claim to the PBM and was reimbursed according to an agreed-upon dispensing fee and discounted price for the drug. The PBM then submitted invoices for its own reimbursement plus a small administrative fee to the plan sponsors (eg, the insurer). The patient was no longer required to file paper claims and the pharmacist was paid quickly. Working on behalf of their customers, typically employers and/or their MCOs, the PBM's goal was to reduce the cost and optimize the use of medications, while maintaining quality.

The PBMs then added functions over time including (1) the delivery of drugs to patients via mail order and pharmacy networks in the 1970s and (2) integrating with physicians via e-prescribing in the 1980s. Major changes occurred in the late 1980s and early 1990s as PBMs helped to achieve lower drug costs via formulary management, generic substitution,

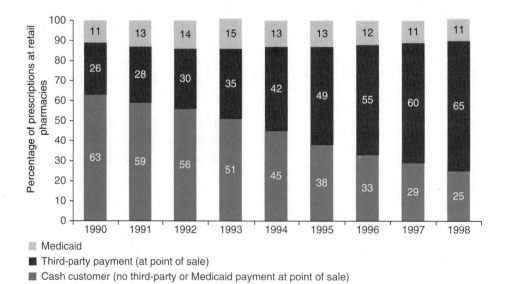

**Figure 16-2** • Growth in Third-Party Coverage for Drugs. (Source: IMS Health Retail Method of Payment Report, 1999.)

**PBM Service Mix by Era**

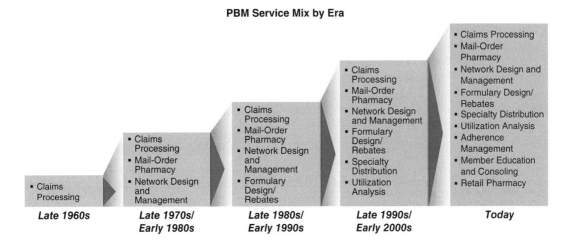

| Late 1960s | Late 1970s/ Early 1980s | Late 1980s/ Early 1990s | Late 1990s/ Early 2000s | Today |

**Figure 16-3** • Progression of Pharmacy Benefit Manager (PBM) Service Offerings.

and (most importantly) negotiating drug prices and rebates with drug manufacturers. In this manner, the PBMs acted as group buyers for drugs on behalf of (1) self-insured employers or (2) health insurers contracting with fully insured employers, offering scale economies in drug purchasing. Later in the 1990s, PBMs took on additional functions that improved the effectiveness and efficiency of drug prescribing via disease management programs, medication therapy management, physician profiling, and drug utilization review. The evolution of PBM services is depicted in Figure 16-3.

Needless to say, as third-party insurance coverage expanded in the 1990s, so did the number of people covered by PBMs. In 1989, the top 7 PBMs covered an estimated 48 million lives; by 1999, the top 7 PBMs covered an estimated 234 million lives. Compared to less than 25% market penetration in 1989, PBMs now administered pharmaceutical benefits to over 50% of the population. This gave them greater leverage in the marketplace.

## THE NEED FOR COST CONTROL OVER THE DRUG BENEFIT

The 1980s witnessed high inflation in drug prices, for both new and existing drugs. The decade marked the beginning of the "blockbuster drug" era (ie, drugs with global sales >$1 billion), with many new drugs targeting widespread, chronic conditions. Tagamet and Zantac hit the market in the late 1970s and 1980s to treat ulcers and gastrointestinal problems. Drug manufacturers expanded their forces of sales representatives to market their new products to physicians. With growing insurance coverage, patients were shielded from their cost. Pharmaceutical manufacturers were not yet threatened by generic drugs and were not yet opposed by any large, organized buyers. It was thus an era of high demand and high supply.

This turned the plastic drug identification card's role as an expanded benefit into a burden for employers. They began to pressure their HMOs and their PBMs in the late 1980s to use their clout to lower drug costs in 2 ways: (1) by reducing dispensing fees at retail pharmacies and (2) by discounting the prices charged by drug manufacturers. The Clinton Health Plan also attacked drug companies as price-gougers.

While initially focused primarily on claims processing, PBMs developed mechanisms by the early 1990s to control drug costs. The major techniques (profiled in depth later) included negotiated discounts with pharmacy networks, development and management of drug formularies, and contracts with brand name drug makers for discounted rebates off their list prices. A full service PBM became responsible for the design, implementation, and administration of pharmacy benefit programs and had 4 defining characteristics: claims processing and adjudication, pharmacy network management, formulary development and management for/with clients, and rebate negotiations with pharmaceutical manufacturers.

While the PBMs exerted some moderating impact on drug prices, drug volume was a different matter. During the period from 1992 to 2002, the expansion in drug coverage (as well as the rise of blockbuster drugs for chronic conditions) led to a massive 74% increase in prescription volumes, a 59% increase in prescriptions filled per person, and a tripling in aggregate US spending on drugs. Price hikes accounted for only 29% of the increase in spending.[5] As a percentage of national health expenditures, retail prescription drug costs rose from 6% in 1990 to 9% by 2000 and 10% by 2005. The consumer price index (CPI) for prescription drugs outpaced the CPI for all medical care and the CPI for all items. Health insurance costs were much more volatile than the costs of benefits and the cost of wages and salaries.

As a result of the rising utilization of drugs, the rising price of drugs, and their rising share of national health expenditures, drug benefits have become of major interest to employers. Employer interest was not confined to coverage of employees. Employers were also the largest source of benefits for the Medicare population due to their coverage of retiree health benefits; in 1996, 32% of Medicare beneficiaries had drug coverage. At that time, Medicare did not include coverage for outpatient drugs that were self-administered by the patients.[6]

Employers have undertaken several strategies to manage their drug benefits, including how they interact with their health insurers and PBMs. The remainder of this chapter reviews

these interactions. This is arguably the most opaque and difficult part of the US healthcare ecosystem to understand. So, please, bear with me, as I attempt to unpack it.

## MEDICAL AND PHARMACY BENEFIT CONTRACTING BY EMPLOYERS

Regardless of whether they are fully insured or self-insured, employers can arrange for the management of drug benefits in 2 different ways. First, they can assign the management of both benefits to a health insurer; the insurer usually manages the medical benefit and contracts with a PBM for the drug benefit (Figure 16-4). Second, employers can contract with health insurers for the medical benefit and contract separately with PBMs for the pharmacy benefit—this arrangement is referred to as a "carve-out" (Figure 16-5).

A majority (81%) of smaller employers (<1,000 employees) contract for both benefits with their health insurer; a near majority of medium-sized employers (1,000-5,000 employees) contract for both benefits with their health insurer; a majority (59%) of large employers (5,000+ employees) contract separately and directly with a PBM for the pharmacy benefit (data for 2017).[7]

Some large insurers have kept the PBM function in house or vertically integrated to

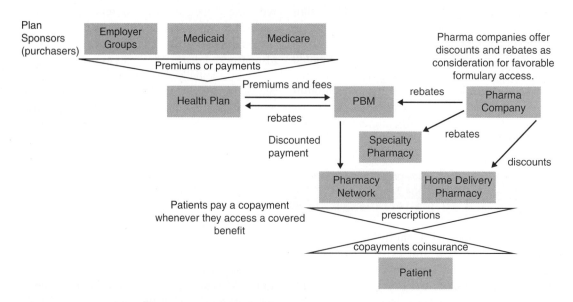

**Figure 16-4** • "Carve-in" Drug Benefit Coverage to Health Plan, which then Contracts with Pharmacy Benefit Manager (PBM). (Source: Robert Navarro, Craig Stern, and Rusty Hailey. "Prescription Drug Benefits in Managed Care," in Peter Kongstvedt [Ed.], *Essentials of Managed Care.* New York, NY: Jones and Bartlett, 2012: 257-282.)

acquire a PBM. This is evident from the recent mergers of CVS with Aetna and Express Scripts with Cigna. Many larger insurers perform several PBM functions in house (eg, formulary management) while outsourcing others.

Thus, there is considerable variability among Employee Retirement Income Security Act (ERISA) plan sponsors in the degree to which they contract with health insurers and PBMs for the medical and pharmacy benefits offered to employees. Some of this variability is detailed in the box titled "Variation Among ERISA Plan Sponsors in Insourcing/Outsourcing PBM Contracting."

---

### Variation Among ERISA Plan Sponsors in Insourcing/Outsourcing PBM Contracting

One of the basic building blocks of drug benefit design is deciding whether, and how, to integrate drug benefits with the medical benefit. When the drug benefit is carved-in, the employer contracts directly with their health plan for both medical and drug benefit management and administration. The drug benefit may be administered directly by the health plan–owned PBM, or the health plan contracts with a PBM to handle the drug benefit administration. Conversely, when the drug benefit is carved-out, the employer contracts with the PBM to administer the drug benefit, either directly or via their health plan, but under a separate contract.

According to the 2018 PBM Customer Satisfaction Report conducted by the Pharmacy Benefit Management Institute (PBMI),[8] the majority of employers (72%) contract with their PBM directly, and 75% reported having a self-insured plan. Self-insured employers have more financial risk and responsibility and usually play a more active role in the day-to-day management of their pharmacy benefit programs. Insurance carriers and MCOs hold most of the financial risk for fully insured pharmacy benefit plans.

Sixty-three percent of firms carved-out the drug benefit. That is, the management of the drug benefit is separate from the management of the medical benefit, using 2 different entities or 2 separate contracts to administer the benefits. Irrespective of whether employers chose a carved-in or a carved-out drug benefit, one thing is clear—most respondents had no plans to change their carve-in or carve-out status. Large employers were more likely to carve out pharmacy benefits than were smaller employers (74% and 56%, respectively). However, there were no differences by employer size in plans to make changes to what was currently in place.

Sixty percent of employers reported carving out their pharmacy benefit to a different vendor from their medical benefit, and the remaining 40% said that they procure pharmacy and medical benefits from the same vendor. Additionally, most (74%) offered a specialty drug benefit managed by the same PBM that provides traditional pharmacy benefit management services.[9]

According to PBMI, consultants are rated by 26% of employers as being the most influential in evaluating drug benefit design. This represents a small decline over the past few years of consultants being reported as most influential (36% in 2016, 30% in 2017). There is no discernible pattern in others that might be gaining or losing influence. There are differences in the most influential group by employer size. Large employers more frequently reported consultants, their PBM, their health plan, and employee benefits committee as most influential when compared to smaller employers. Smaller employers were more likely to report brokers, senior management, and finance as influential.

---

Regardless of whether pharmacy benefits are "carved into" the health plan or "carved out" separately to a PBM, the goals of the ERISA plan sponsor are the same: reduce overall cost, improve quality of care, and increase access to services. However, different ERISA plan sponsors may weight these goals differently and may design health plan options that assign different weights to these goals. As outlined later, some health plan options for the medical benefit may focus on broader access to providers but with higher costs to enrollees; other health plan options may focus on narrower provider network access but with lower costs

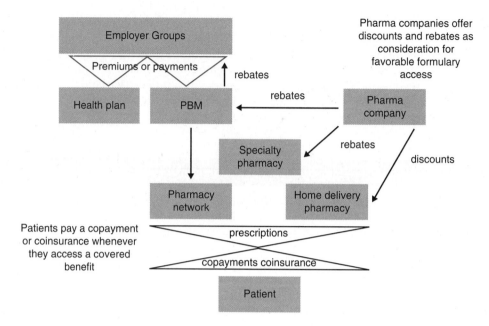

**Figure 16-5** • "Carve-out" Drug Benefit Coverage Directly to Pharmacy Benefit Manager (PBM). (Source: Robert Navarro, Craig Stern, and Rusty Hailey. "Prescription Drug Benefits in Managed Care," in Peter Kongstvedt [Ed.], *Essentials of Managed Care*. New York, NY: Jones and Bartlett, 2012: 257-282.)

to enrollees. The same trade-off may be found in the pharmacy benefit. Some sponsors may try to limit access to certain drugs and increase enrollee cost sharing in order to reduce expenditures, whereas other sponsors (eg, unions) may broaden access to more drugs and limit cost sharing while incurring higher expenditures.

Since the advent of managed care in the 1980s and 1990s, ERISA plan sponsors and health insurers have focused much of their efforts on cost containment. Both parties seek to manage drug expenditures using 2 similar techniques: management of supply costs both upstream and downstream and management of utilization demand downstream. The former includes the negotiation of discounts with pharmaceutical manufacturers and retail pharmacies for drug costs. The latter includes cost-sharing mechanisms for ERISA plan participants, including deductibles, coinsurance, and HDHP plans; these represent the major changes in pharmacy benefit design over the past 2 decades.

Pharmacy benefit management activities have grown in importance as the share of national healthcare expenditures paid out of pocket by consumers has decreased and the share paid by third-party payers (both public and private insurers) has increased. Moreover, ERISA plan sponsors implement and enforce

the pharmacy benefit design using a host of additional techniques, including pharmacy and therapeutics (P&T) committees and formulary development and management practices. For example, the advent of expensive specialty pharmaceuticals has led some employers to delay placing them on their formularies (until their PBM partners can vet them), whereas others, particularly the self-insured employers, have purchased "stop-loss" insurance to protect against catastrophic financial losses.[10] However, the implementation of these pharmacy benefit management techniques differs across ERISA plan sponsors and the health insurers and PBMs with whom they partner, depending on the trade-offs they wish to make in cost, quality, and access.[11] These variations are documented in detail in the following section.

## PRESCRIPTION DRUG BENEFIT DESIGN IN ERISA HEALTH PLANS

Nearly all (99%+) covered workers today are at firms that provide prescription drug coverage in their largest health plan. Many employer plans have increasingly complex benefit designs for prescription drugs, as employers and insurers expand the use of formularies with multiple cost-sharing tiers as well as other management approaches. Cost-sharing tiers generally refer to a health plan placing a drug on a formulary or preferred drug list that classifies drugs into categories that are subject to different cost sharing or management.[12]

Drug benefit plans include several fundamental services. These include[13]:

- Plan design and administration
- Formulary development and management
- Rebate negotiation
- Enrollment and member services
- Utilization management
- Claims adjudication
- Reporting

These services can be performed by several parties within the drug channel system that spans ERISA plan sponsors, health insurers, and PBMs. The PBMI refers to a subset of these activities as "core PBM functions." These include account management, claims processing, eligibility data management, mail-order pharmacy, member services, plan implementation and changes, retail network options, utilization management programs, and the hosting of a member website. Other activities are labeled "noncore PBM services": benefit design consulting, clinical consulting, consumer education tools, formulary management, management reports, medication adherence programs, medication therapy management, trend management programs, and rebates.[14]

Some of these activities (eg, formulary development and management, rebate negotiation) are covered separately in detail later. The prevalence of utilization management tools to manage drug costs has increased over time.[15] Examples of utilization management protocols common within drug formularies include the following:

- *Coverage Restrictions:* Determine the medications that are included within a formulary. Formulary exclusions block access to specific products.
- *Step Therapy:* More expensive drugs are not authorized unless patients do not respond to less expensive therapeutic alternatives.
- *Drug Utilization Review:* Ongoing review of the prescribing, dispensing, and taking of medications.
- *Therapeutic Interchange Programs:* Encourage patients to use preferred formulary products. Pharmacists may substitute one brand name drug for another only with prior physician authorization.
- *Narrow Pharmacy Networks:* Encourage or require patients to use designated pharmacies or dispensing channels instead of allowing them to select from an open network of pharmacies.
- *Quantity Limits:* Establishes limits on the amount of medication a patient may receive during a designated period or in a single refill, such as a 30-, 60-, or 90-day supply.
- *First Fail Protocols:* Require a demonstration that a generic drug, lower level of treatment, or lower-cost drug fails to work for the patient before a health plan will approve a more expensive medication or treatment.
- *Prior Authorization Criteria:* Require the submission and approval through the telephone, an online portal/website, or written coverage request for the health plan to cover the drug.
- *Mail-Order Criteria:* Require a higher copay if the patient obtains the drug from a retail pharmacy versus the PBM's mail-order pharmacy.

## Drug Benefit Design

Drug benefit design typically starts with the ERISA plan sponsor and its team of human resources and benefits professionals. They are responsible for developing and managing employee benefits that make their firm an employer of choice as well as one that provides for the health needs of its workforce. Most of these professionals juggle drug benefit design and management with their other job responsibilities. According to 2018 survey data gathered by PBMI,[16] 62% of respondents reported that 25% or less of their job was focused on designing and managing the drug benefit.[17]

Although the process of designing and evaluating drug benefits differs by employer, the basic components include collaboration with key influencers and advisers, determination of benefits funding, and deciding whether to purchase stop-loss insurance. Most employers rely on experts to help them design and purchase drug benefits. According to PBMI, 83% use a benefits consultant, up from 76% in the prior year. Use of benefits consultants is virtually identical for large and smaller employers (86% large; 81% smaller).

Of those using a consultant, 66% use the same person to evaluate and design the medical benefit. Here, differences by employer size are more striking. Smaller employers are much more likely to use the same person to design both pharmacy and medical benefits (75%) than large employers (53%). Sixty-two percent of employers reported that the drug benefit and medical benefit are designed in concert.

Designing the drug and medical benefit together does not imply that the drug benefit is carved into the medical benefit plan. Rather, the designs on both benefits are done together but may ultimately fall under separate contracts and perhaps through different vendors. Given that smaller employers are more likely to use the same consultant to design both pharmacy and medical benefits, it is not surprising that they are also more likely to report designing both benefits together (66% compared to 56% of large employers).

Employers must also decide how to fund medical and pharmacy benefits. The clear majority (83%) of employers self-insure both pharmacy and medical benefits. Self-insured plans take on more financial risk but may have lower overall costs when they manage benefits effectively.

## Prescription Drug Formulary Overview

A prescription drug formulary is a list of approved drugs that a health plan, often through the help of a PBM, has agreed to cover. The formulary defines the prescription drug benefit. The purpose of using a drug formulary is to provide high-quality care using the most cost-effective medications. Typically, a drug formulary is developed by physicians, nurses, and pharmacists using clinical evidence. PBMs may also design and manage the prescription drug benefit for health plans via a P&T committee, consisting of an outside group of clinicians and tasked with selecting the medications included within a formulary. The P&T committee develops, reviews, and updates the formulary so it reflects the most current clinical guidelines, US Food and Drug Administration (FDA)-approved prescribing protocols, published literature, and clinical trial results. Although the design of the cost-sharing tiers is typically left up to the health plan sponsor or insurer, the information submitted by the P&T committee is valuable in determining the final formulary structure.

The P&T committee recommendations extend beyond the drugs to be included in the formulary. They are also responsible for designing and implementing formulary policies that address utilization and access to medications. These policies aim to promote appropriate use, enabling patients to receive necessary services while limiting overutilization of medical resources.

A drug formulary usually consists of 2 to 5 groups of drugs—called tiers—with different levels of copayments or coinsurance by tier. The drugs in the lowest tier will have the smallest patient cost sharing, whereas the drugs in the highest tier will have the highest patient cost sharing. Generic drugs (medications that are essentially copies of brand name drugs with similar dosage, intended use, and side effects) are often assigned to the lowest tiers, with brand name and "specialty" drugs (ie, high-cost drugs for small patient populations) occupying the higher tiers.

## Variation in Formulary Decision Making

Formulary decisions are an important aspect of drug benefit management, from the perspective of both rebate contracting (ie, rebates may influence or be influenced by formulary placement) and member cost sharing. Plan sponsors can choose to use the PBM's standard national/preferred formulary, develop a custom formulary, or use some other formulary such as that developed by their health plan. According to PBMI, 70% used the PBM's national/preferred formulary, whereas 27% had a custom formulary. A small percentage (3%) used formularies developed by their health plan or medical third-party administrator.

To provide some insight into the decision-making process to choose either the PBM's national/preferred formulary or to use a custom formulary, the PBMI Survey asked an open-ended question on why the employer chose the formulary they did. Common responses from plan sponsors choosing the PBM's national/preferred formulary included the following:

- "We prefer to have a formulary that is consistent, and we can follow recommendations/changes of that formulary made by the PBM."
- "Recommendation by consultant."
- "It was the easiest choice and we feel very comfortable with their formulary development methodology."
- "We do not have the expertise to customize the formulary. That is one of the reasons we hire a PBM."

Among those choosing a custom formulary, reasons included the following:

- "Better control of costs."
- "Greater flexibility and autonomy."
- "Flexibility combined with a focus on clinical outcomes/efficacy first and foremost."
- "Being a faith-based institution, some of the drugs on the standard formularies need to be included or excluded. The result is a custom formulary, although it's not very different."

The practice of excluding specific drugs from the formulary ("formulary exclusions") has emerged as a powerful tool used by PBMs to gain bargaining leverage over pharmaceutical manufacturers. PBMs force manufacturers of therapeutically comparable drugs to offer larger rebates to avoid exclusion from the formulary. Such exclusions are a major factor behind the growth in the "gross-to-net discounts" in the price of branded drugs.[18]

These formulary exclusions influence the national formularies recommended by the PBMs to the ERISA plan sponsors and insurers they contract with. These are recommendations, not requirements or mandates. Plan sponsors and insurers that adopt the recommendations earn higher rebates and face lower plan costs; those that do not adopt the recommendations earn lower rebates and face higher plan costs. Thus, ERISA plan sponsors, like their employees and health insurers, face a trade-off between access and cost. However, a drug's presence on a given formulary does not mean that consumers are denied access to that drug. Employers are constrained in their use of formulary exclusions by the dissatisfaction of their own employees with such exclusions. Nevertheless, the threat of exclusions leads manufacturers to offer steeper rebates.[19] The number of drugs on PBM formulary exclusion lists has grown steadily since 2013 and 2014 (see below).[20]

## ERISA Plan Sponsors' Management of Drug Rebates

Rebates are percentage discounts off the manufacturer's list price paid to the PBMs. Manufacturers lower their list prices in order to gain access to the PBM's formulary for their drugs. These rebates and their percentage levels are typically based on (1) placement of the drug on the PBM formulary, (2) more favorable placement (ie, lower-cost tier) on the formulary, and (3) exclusive placement on the formulary (ie, comparable drugs made by a competing manufacturer are either not on the formulary or placed disadvantageously on a higher-cost tier). These arrangements essentially trade volume for price and serve to reduce the actual price of the drugs for employees with drug coverage.

Rebate terms for employers vary based on how their PBM contract is written. Contracts may guarantee a flat dollar amount or a percentage share of rebates (with or without minimum guarantees), on a "per-prescription," "per-rebatable drug," or brand and generic utilization basis. The payment of rebates is often conditioned on the volume of drugs purchased through the PBM and the latter's ability to move market share for the drug manufacturer paying for formulary access.

Rebates are typically negotiated as part of formulary contracting agreements; depending on the contract, some or all of the savings are passed on to the employer. Some employers are concerned that insurers and PBMs may not be passing on all of the rebates they collect. Data from Kaiser (Figure 16-6) indicate the percentage of rebates received back by the ERISA plan sponsor (employer) among larger firms. One-quarter for large employers report they receive "most" of the rebates; another third report they receive "some" of the rebates. More specific data on the rebates passed along to ERISA plan sponsors are collected by PBMI, which found that 83% of respondents reported that they received rebates on traditional (non-specialty) drugs. The most frequent arrangement was 100% of rebates being passed through to the employer, either with a minimum guarantee (31%) or with no guarantee (27%).

According to PBMI, rebate arrangements are more common for large employers, with 87% reporting receiving rebates versus 80% of smaller employers. Differences by employer size are also seen when looking at receipt of 100% of rebates. Large employers were more likely to receive 100% of rebates with a minimum guarantee than were smaller employers (39% vs 26%), whereas smaller employers were more likely to receive a flat dollar guaranteed amount (17% vs 7%).

Price protection provisions are sometimes included in PBM contracts as a way to provide

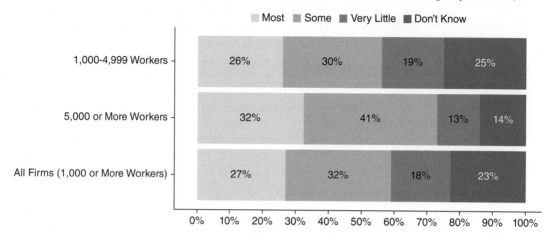

**Figure 16-6** • Percentage of Pharmacy Benefit Manager (PBM) Rebates Passed on to Employers. (Source: KFF Employer Health Benefits Survey, Kaiser Family Foundation, 2019.)

some cost stability. The provisions put a ceiling or cap on the amount manufacturers can increase the cost of a medication during the life of the rebate contract with the PBM. According to PBMI, 31% of respondents reported that they had price protection (inflation cap provisions) in their PBM contract. Large employers were more likely than smaller employers to have price protection provisions (38% vs 26%, respectively). Of those with such provisions, 98% reported that the revenue from them gets passed back to the plan. Nearly all surveyed employers (87%) felt that their plan benefits from price protection provisions.

## Retail Pharmacy Contracts and Reimbursement

PBMs also contract with a network of retail pharmacies where employees can get their prescriptions filled at the negotiated price. PBMs may assemble a large pharmacy network to increase patient access and convenience or a smaller network to reduce the price paid at the pharmacy counter by extracting further discounts from the dispensing pharmacy. The latter is akin to the preferred provider model of MCOs.

PBM contracts with pharmacies may include either traditional markup (often called "spread" pricing) or pass-through pricing. In traditional/spread pricing, PBMs pass along some of the savings negotiated to plan sponsors, retaining some of these savings as compensation

for PBM services. The "spread" is the difference between the amount charged to the plan sponsor by the PBM and the amount the PBM pays the pharmacy that dispenses the drug to the consumer. On the other hand, pass-through pricing passes all pharmacy pricing (including discounts, rebates, other revenues) negotiated by the PBM on to the plan sponsor; the PBM is paid an administrative fee by the plan sponsor for its services. That is, there is no difference in the amount paid by the plan sponsor to the PBM and the amount paid by the PBM to the pharmacy. Smaller PBMs are more likely to contract based on pass-through pricing.[21]

According to Drug Channels data from 2017, 41% of employers reported using spread pricing, while 59% of employers reported using pass-through pricing. Similar data are reported in the PBMI 2018 Survey: 37% of respondents indicated that they received traditional/spread pricing, and 63% reported pass-through pricing. The use of pass-through pricing has increased slightly from last year. Large employers were more likely to report pass-through pricing (71%) than were smaller employers (57%). Discounts on drug ingredient costs are typically expressed as a percentage off the average wholesale price (AWP), a list price benchmark for many drug transactions. According to PBMI, 77% reported a guaranteed discount applied to all generic medications, and 56% reported a guaranteed discount applied to all brand medications. Guaranteed discounts are those that the PBM is contractually obligated to provide to the plan.

Other discounts may also be offered but are not guaranteed. The average discount off AWP varied by channel. For generic drugs, average AWP discounts ranged from 56% at retail to 63% for mail order. Discounts on brand name drugs were much lower with averages between 19% and 25% depending on channel.[22]

## COST SHARING FOR DRUGS

### Cost-Sharing Data From Kaiser

The vast majority of covered workers (91%) are in a plan with tiered cost sharing for prescription drugs; 84% of covered workers are in a plan with 3+ tiers of cost sharing for prescription drugs (Figure 16-7).

High-deductible health plans (HDHPs) with a savings option (SO) have a different cost-sharing pattern for prescription drugs compared to other plan types. Enrollees in HDHP/SOs are more likely to be in a plan with the same cost sharing regardless of drug type (10% vs 3%) or in a plan that has no cost sharing for prescriptions once the plan deductible is met (9% vs 1%; Figure 16-8).

For covered workers in a plan with 3+ tiers of cost sharing for prescription drugs, copayments

are the most common form of cost sharing in the first 3 tiers, with coinsurance as the next most common. These percentage distributions vary by size of the employer and by whether the plans are HDHP/SOs. The average copayments are $11 for first-tier drugs, $33 for second-tier drugs, $59 for third-tier drugs, and $123 for fourth-tier drugs; the average coinsurance rates are 18% for first-tier drugs, 24% for second-tier drugs, 34% for third-tier drugs, and 29% for fourth-tier drugs. Twelve percent of covered workers are in a plan with 2 tiers for prescription drug cost sharing (excluding tiers covering only specialty drugs). For these workers, copayments are more common than coinsurance for first-tier and second-tier drugs. The average copayment for the first tier is $11, and the average copayment for the second tier is $31. Five percent of covered workers are in a plan with the same cost sharing for prescriptions regardless of the type of drug (excluding tiers covering only specialty drugs). Among these workers, 25% have copayments and 75% have coinsurance. The average coinsurance rate is 22%.

Coinsurance rates for prescription drugs often include maximum and/or minimum dollar amounts. Depending on the plan design, coinsurance maximums may significantly limit the amount an enrollee must spend out of pocket

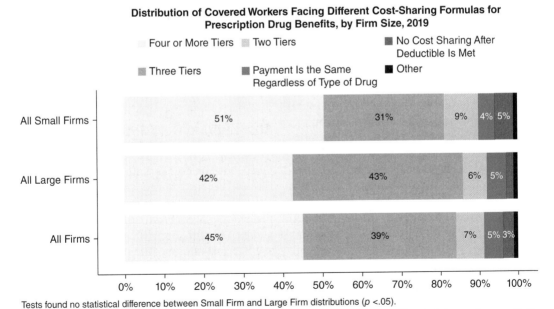

**Distribution of Covered Workers Facing Different Cost-Sharing Formulas for Prescription Drug Benefits, by Firm Size, 2019**

Legend: Four or More Tiers | Two Tiers | No Cost Sharing After Deductible Is Met | Three Tiers | Payment Is the Same Regardless of Type of Drug | Other

| Firm | Four or More Tiers | Three Tiers | Two Tiers | No Cost Sharing After Deductible Is Met | Other |
|---|---|---|---|---|---|
| All Small Firms | 51% | 31% | 9% | 4% | 5% |
| All Large Firms | 42% | 43% | 6% | 5% | |
| All Firms | 45% | 39% | 7% | 5% | 3% |

Tests found no statistical difference between Small Firm and Large Firm distributions (*p* <.05).

NOTE: Small Firms have 3-199 workers and Large Firms have 200 or more workers. Number of tiers includes any tiers specifically for specialty drugs. Excluding tiers specifically for specialty drugs, 64% of covered workers with prescription drug coverage are enrolled in a plan with four or more tiers, 12% have 3 tiers, 5% have 2 tiers, 4% have the same cost sharing regardless of the drug, and 1% have no cost sharing after the deductible is met. For more information on the definition of specialty drugs and how this survey defines drug formulary tiers, see Section 9.

**Figure 16-7** • Percentage of Health Plans With Cost-Sharing Tiers. (Source: KFF Employer Health Benefits Survey, Kaiser Family Foundation, 2019.)

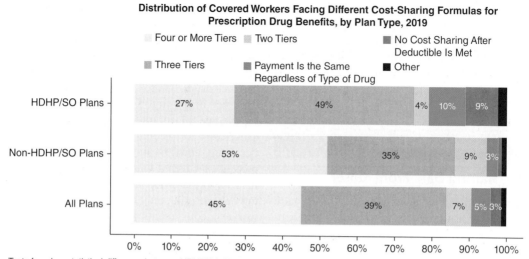

Distribution of Covered Workers Facing Different Cost-Sharing Formulas for Prescription Drug Benefits, by Plan Type, 2019

Tests found no statistical difference between HDHP/SO Plan and Non-HDHP/SO distributions (*p* <.05).

NOTE: Number of tiers includes any tiers specifically for specialty drugs. Excluding tiers specifically for specialty drugs, 64% of covered workers with prescription drug coverage are enrolled in a plan with 4 or more tiers, 12% have 3 tiers, 5% have 2 tiers, 4% have the same cost sharing regardless of the drug, and 1% have no cost sharing after the deductible is met. For more information on the definition of specialty drugs and how this survey defines drug formulary tiers, see Section 9.

**Figure 16-8** • Cost-Sharing Tiers in High-Deductible Health Plan With a Savings Option (HDHP/SO) Plans. (Source: KFF Employer Health Benefits Survey, Kaiser Family Foundation, 2019.)

for higher cost drugs. These coinsurance minimum and maximum amounts vary across the tiers. Among covered workers in a plan with coinsurance for the first cost-sharing tier, 16% have only a maximum dollar amount attached to the coinsurance rate, 6% have only a minimum dollar amount, 18% have both a minimum and maximum dollar amount, and 58% have neither. For those in a plan with coinsurance for the fourth cost-sharing tier, 40% have only a maximum dollar amount attached to the coinsurance rate, 2% have only a minimum dollar amount, 13% have both a minimum and maximum dollar amount, and 43% have neither.

Many plans allow enrollees to fill prescriptions through the mail. In some cases, there may be a financial incentive, such as lower cost sharing, for enrollees to use this process. In 2019, a very small share of workers (2%) were in plans that only covered prescription drugs provided through the mail and 4% were in plans that only covered some prescriptions through the mail. For these workers, the plan would generally not pay anything for a prescription if the enrollee visited a physical pharmacy. Among workers at firms with 50+ employees that offer coverage for prescription drugs, 58% have a financial incentive for enrollees to fill some or all prescriptions through a mail-order pharmacy.

Among covered workers in a plan with coverage for prescription drugs, 13% are enrolled

in a plan that has a separate annual deductible that applies only to prescription drugs. Covered workers in small firms are less likely than those in large firms to be enrolled in a plan with a separate annual deductible for prescription drugs (9% vs 14%). For covered workers in a plan with a separate annual deductible for prescription drugs, the average prescription drug deductible is $194. Sixty-nine percent of covered workers in a plan with a separate annual deductible for prescription drugs are in a plan that applies the deductible to all covered drugs.

## Cost-Sharing Data From PBMI

The PBMI 2018 survey offers a slightly different perspective on cost sharing for drugs. The structure of this cost sharing encompasses at least 5 types of mechanisms: a flat dollar amount and a percentage share (1) with or without a minimum and/or (2) with or without a maximum. The average cost-sharing amounts can vary depending on the choice of retail or mail-order fill.

Employer plans also vary in their use of drug deductibles and whether they are combined (shared) with the medical deductible. Finally, employers report that the biggest influence on the cost-sharing decision is exerted by consultants and brokers, claims history, recommendations by health plans and PBMs, and a host of corporate factors and industry benchmarks.

## THE BROUHAHA OVER THE GROSS-TO-NET PRICE DISPARITY

Over the past few years, observers have noted not only the rise in drug list prices but also the growing disparity between gross and net prices for pharmaceutical products (Figure 16-9). As a percentage of drug price growth, rebates accounted for only 6% to 9% during 2011 to 2012 but then accounted for 57% to 77% during 2013 to 2015. Some mistakenly believe that the rise in list prices is partly caused by the higher rebates (and other payments made by manufacturers to PBMs), which are represented by the gap between gross and net price. In their view, the fact that higher rebates and other fees account for a higher percentage of the drug's list price increase is evidence of causation.

The error in this causal logic is shown by several pieces of evidence. Drug manufacturers raise prices several times a year, whereas PBMs negotiate contracts and rebates every 2 to 3 years, with the rebates remaining constant during the duration of each contract. Moreover, drug manufacturers raise prices in anticipation of losing patent protection (and thus market share), in the event of filing patent lawsuits against competitors (potentially gaining share), in anticipation of a generic product entering the market (losing market share), in anticipation of new competitors entering the market (and thus losing market share), or in the event that an existing competitor pulls their product from the market (gaining market share). In general, drug manufacturers raise prices because they can (eg, when they enjoy more of a monopoly position in their therapeutic category, when they have superior marketing, when their product is the physician preference item, and when their product has brand preference among patients).

Multiple factors have contributed to the growing spread between gross and net drug prices (known as the gross-to-net disparity). *First* is the growing consolidation of the PBM sector. PBM consolidation was legitimated by the Federal Trade Commission's (FTC) sign-off on ESI's acquisition of WellPoint's Next Rx in-house PBM in 2009 and the market valuation placed on Next Rx's business.[23] This consolidation accelerated in the 2012 to 2015 period (Figure 16-10), led by ESI's acquisition of Medco (2012), Catamaran's acquisition of ReStat and TPBG's acquisition of EnvisionRx (both in 2013), and then Optum's acquisition of Catamaran (2015). By 2017, the top 3 PBMs commanded 71% of the market: CVS (25%), ESI (24%), and Optum (22%). The top 7 PBMs controlled 95% of the market. This market concentration of buyers allows PBMs and health

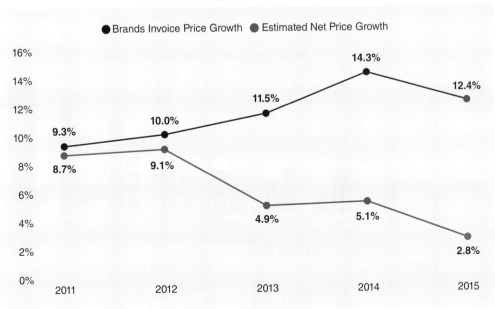

**Figure 16-9 •** Growing Divergence Between Gross Sales Price and Net Sales Price. (Source: IMS Health, National Sales Perspectives, IMS Institute For Healthcare Informatics, March 2016.)

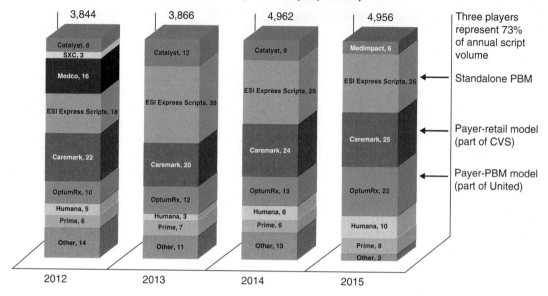

**Figure 16-10** • The Pharmacy Benefit Manager (PBM) Industry Has Consolidated to 3 Key Players, Each With a Unique Model in the Healthcare Value Chain. (Source: Karl Kellner/McKinsey & Company Analysis, Company Filings & Brochures, WellsFargo Report 2015, Pembroke Report 2016.)

insurers to extract large discounts in price from manufacturers in exchange for a drug's position on the formulary. This is a major driver of drug rebates (discounts on list price) paid to the PBMs.

*Second*, complementing the growing concentration on the buyer side (PBM market), there can be growing competition on the supplier side in the form of competing pharmaceutical products. This is also referred to as "crowded therapeutic categories." Such product competition gives PBMs and health insurers great power over manufacturers by virtue of playing one manufacturer off another and threatening to move market share to the manufacturer who offers better terms (including higher rebates).

*Third*, beginning around 2012, but picking up around 2014 (Figure 16-11), PBMs began

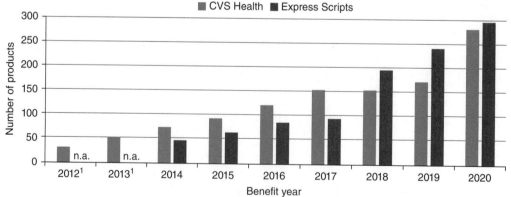

**Figure 16-11** • Number of Products on Pharmacy Benefit Manager (PBM) Formulary Exclusion Lists, 2012 to 2020. (Source: Adam Fein. *The 2020 Economic Report on U.S. Pharmacies and Pharmacy Benefit Managers*. Philadelphia, PA: Drug Channels Institute, 2020.)

to use the strategy of "formulary exclusion" whereby manufacturers are threatened with product removal from the PBM's national formulary. CVS/Caremark removed 34 brand name drugs from its standard national formulary in January 2012 and added another 17 drugs to the exclusion list in 2013; ESI followed CVS's example in 2014. Both PBMs have added more drugs to the list over time. Optum, Prime Therapeutics, Aetna, and Cigna embraced drug exclusions by 2016.

Such a strategy works in the presence of therapeutically comparable brand name drugs. In 2016, more than 50% of the commercial market was covered by plans with formulary exclusions. Note that exclusions block access to specific products on a PBM's recommended national formulary; they are thus suggestions rather than mandates. ERISA plan sponsors and health insurers can ignore the PBM's national formulary but then face reduced rebates and/or higher plan costs. They, thus, trade off higher access to drugs for higher costs incurred, much in the way that formularies financially reward patients for selecting generic and lower-tier drugs with lower costs, while allowing access to additional drugs on higher tiers but requiring patients to face higher costs via higher copays or coinsurance. Nevertheless, the prospect of exclusion leads manufacturers to offer larger rebates. A precipitating event here was the introduction of AbbVie's hepatitis C drug Viekira Pak to compete with Gilead's Sovaldi and Harvoni. The number of products on the formulary exclusion lists for 2 PBMs (CVS and ESI) has grown steadily since 2012.[24]

*Fourth*, statutory rebates are another large driver of gross-to-net discounts. The Patient Protection and Affordable Care Act (2010) increased the mandatory rebates that pharmaceutical manufacturers must pay under the Medicaid program. For single-source (nongeneric) drugs, the unit rebate amount increased from 15.1% of a product's average manufacturer price (AMP) to 23.1% of AMP. It also required manufacturers to provide rebates in the Medicare Part D coverage gap. The Bipartisan Budget Act, signed into law in February 2018, increased these discounts. Rebates and other channel discounts to PBMs and pharmacies constitute "direct and indirect remuneration" (DIR) payments made to Part D plan sponsors. These payments were stable from 2010 to 2012 but began to accelerate beginning in 2013. DIRs help to create a gap between list and net prices.

*Fifth*, the pharmaceutical industry experienced steep patent cliffs in 2012 and 2015 and a much higher level of patent expiries in the period from 2013 to 2019 compared to earlier levels (eg, 2010) (Figure 16-12). Attending these patent expiries was a wave of new generic drugs entering the market. Research documents that drug prices decrease markedly after patent expiration.[25] In 2017, the generic dispensing rate—the percentage of drug prescriptions dispensed with a generic drug instead of a branded drug—was 90%. The rise in generics and generic dispensing rates occasioned a slowdown in the price growth of branded drugs.

All of these factors contribute to gross-to-net discounts. These discounts accelerated from 2012

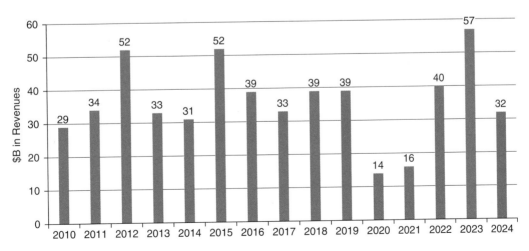

**Figure 16-12 •** Worldwide Total Prescription Drug Revenue at Risk From Patent Expiration From 2010 to 2024 (in Billion US Dollars). (Source: EvaluatePharma. World Preview 2019, Outlook to 2024, Page 9.)

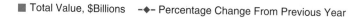

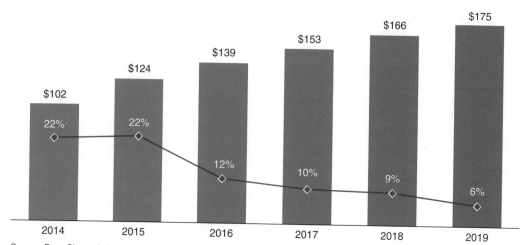

Source: Drug Channels Institute analysis of IQVIA Institute data; Drug Channels Institute estimates. Gross-to-Net Reductions include the total value of rebates, off-invoice discounts, copay assistance, price concessions, and such other reductions as distribution fees, product returns, the 340B Drug Pricing Program, and more.

**Figure 16-13** • Total Value of Pharmaceutical Manufacturers' Gross-to-Net Reductions for Brand Name Drugs, 2014 to 2019. (Source: Adam Fein. *The 2020 Economic Report on U.S. Pharmacies and Pharmacy Benefit Managers.* Philadelphia, PA: Drug Channels Institute, 2020.)

through 2016 (Figure 16-13). Industry analysts estimate that roughly two-thirds of these discounts are attributable to rebates paid to public and private payers; another quarter of these discounts reflect contract administration fees, discounts to wholesalers and pharmacies, discounts to providers under the 340B Drug Pricing Program, and other off-invoice discounts; the remainder reflect patient assistance and copayment support, which are covered later (Figure 16-14).

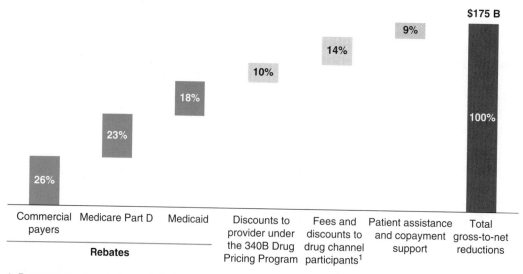

1. Payments by manufacturers include: admin fees to PBMs; fees and discounts to pharmacies and wholesalers; and all other off-invoice discounts and rebates.

Source: Drug Channels Institute estimates. Percentage figures show each category's share of total gross-to-net reductions.

**Figure 16-14** • Total Value of Pharmaceutical Manufacturers' Gross-to-Net Reductions for Brand Name Drugs, by Source, 2019. (Source: Adam Fein. *The 2020 Economic Report on U.S. Pharmacies and Pharmacy Benefit Managers.* Philadelphia, PA: Drug Channels Institute, 2020.)

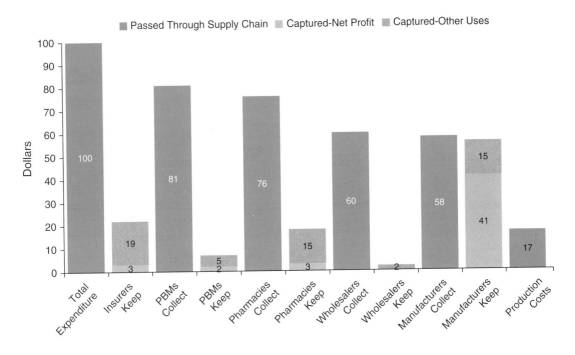

Legend: ■ Passed Through Supply Chain ■ Captured-Net Profit ■ Captured-Other Uses

**Figure 16-15** • Flow of a Hypothetical $100 Expenditure on Prescription Drugs Covered Under Private Insurance Through the US Retail Distribution System. (Source: Neeraj Sood.)

Most of these gross-to-net discounts were not realized by PBMs and other drug channel participants such as wholesalers and pharmacies (which accounted for only 26%), but rather were realized by public and private payers (67%). Researchers estimate that pharmacies capture the bulk (15%) of this 26%, with PBMs (5%) and wholesalers (2%) capturing much less (Figure 16-15).[26]

This means that ERISA plan sponsors and the health insurers they contract with realized large discounts off of drug list prices, which accounts for the majority of the growing gross-to-net disparity. This is reflected in data for both small and large employers that capture the trend in rebates flowing back to the ERISA plan sponsors between 2014 and 2018 (Figure 16-16).

The data indicate that a growing percentage of both smaller and larger employers are receiving 100% of the rebates negotiated by their PBMs. Among larger employers, the 100% pass-through is by far the most common rebate arrangement; a slight majority of smaller employers also received 100% pass-throughs, but nearly one-third receive a percentage share of rebates.

The question is: What did ERISA plan sponsors and health insurers do with the discounts (savings)? PBMI survey data suggest that the vast majority of employers (68%) use

the rebates to offset the overall plan costs to the employer, especially their own spending on drugs.[27] By contrast, a smaller percentage of employers (11%) use the discounts to reduce the premiums of their employees (11%), a strategy that benefits all workers. A small percentage of employers (15%) split the savings with employees or reduce employee out-of-pocket costs at the point of sale (4%). This means that employers use the discounts generated by their employees with more severe illnesses that require expensive drugs (which earn higher rebates) to cover their overall health expenditures rather than benefit the employees who generate the rebates. The irony, according to industry analysts, is that the employees' actual out-of-pocket costs are set by their insurer and ERISA plan sponsor. It is not the PBMs but rather the plan sponsors and health insurers who elect not to share the rebates directly with employees.[28]

Over time, employers' drug benefit designs have shifted out-of-pocket spending from flat copayments to deductibles and coinsurance arrangements. By 2019, more than half of all consumer out-of-pocket spending on prescription drugs was for coinsurance or deductibles, both of which are tied to list price.[29] A comparison of Figures 16-17 and 16-18 shows the decline in cost sharing using copayments and

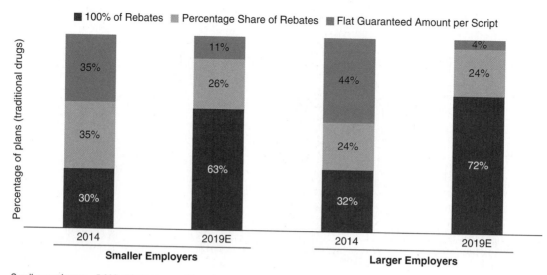

Smaller employers = 5,000 or fewer covered lives; Larger employers = more than 5,000 covered lives. Number of covered lives includes employees and dependents.

Source: Drug Channels Institute analysis of *Trends in Drug Benefit Design*, PBMI, various years; Drug Channels Institute estimates. Data include only responding firms that receive rebates for traditional drugs. 2014 figures recomputed to exclude those who were not sure about their company's rebate arrangements.

**Figure 16-16** • Pharmacy Benefit Manager (PBM) Rebate Arrangements for Traditional Medications in Employer-Sponsored Plans, by Employer Size, 2014 Versus 2019. (Source: Adam Fein. *The 2020 Economic Report on U.S. Pharmacies and Pharmacy Benefit Managers*. Philadelphia, PA: Drug Channels Institute, 2020.)

the rise in cost sharing using coinsurance when employer plans include high deductibles, by drug tier. Figure 16-19 shows the dollar amount of cost sharing by drug tier for both copayment and coinsurance.

Moreover, over time, the percentage of ERISA sponsor plans with pharmacy benefit

deductibles has risen (Figure 16-20). These deductibles can be separate from or combined with the medical deductible.

A recent survey of large employers by the National Business Group on Health suggests some change in employer sentiment here. In 2019, 18% of employers reported having a

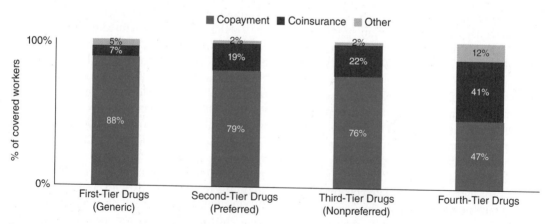

Source: Drug Channels Institute analysis of *2019 Employer Health Benefits Survey*, Henry J. Kaiser Family Foundation. Percentages do not sum to 100% for each tier because other plan designs are excluded for the purposes of presentation. Data presented for covered workers (1) with 3 or more tiers of prescription cost sharing, and (2) who do not have a High-Deductible Health Plan with a Savings Option (HDHP/SOs).

Published on *Drug Channels* (www.DrugChannels.net) on November 13, 2019.

**Figure 16-17** • Type of Cost Sharing for Prescription Drug Benefits, Employer-Sponsored Plans Without High Deductibles, by Benefit Tier, 2019. (Source: Adam Fein. *The 2020 Economic Report on U.S. Pharmacies and Pharmacy Benefit Managers*. Philadelphia, PA: Drug Channels Institute, 2020.)

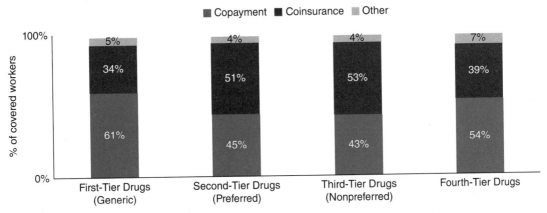

Source: Drug Channels Institute analysis of *2019 Employer Health Benefits Survey*, Henry J. Kaiser Family Foundation.
Percentages do not sum to 100% for each tier because other plan designs are excluded for the purposes of presentation.
Data presented for covered workers (1) with 3 or more tiers of prescription cost sharing, and (2) who have a High-Deductible
Health Plan with a Savings Option (HDHP/SOs).

Published on *Drug Channels* (www.DrugChannels.net) on November 13, 2019.

**Figure 16-18** • Type of Cost Sharing for Prescription Drug Benefits, Employer-Sponsored Plans With High Deductibles, by Benefit Tier, 2019. (Source: Adam Fein. *The 2020 Economic Report on U.S. Pharmacies and Pharmacy Benefit Managers*. Philadelphia, PA: Drug Channels Institute, 2020.)

point-of-sale rebate program in place, 2% said they were implementing a program in 2020, and another 40% were considering such a program for 2021 to 2022.[30] Such programs pass the rebates directly to the employee at point of purchase. Such point-of-sale programs are most appropriate when the employee is filling a prescription during the deductible phase of coverage or when paying a coinsurance.

As industry analysts make clear, this decision about point-of-sale programs is at the

discretion of ERISA plan sponsors and the health insurers with which they contract. These 2 parties choose the overall prescription drug benefit that is offered to plan participants, which can include which drugs are covered, the different levels of cost sharing, the number of pharmacies available to participants, and the incentives for using certain network pharmacies. As far back as 2011 to 2012, PBMI survey data indicate that ERISA plan sponsors, their benefits consultants, and their insurers shoulder

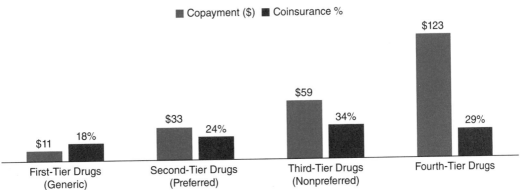

Source: Drug Channels Institute analysis of *2019 Employer Health Benefits Survey*, Henry J. Kaiser Family Foundation.
Percentages do not sum to 100% for each tier because other plan designs are excluded for the purposes of presentation.
Data presented for covered workers with 3 or more tiers of prescription cost sharing.

Published on *Drug Channels* (www.DrugChannels.net) on November 13, 2019.

**Figure 16-19** • Average Cost Sharing by Prescription Drug Tier, Employer-Sponsored Plans, 2019. (Source: Adam Fein. *The 2020 Economic Report on U.S. Pharmacies and Pharmacy Benefit Managers*. Philadelphia, PA: Drug Channels Institute, 2020.)

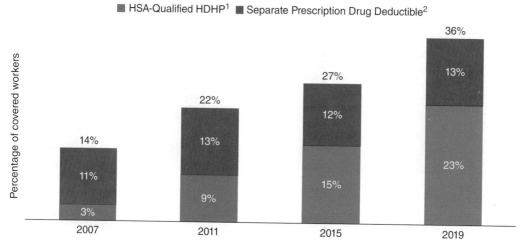

1. HSA-qualified HDHPs are high-deductible health plans that meet the federal legal requirements to permit an enrollee to establish and contribute to a health savings account (HSA). Enrollees are subject to the general annual deductible amounts for all services, including prescription drugs.
2. Includes plans with a separate annual deductible that applies only to prescription drugs.

Source: Drug Channels Institute analysis of *2019 Employer Health Benefits Survey,* Henry J. Kaiser Family Foundation.

**Figure 16-20** • Percentage of Covered Workers With Pharmacy Benefit Deductibles, 2007 to 2019. (Source: Adam Fein. *The 2020 Economic Report on U.S. Pharmacies and Pharmacy Benefit Managers.* Philadelphia, PA: Drug Channels Institute, 2020.)

the responsibility for pharmacy benefit designs offered to employees.[31] These choices reflect the trade-offs that ERISA plan sponsors and health insurers make between access, quality, and cost. These 2 parties then contract with PBMs to *administer* their prescription drug plans and *implement* the choices made by plan sponsors. This means the PBMs process and pay prescription drug claims, secure discounts and rebates from manufacturers, and manage networks of retail, mail, long-term care, and specialty pharmacies. Even in cases of self-funded employers outsourcing their drug plan coverage to PBMs, the PBMs "can provide advice and guidance as pharmacy benefits experts," but ERISA plan sponsors retain control.[32] This has been true for some time. Data from 2012 to 2013 indicate that HMO plans, the most widespread plan option across public and private insurers, rarely adopt a PBM's formulary even though they increasingly outsource pharmacy benefit management services to the PBMs. According to survey data, 80% of HMOs create proprietary formularies rather than adopting the PBM's formulary; only 14% rely on the PBM's formulary.[33]

Beyond the PBMs, ERISA plan sponsors rely on a host of pharmacy benefits consultants to help them analyze PBM relationships, advise on PBM contracting, and assist with the negotiations. Such consultants can include business groups on health as well as employer coalitions (eg, the Health Transformation Alliance).[34] Such coalitions represent large buying hubs that aggregate their purchasing power to extract contract concessions from the PBMs as well as the drug manufacturers with which they contract.

Employers have been criticized for their lack of sophistication and inadequate management of their drug benefits plans, their lack of engagement with the parties they contract with in the pharmaceutical distribution chain, and their reliance on in-house human resources specialists to manage their healthcare and pharmacy benefits, as noted earlier.[35] One reason may be their emphasis on employee compensation (relative to the market) rather than health benefits.[36] The following quotations by employers and employer business group representatives squarely put the responsibility on the employers, the ERISA plan sponsors.

*"The majority of employers are still using HR [human resources] specialists to do negotiations and manage health care plans. Formularies are mostly based off of cost savings not clinical outcomes and most employers don't know how to ask the PBM the right questions. Contracts need to be reworded. What does it really say? How is it helping my business/member?*

*Employers should not engage in contracts they do not understand."*

*"Our 'suppliers' don't share contracts or disclose fees. Employers are starting to notice and wondering why they are paying so much. We need to ask intermediaries what they are paying each other and how they spent the money."*

*"We don't talk to employers about the concept of fiduciary responsibility; in this health care environment, employers will have to make ethical decisions about which drugs to cover that will require making difficult choices."*

*"As a fiduciary, an employer is responsible for reviewing the quality of its vendor and its products; they need to gather information, compare data points among vendors, document the process and why they made the decision."*

*"Employers haven't felt there is a problem (with pharmacy benefits) and have been told by consultants and partners that everything is under control and they are getting the best deal possible. We want to trust our partners, but don't know what questions to ask or what to include in the RFP [request for proposals]. Employers need help!"*

*"Manufacturers can tell you what they charge the wholesaler but they can't talk about rebates with the PBM because of required confidentiality clauses between the two."*

*"When you pay a PBM a PMPM [per member per month] fee, any revenue or rebate derived by adjudicating your formulary should get passed back to you. PBMs have lots of ways to hide revenue streams so it doesn't always happen."*

*"Transparency standards have been in place for a long time but you still need to negotiate with suppliers. Today, employers are not allied and have no common agenda (to drive change). The people you're buying benefits from know it. You have to stand up and ask (your vendors) for accountability."*

*"Include questions in your RFP that ask intermediaries what they have been paid by partners in the supply chain (and indicate they will be audited—you have a fiduciary duty)."*

*"Don't accept the status quo. There is a lack of willingness to change and employers need disruption and transformation. The easiest way to do this is through pharmacy benefits. If one PBM doesn't want to play, there are others waiting."*

---

### Critical Thinking Exercise: The Brouhaha Over Epi-Pens

In litigation brought in US District Court in Minneapolis,[37] plaintiffs alleged that the major PBMs leveraged their role in the pharmaceutical supply chain to collude with a pharmaceutical manufacturer (Mylan), jointly conspire to hike list prices on Mylan's Epi-Pen, and earn kickbacks from the higher rebates that derive from the higher list prices. The higher prices hurt employees in employer plans that enrolled in HDHPs, who thus had to cover huge deductibles calculated as a percentage of the list price. These employees served as the plaintiffs. Based on what you now know, how plausible is the plaintiff's argument? Is there any reason why Mylan's list price might have risen besides the alleged conspiracy with the PBMs?

---

## THE PHARMA MANUFACTURERS STRIKE BACK

Pharmaceutical manufacturers have not sat by idly and watched PBMs, health plans, and employers engage in all of the strategies discussed earlier to manage the cost and utilization of drug benefit coverage. In general, manufacturers have historically resisted discounting the prices of their drugs and have engaged in various efforts of their own. Three of these efforts are briefly detailed in the following sections.

### Co-optation of the PBMs via Ownership

When manufacturers realized that the price discounting by PBMs was a fact of life, they decided to co-opt the PBMs by owning them or allying with them. The 1993 to 1994 period witnessed 3 large-scale mergers of pharmaceutical companies and PBMs: Merck-Medco, Lilly-PCS Health Systems, and Glaxo-Diversified Pharmaceutical Services. One strategic intent here (there were others) was to ensure favorable formulary access on the PBM's formulary for the manufacturer's drugs. The FTC stepped in and made the manufacturers construct a "firewall" between the 2 operations. The firewall stipulated that the manufacturer would not have access to confidential pricing information on its rivals, would not be able to unduly influence the formulary of its (now) in-house PBM, and would allow competing manufacturers access to the same formulary. This put the "kibosh" on such mergers. Two of the 3 mergers unwound within 5 years, with the manufacturer selling off its PBM at a huge loss; the third dissolved years later.

## Disease Management

A second strategy was to avoid paying discounts and ensure formulary access by partnering with health plans on disease management programs for the plans' enrollees. In such programs, the manufacturer stated that it would go "at risk" with the plans, guarantee the clinical benefits of its drugs, and pay back any savings not realized if the drugs did not work—*if* the plan formularies included the manufacturer's drugs. As one prominent example, Pfizer struck such a deal with the State of Florida and its Medicaid program. Disease management programs in general, and the Pfizer-Florida experiment in particular, did not demonstrate positive results.

## Use of Coupons and Patient Assistance Programs

Drug manufacturers operate or fund programs to reduce the costs of prescriptions for patients. Some are aimed at lower-income or uninsured patients, while others assist people with coverage who still may face high out-of-pocket costs. Some drug manufacturers provide coupons to patients who are prescribed their drugs. Coupons are discounts that prescription users can present at the pharmacy that reduce their cost-sharing liability. Payers are concerned that coupons and some patient assistance programs affect the incentives employees otherwise may have to use lower cost drugs.

## SUMMARY

The pharmaceutical supply chain depicted here is easily the most complex and least understood portion of the US healthcare system. It is worthy of an entire volume. The drug benefits covered by health insurance that are managed by this chain are becoming increasingly important, particularly as more and more of the population receives coverage under HDHPs. The rebate portion of this supply chain has prompted many policy makers to subject the PBMs to greater transparency or eliminate the rebates they charge.

## QUESTIONS TO PONDER

1. A drug benefit is a recent addition to coverage by employers. Why did employers add it?
2. A drug benefit is an even more recent addition to coverage by the Medicare program (Part D, 2003). Why didn't Medicare include it back in 1965 when Medicare was passed?
3. Why did the drug benefit in EBHI become so expensive?
4. What employer strategies in managing this high-cost benefit seem to have had the biggest impact?
5. Why have employers traditionally kept their medical benefits separate from their pharmacy benefits?
6. What is (are) the advantage(s) of integrating the medical and pharmacy benefits?

## REFERENCES

1. Robert Cunningham III and Robert Cunningham Jr. *The Blues: A History of the Blue Cross and Blue Shield System* (De Kalb, IL: Northern Illinois University Press, 1997).
2. Office of the Assistant Secretary for Planning and Evaluation. *Report to the President: Prescription Drug Coverage, Spending, Utilization, and Prices* (Washington, DC: ASPE, 2000).
3. Thomas Oliver, Philip Lee, and Helene Lipton. "A Political History of Medicare and Prescription Drug Coverage," *Milbank Q.* 82 (2) (2004): 283-354.

4. Marsha Gold, Mark Joffe, Timothy Kennedy, et al. "Pharmacy Benefits in Health Maintenance Organizations," *Health Aff.* 8 (3) (1989). Available online: https://www.healthaffairs.org/doi/full/10.1377/hlthaff.8.3.182. Accessed on August 4, 2020.

5. Elizabeth Dietz. "Trends in Employer-Provided Prescription-Drug Coverage," *Monthly Labor Review* (August 2004): 37-45.

6. Medicaid, by contrast, did not make drug reimbursement mandatory, but all states elected to include outpatient drug coverage. Private insurers tended to follow the lead of Medicaid in setting their own drug coverage policies. Kathleen Gondek. "Prescription Drug Payment Policy: Past, Present, and Future," *Health Care Financ Rev.* 15 (3) (1994): 1-7.

7. Drug Channels. *The 2018 Economic Report on U.S. Pharmacies and Pharmacy Benefit Managers*. Available online: https://www.drugchannels.net/2018/02/new-2018-economic-report-on-us.html. Accessed on November 13, 2020.

8. The 2018 survey respondents included 466 plan sponsors representing more than 85 million members. Not all respondents provided demographic information, but results are reported for those who did complete this section of the survey. As shown in Figure 40, employers constitute 68% of the respondents, followed by health plans (26%) and union groups (6%). For respondents reporting group size, the median size group represented in the survey was 8,100 members, with a mean of 184,540 (minimum = 5; maximum = 5 million). PBMs with more than 20 million lives include sponsors with a significantly higher mean number of lives (231,769) compared to PBMs with 20 million or fewer lives (25,249). Respondents represented a range of job titles, including pharmacy benefits director (26%), pharmacy benefits manager (15%), and vice president (12%). The primary source for this research was the proprietary database of drug benefit decision makers developed and maintained by PBMI. This database was supplemented with client lists voluntarily provided by PBMs who chose to participate in the sampling process. PBMI conducted its PBM customer satisfaction survey of employers from June 11 to July 9, 2018. PBM employees, as well as brokers and consultants, were excluded from the survey. The survey sample included 466 benefit leaders representing employers providing drug benefit coverage for more than 85 million covered members. As in past years, results for PBMs with more than 20 million reported members and PBMs with 20 million or fewer reported members are presented separately.

9. Employers may also choose to work with a coalition or other group purchasing organization. Coalitions and group purchasing organizations are entities that leverage group purchasing and contracting to obtain better pricing and terms than an individual member of the coalition/group might be able to secure on their own. They may be employer-led, consultant-led, or organized by common interest, industry, or geography. As shown in PBMI Figure 5 (data not presented here), 27% reported that they purchase their PBM services via one of these organizations. This is an increase from the 21% reporting use in 2017. No differences were seen by employer size. Other data suggest that the percentage of employers using such coalitions is smaller (10% or less), with greater use by large employers (5,000+ workers). Drug Channels. *The 2018 Economic Report on U.S. Pharmacies and Pharmacy Benefit Managers.* Exhibit 73: 108. Available online: https://www.drugchannels.net/2018/02/new-2018-economic-report-on-us.html. Accessed on November 13, 2020.

10. Ed Silverman. "Employers Are Planning How to Blunt the Cost of Gene Therapies, Pricey New Specialty Drugs," *Stat+* (August 27, 2020). Available online: https://www.statnews.com/pharmalot/2020/08/27/employers-gene-therapy-drug-prices-insurance/. Accessed on November 13, 2020.

11. Drug Channels. *The 2018 Economic Report on U.S. Pharmacies and Pharmacy Benefit Managers*: 106. Available online: https://www.drugchannels.net/2018/02/new-2018-economic-report-on-us.html. Accessed on November 13, 2020.

12. It is common for there to be different tiers for generic, preferred, and nonpreferred drugs.

13. Drug Channels. *The 2018 Economic Report on U.S. Pharmacies and Pharmacy Benefit Managers*: 107. Available online: https://www.drugchannels.net/2018/02/new-2018-economic-report-on-us.html. Accessed on November 13, 2020.

14. Pharmacy Benefit Management Institute. *Pharmacy Benefit Manager Customer Satisfaction Report 2018*. Available online: https://www.pbmi.com/ItemDetail?iProductCode=CSR_2018&Category=CSR. Accessed on January 19, 2020.

15. Drug Channels. *The 2018 Economic Report on U.S. Pharmacies and Pharmacy Benefit Managers.* Exhibit 74: 111. Available online: https://www.drugchannels.net/2018/02/new-2018-economic-report-on-us.html. Accessed on November 13, 2020.

16. The PBMI survey respondents encompassed 273 benefit leaders representing an estimated 61.6 million covered lives. Respondents included employers, unions, or the person designated to provide responses on their behalf, such as their health plan representative. All respondents offer prescription drug benefits for active employees. To qualify for the survey, respondents had to report being responsible for the organization's prescription drug benefit. Respondents reporting retiree only, workers' compensation, and publicly covered groups (ie, Medicare, Medicaid) were excluded from this survey. All 273 respondents of this year's *Trends in Drug Benefit Design* report

stated that they were responsible for managing the drug benefit for their organization. This group of primarily human resources professionals manages the challenging job of working through both the strategic considerations and budget implications of an ever-changing drug benefit landscape. More than three-quarters (76%) reported they worked directly for the employer who sponsored the drug benefit. The remaining 24% were employed by the employer's health plan (21%) or by a union, union health fund, broker, coalition or group purchasing organization, consulting company, or third-party administrator.

17. Pharmacy Benefits Management Institute. *Trends in Drug Benefit Design 2018* (Plano, TX: PBMI, 2018).

18. Drug Channels. *The 2018 Economic Report on U.S. Pharmacies and Pharmacy Benefit Managers.* Available online: https://www.drugchannels.net/2018/02/new-2018-economic-report-on-us.html. Accessed on November 13, 2020.

19. Adam J. Fein. *The 2018 Economic Report on U.S. Pharmacies and Pharmacy Benefit Managers* (Philadelphia, PA: Drug Channels Institute, 2018): 126.

20. Adam J. Fein. *The 2018 Economic Report on U.S. Pharmacies and Pharmacy Benefit Managers* (Philadelphia, PA: Drug Channels Institute, 2018), Exhibit 85: 127.

21. Adam J. Fein. *The 2018 Economic Report on U.S. Pharmacies and Pharmacy Benefit Managers* (Philadelphia, PA: Drug Channels Institute, 2018): 135.

22. Another pricing metric is the maximum allowable cost (MAC) price. MAC prices represent the maximum payment amounts for generic medications. Because they provide consistent pricing for generic drugs of the same strength and dosage made by multiple manufacturers (eg, multisource generics), MAC prices offer an important source of discounts for plan sponsors. PBMs generally consider their MAC lists to be proprietary, and it is common for PBMs to use different MAC lists within their book of business. Like AWP, there is no standard definition for MAC.

23. Andrew Ross Sorkin and Michael J. de la Merced. "Drug Benefit Unit in $4.7 Billion Deal" (April 13, 2009). Available online: https://www.nytimes.com/2009/04/14/business/14deal.html. Accessed on February 3, 2020.

24. Drug Channels. *The 2018 Economic Report on U.S. Pharmacies and Pharmacy Benefit Managers.* Exhibit 85: 127. Available online: https://www.drugchannels.net/2018/02/new-2018-economic-report-on-us.html. Accessed on November 13, 2020.

25. Gerard Vondeling, Qi Cao, Maarten Postma, et al. "The Impact of Patent Expiry on Drug Prices: A Systematic Literature Review," *Appl Health Econ Health Policy.* 16 (2018): 653-660.

26. Neeraj Sood, Tiffany Shih, Karen Van Nuys, et al. *The Flow of Money Through the Pharmaceutical Distribution System* (Los Angeles, CA: University of Southern California, Leonard D. Schaeffer Center for Health Policy and Economics, 2017).

27. Pharmacy Benefit Management Institute. *2017 Trends in Drug Benefit Design* (Plano TX: PBMI, 2017).

28. Drug Channels. *Employers Are Getting More Rebates Than Ever—But Sharing Little With Their Employees* (January 18, 2018). Available online: https://www.drugchannels.net/2018/01/employers-are-getting-more-rebates-than.html. Accessed on February 1, 2020.

29. IQVIA. "Patient Affordability Part One" (May 18, 2018). Available online: https://www.iqvia.com/locations/united-states/library/case-studies/patient-affordability-part-one. Accessed on August 4, 2020.

30. Drug Channels. *Employers Slowly Warm to Point-of-Sale Rebates—But Most Move Faster for Insulin (rerun)* (September 19, 2019). Available online: https://www.drugchannels.net/2019/09/employers-slowly-warm-to-point-of-sale.html. Accessed on February 1, 2020.

31. Drug Channels. *More Formulary Exclusions for Many Drug Therapies.* Available online: https://www.drugchannels.net/2011/10/more-formulary-exclusions-for-many-drug.html. Accessed on February 2, 2020.

32. Drug Channels. *If Employers Are So Unhappy With Their PBMs, Why Can't They Change the Model?* (November 15, 2017). Available online: https://www.drugchannels.net/2017/11/if-employers-are-so-unhappy-with-their.html. Accessed on February 1, 2020.

33. Drug Channels. *A New Peek at HMO-PBM Relationships* (December 5, 2012). Available online: https://www.drugchannels.net/2012/12/a-new-peek-at-hmo-pbm-relationships.html. Accessed on February 3, 2020.

34. Health Transformation Alliance. Available online: http://www.htahealth.com. Accessed on August 4, 2020.

35. Midwest Business Group on Health. *Drawing a Line in the Sand: Employers Must Rethink Pharmacy Benefit Strategies.* No date. Available online: https://www.specialtyrxtoolkit.org/sites/www.specialtyrxtoolkit.org/files/assets/SP%20Line%20in%20the%20Sand%20Final%20.pdf. Accessed on February 1, 2020.

36. *Health and Well-Being Touchstone Survey Results 2019* (PriceWaterhouseCoopers, June 2019). Available online: https://www.pwc.com/us/en/services/hr-management/assets/pwc-touchstone-2019.pdf. Accessed on February 3, 2020.

37. Litigation available online: https://krcomplexlit.com/wp-content/uploads/2017/09/Pltfs-Consolidated-Complaint.pdf. Accessed on August 6, 2020.

# Private Health Insurance and Managed Care Organizations

17

## TAXONOMY OF INSURANCE

There are 2 main branches in the US health insurance industry: the private sector and the public sector. These are comprised of the following:

**Private Insurers (voluntary health insurance)**

- Blue Cross/Blue Shield plans
- Commercial for-profit insurers
- Self-funded employers
- Individuals/self-pay

**Public Insurers (social health insurance)**

- Medicare
- Medicaid
- Other public programs (State Children's Health Insurance Program)
- Veterans Administration, Department of Defense, Public Health Service

This chapter deals with the private insurers, who can also offer plans that cover many of the beneficiaries of public insurance programs. Chapters 18 and 19 deal with Medicare and Medicaid, respectively.

## WHAT DO INSURERS DO?

Insurers perform several core functions in the healthcare value chain. They insulate their "members" (enrollees) against the unexpected burden of medical care costs; they contract with providers; they pay providers' claims; they offer a variety of member services; they design, price, and then sell the insurance product; and they assume the underwriting risk for that product. Insurance is thus a mechanism to protect people from risk. Risk is defined as the possibility of substantial financial loss from an event whose probability of occurrence is relatively small in the case of a specific individual. For example, hospitalization is a high-loss, low-probability event, whereas dental care is a low-loss, high-probability event. That explains why there is more coverage of the former than the latter. Hospitalization is also more rare and riskier than a physician office visit, which helps to explain why hospitalization coverage has historically outstripped physician coverage: Between 1940 and 1965, the percentage of the population with hospital coverage rose from 9.3% to 80.6%, whereas the percentage with physician coverage rose from 2.3% to 58.8%.

A more fundamental answer to what insurers do is that their insurance coverage enables enrollees to access and use the healthcare system and to develop a regular source of care. All of these have demonstrated beneficial downstream effects on patients' health status and survival.[1]

An insurer, also known as a "health plan" or a "payer," is the firm writing the insurance. It is also known as a "third-party payer" that intermediates and links the provider with the patient (the first 2 parties). Reimbursement is what providers get paid by the health plan for treating the patient. In the private sector, health

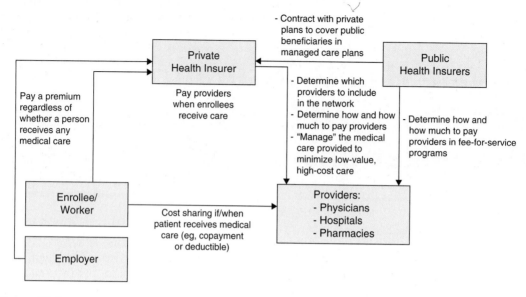

**Figure 17-1** • Schematic on What a Health Insurer Does. (Source: Sean Nicholson, Cornell University.)

insurers are intermediaries in the healthcare value chain that link (1) employers and their employees with (2) provider networks who render care (Figure 17-1). The insurer receives a (usually monthly) premium from the employer to cover the care of employees and then uses those monies to process and pay the claims submitted by network providers for treating them. The insurer also determines which providers to include in the network, how much to pay them and which payment methods to use, and how to "manage" the medical care provided to minimize low-value, high-cost care.[2]

## BRIEF HISTORY: RISE OF HEALTH INSURANCE

The insurance sector got its start in the 1930s with the establishment of the first Blue Cross plans (for hospital services) and Blue Shield plans (for physician services). The first hospital insurance plan was developed by Baylor University Hospital (1929) to cover Dallas teachers for a prepaid amount of 50 cents a month for hospital care when needed. The Baylor prepaid model was quickly copied by others in the 1930s. By 1933, the American Hospital Association (AHA) adopted its own approach for developing hospital insurance, rejecting the Baylor model, which limited consumer choice to only

1 hospital. The AHA sought to create insurance plans that were nonprofit, emphasized the public welfare, and limited themselves to "dignified promotion" (no advertising). As more local hospitals and communities initiated plans, the AHA's Special Commission on Hospital Service, created in 1937, determined that it would offer membership to any nonprofit organization that met specific standards. This marked the founding of Blue Cross. The first Blue Cross plan was established in 1932 in Sacramento; by 1937, there were 26 such plans with more than 600,000 members.

With the growing public reliance on prepaid hospital plans, there also rose a demand for coverage for medical services. Physicians, however, were more resistant than hospitals to the concept of prepaid plans, proposals for national health insurance, the threat of hospital insurance, and the threat prepaid plans posed to the patient-physician relationship. Yet the public continued to feel the financial burdens of paying for medical care that they otherwise could not afford. In response to growing public pressure throughout the country, select physicians and medical groups began to develop special contracts with employers and employees to cover medical services. The California Medical Association launched its own voluntary prepayment plan by 1938-1939, with 20,000 enrollees and 5,000 physicians.

The American Medical Association (AMA) began to seriously consider, rather than outright resist, the concept of prepaid medical care; in 1946, the National Association of Blue Shield Plans was launched. The California Blue Shield plan organized as a nonprofit organization, like its sister hospital plans. Soon thereafter, physician plans quickly flourished in other states and became substantially similar to the Blue Cross plans, giving rise to Blue Shield.[3] The Blue Shield plans preempted the hospital-oriented Blue Cross plans from entering the physician services space, which they were loath to do anyway.[4]

Several features of Blue Cross plans are noteworthy given their endurance over time and imprint on the industry. Blue Cross plans were originally nonprofit plans and exempt from state insurance laws and state premium taxes. The national association of Blue Cross plans also mandated no competition among Blue Cross plans (using the Blue Cross name), assigning them an exclusive geographic market area to serve. Blue Cross plans initially paid hospitals their charges on a fee-for-service (FFS) basis and allowed Blue Cross enrollees freedom of choice among community hospitals, with no patient steerage or restricted networks. They also charged all residents in a community the same premium ("community rating") regardless of the enrollee's health status. Finally, it is important to point out that the Blue Cross plans offered a "service benefit," which guaranteed full payment of all treatment and services specified in the subscriber's contract. Often, these benefits only covered hospitalization expenses (eg, room, board, nursing, ancillary services) and the services of surgeons rendered in the hospital; they did not always cover outpatient care. Nevertheless, their subscribers developed a strong preference for this type of benefit. Moreover, they had maximum limits and did not cover catastrophic expenses.[5]

Blue Shield plans were hampered in setting service benefits due to physicians' traditional fee-setting practices. Data from 1947 indicate that only 4 plans offered service contracts, while 23 offered "indemnity coverage" (ie, guaranteed amount of cash reimbursement) in the event of a covered illness, and the remaining 17 offered a mixture of the two. They typically covered only major surgery and hospitalization due to serious illness.

Blue Cross and Blue Shield plans worked out a variety of arrangements for working together. In some cases, they were totally independent; in other cases, they retained separate governing boards but cooperated on enrollment; in still other cases, they retained separate boards but employed a common staff. Eventually, Blue Cross merged with Blue Shield at the national level, but their plans often remained separate at the local level.

It is also important to note that Blue Cross and Blue Shield were both covered under employer-based health insurance plans but paid hospitals and physicians separately. Figure 17-2 provides a flow chart of how Blue Cross and Blue Shield worked in tandem when a patient needed care.

The Blue Cross plans were quite popular and grew substantially in enrollment during the 1930s; the Blue Shield plans, which formed during the late 1930s, saw substantial growth during the 1940s. The growth of both was aided by economic growth in the late 1930s and then falling unemployment from 17% in 1939 to 1% in 1944 as part of the wartime effort. This bolstered the available pool of labor force participants eligible for insurance coverage. Blue Cross enrollment rose from 4.4 million in 1940 to 15.7 million by 1945 and then 24.2 million in 1947. Blue Shield had 4.4 million enrollees in 1946.

The rapid growth of the Blues attracted competitors. The commercial insurers (who were for-profit) who sold life and casualty coverage to employee groups saw health insurance as a new market to enter. They began to enter the market to compete with the Blues in several ways. First, like some Blue Shield plans, they offered an indemnity benefit. Second, they sometimes offered "1-stop shopping" by combining health coverage with life and casualty coverage. Third, they priced their coverage on the basis of "experience rating" (ie, charging lower premiums for healthier risks who used less medical care). Their offerings were also quite popular. Between 1940 and 1946, they increased their hospitalization enrollees from 3.7 million to 14.3 million and their surgical indemnity coverage from 2.3 million to 10.6 million.[6]

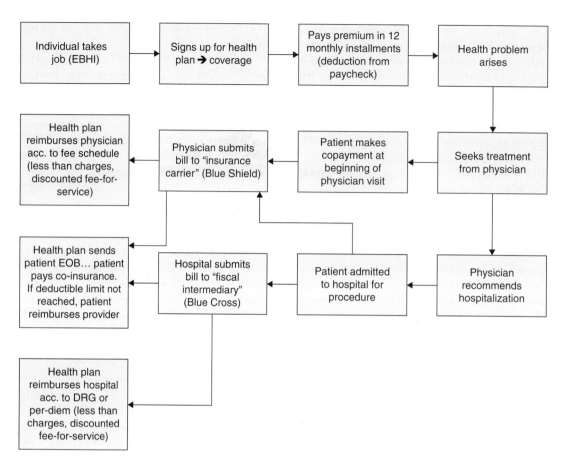

**Figure 17-2** • Fee-for-Service Flows in Blue Cross and Blue Shield. acc., According; EBHI, Employer-Based Health Insurance; EOB, Explanation of Benefits.

Overall, health insurance became an increasingly popular product with growing market penetration, rising from 10% of the population with hospital coverage in 1940 to nearly 70% by 1955. During the 1950s, the number of people with hospital insurance rose from 77 million to 132 million; the number with surgical coverage grew from 54 million to 121 million. Blue Cross had 50% of the market in 1958; Blue Shield had 44%.

The commercial insurers' practice of experience rating threatened to "cherry pick" the healthiest enrollee groups from the Blues plans. This forced the Blues plans to switch away from community rating to experience rating. By 1957, 16 of 77 Blue Cross plans used experience rating, and another 26 used it in conjunction with community rating.

Increasing insurance coverage meant greater hospital utilization and hospital costs; much in the manner of the healthcare quadrilemma (see

Chapter 2), consumers demanded richer benefit packages to cover the costs they were now incurring. The commercial insurers offered a new, competing product during the 1950s: major medical insurance. This product extended the traditional Blue Cross/Blue Shield coverage to include care provided outside of the hospital by doctors, outpatient procedures, diagnostic tests, catastrophic care, and higher maximums—hence the term *major medical*. It thus offered more comprehensive coverage (up to $10,000 in expenses). The product was introduced to meet the demands of particular customers (eg, labor unions). However, in order to compete with the Blues on price, the major medical plans resorted to a tool used by auto insurers—the deductible—which reduced the dollar liability of the insurer, reduced the cost of the premium to the insured, and (hopefully) reduced "moral hazard" (purchased insurance gets used). The major medical insurance product was initially quite popular among employers who liked the lower premiums and cost sharing, but not so much among the employees who did not like the cost sharing. Major medical plans grew in enrollment from 100,000 in 1951 to 34 million by 1961, and then to 39 million by the late 1960s. Such plans were often offered as a supplement to basic Blue Cross policies but began to steal market share away from the Blues. As a result, the Blues began to adopt cost sharing.

The Medicare and Medicaid legislation enacted in 1965 included coverage of doctors, services, outpatient care, drugs, diagnostic tests, and ambulance services. To control the costs of Medicare, patients were charged a deductible. Both practices—extended benefits and patient cost sharing—had now been introduced into the market by major medical and Medicare coverage. The Blues plans would follow suit.

As a result of Medicare and Medicaid, healthcare costs skyrocketed beyond their sharp rise resulting from the expansion of private insurance. In 1973, President Nixon signed the HMO Act, which legitimated the health maintenance organization (HMO) model and provided planning grants for their development. HMOs were viewed as a cost containment vehicle that relied on market competition rather than regulation. HMOs, as noted in earlier chapters, were already in existence (the early prepaid group models like Kaiser) but now got a lift. They expanded their numbers and enrollments in the 1970s and 1980s, posing a competitive challenge to both the Blues plans and the commercial insurers. Both nonprofit and for-profit insurers responded in 2 ways: First, they developed chains (multistate Blues plans, national commercial plans); second, they developed their own HMO (and preferred provider organization [PPO]) models in the late 1980s and early 1990s. The managed care revolution was on!

## CHANGING ROLE OF INSURERS: FROM INDEMNITY TO MANAGED CARE

Through the 1970s and into the early 1980s, most of the insured, nonelderly population in the United States were enrolled in indemnity plans that paid providers claims (with little oversight) and engaged with their members on a minimal basis. Also known as "FFS plans," they allowed members free choice of physician and hospital, used little cost sharing (beyond small deductibles), and collected providers' claims data without analyzing them. The insurer paid a predetermined percentage of the physician's "usual, customary, and reasonable" (UCR) charge for a given service, leaving the enrollee to pay the balance.

As noted in prior chapters, this situation began to dramatically change in the late 1980s and 1990s with the support of employers for a new type of health plan—what is now collectively known as the "managed care organization" (MCO). The contrast between the indemnity and MCO plans could not have been starker (Figure 17-3). The essence of managed care can be summed up as a system to manage the quality of healthcare, access to that healthcare, and (in particular) the cost of that care. Common denominators across the various managed care plans included (1) a network of contracted providers (not every doctor or hospital); (2) limitation on benefits for using noncontracted providers (those not in the network); (3) methods to measure utilization, referral patterns, and quality of care; and (4) programs to improve the health status of members. Overall, the focus was to reduce the underuse, overuse, or misuse of medical services (see Figure 2-4).

The managed care plans sit in a wider value chain of activity, depicted in Figure 17-4. They contract with employers, individuals, and public purchasers of healthcare (Medicare, Medicaid) as well as with providers and the integrated delivery networks of providers covered in Chapter 12. Managed care plans can also choose to outsource certain functions (eg, the pharmacy benefit managers [PBMs] covered in Chapter 16, disease management) to carve-out vendors or perform them in-house.

## TYPES OF MANAGED CARE HEALTH PLANS

The table on page 326 provides a thumbnail sketch of the major managed care plans.[7]

| | Indemnity | Managed Care |
| --- | --- | --- |
| Provider access | • Any healthcare professional provides care | • Network of credentialed healthcare professionals provide care |
| | • Unlimited access to specialty providers | • Restricted access to specialty providers |
| Covered benefits | • Coverage for acute illness or injury only | • Coverage for primary and preventive care as well |
| Coordination of care | • Multiple providers deliver care without knowledge of total patient health | • PCP usually designated to manage and coordinate all patient care |
| Provider relations | • Relationship limited to reimbursing providers for services rendered | • Extensive relationships with providers—practice management tools and incentives to manage care |
| Quality management | • No health promotion programs | • Programs to encourage patients to maintain good health |
| | • Collection of claims data only | • Tracking and analysis of data on costs, utilization, and quality |
| Cost control | • Limited financial controls | • Financial controls on care |
| | • Assumption of all financial risk | • Some transfer of risk to providers |
| | • Retrospective audit of claims | • Prospective review of treatment |
| Locus of risk | • Payer | • Provider |
| Hospital and specialists | • Revenue center | • Cost center |
| | • Piece work | • Fixed income |
| Provider incentive | • Maximize utilization | • Manage utilization |
| | • Individual | • Team |
| Payer concern | • Overutilization | • Underutilization |
| | • Small provider groups | • Large integrated groups |
| PCPs | • Less influence | • More influence |
| | Less relative income | More relative income |

**Figure 17-3** • Indemnity Versus Managed Care. PCP, Primary Care Physician.

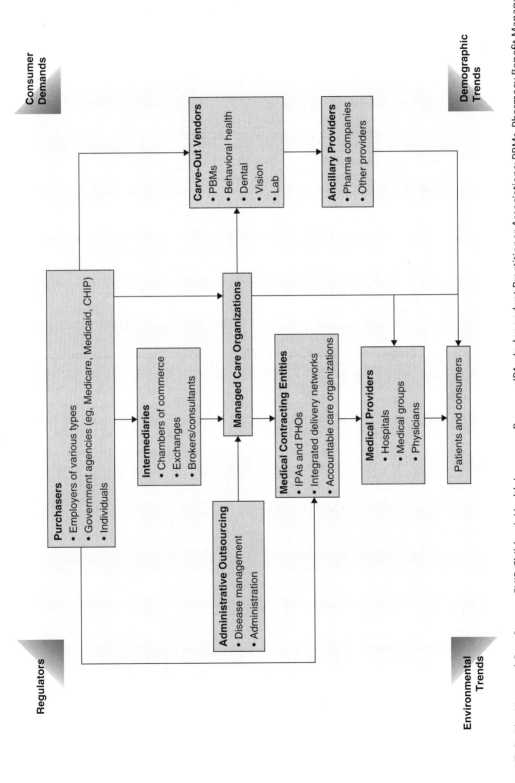

**Figure 17-4 •** The Managed Care System. CHIP, Children's Health Insurance Program; IPAs, Independent Practitioner Associations; PBMs, Pharmacy Benefit Managers; PHOs, Patient-Hospital Organizations. (Source: Brad Fluegel, Presentation to Wharton School, 2017.)

| Type of Plan | Description |
|---|---|
| Health maintenance organization (HMO) | An HMO plan provides coverage for healthcare services received from providers directly employed by the plan or contracted with it. HMO plans generally require enrollees to select a primary care physician who manages their care and serves as a gatekeeper for other health services: Enrollees must obtain a referral from their primary care physician before receiving care from another in-network provider. An HMO plan typically does not cover any costs associated with services obtained outside of its network. For services obtained in the network, the enrollee incurs minimal cost sharing. Provider networks are small relative to the other models. |
| Point-of-service (POS) | A POS plan is similar to an HMO in that an enrollee is typically required to designate a primary care physician and obtain a referral prior to receiving care from a network specialist. Unlike an HMO plan, a POS plan provides benefits for services received out of network, although usually with higher cost sharing. It is basically an HMO with a parachute. |
| Exclusive provider organization (EPO) | An EPO plan provides coverage through a network of contracted providers. An EPO plan allows enrollees greater flexibility to visit in-network providers than do HMO plans: EPO plans do not require designation of a primary care physician or referrals to specialists. But, like an HMO, an EPO plan does not provide any coverage for care received out of network. |
| Preferred provider organization (PPO) | A PPO plan provides coverage through a network of contracted providers that is usually much larger than the network found in HMOs. PPO plans generally provide enrollees the greatest level of flexibility to visit a desired provider. Plans do not require designation of a primary care physician or referrals to specialists, and they do include coverage for care received outside of the network, although usually with higher cost sharing. The reason why the providers in such models are called "preferred" is that they have voluntarily elected to receive lower reimbursements from the managed care plan in exchange for seeing their enrollees (and hopefully garnering higher patient volumes). |
| High-deductible health plan (HDHP) | An HDHP is a plan with a high deductible and maximum out-of-pocket limits as defined by the Internal Revenue Service (IRS). Other than certain preventive services, all medical care must be paid for out of pocket until the deductible is met. The HDHP network can be based on either a PPO or POS chassis. They can have a savings option (health savings account [HSA]) or a health reimbursement arrangement (HRA). The HDHP differs from the above models in terms of having specific IRS guidelines governing the tax deductibility of the HSA, as well as limited first-dollar coverage of the employees' health expenses. |

Source: Justin Giovannelli, Kevin Lucia, Sabrina Corlette, et al. "Regulation of Health Plan Provider Networks," Health Affairs – Health Policy Brief (July 28, 2016).

These plans are similar on some important dimensions, including the use of defined provider networks, the use of medical management tools, and the discounting of the fees that providers charge. These plans also differ on many important dimensions, including the use of primary care physicians (PCPs) who act as gatekeepers to seeing specialists, the methods by which they pay providers in the network, and their reimbursement of care rendered by non-network providers. For example, the HMO and point-of-service (POS) plans are most likely to employ gatekeeping PCPs, to use capitation and other risk-sharing mechanisms to pay their physicians, and to have lower tolerance for out-of-network care.

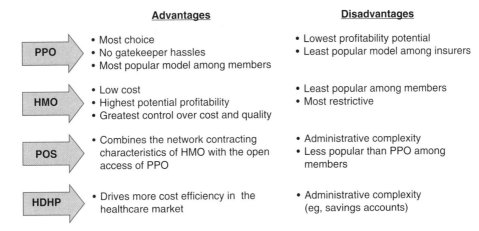

**Figure 17-5** • Managed Care Organization Health Plans: Advantages and Disadvantages. HDHP, High-Deductible Health Plan; HMO, Health Maintenance Organization; POS, Point-of-Service; PPO, Preferred Provider Organization. (Source: Brad Fluegel, Presentation to Wharton School 2017.)

There is a major trade-off taking place as one moves from indemnity plans to PPOs, POS plans, and then to HMOs: The enrollee gives up open provider networks and free choice of provider in exchange for lower premiums (the iron triangle: access vs cost). There are, nevertheless, trade-offs involved in all of these managed care options. The advantages and disadvantages of each are portrayed in Figure 17-5.

Turning back to Figure 15-5, the HMO model achieved its zenith in terms of market penetration in 1996, with enrollments increasing throughout the decade. The PPO model gained ascendance in the late 1990s in the wake of the consumer backlash against HMOs and their restrictive policies regarding narrow provider networks (who you could see) and benefits (what services were covered). Although the PPO premium was higher than the HMO or POS premium, consumers wanted greater access and were willing to pay for it (part of the iron triangle). PPOs also fit with the robust economy and full employment model of the late 1990s. Employers wanted workers and were willing to offer the open-network PPO plans that consumers wanted.

Although the PPO model is still the most prevalent, it has ceded market share to the high-deductible health plan (HDHP) model. The HDHP model has its roots in (1) the health reimbursement accounts (HRAs) that were first included in benefit plans in the 1960s to reimburse employees for those health expenses outside traditional employer-sponsored coverage; (2) the Internal Revenue Service's creation of a health version of the flexible spending account

(FSA) in the 1970s to address tax issues arising from increasing deductibles and copays, which began in the 1950s—a precursor to the health savings account (HSA); (3) the growing consumerism movement that burgeoned in the 1970s; and (4) the Health Insurance Portability and Accountability Act (HIPAA, 1996), which allowed demonstrations of "medical savings accounts" (MSAs), another forerunner of the HSA. The HDHP model was originally introduced in the early 2000s under its former moniker, the consumer-driven health plan (CDHP). Federal legislation (Medicare Prescription Drug, Improvement, and Modernization Act of 2003) then encouraged the spread of the HDHP model. Employers and employees alike viewed the HDHP model favorably because of the lower cost of their premiums compared to the other models. Enrollment in HDHPs with an HSA rose from 4.2% to 18.9% between 2007 and 2017; enrollment in HDHPs without an HSA rose from 10.6% to 24.5%.

There is considerable irony here. The managed care plans generally offered comprehensive care, hoping to use coverage for physician office visits, prescription drugs, and prevention to avert and/or substitute for the more expensive types of care, such as hospitalization and emergency department (ED) visits. HMOs and PPOs included first-dollar coverage; HMOs had minimal cost sharing, whereas PPOs traded off higher premiums and more cost sharing for wider provider access. The HDHPs, by contrast, were high-deductible insurance—a return to the past practice of major medical plans.

## Types of HMOs

Not only are there types of MCOs, there are subtypes of the HMO.[8] In the early 1970s, there were 4 main HMO types: staff, group, independent practitioner association (IPA), and network. The staff model is characterized by HMO ownership of the delivery system facilities (eg, a hospital) and the employment of salaried physicians who serve the HMO members exclusively. In the group model, the HMO contracts with (rather than employs) a medical group to serve the HMO's members; typically, the medical group serves the HMO's members exclusively and are paid on either a capitation or FFS basis. In the IPA model, the HMO contracts with individual FFS physicians to provide services to HMO members in the physicians' private offices. These physicians are generally paid on a discounted FFS basis, while some could be capitated (eg, West Coast IPAs). They may also be at financial risk to the extent of a withhold from their FFS payments. The network model combines both group practices and individual physician practices, thereby maximizing its geographic footprint.

The rapid growth in the number of HMOs occurred primarily through the development of new IPA and network-model HMOs that contracted with medical groups that serve both FFS and prepaid patients. The development of a staff model or group model HMO that contracts with a medical group to serve exclusively prepaid patients required substantial capital investment for facilities and physician recruitment and salaries. In contrast, the development of an IPA or network required minimal capital investment because the physicians' existing private offices are to be used for serving prepaid patients.

## HMO Versus PPO

For some years dating back to the late 1980s, the HMO and PPO models were the 2 dominant forms of managed care. It is instructive to point out their differences, since both models are used in covering the Medicare Advantage population (see Chapter 18). How do HMOs work? HMOs wield purchasing power over providers by using "selective contracting" (ie, contract with only a small subset of local providers) and thereby concentrated buying power. They compensate physicians based on capitation, thereby rewarding them for efficiency and parsimony in patient treatment. With regard to hospitals, HMOs employ prior authorization and pre-utilization review of patient stays in order to keep patients out of the hospital and decrease admissions; they also use concurrent and retrospective utilization review to decrease length of stay (if patients do get admitted) and deny payments for excessive stays. Their approach helped to retard diffusion of costly new technologies in local communities. The rise of HMO payments in a physician's patient panel also exerted "spillovers" in terms of how they treated their FFS patients. Overall, HMOs saved on hospital admissions, lengths of stay, and costs without harming quality or leading to adverse outcomes.[9]

By contrast, PPOs incur higher costs and utilization. They have broader provider networks and thus less ability to steer patients. Without steerage, they have less bargaining power and thus cannot get the providers they contract with to accept the low reimbursements that HMO providers accept. Moreover, their open networks attract higher-risk, higher-cost enrollees, who self-select into PPOs. So why were PPOs so much more popular over time? They gave enrollees greater access and choice of provider.

## MANAGED CARE LINES OF BUSINESS

MCOs not only offer various products (health plans), but they also offer them to various customers—known as "lines of business." These lines are usually broken out by insurers into (1) group and specialty, (2) retail, and (3) healthcare services. These include the following:

**Group and Specialty Line of Business**
- Fully insured risk contracts with employers (large group, small group)
- Federal Employees Health Benefits Program (FEHBP)
- Administrative services only (ASO) contracts with employers
- ASO contracts with Defense Department to cover TriCare (active military dependents)

**Retail Line of Business**
- Medicare Advantage (HMOs and PPOs for the elderly enrolled in Medicare)
- Medicare stand-alone prescription drug plans (PDPs)
- Medicare supplement plans (MediGap)
- State Medicaid programs
- Individual market

### Healthcare Services Line of Business

- Predictive modeling and informatics services
- Provider care delivery (owned or allied medical practices)
- Clinical care services (home-based care management, population health)
- Wellness services (eg, employee assistance programs)
- Pharmacy benefit management and mail-order pharmacy

MCOs thus offer a complex, matrix-based menu of health plans to a host of customers (Figure 17-6). Moreover, because "all healthcare is local" (see Chapter 2), these plans are sold in different markets (metropolitan areas).

In late 2018, 265 million Americans had health insurance. Over time, much of the MCO's business has shifted from employers to public managed care plans offered to Medicare and Medicaid enrollees. Among employers, the MCO's business has shifted from fully insured to self-insured customers (ASO contracts). Instead of taking risk on these contracts, insurers receive fees from employers for providing administrative services, such as the following:

- Adjudication of claims and benefits processing
- Eligibility and enrollment determination and reporting
- Communications and customer service
- Employer and government report preparation
- Assistance with stop-loss coverage
- Actuarial and underwriting advice
- Cost-containment services

Overall, the employer ASO market accounted for the largest share (46%) of health enrollment during the fourth quarter of 2018, followed by the employer risk market (22%; including FEHBP), Medicaid (19%), Medicare Advantage (8%), and the individual market (5%). The fastest growing segment has been Medicare Advantage (+3.6% from 2017-2018), with the employer ASO market growing slightly (+0.7%); the largest decrease has been in the individual market (–6.7%), due to declines in enrollment on the Patient Protection and Affordable Care Act (PPACA) market exchanges (see later discussion and Chapter 19). The absolute enrollment numbers and their changes between 2017 and 2018 are presented in Figure 17-7.[10] Between 2010 and 2016, the proportion of health plan revenues from premiums and ASO contracts coming from the government rose from 44% to 59%.[11]

The distribution of health plans by enrollment size (for fully insured and self-insured plans in 2016) is presented in Figure 17-8.[12] Data are presented for 56,000 plans that covered more than 75 million participants, based

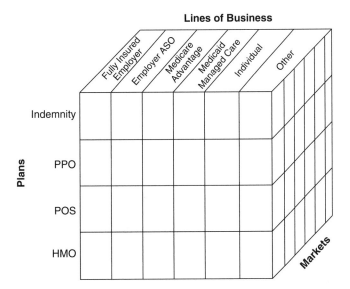

**Figure 17-6** • Lines of Business. ASO, Administrative Services Only; HMO, Health Maintenance Organization; POS, Point-of-Service; PPO, Preferred Provider Organization.

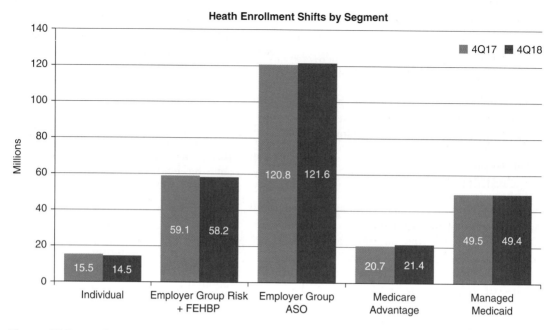

**Figure 17-7** • Heath Enrollment Shifts by Segment. ASO, Administrative Services Only; FEHBP, Federal Employees Health Benefits Program. (Source: Mark Farrah Associates. "Health Insurance Enrollment Trends for Year-End 2018." https://www.markfarrah.com/mfa-briefs/health-insurance-enrollment-trends-for-year-end-2018/.)

on having at least 100 enrollees. The data show that the majority of plans have medium-sized enrollments (100-500 members), whereas the majority of enrollments are in large plans (5,000+ members). Of these 56,000 plans, 42% were self-insured, 51% were fully insured, and 7% had a mix (eg, employer offered both a fully insured HMO and a self-insured PPO); enrollees were distributed as 46% self-insured, 18% fully insured, and 37% mixed.

| Participants in plan | Plans | Percent | Participants (millions) | Percent |
|---|---|---|---|---|
| 0 | 1,859 | 3.3% | 0 | 0% |
| 1-99 | 3,914 | 7% | 0.2 | 0.2% |
| 100-199 | 18,127 | 32.2% | 2.6 | 3.5% |
| 200-499 | 17,098 | 30.4% | 5.3 | 7.1% |
| 500-999 | 6,520 | 11.6% | 4.5 | 6% |
| 1,000-1,999 | 3,774 | 6.7% | 5.3 | 7.1% |
| 2,000-4,999 | 2,749 | 4.9% | 8.5 | 11.3% |
| 5,000+ | 2,170 | 3.9% | 48.7 | 64.8% |
| **Total** | **56,211** | **100%** | **75.2** | **100%** |

**Figure 17-8** • Distribution of Health Plans by Enrollment Size. (Source: Advanced Analytical Consulting Group. "Self-Insured Health Benefit Plans 2019." https://www.dol.gov/sites/dolgov/files/EBSA/researchers/statistics/retirement-bulletins/annual-report-on-self-insured-group-health-plans-2019-appendix-b.pdf.)

## THE INTERNAL VALUE CHAIN OF A MANAGED CARE ORGANIZATION

A more expansive view of what MCOs do is presented in Figure 17-9, which depicts the health plan's "internal value chain." Starting on the left of the diagram, insurers develop "products" and then price them. These products are the MCO plans that they offer to employers and public sector insurance beneficiaries. The health plans of the past (indemnity, FFS plans) are nearly extinct; today, insurers offer a range of "managed care" plans that seek to manage the quality and cost of care provided. These managed care plans encompass the HMOs, PPOs, POS plans, and exclusive provider organizations (EPOs) described earlier. Insurers also develop the provider networks for the HDHPs described in Chapter 15.

In order to price these products, insurers need to employ actuaries and underwriters. These staff estimate the likely cost of a given plan (based on the utilization of its enrollees) over a future period and then derive an annual premium to cover the plan's cost (medical and administrative) along with a small profit margin. Insurers start with the prior experience of enrollees in a "base period" and then make projections for a future period that capture changes in utilization, unit costs (eg, price increases in provider contracts), service intensity, and population mix. For large group customers (500+ employees), insurers rely on pure "experience rating" to estimate these costs; for smaller groups (100-500 employees), they use a "blended rate" that combines the group's experience with a "manual rate" where there are reliable statistics that can predict future losses.

Insurers then need to market these plans. In the private sector, the market segments include (1) the large group market that serves large employers, (2) the small group market that serves small firms, and (3) the individual market (eg, the self-employed, employees of firms that do not offer insurance, early retirees) and those on the insurance exchanges. Large employers can contract directly with insurers as "national accounts"; smaller employers may use intermediaries such as brokers, consultants, digital insurance companies, and local chambers of commerce to help them find the proper insurance coverage. To attract Medicare Advantage and Medicare Part D (PDP) enrollees, insurers require the use of sales representatives, telemarketing representatives, and brokers to help link them to individual seniors through any number of venues (eg, community centers).

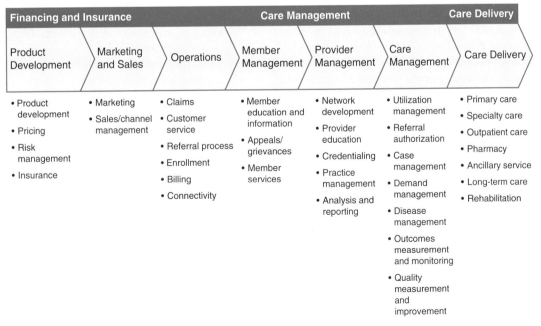

**Figure 17-9** • Value Chain Activities of a Health Plan. (Source: Brad Fluegel, Presentation to Wharton School, 2017.)

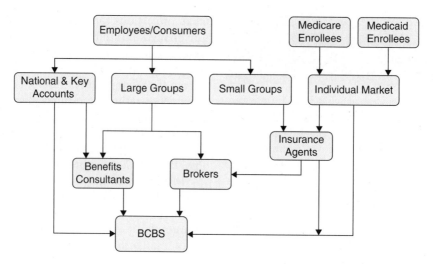

**Figure 17-10** • Health Plans' Downstream Channel Complexity. BCBS, Blue Cross/Blue Shield.

Some insurers also partner with retail chains (eg, Walmart) to market to seniors. Figure 17-10 shows some of the channel complexity facing insurers in their different lines of business.

After marketing and selling the health plan products, insurers then need back-office operations to support them. These include enrollment, claims processing, customer service, referral processes, billing, and connectivity with members. They also need a host of member services that include education, information, and handling of appeals and grievances.

In addition to member management, insurers need personnel and systems for provider management (ie, managing the providers in the networks offered by their health plan products). Management issues concern utilization management, case management, disease management, demand management, referral authorizations, outcomes measurement and monitoring, and quality measurement and improvement. These are briefly defined in the following list:

- **Utilization management:** The evaluation of the medical necessity, appropriateness, and efficiency of the use of healthcare services, procedures, and facilities under the provisions of the health benefits contained in the enrollee's chosen plan. This is usually administered under the auspices of a medical director and includes one or more of the following services: (1) preadmission review; (2) concurrent hospital review; (3) second surgical opinions; (4) specialty and/or out-of-network

referral authorizations; (5) retrospective review of services; (6) bill audit; and (7) remedial action for providers suspected of fraud or noncompliance with utilization review or referral procedures.
- **Case management:** A subset of utilization management that includes the utilization review of high-cost cases, usually by a nurse case manager.
- **Disease management:** Identification of segments of the enrolled population with specific chronic conditions (eg, asthma, diabetes), targeting them for health promotion and prevention efforts, encouraging providers to follow evidence-based protocols in treating them, and developing patient registries for each of these chronic conditions to track the chronically ill.
- **Demand management:** Tools used to moderate patients' demands for (especially expensive) healthcare services. At one extreme, these can include telephone triage and ED nurse screening. At the other extreme, they can include methods used to monitor, direct, or regulate patient referrals from PCPs to specialists.
- **Referral authorization:** Previously known as "precertification," the process by which the enrollee's PCP must authorize a referral to see a specialist or obtain a specific diagnostic test. Found most commonly in HMO and POS models of managed care.
- **Quality measurement and management:** Previously known as quality assessment, this function evaluates quality of care

through structure, process, and outcome measures, as well as takes corrective action for identified deficiencies. In its broadest sense, quality management includes diverse activities such as credentialing of providers, measuring the quality of care they provide, evaluating physician performance on these criteria, disciplining poor performers, continuing education, tracking malpractice claims, collecting grievance information, conducting member satisfaction surveys, and performing facilities review.

- **Outcomes measurement:** A subset of the quality measures that deal with the patient's functional health status, morbidity, and mortality levels.

Finally, some MCOs operate in the "care delivery" business, owning their own hospitals and employing their own physicians (the Kaiser model). Many commercial insurers employed physician networks in the 1980s but quickly exited this business line in the early 1990s due to financial losses. In recent years, the MCOs have returned to this strategy. As noted in Chapter 13, WellPoint acquired CareMore's 26 clinics in California in 2011; Humana acquired a chain of occupational medicine clinics (Concentra) in 2010; and UnitedHealth/Optum acquired the Monarch medical group in 2011 and its network of 425 "affiliated" (eg, employed) physicians.

There are several rationales for these acquisitions. First, the MCOs are positioning themselves for increased enrollment in Medicare Advantage plans and the growth in Medicaid enrollment following the implementation of PPACA in 2014. Second, MCOs want to develop networks to help manage the care of the sickest patients, such as the chronically ill, the dual eligibles, and those with preexisting conditions, who are the target of several initiatives in the PPACA. Third, MCOs believe that the only way to manage risk contracts and satisfy the dictates of value-based contracting is by owning the front end of (ambulatory) care and incentivizing their employed physicians to treat enrollees cost-effectively. Fourth, and finally, MCOs are responding to the threat posed by hospital efforts to develop captive physician networks and accountable care organizations (ACOs) that might have as their real goal limiting insurer contracting options and increasing the prices charged them. Insurers may be

vertically integrating back into the physician market to develop countervailing power and/or avoid being locked out.

## BUSINESS MODELS OF MANAGED CARE ORGANIZATIONS

### Sources of Revenues and Types of Expenses

MCOs have 2 major drivers of revenue: enrollments multiplied by the premiums paid. MCOs also have 2 major drivers of expenses: administrative costs and medical costs. The rough mix between the 2 types of cost is 15% administrative and 85% medical. Administrative costs include many of the chevrons of Figure 17-9: marketing and sales, operations, medical administration, and general administration. The types of medical costs and their distribution are depicted in Figure 17-11. Clearly, the most important expense items to manage are inpatient hospital utilization and the use of specialists.

MCOs may have other revenue sources as well, such as fees earned from ASO contracts with self-insured employers. MCOs can also operate other lines of business (described earlier); some, like PBMs and services provided to other insurers, can earn substantial revenues.

MCOs are a variable cost business. The vast majority (~85%) of expenses are medical costs, which, by definition, are variable; only approximately 12% of expenses are "sales, general, and administrative" (SG&A), which are largely fixed costs. MCOs are also a low-margin business, with profits ranging from 2% to 5%; they are slightly higher for the commercial insurers (roughly 50% of market revenues) than for nonprofit Blues plans.[13] The margins also vary by line of business, being higher (at least historically) for ASO contracts and large group employer risk contracts.

Over time, however, largely due to PPACA (covered later), the underwriting margins on fully insured business lines have fallen for both nonprofit and for-profit plans to 1% to 3% (2016 average = 1.6%, down from 3.5% in 2011), even as revenues rose 55% and enrollments rose 29%.[14] By 2016, nearly half of the fully insured plans were reporting losses, with growing volatility and wide dispersion in plan margins. The 3 largest plans (United, Kaiser, and Anthem) captured 34% of revenues and 30% of enrollments but 84% of underwriting gains; the top 10 plans

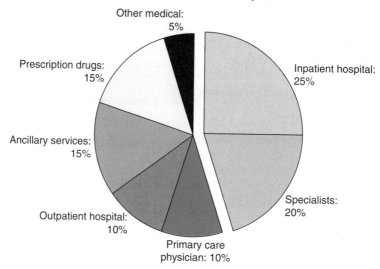

**Components of Medical Expense**

Other medical: 5%

Prescription drugs: 15%

Inpatient hospital: 25%

Ancillary services: 15%

Specialists: 20%

Outpatient hospital: 10%

Primary care physician: 10%

**Figure 17-11** • Largest Portion of Medical Costs Comes From Inpatient Hospital and Specialist Services. (Source: Brad Fluegel, Presentation to Wharton School 2017.)

captured 61% of revenues, 58% of enrollments, and 92% of underwriting gains. This suggests that most fully insured plans are small, and most are break-even or close to break-even.

## Medical Loss Ratio

The ratio of medical costs to total expenses is known as the medical loss ratio (MLR; ie, how much of the premium dollar is "lost" to paying for healthcare utilization). PPACA mandated minimum MLR levels for insurers: Large group insurers must spend at least 85% of their premiums to improve healthcare quality, while small group insurers and individual plans must spend at least 80%. The MLR rule ensured that enrollees got more value from their insurance premiums; it also led insurers to reduce their administrative costs such as advertising and broker commissions. However, there is no evidence that the MLR rule led insurers to reduce premiums or increase spending on quality improvement (only 1% of insurer premiums). It may have inadvertently prompted insurers to merge in an effort to achieve some scale economies.

To manage the MLR, which is a key metric used by investors to evaluate the MCOs, insurers must use strategies that address both medical expenses and premium revenues. These strategies are portrayed in Figure 17-12. Chapters 15 and 16 have already dealt with strategies to shift more risk to enrollees via

cost sharing (deductibles and copayments), use of hospital tiers and selective contracting, and management of the pharmacy benefit. Four other strategies are discussed in the following sections: diversification into new lines of business, consolidation to leverage providers, shifting risk to providers, and managing specialty pharmacy costs.

## Managed Care Diversification of Business Lines

MCOs can diversify in several different ways. First, they can diversify their mix of health plans

- Narrow networks
- Reduce physician/hospital fees via bargaining power
- Restrict access to expensive medical technology
- Disease management
- Utilization management (restrict low-value care)
- Shift costs to enrollees (eg, copayments)
- Preventive medicine
- Shift risk to providers

**Full-Risk Enrollees' Medical Expenses**

**Premium Revenue**

- Raise premiums
- Accurate underwriting: base premiums on expected costs

**Figure 17-12** • Various Methods to Control Expenses and Increase Revenues. (Source: Sean Nicholson. Cornell University.)

offered (eg, HMO, PPO, POS) to appeal to more customer segments. Second, they can diversify into new geographic markets that move them from local to state to multistate to national competitors. Third, they can diversify the lines of business they serve (eg, commercial, Medicare, Medicaid). The goal of diversification is to grow; revenue growth is a major metric (along with the MLR) by which investors evaluate the prospects of the commercial insurers. Another hoped-for result of diversification is *scope economies* (ie, spreading fixed costs across multiple lines of business to lower overall costs). Such economies may be limited in health insurance due to the different back-office activities (eg, sales and marketing) needed to service different customer segments.

## Consolidation Strategy to Leverage Providers

Figure 17-13 shows the long-term trend in the consolidation of health plans. Such consolidation can confer leverage for MCOs when they contract with employers downstream (charge higher premiums) and with providers upstream (pay lower reimbursement rates). Both help the

MCOs lower their MLRs and thereby improve their profitability. Research evidence suggests that MCOs operating in concentrated markets (small number of large MCOs with large market share) charge higher premiums to fully insured, small group employers.[15] MCOs also hope that through consolidation they can reap *scale economies*—that is, spread fixed costs over larger volume (eg, customers served or services rendered). Unfortunately, the evidence suggests that such economies of scale are limited.[16]

There are many other rationales for consolidation (Figure 17-14). Among all of these rationales, "growth" may dominate. As evidence, consider the proposed 2016 merger of Aetna and Humana. Aetna stated that the purpose of the merger was to diversify into the Medicare Advantage market, where Humana enjoyed sizeable market share. The merger was successfully opposed by the Department of Justice in early 2017 on the grounds that it was anticompetitive. Immediately afterward, Aetna entered an agreement to merge with CVS Health (a PBM and pharmacy business), while Humana developed a deal to merge with Kindred (a post-acute care business). Both mergers could be

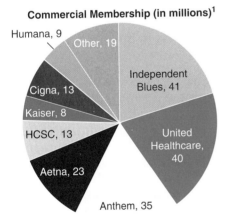

**Commercial Membership (in millions)[1]**

**Consolidation Drivers:**

- Economies of scale
- Demand for new products and services (HDHP)
- Infrastructure and tools (transparency, analytics)
- Cost of care capabilities
- Network size and scale
- Regulatory mandates

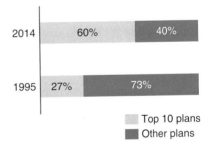

**Percentage of US Health Insurance Market (based on membership)[2]**

1. Enrollment includes commercial fully insured (PPO, HMO, POS), and commercial self insured (employer sponsored/ASO)
2. 2014 estimated total with coverage : Commercial + Medicare + Medicaid—Dual Eligibles based on managed care lives, excludes non-managed Medicaid

**Figure 17-13 •** Trends in Managed Care Organization Consolidation. ASO, Administrative Services Only; HDHP, High Deductible Health Plan; HMO, Health Maintenance Organization; POS, Point-of-Service; PPO, Preferred Provider Organization. (Source: Brad Fluegel, Presentation to Wharton School 2017.)

- Growth
- Employers' use of HDHPs and private exchanges ➔ full-risk market shrinks
- Pressure on HI margins due to state scrutiny of rate increases
- PPACA placed limits on favorite MCO strategies used in the past:
  - *Favorable risk selection*
  - *Profits* (via minimum MLR)
- Easy access to cheap debt and high market valuations ➔ Attractiveness of M&A
- Combine insurers to pool their PBMs to gain bigger price discounts on drugs
- Curb negotiating leverage of hospitals
- Leverage hospitals to accept value-based payments
- Counter hospital consolidation over time ➔ restore "balance" in buyer-supplier bargaining
- Achieve broad national presence
- Increase ability to sell insurance directly to consumers online (and not through employers, brokers)
- Larger scale that makes it easier to assemble dedicated provider networks
- Larger scale to invest in new capabilities (IT, care management, analytics, etc.)

**Figure 17-14** • Rationales for Insurer Consolidation. HDHP, High-Deductible Health Plan; HI, Health Insurance; IT, Information Technology; M&A, Mergers and Acquisitions; MCO, Managed Care Organization; MLR, Medical Loss Ratio; PBM, Pharmacy Benefit Manager; PPACA, Patient Protection and Affordable Care Act.

considered unrelated diversification or vertical integration, rather than horizontal integration; both mergers were also growth initiatives.

Of course, there is a major policy issue here: Is MCO consolidation good or bad for the public's welfare? There are arguments on both sides. On the "plus" side, larger MCOs can serve as a potential counterbalance to the hospital systems described in Chapter 12 and hopefully restrain their price increases. Given that hospitals account for nearly one-third of national health expenditures, the fact that only 1 or 2 hospitals operate in many communities, and that their rate hikes play a large role in driving healthcare cost inflation, this may not be a bad rationale. Any savings achieved by larger insurer bargaining may get passed on to consumers due to PPACA requirements regarding MLRs.[17] Larger MCOs may also be able to serve as a counterbalance to rising prices of specialty pharmaceuticals. More concentrated insurance markets are also associated with greater patient experience of care, particularly in the face of concentrated hospital markets.[18] Finally, according to a recent academic study, the average pretax operating margins of MCOs in Covered California (the state's Medicaid program) were only 1%, compared to 24% among the top 151 biopharma firms and 23% among the top biotech firms.[19]

On the "minus" side, MCO consolidation can spur some potentially negative developments, such as more hospital consolidation, more hospitals starting their own health plans, higher MCO costs due to mergers, higher MCO market power and thus higher premiums, reduced payer incentives to innovate, and higher payer-provider tensions.

## Payment Models to Shift Risk to Providers

A major strategy underway over the past 2 decades to control costs in managed care is to shift more risk to providers for the costs of the care they provide. For hospitals, MCOs have followed the lead of Medicare and paid on the basis of diagnosis-related groups (DRGs; fixed amount for a patient with a given admitting diagnosis), as well as on the basis of per diems (fixed amount per day), case rates (eg, fixed amount for a given procedure), or capitation. For physicians, MCOs have followed the lead of Medicare and paid them a percentage of the Resource-Based Relative Value Schedule (RBRVS) used by Medicare, as well as case payments and capitation.

In recent years, with prodding by the Department of Health and Human Services (DHHS), MCOs have tried to migrate their provider payments from FFS to value-based purchasing payments. By the end of 2018, many of the largest insurers had moved to 50% value-based payments. The definition of such payments is quite loose and variable, but they usually encompass alternative payment models (APMs) linked to health outcomes, quality of care, and cost (eg, pay-for-performance contracts [P4P] and shared savings payments to ACOs).

It is unclear how much these APMs have penetrated provider reimbursement. First, physicians and hospitals are reimbursed by multiple insurers using multiple payment methods; what constitutes an APM payment and its linkage to cost and quality may differ across insurers. Moreover, the percentage of providers receiving some APM payment differs from the percentage of reimbursements based on APMs. Second, the reported percentage of payer reimbursement to provider groups based on APMs often exceeds the percentage of reimbursement to individual physicians in the group based on APMs. Payers report greater readiness to embark on APMs, greater progress toward value-based payment, greater (perceived) positive financial impact of APMs on profitability, and greater provider readiness to implement APMs, compared with what providers report. Third, any payment system can be made attractive to providers if the payment rate is set high enough, but then it will be unattractive to payers. Hence, overall views depend on the level as well as the form of payment under one arrangement compared to another.

The evidence on the penetration of APMs is all over the map.[20] To wit:

- Data from 2015 showed that 62% of insurer payments are based on FFS, 15% are based on FFS linked to quality or value performance metrics (akin to P4P), and 23% are based on APMs with an FFS chassis or population-based payment.
- Other 2015 data showed that payments from commercial payers were heavily dominated by FFS (78%), with small percentages coming from shared savings/ACO models (7%), shared risk (5%), and partial capitation (4%).
- Data from 2016 reported 55% reimbursement based on FFS, 14% based on capitation, 13% based on episodes or bundles, 9% based on P4P, and 8% based on shared savings models (4% each for upside and downside risk).
- Other 2016 data showed that only 12% of provider organizations had more than 25% of patient care revenues tied to risk sharing with payers. A majority

(56%) reported risk-sharing revenues below 25%; 20% reported it was 0%. Surprisingly, 32% of providers did not know what the amount of risk sharing was. With regard to revenues tied to quality improvement, only 15% said that 25% or more of revenues were so linked; 12% reported it was zero.

- More 2016 data showed that only 30% of physicians reported receiving any value-based payments, broken out as follows: episode-based payments (16% of physicians), bundled payments (13%), shared savings (10%), capitation (10%), and shared risk (4%). More than half of physicians indicated that less than 10% of their personal compensation derived from incentive payments tied to cost and quality goals; one-third said they were not eligible; only 6% said they derived more than 20% of compensation from APMs.
- Among 33 large and advanced multi-specialty groups, 66% of payments were FFS, while 34% of payments were "at risk": 2% P4P, 4% shared savings, 2% partial capitation, 3% shared risk, 16% global capitation, and 7% payments from an owned health plan.

These data beg the question: Why is the proportion of physician compensation based on APMs apparently so low, given the high percentages of reimbursements based on APMs reported by insurers? Interviews at 34 medical practices offered one explanation: Payers' incentives to the group were not passed on to the individual physicians within it, thereby shielding them from direct exposure to payer risk or reward. Moreover, financial incentives passed on to the group were translated into nonfinancial incentives for the individual physician. The biggest financial incentive for physicians—even in those groups with heavy APM exposure—was to increase FFS productivity by paying based on relative value units (RVUs). In summary, it appears that APMs have had (1) relatively little impact on physician incomes or how they deliver patient care (covered later), and (2) a smaller impact on physician rewards than on rewards to the larger organization in which they practice.

Since the mid-1990s, the percentage of the commercially insured population enrolled in HMOs has fallen, from 31% in 1996 to 15% in 2016. Not surprisingly, the percentage of office

| | 2013 | 2014 | 2015 | 2016 | 2017 | 2018 |
|---|---|---|---|---|---|---|
| **Reimbursement Methods (% of net patient revenue)** | | | | | | |
| Traditional capitation (per member per month) (%) | 1.1 | 1.5 | 1.5 | 1.5 | 1.6 | 1.8 |
| DRG (%) | 41 | 40.5 | 40.2 | 40.6 | 41 | 41 |
| Percentage of charges (%) | 18.6 | 18 | 17.9 | 17.2 | 17 | 16 |
| Fee schedule (%) | 23.3 | 25.9 | 26.1 | 27.4 | 28 | 29.8 |
| Per diem (%) | 4 | 3.3 | 3.4 | 3.3 | 2.8 | 2 |
| Risk based (%) | 1 | 1 | 1.5 | 1.3 | 1.2 | 1.9 |
| Other (%) | 5.8 | 5 | 4.5 | 4.6 | 4.3 | 3.9 |

**Figure 17-15** • Reimbursement Methods. DRG, Diagnosis-Related Group. (Source: Moody's Investors Service, "Medians – Revenue Growth Rate Inches Ahead of Expenses as Margins Hold Steady," September 3, 2019.)

visits covered by capitation has also dropped to below 10% across public and private payers. In sum, FFS payment remains the predominant payment model for providers, while APMs are struggling to gain traction and make a difference (Figure 17-15).

Similarly, among hospitals, survey research suggests that only 13 of 80 hospital systems derived more than 10% of net patient revenue from risk-based contracts in 2015. AHA data show the percentage of hospitals reporting any capitated revenue fell from 12.6% to 8.0% between 2003 and 2014. Two-thirds of hospitals reported that they derived less than 1%. Why was the percentage so low? One possibility is that

economic surpluses from commercial (and likely non–risk-based) contracts make risk-based contracts less attractive, so hospitals with little excess capacity decline to participate in the latter.

There are some other possible reasons for the headwinds confronting these new payment models. First, many physicians are not very willing to change their decisions or actions that would alter utilization. Second, many physicians do not feel they are able to control healthcare waste. Third, many physicians do not feel that it is their responsibility to do so. Fourth, many physicians do not see their compensation as the best lever to use to get them to change their practice patterns.[21]

## Critical Thinking Exercise: Aetna and ACOs

By 2012, Aetna had developed partnerships with more than 100 provider organizations to help manage their Medicare Advantage plan enrollees. These partnerships were subsumed under Aetna's Medicare Physician Collaboration Program; the performance results from the first such partnership were depicted in a September 2012 article in *Health Affairs*.[22] Aetna's Collaboration Model included 3 components: Medicare risk adjustment, a host of quality measures, and a collaborative care management approach using embedded case managers. The quality measures included acute admissions and days (per 1,000), sub-acute admissions and days (per 1,000), ED

visits (per 1,000), readmission rates (as a percentage of discharges), and the percentage of hospital stays greater than 15 days. The third component is where much of the collaboration with the provider group occurred.

Aetna experienced wide variations in their success in hitting these quality metrics in their partnerships with providers. Aetna has asked you to develop a research proposal to investigate the reasons for this variability in performance across all of its Medicare Advantage collaborations. What characteristics of the provider organizations would you want to look at? What would you want to know about the history of Aetna's relationships with those providers?

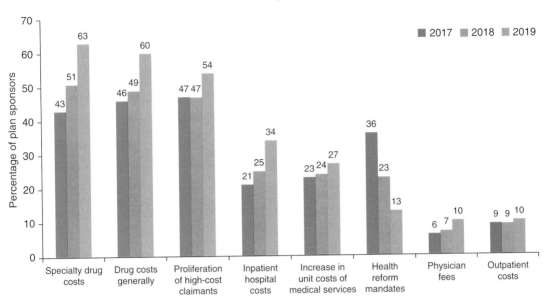

**Figure 17-16** • Most Important Drivers of Year-over-Year Medical Cost Increases, According to ERISA Plan Sponsors. (Source: UBS Evidence Lab.)

## Managing Specialty Pharmacy Costs

According to Employee Retirement Income Security Act plan sponsors, their number 1 challenge in managing their costs is control over rising costs of specialty drugs (Figure 17-16), a problem that is becoming more acute (Figure 17-17). Specialty drugs are used to treat complex, chronic conditions (eg, cancer) and are among the most expensive medicines on the market. They are typically biologics with few or no competitors. In 2017, retail prices for 97 of those widely used medications increased by an average of 7%, greater than 3 times the overall inflation rate. The average annual price for a specialty medication was $78,781. Patients usually pay either a flat copay or a percentage coinsurance of the drug's retail price. Out-of-pocket costs for specialty drugs typically require coinsurance, which can mean thousands of dollars.

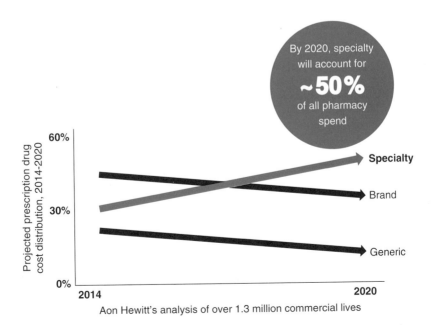

**Figure 17-17** • Projected Pharmacy Costs, 2014 to 2020. (Source: Mike Taylor. Adapted from Aon Hewitt, 2015.)

The $78,781 annual average cost for one of these medicines is more than 3 times the median income for Medicare beneficiaries ($26,200), and $20,000 more than the median income for all US households ($60,336).[23]

Kaiser data indicate that 97% of insured workers at large firms have coverage for specialty drugs. Among these workers, 45% are in a plan with at least one cost-sharing tier just for specialty drugs; among them, 45% have a copayment (average = $109) and 52% have coinsurance (average = 24%). MCOs and the employers they represent have sought to address the high prices and level of specialty drug spending in a number of ways beyond drug formularies and cost sharing. These include additional formulary tiers to drive higher member contributions for targeted drug classes, value-based copay structures, and managing the site of care (physician office preferred over hospital outpatient department).

MCOs and employers are pursuing other avenues besides cost sharing to control specialty drug spending. These include managing the sites of specialty drug infusion, directing patients to specific infusion sites, ensuring clinically appropriate use of such drugs, determining the "value" (quality vs cost) of specialty drugs, outcomes-based contracting for such drugs, examining different ways to reimburse specialty drugs (eg, bundled payment), use of prior authorization and other utilization management programs, use of clinical pathways, and choice of specialty pharmacy providers (SPPs) for the MCO's network.

Finally, some MCOs are moving to integrate the medical and pharmacy benefits (discussed earlier in Chapter 15). Studies conducted in house by several MCOs suggest there may be cost savings in integrating benefits by virtue of being able to substitute drug therapies for more expensive physician and hospital utilization. The reported savings are actually greater when the patient has a condition requiring specialty drugs.[24]

## NEW HORIZONS IN PRIVATE HEALTH INSURANCE

For much of its history, health insurance was a fairly boring segment of the healthcare ecosystem with not much innovation. That changed at the turn of the millennium with the development of CDHPs and then HDHPs. Since then, there have been several new developments worth discussion: the rise of the small and medium business segment, the Alternative Quality Contract (AQC) in Massachusetts, new start-ups such as Oscar (and others), and short-term plans. These are covered in the following sections.

## Small and Medium Business Segment

One segment of health plans now contesting for share is the small and medium business (SMB) market, which is defined as payers with less than 500,000 enrollees. This is a very competitive sector of the health insurance sector. Between 2013 and 2018, there were 111 new entrants to the SMB market and 104 exits (mostly due to mergers or ceasing operations).

This market composes 83% of all available insurance plans but only 11% of covered lives in the United States (~36 million in 2018); the plans thus have lots of competition (estimated at 409 payers in 2018) and small enrollments. Of the 409 plans, 240 are small (<50,000 enrollees), whereas the remainder are medium (50,000-499,000 enrollees). These payers offer all lines of business (eg, fully insured employer, ASO employer, managed Medicare and Medicaid, State Children's Health Insurance Program [CHIP], and dual eligible); however, the government lines of business account for the majority (64%) of their enrollees.

Nearly half of the plans (216 plans, 46%) targeting the SMB market are provider-sponsored health plans; commercial risk and ASO plans compose 51%. The provider-sponsored plans account for 53% of the SMB plans and have experienced the largest growth (34% increase in plans since 2013), due to federal government impetus behind payment reform (eg, PPACA, Medicare Access and CHIP Reauthorization Act) and value-based purchasing.[25] Of the 216 provider plans, 143 are small health plans with an average number of enrollees per plan of 10,000. Combining both small and medium plans, the average provider plan has 71,000 enrollees. Only 13 Blue Cross and Blue Shield plans fall in the SMB market.

## Alternative Quality Contract

In 2009, the leaders of Blue Cross and Blue Shield of Massachusetts (BCBSMA) developed a new value-based contracting approach to improve quality and outcomes while also reducing the rate of growth in healthcare costs. The AQC used a global budgeting approach and paid contracting provider organizations on a capitated, per-member-per-month (PMPM) basis for the total cost of care, annually adjusted for inflation and patient health status, with providers having real 2-sided risk (for both surpluses and losses).

The AQC model contained a *unique contract model* that included accountability for quality and resource use across a full care continuum (inpatient, outpatient, pharmacy, behavioral health) over the long term (5 years); *control over cost growth* (via a global population-based budget, shared 2-sided symmetrical risk with providers, adjustments for enrollee health status, and annual inflation targets set at baseline for each year of the contract and designed to significantly moderate cost growth); and *improved quality, safety, and outcomes.* With regard to the latter, the model included process measures, outcome measures, and patient experience measures on both the inpatient hospital side and the ambulatory physician office side. It also included a performance payment incentive whereby improvements in provider quality performance were met with higher sharing of surpluses (or lower sharing of deficits).

The AQC program delivered on its outcome goals while, at the same time, lowering the cost trend 6% to 8% relative to competitors in the state (2013-2016). These results are both impressive and hopeful. One should bear in mind that they were achieved in one state by the largest insurer in that state using its HMO health plan; BCBSMA is now trying to replicate these results in their PPO plan. The key elements employed here are (1) a total cost approach that spans accountability for the continuum of care, (2) focus on process and outcome measures used in both inpatient and outpatient settings, (3) a long-term approach, and (4) considerable BCBSMA support to contracting providers (including consultation, sharing of best practices, approaches to patient engagement, staffing models, data and actionable reports, practice pattern variation analysis, and training). As with other value-based approaches, individual providers are still paid on a FFS basis.

## Health Insurance Start-Ups

### Oscar Health

Oscar was cofounded in 2012 by a Stanford-trained data scientist, Mario Schlosser, and Joshua Kushner (Jared's younger brother). Mr. Schlosser started the company after he saw how complicated it was to find the right care and physician for his wife's first pregnancy. They focused on making it easier for Millennial consumers to navigate healthcare, as well as providing more affordable and convenient care. Part of this was achieved through their user-friendly website, online medical history, unlimited free phone calls with a physician 24/7, and (later) free and unlimited generic prescriptions.[26]

Initially, Oscar Health sought to take advantage of the PPACA's creation of new marketplaces for individuals to buy health insurance on state-run exchanges. Such exchanges sold approximately 43% of individual policies, offering a large potential market to serve. Moreover, PPACA prohibitions and restrictions on prior MCO strategies (cherry-picking the healthy, limiting spending on the unhealthy, exclusions of bad risks) forced plans to compete in new ways. The exchanges allowed consumers to compare plans side by side (including their price/cost), which might influence the choice of the new, price-sensitive enrollees who previously did not purchase (or could not afford) health insurance.

The company had some initial enrollment success in its state exchange products, reaching 40,000 in New York by 2015. However, due to large start-up costs, it lost $115 million in 2015, $205 million in 2016, and then another $127 million in 2017 (on $229 million in revenues). In 3 states in which it operated, it had an MLR of 94%; administrative costs reportedly consumed more than half of the company's revenues. Moreover, the PPACA did not contain enough penalties to compel Millennials to sign up, and they didn't; then, in December 2017, Congress repealed the tax penalty associated with the individual mandate. The state insurance exchange market was no longer growing.

The company has since pivoted away from a sole reliance on the insurance exchanges to focus on growing markets, such as Medicare Advantage and the small business market. Oscar partnered with Cleveland Clinic on a co-branded health plan, launched in 2018, to offer individual coverage to 5 counties in northeast Ohio. Enrollees get access to Cleveland Clinic PCPs and care managers, as well as an Oscar concierge nurse and 3 care guides, and 24/7 access to telemedicine. The plan enrolled 11,000 members for 2018 and is now engaged in rolling it out to additional counties in Ohio. Oscar also announced partnerships with both Humana and Cigna to provide services to small business owners. Essentially, Oscar can bring its technology-enabled healthcare services to small businesses in concert with the large healthcare networks that employers are used to working with. For 2020, Oscar plans to expand into 19 new markets and 4 new states, which would bring its total footprint to 47 markets in 19 states. Part of the expansion will rest on Oscar's "Virtual Primary Care" that offers digital and in-home services (eg, lab draws) at no cost in selected markets to respond to the COVID-19 crisis.

Oscar faces stiff competition in all of the new markets it is trying to enter. Medicare Advantage (MA) is an increasingly saturated market, with an estimated 2,700 MA plans open for enrollment in 2019; this is 18% higher than the 2,300 offered in 2018. Over the same period, MA enrollment is projected to grow 11.5%. If growth in new plans continues to outpace growth in new enrollees, Oscar may struggle to grab any market share. Oscar also has to compete with the largest insurers, which account for a large share of MA enrollees and have disproportionate underwriting gains. Oscar may not find the SMB market any easier, given the large number of players.

Ultimately, Oscar envisions a healthcare market where employer-defined plans will disappear as more consumers turn to individual coverage, HDHPs, and health reimbursement arrangements (HRAs). From a small base of only 70,000 enrollees several years ago after retrenchment and withdrawal from several markets (Dallas, New Jersey), Oscar Health has grown to roughly 400,000 enrollees by 2020, including around 375,000 individual members and another 20,000 coming through small-group insurance and MA. Fueling this expansion is a massive capital infusion of $540 million raised from Alphabet, Founders Fund, Capital G (Alphabet's later-stage investment firm), and Verily (Alphabet's investment firm focused on life sciences). Overall, Oscar has raised $1.3 billion. In this manner, Oscar resembles some of the innovative primary care network start-ups profiled in Chapter 13.

## Haven

In January 2018, Amazon, Berkshire Hathaway, and JP Morgan Chase announced a joint venture to revolutionize healthcare delivery and lower healthcare costs. The 3 companies would reportedly pool their 1.2 million workers in new plans using sophisticated technology and transparency. That venture, Haven, was officially launched in March 2019. The company hopes to improve healthcare services and lower costs for the 3 companies' employees, make insurance benefits easier to understand, make primary care easier to access, and make drugs more affordable. Amazon and JP Morgan will offer new plans to employees in 2020 that feature wellness incentives, no deductibles or coinsurance, flat copays, and out-of-pocket maximums; Berkshire is testing a similar pilot in a few of its companies. The plans will be administered through the major MCOs (eg, Cigna, Aetna).

Haven's early history has been rocky. In its first 3 years of operation, it has seen the turnover of its chief executive officer (CEO; Atul Gawande), its Chief operating officer, its chief technology officer, and its data scientists and software engineers—in all, about 14% of the workforce with public profiles on LinkedIn. The CEO said he wanted to spend more time on policy and advocacy work (eg, COVID-19), which is perhaps not too surprising, given that he never left his academic position at Harvard. Haven's ambitions to shake up health insurance likely exceeded its ability, especially given the geographic dispersion of the 3 founding companies' workforces, the lack of any concentrated presence of these employees among any set of providers, and the numerous stakeholders in the US healthcare ecosystem that they would need to engage. It also did not help that Amazon has pursued its own provider initiatives (eg, virtual care; see Chapter 24).

## Other New Entrants

The private insurance sector witnessed some newer entrants in late summer 2020. In July 2020, Walmart unveiled its "Walmart Insurance Services" to accompany its already existing education program ("Healthcare Begins Here") to help consumers find the right health plan. The new subsidiary will reportedly sell MA plans, a growth sector. Then, in August 2020, Google announced a new subsidiary, "Coefficient Insurance" (backed by a large Swiss reinsurance firm), to assist self-insured employers with stop-loss protection against unexpected, large claims.

## Short-Term Health Plans

Short-term plans were defined in 1997 regulations (pursuant to HIPAA) as health insurance coverage with a term of less than 1 year. HIPAA exempted these plans from federal regulation. In 2016, the Obama administration changed the definition, limited the plans to no more than 90 days of coverage, and denied consumers the opportunity to renew coverage. The Trump administration reversed the Obama-era changes in 2018. Moreover, there has been a heated, partisan political exchange in mid-2020 about the utility of these plans—even though the number of people covered by them is roughly just 1 million. What's going on here?

The short-term plans compete with plans offered on the health insurance exchanges ushered in by President Obama's PPACA (see Chapter 19). Many middle-income individuals find the insurance plans offered on the exchanges to be out of their price range; those who do not qualify for premium subsidies often drop individual market coverage and typically buy short-term plans instead. They thus function as a safety net for many of the roughly 30 million uninsured (eg, people between jobs, retirees looking for coverage before Medicare kicks in, the self-employed, and workers in the "gig economy"). They also feature deductibles that are much (up to 60%) lower than the exchange plans. Opponents charge these plans with avoiding PPACA regulations regarding underwriting and some benefit limitations (eg, maternity), as well as with misleading marketing and sales practices. This "hot potato" issue has interesting arguments on both sides for you to consider.[27]

## SUMMARY

Like the PBMs portrayed in the prior chapter, the MCOs depicted here are complex and confusing critters. The 3-letter acronyms introduced here that capture their variety are both mind-boggling and essential to master. They serve as the system's shorthand for some very impenetrable models. Virtually the entire universe of insurers in the United States, both public and private, operate in the managed care world. In terms of the iron triangle discussed in Chapter 5, the MCOs have historically focused on cost containment but are trying to manage quality as well.

### QUESTIONS TO PONDER

1. What are the major trade-offs associated with selecting among the different MCO health plans (HMO, PPO, POS, HDHP)?
2. What are the major differences among the different types of HMOs (group, staff, IPA)?
3. How do you measure the success of an MCO?
4. How well have MCOs performed in solving the iron triangle?
5. Can providers who set up health plans develop the same managed care infrastructure depicted in Figure 17-9?
6. What are the major ways in which MCOs manage their expenses?
7. How successful have APMs been?
8. How successful have new entrants into the health insurance market been?

## REFERENCES

1. Benjamin Sommers, Atul Gawande, and Katherine Baicker. "Health Insurance Coverage—What the Evidence Tells Us," *N Engl J Med.* 377 (2017): 586-593. Steffie Woolhandler and David Himmelstein. "The Relationship of Health Insurance and Mortality: Is Lack of Insurance Deadly?" *Ann Intern Med.* 167 (2017): 424-431.
2. Insurers play somewhat similar roles in the public sector. For beneficiaries enrolled in managed care plans (HMOs, PPOs), state Medicaid plans and federal Medicare Advantage plans contract with private insurers (usually on a capitated basis) to care for their beneficiaries. For Medicaid and Medicare beneficiaries in fee-for-service plans, the private insurers serve as claims processors and conduits of government monies to pay providers.
3. *Blue Cross and Blue Shield: A Historical Compilation.* Available online: https://advocacy .consumerreports.org/wp-content/uploads/2013/ 03/yourhealthdollar.org_blue-cross-history-compilation.pdf. Accessed on April 3, 2020.
4. George Moseley. "The U.S. Health Care Non-System, 1908-2008," *Am Med Assoc J Ethics.* 10 (5) (2008): 324-331.
5. Beatrix Hoffman. "Restraining the Health Care Consumer: The History of Deductibles and Co-Payments in U.S. Health Insurance," *Soc Sci Hist.* 30 (4) (2006): 501-528.

6. Robert Cunningham III and Robert M. Cunningham, Jr. *The Blues: A History of the Blue Cross and Blue Shield System* (DeKalb, IL: Northern Illinois University Press, 1997).

7. Adapted from: Justin Giovannelli, Kevin Lucia, Sabrina Corlette, et al. "Regulation of Health Plan Provider Networks," *Health Affairs Health Policy Brief* (July 28, 2016).

8. Kathryn Langwell. "Structure and Performance of Health Maintenance Organizations: A Review," *Health Care Financ Rev.* 12 (1) (1990): 71-79.

9. David M. Cutler, Mark McClellan, and Joseph P. Newhouse. "How Does Managed Care Do It?" *RAND J Econ.* 31 (3) (January 2000): 526-548.

10. Mark Farrah Associates. "Health Insurance Enrollment Trends for Year-End 2018 (May 1, 2019). Available online: https://www.markfarrah.com/mfa-briefs/health-insurance-enrollment-trends-for-year-end-2018/. Accessed on April 3, 2020.

11. Data from 5 largest insurers. Cathy Schoen and Sara Collins. *The Big Five Health Insurers' Membership and Revenue Trends: Implications for Public Policy* (New York, NY: Commonwealth Fund, December 4, 2017).

12. Constantijn Panis and Michael Brien. *Self-Insured Health Benefit Plans 2019: Based on Filings Through Statistical Year 2016* (Deloitte, January 7, 2019). Available online: https://www.dol.gov/sites/dolgov/files/EBSA/researchers/statistics/retirement-bulletins/annual-report-on-self-insured-group-health-plans-2019-appendix-b.pdf. Accessed on April 4, 2020.

13. Greg Scott, Andrew Davis, Andreea Balan-Cohen, et al. *Health Plan Financial Trends, 2011-2016* (Washington, DC: Deloitte Center for Health Solutions, 2017).

14. Greg Scott, Andrew Davis, Andreea Balan-Cohen, et al. *Health Plan Financial Trends, 2011-2016* (Washington, DC: Deloitte Center for Health Solutions, 2017).

15. Erin Trish and Bradley Herring. "How Do Health Insurer Market Concentration and Bargaining Power With Hospitals Affect Health Insurance Premiums?" *J Health Econ.* 42 (2015): 104-114. This is particularly true in markets with high levels of fully insured firms and highly concentrated providers.

16. Douglas Wholey, Roger Feldman, Jon Christianson, et al. "Scale and Scope Economies Among Health Maintenance Organizations," *J Health Econ.* 15 (6) (1996): 657-684. Douglas Wholey, Roger Feldman, and Jon B. Christianson. "The Effect of Market Structure on HMO Premiums," *J Health Econ.* 14 (1) (1995): 81-105. Ruth Given. "Economies of Scale and Scope as an Explanation of Merger and Output Diversification Activities in the Health Maintenance Organization Industry," *J Health Econ.* 15 (6) (1996): 685-713.

17. Victor Fuchs and Peter Lee. "A Healthy Side of Insurer Mega-Mergers," *Wall Street Journal* (August 26, 2015).

18. Caroline Hanson, Bradley Herring, and Erin Tosh. "Do Health Insurance and Hospital Market Concentration Influence Hospital Patients' Experience of Care?" *Health Serv Res.* 54 (2019): 805-815.

19. See: Victor R. Fuchs and Peter V. Lee. "A Healthy Side of Insurer Mega-Mergers." Available at: https://www.wsj.com/articles/a-healthy-side-of-insurer-mega-mergers-1440628597. Accessed on August 6, 2020.

20. Lawton R. Burns and Mark V. Pauly. "Transformation of the Healthcare Industry: Curb Your Enthusiasm?" *Milbank Q.* 96 (1) (March 2018): 57-109.

21. McKinsey & Company. *2011 McKinsey Physician Survey* (2011).

22. Thomas Claffey, Joseph V. Agostini, Elizabeth N. Collet, et al. "Payer-Provider Collaboration In Accountable Care Reduced Use And Improved Quality In Maine Medicare Advantage Plan," *Health Aff.* 31 (9) (2012): 2074-2083.

23. Dena Bunis. "Specialty Drug Prices Soar to Nearly $79,000 a Year," *AARP.com* (June 25, 2019). Available online: https://www.aarp.org/politics-society/advocacy/info-2019/specialty-drug-prices-rise.html. Accessed on April 3, 2020.

24. EMD Serono. *EMD Serono Specialty Digest: Managed Care Strategies for Specialty Pharmaceuticals* (Darmstadt, Germany: EMD Serono, 2017).

25. Chuck Green. "Health Payers Contend for Share of SMB Health Insurance Market," *Health Payer Intelligence* (November 29, 2018). Available online: https://healthpayerintelligence.com/news/health-payers-contend-for-share-of-smb-health-insurance-market. Accessed on April 4, 2020. Mary Swaykus. *Insights Into the Small and Medium Health Insurance Market* (Bellevue, WA: Edifecs Corporation, 2018).

26. Leemore Dafny. *Oscar Health Insurance: What Lies Ahead for a Unicorn Insurance Entrant?* (Boston, MA: Harvard Business School, August 5, 2019). Case 9-319-025.

27. Brian Blasé and Doug Badger. "The Value of Short-Term Health Plans: Rebutting the Energy and Commerce Democratic Staff Report," *Health Affairs Blog* (August 17, 2020). US House of Representatives. *Shortchanged: How the Trump Administration's Expansion of Junk Short-Term Health Insurance Plans Is Putting Americans at Risk* (Washington, DC: Committee on Energy & Commerce, June 2020).

# 18

# Medicare

## INTRODUCTION

Medicare was enacted in 1965 as Title XVIII of the Social Security Act. Medicare covers the elderly population (65+ years old) regardless of income or health status and represents the country's only version of national health insurance. The program was expanded twice: (1) in 1972 to include individuals under 65 suffering from end-stage renal disease (ESRD) and the disabled who received Social Security Disability Insurance (SSDI) payments, and (2) in 2001 to cover people with amyotrophic lateral sclerosis (ALS, or Lou Gehrig's disease).

Medicare (along with Medicaid) is one of the country's largest "entitlement" programs (see Chapter 6). To be entitled to Medicare, an individual (or spouse) must have contributed payroll taxes into the Social Security system for at least 10 years. To some, the elderly are thus "deserving" and "worthy" of receiving Medicare benefits because they have already "paid into the system." Moreover, the elderly have the highest level of voting participation in the country (Figure 18-1) and vote their interests (which include protecting Medicare and Social Security). That is why Medicare is often called "the third rail in American politics": Touch it and you die instantly.

When seniors qualify for Medicare, they have several options (Figure 18-2). First, they can register for "traditional" Medicare, also known as fee-for-service (FFS) Medicare. This includes Part A and Part B (covered later), which provide hospital and medical services, respectively, on an FFS basis. Second, they can enroll in FFS Medicare with or without supplemental coverage (Medigap) and/or prescription drug plan (PDP) coverage.

Third, seniors can also enroll, if they choose not to register for FFS Medicare, in a Medicare Advantage (MA) plan offered to seniors through private insurers. MA plans cover Medicare Part A and Part B services and may also cover prescription drugs through an MA prescription drug (MA-PD) plan. Many MA plans offer additional benefits such as dental and vision coverage.

## MEDICARE BENEFITS AND COMPONENTS

### The Two Wilburs

Medicare and Medicaid emerged as part of President Johnson's "Great Society" program in 1965 and, specifically, its "war on poverty." Medicare and Medicaid were not designed in any rational way. Rather, they reflected a political compromise brokered in Congress by Wilbur Mills, Chairman of the House Ways and Means Committee. Wilbur Cohen, a leader in the Social Security Administration, called it a "3-layer cake" that encompassed 3 bills floating around Congress sponsored by the 2 parties: hospital insurance paid for by Social Security taxes, a voluntary program covering physicians' costs paid for by a contribution from beneficiaries and general revenues, and an expanded version of the Kerr-Mills Act (which provided medical assistance to the aged). The first 2 parts constituted Medicare; the third became Medicaid. In 1965, Medicare did not cover pharmaceuticals, catastrophic illness, or all costs; these were not significant issues at the time. These omissions would later call for solutions in the form of Medicare Part D and Medigap plans.

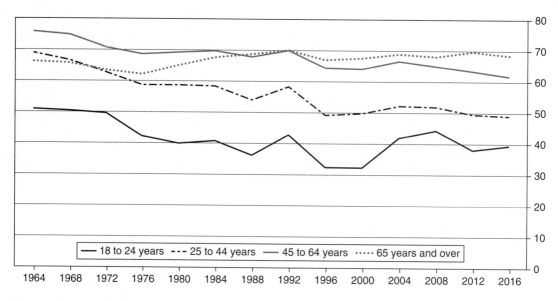

**Figure 18-1** • Voting Participation Rates in Presidential Elections, by Age, 1964 to 2016.

## Parts

The easiest way to remember the benefits and components of Medicare is to recall the 1994 movie, *Four Weddings and a Funeral* (with Hugh Grant and Andie MacDowell). Medicare is "4 parts and a supplement." Parts A and B were in the original Medicare legislation; Part C was added in 1997; Part D was added in 2003. The supplement was first

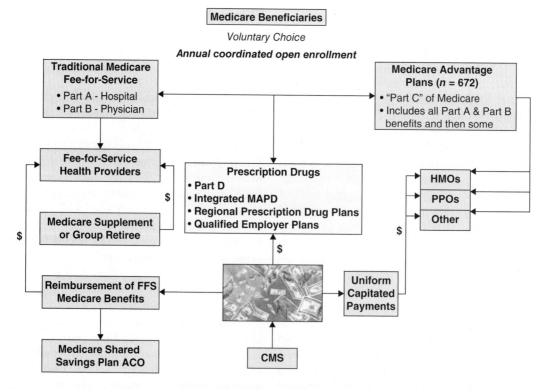

**Figure 18-2** • Medicare Coverage Options. ACO, Accountable Care Organization; CMS, Centers for Medicare and Medicaid Services; FFS, Fee-for-Service; HMOs, Health Maintenance Organizations; MAPD, Medicare Advantage Prescription Drug; PPOs, Preferred Provider Organizations. (Source: Steve Wood, Clear View Solutions LLC. Presentation to the Wharton School, Spring 2017.)

made available in 1980. These parts are briefly described here:

- **Part A—Medicare Hospital Insurance:** Pays for inpatient hospital care (ie, including both acute care and post-acute care facilities), hospice care services for persons with a life expectancy of 6 months or less, and home healthcare services following hospital discharge. Part A also covers drugs used in inpatient hospital and nursing home stays. When beneficiaries reach age 65, they are automatically enrolled in Part A. While enrollees do not pay a premium, they do face cost sharing in the form of a $1,316 deductible (2017 data).
- **Part B—Supplementary Medical Insurance:** Pays for physician care, hospital outpatient care, outpatient renal dialysis, medical supplies and durable medical equipment, emergency room treatment and ambulance, clinical lab and diagnostic tests, home healthcare, prescription drugs that cannot be self-administered,[1] and (due to the Patient Protection and Affordable Care Act [PPACA]) annual wellness visits. There is no automatic enrollment in Part B; beneficiaries must enroll and pay a monthly premium ($134 in 2017). Moreover, they face cost sharing in the form of a $183 deductible and 20% coinsurance. Physicians who accept the Medicare fee as payment-in-full (ie, "accept assignment"), and thereby agree not to balance-bill the patient, get paid electronically by the Centers for Medicare and Medicaid Services (CMS); those who do not accept assignment can bill the patient for an additional fee (up to 15%) but may face slower reimbursement and cost of patient collection.
- **Part C—MA:** Covers benefits under Parts A, B, and D that are provided through a managed care plan like a health maintenance organization (HMO), preferred provider organization (PPO), private FFS (PFFS) plan,[2] or a special needs plan (SNP).[3] Medicare beneficiaries can voluntarily enroll in Part C during an annual enrollment period.
- **Part D—Prescription Drug Benefit:** Provides coverage for prescription drugs either through a freestanding PDP or through an MA-PD plan. PDP is a voluntary program for which beneficiaries pay a monthly premium ($30+).
- **Supplemental Insurance ("Medigap") Plans:** Medicare Parts A, B, and D leave many gaps in the enrollee's coverage. For example, Part A provides less coverage beyond the first 60 days of hospitalization. Parts A, B, and D also entail cost sharing (eg, deductibles, coinsurance). FFS Medicare also does not cover such benefits as vision, dental, and hearing aids. To make coverage more comprehensive and to reduce the amount of cost sharing, the federal government supervises private sector plans that fill in the gaps using 10 different options. This is a voluntary program for which beneficiaries pay the private insurer a monthly premium. Medigap plans are not the only solution to supplemental insurance coverage, however; a large (but shrinking) percentage of retirees get supplemental coverage through their former employer, whereas others get it through Medicaid by virtue of also being poor (Figure 18-3). Of historical note, the American Association of Retired Persons (AARP) built its membership on the basis of selling Medigap coverage.

Medicare bears a striking resemblance to Blue Cross and Blue Shield (Figure 18-4). Blue Cross and Medicare Part A pay the hospital; Blue Shield and Medicare Part B pay the physician. This was intentional. The American Hospital Association and the American Medical Association both opposed the Medicare legislation on the grounds that it was "socialized medicine" and "government intrusion." They relaxed their opposition when the legislation satisfied providers' interests, as follows: (1) providers would be paid cost-plus FFS, (2) hospital and physician payments would remain separate and independent, and (3) the government would reimburse hospitals using local Blue Cross plans as "fiscal intermediaries" and would reimburse physicians using local Blue Shield plans as "fiscal carriers." Figure 18-5 charts the different premium and cost-sharing payments made by a Medicare beneficiary using Parts A and B and how the Medicare supplement fits in.

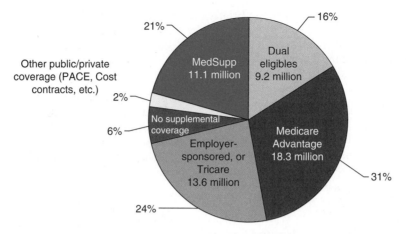

**Total Medicare Beneficiaries, 2017 = 57.9 million**

**Figure 18-3** • Sources of Supplemental Coverage (2017). (Source: 2014 Trustees Report, Medicare and Clear View Solutions estimates.)

## MEDICARE FINANCING

Medicare accounted for 15% of federal spending in 2018, a figure projected to rise to 18% by 2029. Medicare also comprises 20% of national health spending (2017). There has been a notable deceleration in Medicare spending growth (see Figure 6-9). In prior decades, the growth rates in spending per enrollee were comparable for Medicare and private health insurance. Medicare grew at an average annual rate of 5.8% (1990s) and 7.3% (2000s), compared to 5.9% and 7.2% for private insurance spending, respectively. By contrast, the average annual growth in Medicare spending per beneficiary was just 1.7% during 2010 to 2018, compared to

3.8% among private insurers. The slowing rate of growth has been attributed to the PPACA of 2010, which cut payments to MA plans and providers, as well as to the Budget Control Act of 2011 (see Chapter 14), which imposed 2% cuts through the sequestration.

Medicare is financed in a Byzantine manner through a mix of general tax revenues (43%), payroll taxes (36%), and premiums (15%). Each part of Medicare is financed differently, however, as follows:

• Part A is mostly financed (88%) through a 2.9% payroll tax on earnings paid by employers and employees (1.45% each); higher-income taxpayers (earning more than $200,000 per individual and

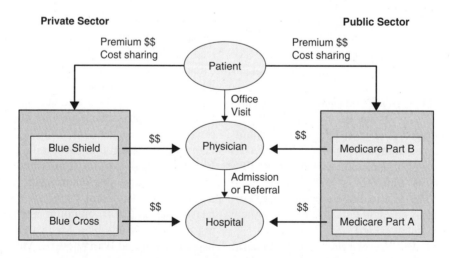

**Figure 18-4** • Blue Cross/Blue Shield Versus Medicare Parts A and B.

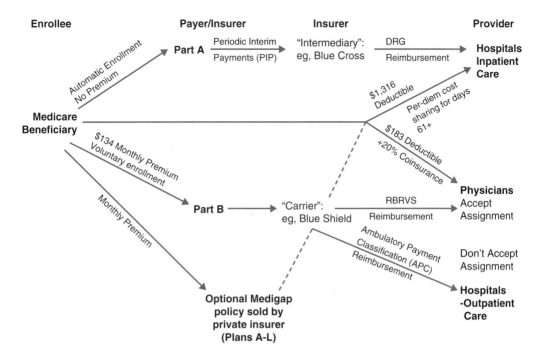

**Figure 18-5** • Payment Flows in Fee-for-Service Medicare (2017). DRG, Diagnosis-Related Group; RBRVS, Resource-Based Relative Value Schedule.

$250,000 per couple) pay a higher payroll tax (2.35%) on earnings.
- Parts B and D are mostly financed through premiums (17%-26%) and "general revenues" (71%-72%), which include individual income taxes, corporate taxes, and excise taxes (data from 2018). Beneficiaries with annual incomes over $85,000 (individual) or $170,000 (couple) pay a higher, income-related Part B premium reflecting a larger share of total Part B spending. Higher-income enrollees pay a larger share of the cost of Part D coverage, as they do for Part B.
- MA plans (Part C) provide benefits covered under Part A, Part B, and (typically) Part D; these benefits are financed primarily by payroll taxes, general revenues, and premiums. MA enrollees generally pay the monthly Part B premium; many also pay an additional premium directly to their plan (averaging $34 per month).

Payroll taxes account for the bulk of the Hospital Insurance Trust Fund's income ($262 million out of $299 million, 2017). The trust fund faces long-term deficits as the number of Medicare beneficiaries increases (from 58.4 million in 2017 to nearly 80 million by 2030), as the number of workers per beneficiary declines

from 3.1 to 2.4 (Figure 18-6), and as the cost of healthcare increases. Hospital insurance trust expenditures exceeded taxes for several years up to 2016, have since stabilized, but are nevertheless projected to be exhausted by 2027. These pressures will force lawmakers to find ways to finance promised benefits or cut services or provider payment rates. Of the $755.7 billion expenditures in 2018, Parts A, B, and D accounted for $306.6 billion, $353.7 billion, and $95.4 billion, respectively.

## MEDICARE BENEFICIARIES

The Medicare beneficiaries include 2 distinct population segments: the elderly over 65 (84% in 2016) and the disabled under 65 (16%). Both segments are growing in numbers (Figure 18-7), but for different reasons. The elderly portion of the Medicare population is growing as the Baby Boomers "age into Medicare" (Figure 18-8). The disabled portion of the Medicare population is growing for several reasons:

- Aging of the population
- Congressionally expanded definition of "disability" in the Social Security Disability Benefits Reform Act (1984), which put greater weight on applicants' own

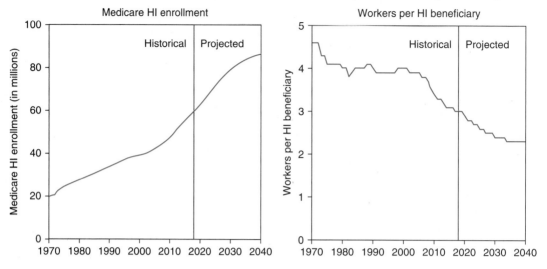

**Figure 18-6** • Medicare Enrollment. (Source: 2019 Annual Report by the Boards of Trustees of the Medicare Trust Funds.)

assessment of their disability (eg, pain, discomfort) and replaced the government's medical assessments with those of the applicants' own physicians

- Loosening of the screening criteria for mental illness
- Recessions, which increase unemployment, which, in turn, lead to more SSDI applications
- Growing economic value of disability payments (which attracts applications)

A large segment of the elderly Medicare population is not in good health: 32% report at least 1 limitation in activities of daily living, 25% report their health is either fair or poor, 22% have 5 or more chronic conditions, and two-thirds have multiple chronic conditions. However, over time, their health status has slightly improved. Between 1991 and 2017, the percentage reporting being in fair or poor health has declined from 26% to 18% (those aged 65-74) and from 34% to 27% (those aged 75+).

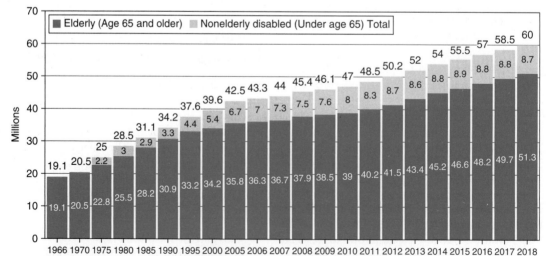

**Figure 18-7** • Medicare Enrollment, 1966 to 2018. (Source: Centers for Medicare and Medicaid Services.)

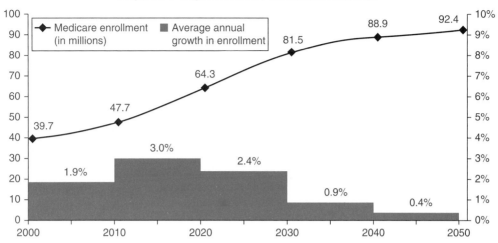

**Figure 18-8** • Boomers Aging Into Medicare. (Source: 2013 Annual Report of the Boards of Trustees of the Federal Hospital Insurance and Federal Supplementary Medical Insurance Trust Funds.)

The elderly are also not a bunch of wealthy "fat cats." Roughly half of the beneficiaries have incomes below $23,000 and savings below $78,000. At the same time, the percentage of beneficiaries living in poverty has fallen over the past 50 years from roughly 25% to just under 10%. This may help to explain the improvement in the health status of the beneficiaries noted earlier.

Nevertheless, the elderly face financial challenges even with Medicare coverage. This is due to Medicare's (as well as employers') increased emphasis on enrollee cost sharing in the form of higher premiums, deductibles, and coinsurance. In 2016, the average out-of-pocket spending by a beneficiary covered by FFS Medicare was $5,806 (see Figure 18-9 for the distribution of this spending across services). This is a sizable portion of spending for the half of the Medicare population with less than $23,000 in income. Thirty-nine percent of beneficiaries earning less than 100% of the federal poverty

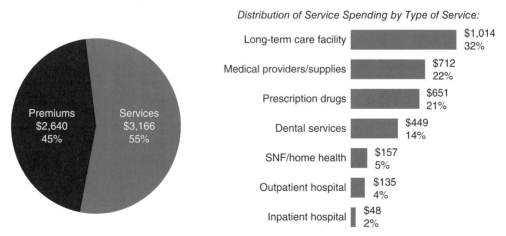

**Figure 18-9** • Average Out-of-Pocket Spending by Medicare Beneficiaries in 2016. SNF, Skilled Nursing Facility. (Source: KFF Analysis of Centers for Medicare & Medicaid Services 2016 Medicare Current Beneficiary Survey.)

level spend 20% or more of incomes on premiums and care; 40% to 41% of those earning between 100% and 200% of the poverty level spend 20% or more.

## MEDICARE ADVANTAGE[4]

In 1997, the Balanced Budget Act (BBA) enacted Part C of Medicare, known at the time as "Medicare+Choice" (M+C), to control the growth of Medicare spending. The BBA of 1997 tried to build upon the foundation established in earlier legislation (the Tax Equity and Fiscal Responsibility Act [TEFRA] of 1982). TEFRA provided incentives for HMOs to enroll Medicare beneficiaries on an at-risk basis, paying them a capitated rate of 95% of the local costs of treating FFS Medicare beneficiaries. BBA now allowed beneficiaries to enroll in more open-panel plans like PPOs (not just HMOs), as well as health plans sponsored by providers. But BBA scrapped the TEFRA payment formula and reduced payments to the private plans. Plans responded by increasing beneficiary cost sharing and cutting benefits; enrollments fell 30% over the next few years and many plans withdrew.

In 2003, the Medicare Modernization Act (MMA) sought to restimulate Medicare risk plan enrollment, raising payments to the managed care organizations (MCOs) by 10% to 11% between 2003 and 2004. Payments to plans averaged 107% of FFS Medicare spending in 2004; by 2009, plans were paid 114% of what FFS Medicare would have spent on the same beneficiaries, amounting to $11.4 billion in excess payments (Figure 18-10).

The MMA also established a mechanism whereby plans submitted a bid representing their estimated costs of providing basic Medicare benefits to enrollees for the coming year (including overhead and profit). If the bid was lower than a county-level benchmark based on FFS Medicare spending per enrollee, the plan was paid most of the difference as a rebate or bonus, which the plan was required to use in offering commensurate additional benefits. Like BBA, the MMA also created new private plan options, such as regional PPOs and SNPs (which served specific vulnerable populations).

The MMA also included coverage for prescription drugs (beyond those infused in a physician's office). Medicare provided such coverage 2 ways: (1) MA plans with such coverage, or (2) PDPs approved by Medicare and

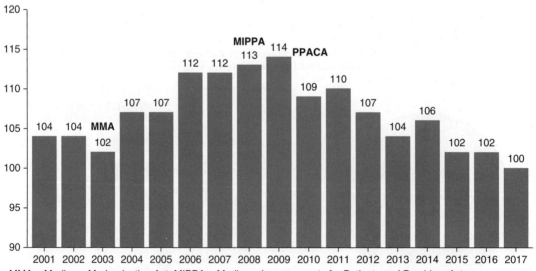

MMA = Medicare Modernization Act; MIPPA = Medicare Improvements for Patients and Providers Act; PPACA = Patient Protection and Affordable Care Act.

Percentages based on the risk-adjustment system used during publication of each MedPAC report. As a result, Medicare Part C payments relative to traditional Medicare are likely much higher than reported from 2001 to 2006 as diagnosis-based risk adjustment had not yet been fully phased in. Payments also are likely higher than reported from 2010 to 2017 because of higher Medicare Advantage risk score growth relative to coding intensity adjustments. MIPPA helped to improve Medicare access and affordability for low-income beneficiaries.

**Figure 18-10 •** Medicare Private Plan Payments Relative to Fee-for-Service Costs. (Source: Commonwealth Fund, Medicare Payment Advisory Commission.)

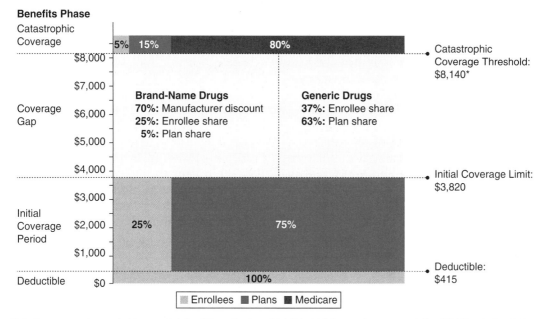

**Figure 18-11 •** Medicare Part D Standard Benefit Design in 2019. (Source: KFF, Based on 2019 Part D Benefit Parameters.)

run by private companies—known as Medicare Part D. The latter plans involve deductibles and cost sharing (Figure 18-11). Part D was the last major change made to the Medicare program.

The impact of MMA was almost immediate. By 2006, 100% of Medicare beneficiaries had access to at least 1 plan; by 2009, beneficiaries had an average of 48 plans to choose from.

With the integration of a standard drug benefit, 94% of beneficiaries had access to an MA-PD plan with zero additional premium. With Parts A, B, and D now available under a single plan, as well as supplementary benefits subsidized by generous payments, MA enrollment skyrocketed (Figure 18-12). Most of the new MA enrollees were beneficiaries who had switched from

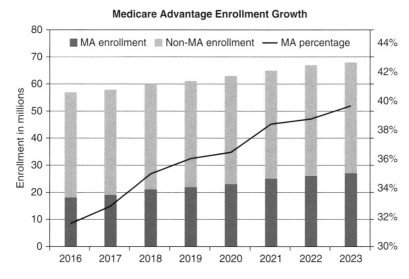

**Figure 18-12 •** Medicare Advantage (MA) Enrollment Growth. (Source: Congressional Budget Office-Medicare Baseline Projections.)

FFS Medicare. By 2017, enrollment reached 19 million, or 33% of all beneficiaries.

The MA market has become less competitive over time. Between 2009 and 2017, the number of MA plans serving a given county has fallen, and the concentration of plans has increased.[5] As a result, 70% or more of MA enrollees are enrolled in markets dominated by 2 or 3 plans, which may retard competition and the ability to reduce premiums. At the same time, researchers have found an average of 6 potential entrants into MA markets, which could increase competition; but, as noted in Chapter 17, many of these are smaller, provider-sponsored plans.

To encourage quality improvement, CMS instituted a 5-star rating for risk plans (covered later) in 2008, using the Healthcare Effectiveness Data and Information Set (HEDIS), a survey used to assess plan performance in the private sector (see Chapter 5). Even without direct financial incentives, plans showed improvement in certain HEDIS measures.

The situation changed after 2008 with the election of Barack Obama as president. Obama ran on a campaign of reducing wasteful spending on insurers; that included the payments to MCOs under MA. Payment provisions in the PPACA (2010) brought MA plan payments closer to FFS Medicare spending levels and reduced rates overall (see Figure 18-10). The reform provisions also required a medical loss ratio, which measures plan spending on medical benefits compared to premiums, of at least 85% to limit administrative overhead—similar to the PPACA requirement for all private health plans (see Chapter 17).

Despite the cuts in payment, enrollments in MA plans have continued to rise. Medicare beneficiaries like the MCO plans because they could:

- Avoid cost sharing in Parts A and B
- Avoid paying premiums for Medicare supplemental coverage
- Enroll in zero-premium MA plans
- Enjoy the possibility of added benefits: drug coverage, vision, and dental
- Enjoy limits on out-of-pocket costs
- Enjoy steady cost of Part D premiums

The 2010 reforms created incentives for enhanced quality. Standard rebates were reduced but were set higher for plans rated above 3.5 stars. Furthermore, plans rated above 4 stars received an "add on" to their benchmarks, and enrollment in 5-star plans was allowed outside the annual election period.

## How CMS Reimburses MA Plans

The amounts that CMS reimburses an MA plan member depends on 4 factors: (1) the county in which the plan is offered; (2) the bid made by the insurer for that plan; (3) the risk of the insured; and (4) the star rating of the plan. For each county, CMS sets "benchmark rates" (ie, the maximum CMS will pay). Insurers who bid above the benchmark rate will have to charge members premiums for basic Part A and Part B coverage. By contrast, plans that bid below the benchmark can earn rebates in the form of a percentage of the difference between their bid and the benchmark. The rebate must be used either to reduce plan cost sharing or to improve plan benefits (eg, dental services, eye exams, fitness benefits). Plans with a 4-star or above rating are able to bid against a higher benchmark. The difference between the higher benchmark and the standard benchmark is often referred to as a "quality bonus payment," which allows plans to receive larger rebates than plans with lower star ratings.[6] All of this means that highly rated plans are reimbursed more generously by CMS and thus able to offer more attractive plans. Plans with 4 or more stars receive larger rebates both because of their higher benchmarks and because of their higher rebate percentages; larger rebates are directly tied to more generous benefit packages.[7]

## How MA Plans Reimburse Providers

MA plans are capitated by CMS. MA plans do not usually capitate providers, however. Instead, they can pay providers in a number of other ways including diagnosis-related group (DRG) payments to hospitals, a percentage of the physician fee schedule (Resource-Based Relative Value Schedule) to physicians, or discounted FFS.

## Competitive Capabilities of MA Plans

MA plans are run by private health insurance companies that compete on cost, star quality ratings, benefits, provider networks, marketing, and brand. In many ways, the individual MA plans compete on the chevrons depicted in Figure 17-9. The competitive capabilities, which are interrelated, are briefly outlined in the following sections.

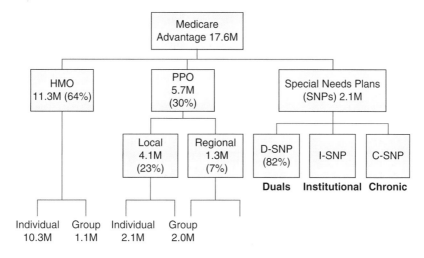

**Figure 18-13** • Managed Care Organization Plans in Medicare Advantage. HMO, Health Maintenance Organization; M, Millions; PPO, Preferred Provider Organization.

## MA Provider Networks

There are both individual and group MA plans. Individual plans are sold directly to seniors, whereas group MA plans are sold to employers and largely cover retiree health benefits. Both sets of plans can utilize HMO and PPO network models; HMOs account for the majority of enrollment (Figure 18-13).

Provider networks are a key factor affecting enrollment in individual MA plans. Having access to their preferred physicians and satisfaction with the choices among doctors in the network are important factors in Medicare beneficiaries' choice of health plan. Conversely, limited access to providers and/or not having one's primary care physician (PCP) in the MA plan network leads to disenrollment. An insurer could offer higher rates to providers as an incentive for them to participate in its networks, but then offering higher rates would reduce its profitability and ability to compete. A geographically broad network is also a competitive advantage for MA plans (eg, by offering a travel benefit that allows MA enrollees to access the same health benefits outside the service area as at home).

## Provider Reimbursement Rates and Other Negotiated Terms

When contracting with providers, an MA plan can obtain better (lower) reimbursement rates if it can advertise a larger number of enrollee members to providers as possible patients. The bigger

its market presence, the more leverage it has in negotiations with providers, and thus the better pricing it can extract from them. Academic research shows that insurers generally pay lower rates to hospitals for their services in markets with higher levels of insurer concentration covering the fully and self-insured population and where their enrollees account for a larger share of the provider's patients.

Rates are not the only factor in provider negotiations. Others include utilization management, customer service, generation of claims data, claims administration, the authorization process for treatment, the period for submitting claims, the time specified for timely payment, the interest due for late payments, processing, and coverage adjudication. Whether insurers can negotiate favorably on these factors depends on the volume of patients that the providers can obtain by contracting with the insurer.

## Value-Based Contracts

As noted earlier, commercial insurers who operate in the MA market have placed heavy emphasis on value-based contracting (VBC). VBC is a new model of reimbursement that gives providers incentives to deliver care at higher quality and lower costs. VBC relies on the use of less-established performance measures, a new emphasis on data collection (eg, cost and quality performance of providers in the networks), the ability to gather and manage these data at the local market level, and data sharing with providers. Moreover, to strike VBC agreements with providers requires considerable trust in the insurer's long-term experience in MA, its commitment to MA, and its technological capabilities to serve that market. Thus, to be successful, VBC depends on the insurer's scale and experience.

## MA Star Ratings

Star ratings are a quality rating system that measures 32 individual metrics for Part C coverage that span 5 criteria: (1) preventative care; (2) chronic condition management; (3) member experience; (4) member complaints and changes in plan performance; and (5) customer service. Star ratings range from 1 to 5, in half-star increments, with 5 stars being the highest possible rating. Star ratings are awarded at the contract level, where a "contract" consists of 1 or more plans from the same insurer all with the same network type (eg, HMO or PPO).

Star ratings affect MA plan enrollment. Insurers who have contracts with high star ratings can offer plans with supplemental benefits (1) at a lower cost to the customer (without raising premiums) and (2) financed through quality bonus payments and rebates. Evidence indicates that plans with higher star ratings have higher enrollment. Each additional star can be associated with a 10% increased likelihood of enrollment for first-time enrollees. For seniors switching from one MA plan to another, each additional star can be associated with a 4% to 5% increased likelihood of enrollment. Research also shows that beneficiaries are willing to pay more in premiums and out-of-pocket costs for higher-rated plans. Conversely, seniors are more likely to disenroll from MA plans with low star ratings.

MA plans need help from providers to improve their star ratings because some of the star rating measures are directly related to quality of care and the provider is the one providing the care. In recognition of this dependency, some MA plans try to incorporate star rating measures into their provider contracts and value-based contracts, paying bonuses to providers who meet or improve star measure targets. Some MA plans utilize multiple initiatives to drive higher star ratings, including distributing provider scorecards, implementing surveys to consumers and providers to gather better insights and make critical improvements, and incentivizing providers to have compliant members.

## Brokers and Marketing

To successfully compete, MA plans need to compete for the attention of brokers. Brokers are an important channel for the sale of individual MA plans. Most consumers who choose a Medicare plan for the first time know very little about Medicare and often rely on independent agents and brokers to help them choose. As a result, the majority of new enrollees come to an MA plan through a broker.

Marketing materials also influence seniors' choices of individual MA plans. A large percentage of seniors reportedly read direct mail from insurers; many also hear the radio ads or see the television commercials for MA plans during open enrollment period during the fall.

## Brand

Seniors often use an individual MA product's brand to infer quality. Enrollees are more likely to choose a plan when they are familiar with the company offering it and feel it has a trustworthy brand. Brand perceptions also influence customer loyalty and retention. Research shows that a very high percentage of MA enrollees remain in their current plan because it has a well-known name that they could trust. Among those switching MA plans, a large percentage list "well-known name" as a key purchase criterion. Brand reputation is important not only for consumers, but also for brokers and network providers.

## Experience Administering PPO Plans

Roughly one-third of MA plans are based on a PPO model. Administering PPO plans requires specialized expertise, not only developing the broader provider networks that PPO enrollees want but also the tools to track and manage out-of-network utilization, reimbursements, and beneficiary cost-sharing payments (eg, copays or coinsurance). This is because MA providers are required to track enrollees' out-of-pocket costs and notify them when they are near the limit. CMS requires PPO plans to reimburse services from out-of-network providers without requiring prior authorization or offering enrollees a cost-sharing discount to do so. This provides greater choice of providers for enrollees but presents a challenge for insurers because they cannot use a gatekeeper to control unit costs and provide a more competitively priced product.

**Critical Thinking Exercise: Molina Healthcare and Medicare Advantage**

In 2016, several large MCOs were involved in merger deals. Aetna sought to acquire Humana, particularly to gain Humana's large presence in the MA market. The Department of Justice (DOJ) sought to block the deal, claiming it was anticompetitive (ie, too much MA business concentrated in the merged firms in select geographic areas around the country). Aetna countered by saying it would allay such concerns by selling off the plans in those areas to a third party, Molina Healthcare, which was prominent in the Medicaid market. The DOJ was concerned that, given its past experience in Medicaid, Molina would not serve as an effective competitor in the MA market. The DOJ has asked you whether Molina would have an easy time of developing the competitive capabilities analyzed above. What do you think?

## EFFORTS TO CONTROL MEDICARE SPENDING

Prior to 1965, individuals paid most healthcare expenditures out of pocket (44% of spending in 1965). With the expansion of insurance coverage to the elderly and the poor in 1965 by Medicare and Medicaid, enrollments in and spending by public insurance programs grew, and out-of-pocket spending as a percentage of the total fell. Medicare spending grew 28.6% *annually* from 1967 to 1973, fueled by lots of factors:

- Pent-up demand
- Greater access to services
- Higher utilization of services
- Substitution of federal spending for out-of-pocket household spending
- Financing of hospital capital spending
- Encouragement of the rise of the investor-owned hospital sector
- Rapid escalation in hospital costs
- Faster price growth for hospital care
- Generous FFS reimbursement mechanisms
- Faster price growth in the economy
- Prohibitions against the government setting provider rates

- Requirement that hospital-based physicians be paid FFS, not hospital salary
- Underestimation of the cost (see later discussion)

Adding more fuel to the fire were Social Security amendments (1971-1972) that expanded both Medicare and Medicaid coverage and high economy-wide inflation from 1974 to 1982 that attended shocks in the oil supply and 3 recessions.

The cost of the Medicare program has exceeded forecasted spending since the program's inception. Prior to passage in 1965, Robert Myers in the Social Security Administration estimated it would cost $3 billion by 1970; it cost twice as much ($6 billion). He also estimated it would cost $12 billion by 1990; it cost nearly 10 times as much ($110 billion). It's hard to blame him—his calculations and forecasts were made with paper and pencil. But more recent forecasting of the cost of federal health programs, even with the aid of computers, has not been any better (Figure 18-14). The lesson is not only that forecasts are usually wrong, but they are exceedingly wrong the farther out one projects. Beginning in the early 1980s, the federal government has applied several remedies to the high levels of Medicare spending, starting first with hospitals (Part A) and then with physicians (Part B)—the 2 biggest buckets of spending.

### Inpatient Prospective Payment System (1984)[8]

As part of the Deficit Reduction Act (1984), Congress mandated the Prospective Payment System (PPS). It was later known as the Inpatient Prospective Payment System (IPPS) to distinguish it from the PPS systems applied to post-acute care, covered in Chapter 14.

IPPS changed the method of reimbursing acute care hospitals under Part A of Medicare from retrospective, cost-based reimbursement to a prospective, budget-based reimbursement. Hospitals were now paid a fixed price for a given patient discharged in a given DRG. This was designed to give hospitals an incentive to be efficient: If they spent more than the budgeted amount, they suffered a portion of the loss; if they spent less than the budgeted amount, they kept the surplus as a profit. As noted in Chapter 2, IPPS decreased admissions, lengths

| Benefit | Estimated cost at time of enactment ($billions per year or for a single specific year) | Actual cost | Difference | Error ratio |
|---|---|---|---|---|
| UK National Health Service (in British pounds) | 0.260 | 0.359 | −0.099 | 1.38 to 1 |
| Medicare hospital insurance | 9 | 67 | −58 | 7.44 to 1 |
| Medicare (entire program) | 12 | 110 | −0.98 | 9.17 to 1 |
| Medicare DSH program | 1 | 17 | −16 | 17.00 to 1 |
| Medicare home care benefit | 4 | 10 | −6 | 2.50 to 1 |
| Medicare catastrophic coverage (multiyear estimate) | 5.7 | 11.8 | −6.1 | 2.07 to 1 |
| Massachusetts Health Reform | 0.725 | 0.869 | −0.144 | 1.20 to 1 |

**Figure 18-14** • Historical Examples of Erroneous Healthcare Estimates, in $ Billions. DSH, Disproportionate Share Hospital. (Source: AEI; Joint Economic Commission, Republican Staff, July 2009.)

of stay, and inpatient Part A spending; part of the savings was counterbalanced by a rise in outpatient spending, physician visits, and Part B costs (squeezing the balloon). It also led to a rise in post-acute care use.

The IPPS is rooted in groupings of patients that reflect differences in their acuity and need. In 2019, under the IPPS, Medicare set national base rates (covering operating and capital expenses), which are then adjusted to reflect the following 2 factors:

1. Per-discharge payment rates for 759 Medicare severity DRGs (MS-DRGs), which are based on patients' clinical conditions (principal discharge diagnosis and secondary diagnoses reflecting comorbidities and complications). Each MS-DRG has a relative weight that reflects the expected relative costliness of inpatient treatment for patients in that group.
2. The hospital's location (local input prices, rural areas) and other characteristics (eg, residency training, disproportionate share hospitals that treat low-income patients). Teaching hospitals receive graduate medical education (GME) payments per resident as well as indirect medical education (IME) payments, based on the number of residents per bed, to cover the costs of training residents.

## Resource-Based Relative Value Schedule (1992)[9]

In 1992, Congress altered the payment mechanism for physicians paid under Part B of Medicare from the usual, customary, and reasonable fee (UCR) approach to a national fee schedule based on the resources used in patient care. The UCR fee system was inserted by Wilbur Cohen into the Social Security Act (1965) to placate the AMA. It led to large variations in spending between physician specialties and geographic regions, as well as the tendency for Medicare to overpay some services (eg, surgery, diagnostic tests) and underpay others (primary care).

Known as the Resource-Based Relative Value Schedule (RBRVS), it focused on 3 component resources needed to generate medical services: total physician work for a given service (time, intensity of effort), practice costs (nonphysician inputs, supplies, equipment), and cost for liability insurance. The relative costliness (or value) of these components is reflected in weights called "relative value units" (RVUs). The values attached to these 3 components are adjusted for local input prices and multiplied by a standard dollar amount (known as the conversion factor, $35 in 2017).[10] The starting point for the RVU is the Current Procedural Terminology (CPT) 5-digit code set up by the AMA in 1966 to classify physician services. Each CPT code has a numeric value assigned to it for the 3 components listed earlier; the sum of the 3 components is the total RVU for each CPT code. The physician work component comprises 50%; practice expenses comprise another 45%.[11] RBRVS also shifted funding from "procedural" to "cognitive" services in an effort to encourage physicians to enter primary care by increasing payments to PCPs and reducing specialist fees.

RBRVS had an enormous impact on Part B payments to physicians. During the period from 1980 to 1990, Medicare payments to physicians, based on charges (UCR fees), grew 13.4% annually. During the 5 years after RBRVS (1992-1997), spending on physician services grew only 1% to 2% annually.

## Balanced Budget Act (1997) and the Sustainable Growth Rate

The BBA, enacted in the fall of 1997, reduced federal spending by $250 billion, balanced the federal budget, and generated budget surpluses over the next 4 years (until President Bush invaded Iraq). However, BBA balanced the budget on the back of the Medicare program. Of the $250 billion in cuts, $119 billion came from Medicare and two-thirds of that from payments to providers. The cuts to hospitals came in the form of a 7% reduction in DRG payments.

BBA revisited physician payment as well, since physicians could collectively increase total Medicare spending even paid on a national fee schedule. BBA stipulated that it would henceforth raise physician payments when physician spending growth fell below growth in gross domestic product (GDP); conversely, it would lower physician payments when physician spending growth exceeded growth in GDP. This became known as the sustainable growth rate (SGR).

For the first few years, everything was fine. In 2002, however, total physician spending under Part B exceeded the GDP target for the first time, triggering a cut in Medicare's base payment rate for physician services by 4.8%. The lower rate caused physicians and their professional association, the AMA, to complain. In response, Congress began to annually block the cuts generated by the SGR formula, a tactic known as the "Doc fix" or "kicking the can down the road." Moreover, the administrator of the CMS turned to pay for performance (P4P) as an alternative approach (and quid pro quo for SGR relief) to improve value in Medicare Part B. In the end, such P4P

programs failed to live up to their promise of reducing costs or improving quality.[12]

In 2008, presidential candidate Barack Obama promised the AMA to correct the problem if elected; in 2015, when the cumulative SGR cuts would have amounted to approximately 25% of physician rates, the "Doc fix" was replaced by the Medicare Access and CHIP Reauthorization Act (MACRA, 2015). MACRA repealed the SGR formula, allowed Medicare to reward clinicians for value over volume, streamlined multiple quality programs under the new Merit-Based Incentive Payments System (MIPS), and gave bonus payments for participation in eligible alternative payment models (APMs).[13]

## Outpatient Prospective Payment System (2000)

The Outpatient Prospective Payment System (OPPS) was designed to cover hospital outpatient services, community mental health centers (CMHCs), partial hospitalization, and other services. The Balanced Budget Refinement Act (1999) mandated that OPPS establish payments in a budget-neutral manner based on estimates of amounts payable in 1999 from the Medicare Part B Trust Fund and patient coinsurance under the system prior to OPPS. The unit of payment under OPPS is the Ambulatory Payment Classification (APC) system. CMS assigns individual services (Healthcare Common Procedural Coding System codes) to APCs based on similar clinical characteristics and similar costs. The APC payment rate and calculated copayment apply to each service within the APC.

## Medicare Innovations and Demonstrations

Finally, Medicare has funded many demonstration programs over the past 20 years (and more) to find ways to improve quality and reduce costs. Demonstrations are mandated by Congress and serve as real-world tests of new ways to deliver health services, pay providers, and design benefits. They serve as laboratories for policy makers to experiment on a low-risk basis, since the demonstrations are time limited (usually 2-3 years) and are confined to limited geographic areas, enrollee subgroups, or provider subgroups.

Some of the earliest programs were demonstrations of "bundled payment"—combining the payment of different providers involved in a patient's episode of care. The original IPPS followed a similar approach, bundling all inpatient hospital services (eg, labor, supplies, facility costs) together under the DRG payment. The first of these was the Medicare Participating Heart Bypass Center Demonstration in 1991, followed by the Acute Care Episode (ACE) Demonstration in 2009 and several additional models over the past few years (eg, Bundled Payment for Care Improvement Initiative [BPCI] and Comprehensive Care for Joint Replacement Model [CCJR]). Medicare has also funded various P4P programs (eg, the Premier Hospital Quality Incentive Demonstration [HQID]), VBP programs for nursing homes, care management programs for high-cost Medicare beneficiaries, hospital gain-sharing programs, and medical home programs. Bundled payment programs have had some positive effects, including consistent, downward effects on both spending (<10%) and utilization (5%-15%); many of the savings are achieved in use of post-acute care and the costs negotiated with product vendors for implantable devices. The results from other demonstration programs are mixed (eg, inconsistent, small impacts on quality).[14]

In 2006, CMS funded the Physician Group Practice (PGP) Demonstration program, contracting with 10 physician groups in 2005 to 2010 on a P4P and "shared savings model." The groups were rewarded for meeting cost and 32 quality targets by keeping a portion of the savings they reaped. The program's goal was to achieve Medicare savings of 2% or more. The groups performed well on the quality metrics; savings were another matter. While 6 of the 10 groups earned savings, the vast majority of savings was earned by just 1 group. The overall savings were also not impressive: $114 per individual. The savings reaped by some groups were offset by the lack of savings by others; most of the savings derived from treating the "dual eligibles." The PGP Demonstration was thus not very successful. Nevertheless, the administration "declared victory" and used the demonstration as "proof of concept" for the launch of accountable care organizations (ACOs) as part of the PPACA.

The federal government has launched many more demonstrations and initiatives beyond these, often using the Center for Medicare and Medicaid Innovation (CMMI) as the test ground. CMMI's agenda is to accelerate the development and testing of new payment and delivery models and then to help speed the adoption of best practices. The array of such initiatives is presented in Figure 18-15.

---

**CMS Innovations Portfolio**

**Accountable Care Organizations (ACOs)**
- Medicare Shared Savings Program (Center for Medicare)
- Pioneer ACO Model
- Advance Payment ACO Model
- PGP Transition Demonstration
- Comprehensive ESRD Care Initiative

**Primary Care Transformation**
- Comprehensive Primary Care Initiative (CPC)
- Multi-Payer Advanced Primary Care Practice (MAPCP) Demonstration
- Federally Qualified Health Center (FQHC) Advanced Primary Care Practice Demonstration
- Independence at Home Demonstration
- Graduate Nurse Education Demonstration

**Bundled Payment for Care Improvement**
- Model 1: Retrospective Acute Care
- Model 2: Retrospective Acute Care Episode & Post Acute
- Model 3: Retrospective Post Acute Care
- Model 4: Prospective Acute Care

**Capacity to Spread Innovation**
- Partnership for Patients
- Community-Based Care Transitions
- Million Hearts
- Innovation Advisors Program

**Healthcare Innovation Awards**

**State Innovation Models Initiative**

**Initiatives Focused on the Medicaid Population**
- Medicaid Emergency Psychiatric Demonstration
- Medicaid Incentives for Prevention of Chronic Diseases
- Strong Start Initiative

**Medicare-Medicaid Enrollees**
- Financial Alignment Initiative
- Initiative to Reduce Avoidable Hospitalizations of Nursing Facility Residents

**Figure 18-15** • Centers for Medicare and Medicaid Services Innovations Portfolio. ACO, Accountable Care Organization; ESRD, End-Stage Renal Disease; PGP, Physician Group Practice.

## OTHER BUDGET REMEDIES GOING FORWARD?

To date, the only policy levers that have successfully moderated the rate of increase in Medicare spending have been draconian: the BBA 1997 cuts, cuts under PPACA, and the 2013 sequester. Other possible avenues that are periodically debated (and then shelved due to a combination of fierce opposition and lack of political will) are to raise the age of Medicare eligibility (eg, from 65 to 67 years), raise the cost-sharing requirements of beneficiaries (eg, increase Part B and Part D premiums), restrict/discourage supplemental coverage, move to more means testing of benefits (which started in 2013 with Part B), raise the payroll tax even further, increase sin taxes on alcohol/tobacco, and/or convert Medicare into a premium support system.

## DUAL ELIGIBLES

A subset of the Medicare population is also poor and, thus, qualifies for Medicaid as well. They are known as the "dual eligibles." There are roughly 9 to 10 million dual eligibles. They compose 20% of the Medicare population, 14% of the Medicaid population, and 34% of spending in each program. They are thus some of the highest health risks in the publicly-insured programs. On average, Medicare FFS per-capita spending is more than twice as high for dual eligibles ($30,619 in 2012) as for non–dual eligibles. Disability is a pathway for individuals to become eligible for both Medicare and Medicaid benefits.

Medicare pays covered medical services first for dual-eligible beneficiaries because Medicaid is generally the payer of last resort. Medicaid may cover medical costs that Medicare may not cover or partially covers (eg, nursing home care, personal care, and home- and community-based services). Medicare and Medicaid dual-eligible benefits vary by state. Some states offer Medicaid through Medicaid managed care plans, whereas other states provide FFS Medicaid coverage. Some states provide certain dual-eligible beneficiary plans that include all Medicare and Medicaid benefits.

## SUMMARY

As a result of Medicare and Medicaid, the US federal government is the single biggest payer of healthcare. One cannot overestimate its impact on the population and the healthcare ecosystem, yesterday and today. For example, the Medicare program has lifted a lot of elderly people out of poverty, alleviated the financial burden of their health expenses, helped them to gain financial access to care, and improved their utilization of needed services from the same set of providers used by those with private health insurance. In this manner, Medicare has helped to "mainstream" the elderly.

Medicare has been a major source of innovation in healthcare financing, provider reimbursement, and provider organization. As one illustration, the IPPS introduced in 1983 has since been extended to outpatient care and post-acute care; the DRG payment system has since become a mainstream form of reimbursement worldwide; its P4P program and RVU system of paying physicians have been copied by the private insurers; and its Medicare ACOs have been copied in the private sector. Compared to private sector insurance, Medicare has been a leader in controlling spending increases over the past several years.

The Medicare program has not been without its problems, however. It failed to build in cost controls at its inception, which fostered huge spending inflation in the United States and led to a long series of "bolt-on" solutions over time, most of which have failed to control escalating costs. Its financing and reimbursement initiatives have made healthcare financing incredibly complex and brought with it massive regulation of payers and providers (which impose huge costs). Its allowance of Medigap plans created a large, powerful block of election voters in the form of AARP. It encouraged seniors to see themselves as a separate, entitled group with interests morally superior to those on Medicaid (since they "paid into the system"), even though they may be unaware of how big a subsidy they have received from younger workers who are really footing the Medicare bill with their payroll taxes. Medicare transfers large amounts of money from the young to the old, which may explain why the elderly love the program. Medicare has also skewed public spending away from social services to health-care spending (ie, medicalization of social welfare expenditures), which has gradually starved other social programs. Medicare was also created to deal with acute care problems, not the chronic illness challenges that we currently face (and that are so expensive to treat).

---

### QUESTIONS TO PONDER

1. What are the major differences between FFS Medicare and managed care Medicare (MA)?
2. Despite government efforts that reduced the rates paid to MA health plans, these plans are flourishing and growing in popularity with seniors. What explains this?
3. How successful has the government been in controlling Medicare spending?
4. In the spring of 2020, several Democratic candidates for president supported "Medicare for All."[15] What would be the benefits of extending Medicare coverage to the entirety of the US population? What might be some of the downsides?
5. Why do the "dual eligibles" have such high expenditures? What are the difficulties in managing the care for this population segment?

---

### REFERENCES

1. Drugs covered under Part B include most injectable and infusible drugs given as part of a doctor's service, drugs and biologicals (eg, those used for the treatment of end-stage renal disease), drugs used at home with some types of Part B–covered durable medical equipment (nebulizers and infusion pumps), and some oral drugs with special coverage requirements like certain oral anticancer and antiemetic drugs, as well as immunosuppressive drugs.
2. According to CMS, PFFS plans pay providers on a fee-for-service basis without placing the providers at financial risk; vary provider payment rates only based on the specialty or location of the provider or to increase utilization of certain preventive or screening services; do not restrict members' choices among providers that are lawfully authorized to furnish services and accept the plan's terms and conditions of payment; and do not permit the use of prior authorization or notification. They can offer full or partial networks of providers, or in certain cases, they may not use a network of providers at all. No matter what kind of network a PFFS plan provides, its enrollees can see any provider who is eligible to receive payment from Medicare and agrees to accept the plan's terms and conditions of payment.
3. According to CMS, a special needs plan (SNP) is a Medicare Advantage (MA) coordinated care plan (CCP) specifically designed to provide targeted care and limit enrollment to special needs individuals. A special needs individual could be any one of the following: an institutionalized individual, a dual eligible, or an individual with a severe or disabling chronic condition, as specified by CMS.
4. This section draws heavily on the excellent summary written by: Yash Patel and Stuart Guterman. *The Evolution of Private Plans in Medicare* (New York, NY: Commonwealth Fund, December 8, 2017). Available online: https://www.commonwealthfund.org/publications/issue-briefs/2017/dec/evolution-private-plans-medicare. Accessed on April 6, 2020.
5. Richard Frank and Thomas McGuire. *Market Concentration and Potential Competition in Medicare Advantage* (New York, NY: Commonwealth Fund, February 2019).
6. If a plan has 4 stars or higher, an insurer can bid at a benchmark that is 5% higher than the standard benchmark for the county. Plans that are new or have low enrollment bid against a benchmark that is 3.5% higher than the standard benchmark. Plans that are rated 3.5 stars or less bid against the standard benchmark. Moreover, the percentage of the difference between the bid and the benchmark that is paid to insurers by CMS is larger for highly rated plans. The percentage of the difference between a plan's bid and its benchmark is 70% for 4.5- and 5-star plans, 65% for 3.5- and 4-star plans, and 50% for plans with 3 or fewer stars. The percentage for new plans is 65%.
7. For instance, a 4.5-star plan can bid against a benchmark that is 105% of the area benchmark, and if the bid is below the benchmark, 70% of the difference will be returned in the form of a rebate payment. A 4-star plan bids against the same benchmark, but only receives a 65% rebate. Plans below 4 stars bid against 100% of the area benchmark and receive a 65% rebate (or less). Thus, having a contract with a rating of 4 or more stars results in substantially larger reimbursements from CMS and gives insurers a competitive advantage. Plans with star ratings of 5 have an additional advantage in that they are allowed to market to and enroll members in their plans year-round.

8. This section draws on MedPAC. *Hospital Acute Inpatient Services Payment System* (Washington, DC: MedPAC, October 2016). Available online: http://www.medpac.gov/docs/default-source/payment-basics/medpac_payment_basics_16_hospital_final.pdf. Accessed on April 7, 2020.

9. This section draws on MedPAC. *Physician and Other Health Professional Payment System* (Washington, DC: MedPAC, October 2016). Available online: http://medpac.gov/docs/default-source/payment-basics/medpac_payment_basics_16_physician_final.pdf?sfvrsn=0. Accessed on April 8, 2020.

10. Under the RBRVS system, CMS assigns a work relative value unit (RVU or wRVU) to each distinct physician service, taking into account factors such as the time, skill, and equipment needed to render that service to a patient. For example, a routine office visit for evaluation and management may have a wRVU of 1.50, whereas a total knee replacement may have a wRVU of 20.72. CMS annually determines the price that physicians are paid for each service by multiplying the wRVU by a set dollar conversion factor (eg, a 1.50 wRVU for an office visit is multiplied by the 2017 CMS conversion factor of $35, rendering a $52.50 fee for that physician service). Under the RBRVS model, physicians are paid based on the volume of services they perform as measured by wRVUs. The wRVU system thus represents the volume, but not the quality or efficiency, of services provided by physicians. This wRVU-based system is the model used by many commercial payers in fee-for-service contracts. Some commercial payers negotiate the reimbursement rate as a different conversion factor ($45 instead of Medicare's $35). Other payers might structure and negotiate the reimbursement rates as a percentage of the Medicare RBRVS fee for a particular year (eg, 110% of 2017 RBRVS, or 110% of the wRVU multiplied by the conversion factor).

11. These RVUs are updated by the AMA/Specialty Society Relative Value Scale Update Committee (RUC). The RUC is an independent group of volunteer physicians exercising its First Amendment right to petition the federal government. The RUC is comprised of 31 members, 28 of whom are voting members (16 of these 28 voting members are from specialties whose Medicare-allowed charges are primarily derived from the provision of evaluation and management services). The RUC is an expert panel. Individuals exercise their independent judgment and are not advocates for their specialty.

12. Aaron Mendelson, Karli Kondo, Cheryl Damberg, et al. "The Effects of Pay-for-Performance Programs on Health, Health Care Use, and Processes of Care," *Ann Intern Med.* 166 (2017): 341-353. Kathleen Mullen, Richard Frank, and Meredith Rosenthal. "Can You Get What You Pay For? Pay-for-Performance and the Quality of Health Care Providers," *RAND J Econ.* 41 (1) (2010): 64-91.

13. MIPS consolidated 3 existing Medicare quality programs that affect FFS payment: meaningful use, value-based payment modifier (clinicians' Part A and B costs), and physician quality reporting system (pay for reporting). Providers were subject to quality reporting requirements. Their reimbursement can be positively or negatively adjusted based on performance in (1) quality (6 measures with 50% weight in 2019); (2) resource use (efficiency; 10% weight); (3) meaningful use of electronic medical records and advancing care information (25% weight); and (4) clinical practice improvement activities (CPIA; 15% weight). MACRA is a "revenue neutral" program: The poorest performer doctors can get payments cut up to 9%, whereas high performers can get increases as high as 27% over time.

14. Congressional Budget Office. *Lessons from Medicare's Demonstration Projects on Disease Management, Care Coordination, and Value-Based Payment.* Issue Brief (Washington, DC: CBO, January 2012).

15. Jonathan Oberlander. "Navigating the Shifting Terrain of US Health Care Reform—Medicare for All, Single Payer, and the Public Option." Available online: https://www.milbank.org/quarterly/articles/navigating-the-shifting-terrain-of-us-health-care-reform-medicare-for-all-single-payer-and-the-public-option/?gclid=EAIaIQobChMIg9jeoL2O6wIViJWzCh3LOQ6MEAAYASAAEgJbSfD_BwE. Accessed on August 9, 2020.

# Medicaid and the Patient Protection and Affordable Care Act

**19**

## OVERVIEW: MEDICARE VERSUS MEDICAID

Medicare and Medicaid were both implemented by Congress in the same year to address the same issue: the War on Poverty. Both programs have also grown in enrollment and spending (Figure 19-1) and now represent the major growth markets for private health insurers.

The 2 programs could not be more different, however, and since 1965, they have taken very different trajectories. In contrast to the national Medicare program that covers all of the elderly and (starting in 1972) the disabled and those with kidney failure, Medicaid has traditionally been an income-based welfare program that sets minimum federal eligibility requirements, has varying state-level eligibility criteria, and historically covered selected (and very diverse) segments of the low-income population. Moreover, many of those eligible for Medicaid were initially "bolted on" over time through a series of program expansions, culminating in a huge increase in eligibility based on income following enactment of the Patient Protection and Affordable Care Act (PPACA) (Figure 19-2).

As briefly noted in Chapter 18, Medicare is a popular and dignified program, partly because it provides insurance to our parents and grandparents, but also because the latter paid into the system through their payroll taxes and are considered "deserving" to be paid back. This is despite the fact that Medicare is largely funded through general tax revenues and higher taxes on higher income earners (to cover Parts B and D). The elderly believe they have paid for their care, but not as much as they think. By contrast,

Medicaid traditionally bore (until recent decades) the stigma of a welfare program that beneficiaries did not pay into and who may not be as deserving. These perceived differences are reinforced by the fact that Medicare serves the elderly and disabled, whereas Medicaid serves young people and racial minorities (Figure 19-3). These perceived differences are further bolstered by the contrast in voting participation between the elderly (high turnout) and the poor (low turnout). They are further reinforced by the relatively high payment rates that Medicare Part B pays physicians (39% more than Medicaid), which elicits high physician willingness to treat Medicare patients, and deters some physicians from seeing Medicaid patients.

Beyond these contrasts, Medicare Part A is a "pay-as-you-go" system based on payroll taxes paid by the working population under 65 that serve as a wealth transfer to the elderly, whereas Medicaid is financed through general federal revenues and state tax revenues. Moreover, Medicare automatically enrolls the eligible elderly in Part A when reaching age 65, whereas some state Medicaid programs pose significant barriers to enrollment and maintaining coverage, including taking off time from work to apply in person, requiring substantial paper documentation of income and other eligibility criteria (employment verification in some states), waiting weeks or months for eligibility determination, misunderstanding official notices due to language or literacy challenges, not receiving notices due to unstable housing arrangements, and repeating these steps at renewal. By contrast, other states make enrollment easier (eg, sometimes by default when the patient is hospitalized).

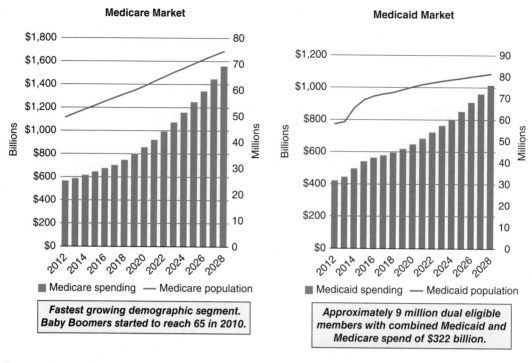

**Figure 19-1** • Medicare and Medicaid Growth Markets. (Source: Centers for Medicare and Medicaid Services.)

## ORIGINS OF MEDICAID

Before Medicaid was enacted, the federal government made limited payments to states for healthcare services they purchased on behalf of public assistance recipients (ie, those "on welfare" receiving cash assistance from local government). For example, the Social Security Act Amendments of 1950 (Title XVI) established a state grant program known as Aid to

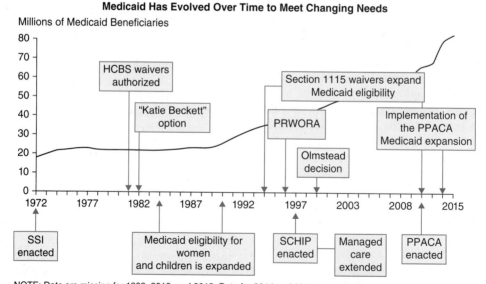

NOTE: Data are missing for 1999, 2012, and 2013. Data for 2014 and 2015 are projections.

**Figure 19-2** • Evolution of Medicaid. PPACA, Patient Protection and Affordable Care Act; HCBS, Home and Community-Based Services; SCHIP, State Children's Health Insurance Program; SSI, Supplemental Security Income. (Source: Robin Rudowitz, Rachel Garfield, and Elizabeth Hinton. "10 Things to Know About Medicaid: Setting the Facts Straight," Kaiser Family Foundation, 2019. Available Online: https://www.kff.org/medicaid/issue-brief/10-things-to-know-about-medicaid-setting-the-facts-straight/.)

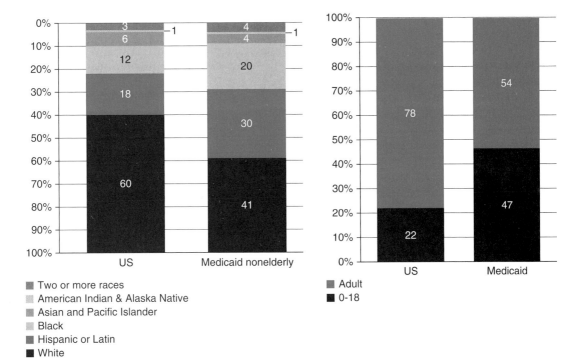

**Figure 19-3** • Medicaid Disproportionately Serves Young People and Racial Minorities. (Source: Centers for Medicare and Medicaid Services, US Census Bureau, Kids Count Data Center.)

the Permanently and Totally Disabled (later replaced by the Supplemental Security Income [SSI] program in 1972) that provided cash payments to the elderly, blind, or disabled with low incomes. In 1960, the Kerr-Mills Act authorized open-ended federal matching payments to states for healthcare provided to the 'medically indigent', ie, elderly not receiving old age assistance cash payments but too poor to pay for needed services. Nevertheless, states varied widely in the scope of the services they funded for their low-income population; some did not even participate.

Medicaid was authorized by Title XIX of the 1965 Social Security Act. When passed, the goal was to consolidate several grant programs already administered by the states. Medicaid's reach was initially limited, however. First, it was designed to provide mostly acute care services to public assistance recipients. Second, the states had discretion over the range of services each would cover. Third, although it was an entitlement program, it was a "means tested and needs based" social welfare program (ie, with income and asset limitations for eligibility), targeting the needs of women and children. Fourth, it confined support to 2 groups of "mandated categorically needy";

that is, those individuals and families receiving cash benefits from 2 programs: (1) poor children and their parents (Aid to Families with Dependent Children [AFDC]), and (2) the aged, blind, and disabled. It also extended coverage to the "medically needy"—families who had incomes above AFDC's income and asset criteria could become eligible if they incurred significant medical expenses that reduced their net income to the Medicaid eligibility limits ("spend down"). In keeping with the welfare principles of the era and budget considerations, enrollment was not encouraged; most low-income families remained uninsured. Fifth, it was a voluntary program; states did not have to participate (but all eventually did).

The federal government established broad requirements for state Medicaid programs that wished to receive federal funding. These included (1) who must be covered, (2) what types of medical services must be offered, and (3) whether beneficiaries can be required to face cost sharing (eg, deductibles, copays). For their part, the states administered their own program and decided (1) whether to make certain types of people eligible beyond what was required by the federal government mandate, and (2) how much to pay physicians, hospitals, and other providers. States had considerable flexibility in setting service and eligibility requirements, which led to considerable variation across state programs and, in the eyes of many, great inequities.

Medicaid is thus a joint federal-state program. There are lots of Medicaid programs—one for each state, the District of Columbia, and US territories. As a federal-state program, there is a division of labor between the 2 levels of government, with the federal government matching state expenditures based on a formula using state per-capita income. The federal contribution to total program costs ranges from approximately 50% (for higher-income states) to 78% (for lower-income states). In fiscal year 2017, the federal government covered about 62% of all Medicaid spending, while the states picked up the remaining 38%. One irony of Medicaid is that the poor are much better off in richer states. The steepest Medicaid benefits per poor person can be found in states (many in the Northeast) with higher-income taxpayers and relatively few poor persons. These states are better equipped to provide generous benefits than are lower-income states with higher poverty levels and fewer rich taxpayers.

## HISTORICAL GROWTH AND EXPANSION

During its first year of operation (1966), 26 states implemented Medicaid; all but one implemented their programs by 1972 (Arizona held out until 1982). The program's initial combined (federal and state) spending for 1966 was only $1.5 billion. Spending and enrollment rose exponentially thereafter. Between 1966 and 1971, average *annual* spending rose by more than 50%, whereas average *annual* enrollment grew by nearly 33%. Rapid growth in covered services resulted in per-enrollee cost growth that exceeded economy-wide inflation by nearly 11%.

By 1971, annual costs reached $6.5 billion, and enrollment reached 16 million. Initial projections of Medicaid spending forecast less than one-half of this amount, largely because they underestimated the extent to which states would offer coverage to optional eligibility groups (eg, the medically needy) and for optional services. A significant benefit expansion occurred with enactment of the Early Periodic Screening

Diagnostic and Treatment (EPSDT) program in 1967, which guaranteed preventive services for eligible children.

More program changes in the early 1970s fueled even greater spending. The 1972 Amendments to the Social Security Act created the SSI program, which federalized existing state cash assistance programs for aged and disabled persons.[1] Nearly all SSI beneficiaries received Medicaid coverage. The implementation of SSI resulted in significant increases in enrollment among the aged and disabled, averaging nearly 8% per year during 1972 to 1976. Other amendments added optional Medicaid benefits that included intermediate care facilities for the mentally retarded (ICF/MR) and inpatient psychiatric services for younger beneficiaries. Residents of these facilities, and the disabled in general, were among the most expensive groups in Medicaid. These amendments fostered 18% average annual expenditure growth (1972-1976) and 5% average annual enrollment growth.

The Reagan administration cut back on Medicaid spending during the early 1980s. The Omnibus Budget Reconciliation Act (OBRA, 1981) cut the federal matching rate for the next 3 years for states whose growth exceeded certain targets. OBRA also reduced eligibility for welfare benefits and made it more difficult to qualify for Medicaid. Along with a decrease in inflation, Medicaid expenditures grew at an annual average rate of less than 8% between 1981 and 1984, whereas Medicaid enrollment remained stable.

To offset reduced federal support, Congress broadened state options for providing and reimbursing Medicaid benefits. Many experimented with prospective payment systems, managed care organization (MCOs; such as health maintenance organizations [HMOs]) under Section 1915(b) waivers, and home and community-based service (HCBS) programs under Section 1915(c) waivers that assisted individuals with disabilities who otherwise require institutionalization to remain in the community (see box titled "Medicaid Program Waivers"). Medicaid's focus shifted from just paying claims to managing costs and services. OBRA also required that states make additional Disproportionate Share Hospital (DSH) payments to hospitals that serve especially large numbers of Medicaid and other low-income individuals to defray the impact of low reimbursements and uncompensated care.

| Medicaid Program Waivers |
|---|

The Social Security Act (SSA) authorized several waiver and demonstration programs to provide states more flexibility to operate Medicaid. Waivers allowed states to disregard certain requirements and operate outside of Medicaid rules. States may try different approaches to healthcare delivery or adapt their programs to the special needs of particular geographic areas or groups of Medicaid enrollees. The primary Medicaid waiver programs include the following:

- **Section 1115 Research and Demonstration Projects**—SSA Section 1115 allows states to (1) waive Medicaid requirements regarding *freedom of choice* of provider, *comparability* of services, and *statewideness,* and/or to (2) allow expenditures that do not otherwise qualify for federal financial aid that permit states to conduct experimental, pilot, or demonstration projects that assist in promoting the objectives of the Medicaid program. States can use waivers to change eligibility criteria to offer coverage to new groups of people, condition Medicaid eligibility on an enrollee's ability to meet work

requirements, provide services that are not otherwise covered, offer different service packages or a combination of services in different parts of the state, cap program enrollment, and implement innovative service delivery systems.

- **Section 1915(b) Managed Care/Freedom of Choice Waivers**—SSA Section 1915(b) waives the provider *freedom of choice* requirement to establish mandatory managed care programs or otherwise limit enrollees' choice of providers.

- **Section 1915(c) Home and Community-Based Services Waivers**—SSA Section 1915(c) waives requirements regarding *comparability* of services and *statewideness* in covering a broad range of HCBSs for certain persons with long-term support services (LTSSs) needs. States also may waive certain income and resource rules applicable to persons in the community, which means that a spouse's or parent's income and, to some extent, resources are not considered available to the applicant for the purposes of determining Medicaid financial eligibility.

In contrast to the first half of the decade, Medicaid made several expansions during the latter half of the 1980s. In 1986, Medicaid funds could be used to cover costs of low-income Medicare beneficiaries; in 1989, Medicaid covered pregnant women and children up to age 6 in families with incomes up to 133% of the Federal Poverty Level (FPL); in 1990, coverage was extended to children up to age 18 in families with incomes at or below 100% of FPL. However, many of these expansions were subject to delayed effective dates or phase-in provisions. Coverage of children below the poverty level, for example, was still phasing in during the 1990s. As a result, the full impact of these expansions was not felt until later.

The 1980s' mandates and the recession of the early 1990s pressured state budgets that were already strained; most were running deficits. Average annual enrollment growth of 12% plus rising expenditures prompted some states to turn to alternative financing mechanisms. One of these involved their DSH payments.

DSH payments were required by law and were not subject to the federal limits that applied to all other types of Medicaid reimbursement. States could thus increase DSH payments to a provider to any level it chose, recoup the increased payment through a donation from or tax on that provider, and thereby receive essentially unlimited federal matching funds with little or no increase in net state spending. By 1992, DSH payments had grown to more than $17 billion, or more than 15% of total Medicaid spending. Congress responded by outlawing the use of most provider donations and placed a statutory aggregate cap on DSH payments at 12% of Medicaid spending. Medicaid spending growth, which averaged over 27% annually between 1990 and 1992, slowed considerably.

During the mid-1990s, states continued experimentation with increased use of Section 1915(b) MCO waivers, as well as demonstrations allowed under Section 1115 of the original SSA in 1965. The 1115 plans permitted mandatory

MCO enrollment and automatic assignment (ie, no choice) to a health plan; there was often only 1 health plan per geographic area.

By the end of 1996, more than 24 states, accounting for over 60% of Medicaid spending, had demonstration projects that were either approved or pending. Two subsequent pieces of federal legislation had a huge impact on the program. The Personal Responsibility and Work Opportunity Reconciliation Act of 1996 (PRWORA; also known as "welfare reform") decoupled Medicaid from cash assistance for low-income families by replacing AFDC with a block grant program known as Temporary Assistance for Needy Families (TANF). The goal was to reduce reliance on welfare and cash assistance and impose work requirements and welfare time limits, but also ensure that very-low-income parents could enroll in Medicaid regardless of their eligibility for cash assistance.

The Balanced Budget Act (BBA) of 1997 gave states freedom to do mandatory enrollment in Medicaid managed care programs for certain eligible categories without the use of waivers; in many states, the managed care enrollment decision was not voluntary but mandatory. Between 1996 and 2003, the percentage of Medicaid beneficiaries in managed care plans grew from 40% to nearly 60%. The most significant provision in BBA for Medicaid was the establishment of the State Children's Health Insurance Program (SCHIP), which authorized nearly $40 billion in federal funding over 10 years (1998-2007) to provide health coverage to low-income children who did not qualify for Medicaid. States could use SCHIP monies to fund coverage of children through expansions of their Medicaid programs or through separate state programs under a new Title XXI of the SSA. The uninsured rates for children fell from 15% in 1994 to 7% by 2013. The effects of welfare reform and a thriving economy resulted in a 0.4% average annual decline in enrollment (1996-1998) and a spending slowdown to an average annual rate of 5.6% (1997-1999).

## OVERVIEW OF PATIENT PROTECTION AND AFFORDABLE CARE ACT

The PPACA was passed in 2010 and implemented in 2014, and represents the signature legislation of President Obama's administration. Historically, Medicaid eligibility generally was limited to low-income children, pregnant women, parents of dependent children, the elderly, and individuals with disabilities. The PPACA threatened states that did not expand their Medicaid programs with losing federal funding for their existing Medicaid populations; in 2012, the US Supreme Court ruled this requirement was unconstitutional. Since then, states have had the option to expand their Medicaid programs to cover nonelderly adults with income up to 138% of the FPL under the PPACA. As of 2019, 14 states had not yet done so. The PPACA promoted Medicaid's transition from a welfare program focused on defined needs-based populations to an insurance-type program for all low-income Americans at or below 138% of the FPL (in states that expanded Medicaid). For the first time, Medicaid coverage was available to all adults in all states based on their income, whether or not they had children.

The administration initially hoped to use it to solve the iron triangle: increase access to insurance and thus healthcare, improve quality, and reduce cost—and do it all in a budget-neutral manner. It had to settle on (and be satisfied with) tackling the first goal and hope to make progress on the second and third goals. PPACA also had 3 pillars: coverage expansion, financing, and reform of the delivery system. These are detailed in the following sections.

## Insurance Expansion

Insurance coverage expansion came through 2 vehicles: expanded Medicaid coverage to 12 million newly eligible enrollees and another 1.7 million who were already eligible in nonexpansion states who now signed up ("welcome mat" effect), and coverage to another 10.6 million people through state-based health insurance exchanges (HIEs) as of 2019. With regard to the former, those earning up to 133% (and then 138%) of the FPL were now automatically eligible for Medicaid nationally; in 2011, that income threshold amounted to $14,484 for an individual and $29,726 for a family of 4. Families without access to employer coverage and with incomes that ranged from 138% to 400% of FPL were eligible for a subsidy to purchase insurance on the HIEs; the premium subsidies were pegged to a fixed percentage of income, not to exceed 10%. Families with incomes over 400% of FPL could also buy coverage on the HIEs but did not get the subsidies. In addition to the premium subsidies, the PPACA also provided subsidies to insurers to provide cost-sharing assistance to those with incomes of 100% to 250% of the FPL. Finally, the law's dependent coverage provision enabled children up to age 26 to stay on their parents' insurance, benefiting between 2 and 3 million young people.

As for the HIEs, the public had a choice among 4 types of plans known as "metal tiers": bronze, silver, gold, and platinum. The tiers varied in the actuarial value of the healthcare services they covered (60% bronze, 70% silver, 80% gold, 90% platinum), the out-of-pocket expense or liability to the insured (40%, 30%, 20%, and 10%), the premium to be paid, and the size of the deductible. Most HIE enrollees chose plans in the bottom 2 tiers—those with lower premiums but higher cost sharing—similar to workers choosing HDHPs. Moreover, at least initially, there was also an "individual mandate" that required people to purchase coverage on the HIEs or face financial (tax) penalties; that penalty was repealed by the Tax Cuts and Jobs Act (2017).

Health plans on the HIEs faced new requirements to provide "essential health benefits" (similar to those provided by employer-based plans) and "preventive services" for all adults. They were also (1) required to cover pre-existing conditions and renew coverage for all who wished to do so, and (2) restricted in the criteria they could use to underwrite insurance premiums to age, family size, geographic area, and smoking status.

## Financing

The PPACA was forecast to cost $1.2 trillion over a 10-year period (2016-2025) to cover an estimated 24 million people. Most of the costs derived from insurance subsidies to join the HIEs and from Medicaid expansions (with the federal government covering 100% of the cost for 2014-2016, and then tapering to 90% by 2020). This compares with the 61% of the bill for fee-for-service (FFS) Medicaid that the federal government now pays for. To finance the insurance expansion and keep PPACA budget neutral, the administration came up with the following sources of funds (in billions of dollars):

| | |
|---|---|
| • Reduced Medicare payments to Medicare Advantage plans, hospitals | $627 |
| • Fines/taxes on individuals ignoring individual mandate | $43 |
| • Fines/taxes on employers ignoring employer mandate | $167 |
| • New fees/taxes on health insurers | $102 |
| • New fees/taxes on pharmaceutical firms | $34 |
| • Excise tax on device firms (2.3% of sales) | $29 |
| • Higher Medicare Part A tax on households making $250,000+/year | $63 |
| • Taxes on "Cadillac" health insurance plans | $87 |

The provider cuts were daunting: Hospitals faced $260 billion in cuts from 2013 to 2022; they also faced an additional $56 billion cut in DSH payments to Medicare and Medicaid, and they were to face another $151 billion in cuts through the sequestration and 2013 budget bill that shortly followed. Many of the other taxes outlined in the previous list, however, were "kicked down the road" and then never tapped. The health insurer tax was deferred to 2017 and subsequently repealed; the medical device firm tax was deferred until 2018 and then repealed altogether; and the Cadillac tax was deferred until 2020 and then repealed altogether.

## Reform of the Delivery System

Finally, PPACA sought to simultaneously improve quality while reducing costs of care by shifting more risk to providers. The signature reforms here were the accountable care organizations (ACOs; covered in Chapter 12), which entailed the largest number of beneficiaries and the largest amount of spending. Another hallmark were the bundled payment and quality improvement efforts embedded in the Centers for Medicare and Medicaid Services (CMS) Center for Medicare and Medicaid Innovation (CMMI) demonstrations covered in the previous chapter. In addition, the administration pursued several pay-for-performance (P4P) and value-based purchasing (VBP) initiatives that included (1) Medicare paying hospitals 2% more if they do well on process measures for cardiac, surgery, and pneumonia care; (2) Medicare reducing payments (up to 3%) for hospitals with high readmission rates; and (3) Medicare reducing payments to the worst-performing hospitals by 1% for hospital-acquired conditions. As of early 2020, it is not clear that the ACO, P4P, or VBP initiatives had worked to either improve quality or save money.[2]

CMMI also attempted to redesign primary care payment and delivery (see Chapter 10) via 8 different initiatives. These initiatives focused on care management, care coordination, patient-centered care, and quality improvement. Analyses suggest how hard it is for such initiatives to control costs and improve patient outcomes on a limited set of quality metrics. What may be lacking is a substantial increase in payments to primary care practices, financial incentives to other providers, and concomitant changes in the staffing, processes, and work flows of primary care practices.[3]

## PPACA IMPACT ON THE IRON TRIANGLE[4]

### Access to Care

The major goal of PPACA was to increase access to health insurance and thus access to care among the nonelderly. It clearly did so. Compared to 2013 (the year before many reforms went into effect), Medicaid coverage in the expansion states increased by 6.5% in 2014, 9.7% in 2015, and 11.8% in 2016. By contrast, the coverage increases in states that did not expand were 3.6%, 5.9%, and 8.3%. The PPACA also reduced reports of cost barriers to seeking care and increased the likelihood of having a primary care physician (PCP), with the effects growing over time; however, the gains were only modestly larger in the expansion states and may thus reflect other ongoing trends. Figure 19-4 shows that on several dimensions, Medicaid beneficiaries enjoy access to care comparable to those with private health insurance.

Overall, since the law's implementation, nearly 14 million new people have become

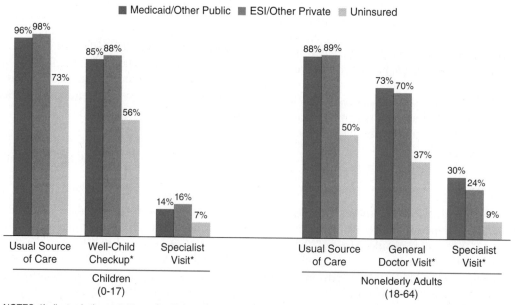

NOTES: *Indicates in the past 12 months. Respondents who said usual source of care was the emergency room are not counted as having a usual source of care. All estimates are statistically significant from the uninsured group (*p* <0.05).

**Figure 19-4** • Access to Care for Those with Medicaid, Private Insurance, or no Insurance. ESI, Employer-Sponsored Insurance. (Source: Robin Rudowitz, Rachel Garfield, and Elizabeth Hinton. "10 Things to Know About Medicaid: Setting the Facts Straight," Kaiser Family Foundation, 2019. Available Online: https://www.kff.org/medicaid/issue-brief/10-things-to-know-about-medicaid-setting-the-facts-straight/.)

enrolled in Medicaid, with another 10 to 11 million enrolled through the HIEs. The number of uninsured people in the country has fallen by 18.6 million from 48.6 million in 2010 to roughly 30 million.[5] According to the Centers for Disease Control and Prevention, the percentage of uninsured decreased from 16% of the population in 2010 to 9.1% in 2017 and 8.5% in 2018, with much of the decrease attributed to the PPACA. The law also reduced the percentage of young adults aged 19 to 25 who were uninsured from over one-third to roughly 15%.

Research demonstrates that Medicaid expansion has improved access to care, the affordability of care, and financial security among the low-income population. It has also led to increased utilization of services. PPACA has also reshaped private insurance by establishing new federal consumer protections (eg, discriminating on the basis of preexisting medical conditions). Additional policies encouraged people to enroll in coverage provided on the HIEs and reduced cost sharing.

Perhaps one of the biggest impacts of PPACA on access occurred following the COVID-19 outbreak in the first half of 2020. The economic shutdown led to layoffs, rising unemployment, and loss of employer-based health insurance for roughly 12.7 million people (includes employees and their dependents). Researchers estimate that roughly 85% of these workers retained coverage, many through the Medicaid PPACA expansions. Along with PRWORA, this served to vitiate the earlier welfare stigma of Medicaid coverage.[6]

## Quality and Health Outcomes[7]

Overall, however, PPACA effects on health status are either mixed or to be determined.[8] Studies show that Medicaid expansion led to improved (self-reported) health status, certain positive health outcomes (eg, reduced number of reported days in poor mental health), improved access to primary care and preventive health services, medication compliance, increased cancer diagnosis rates, improved treatment for diabetes and other prevalent conditions, reductions in mortality from cardiovascular conditions for middle-aged adults, reduced mortality from end-stage renal disease, and better access to medications and services for people with behavioral and mental health problems. A small subset of study findings showed no effects of expansion on certain specific measures within specific access-related categories. The PPACA's impact on health status may likely unfold over time.

## Healthcare Costs and Spending

The implementation of PPACA had an immediate impact on Medicare spending by virtue of several statutory changes reducing the market-basket payment updates to the Prospective Payment System. PPACA also impacted Medicare spending by reducing the rate of increase in future payments to Medicare Advantage plans and reducing payments to hospitals with excessive readmissions. Conversely, PPACA increased Medicaid spending by expanding enrollment and increasing fees paid to PCPs for 2 years.

The impact on overall healthcare costs is less clear. Some have concluded that PPACA helped to reduce national healthcare spending. In March 2019, the Office of the Actuary of the Department of Health and Human Services (DHHS) reported that, cumulatively, PPACA had reduced national healthcare spending by $2.3 trillion between 2010 and 2017. In 2017 alone, health expenditures were $650 billion lower than projected, keeping healthcare spending under 18% of gross domestic product (GDP; just slightly more than the level in 2010 when PPACA was passed). These reported savings were based on initial projections that national expenditures would reach $4.14 trillion per year in 2017 and constitute 20.2% of GDP. It did all of this while expanding health coverage to more than 20 million previously uninsured Americans.

However, healthcare spending may well have decelerated for reasons other than PPACA and its reforms. First, some states did not elect to expand Medicaid coverage. Second, the number of people taking up coverage on the exchanges was lower than anticipated, perhaps due to the small penalty for ignoring the individual mandate. Third, the temporal effects of PPACA overlap with those of MACRA (2015), making it hard to disentangle the two. Fourth, the stabilization of healthcare spending as a percentage of GDP may have resulted from higher GDP growth in 2018, not changes in healthcare.

PPACA did not decrease per-capita spending on healthcare services; it did not even slow down the rate of increase in costs. As shown in Figure 19-5, per-capita expenditures increased more rapidly starting in the first quarter of 2014. An analysis by the CMS suggests that per-capita

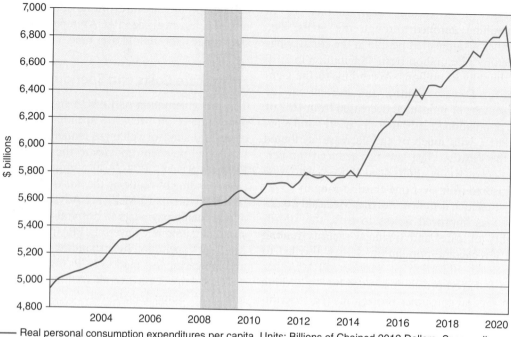

Figure 19-5 • Rise in Personal Spending on Healthcare. (Source: U.S. Bureau of Economic Analysis.)

costs have increased by 2.9% yearly since the PPACA was fully enacted compared with 2.0% before its passage in 2010 (Figure 19-6).

Analyses do suggest beneficial effects of expansion on numerous economic outcomes at the state level, however, including state budget savings, revenue gains, and overall economic growth. Expansion can result in state savings by offsetting state costs in other areas, reductions in uncompensated care costs for hospitals and

| Year | Health expenditures per person (2012 $) | Average yearly growth rate (%) | Policy |
|---|---|---|---|
| 2003 | 7,349 | | |
| 2004 | 7,539 | | |
| 2005 | 7,726 | | |
| 2006 | 7,909 | 2.0 | Healthcare policies before the PPACA |
| 2007 | 8,051 | | |
| 2008 | 8,157 | | |
| 2009 | 8,264 | | |
| 2010 | 8,281 | | |
| 2011 | 8,312 | | |
| 2012 | 8,450 | 0.8 | Increased coverage with the PPACA |
| 2013 | 8,521 | | |
| 2014 | 8,786 | | |
| 2015 | 9,161 | 2.9 | Full PPACA with exchanges |
| 2016 | 9,398 | | |
| 2017 | 9,540 | | |

**Health Expenditures and Average Yearly Growth by Government Policy**

Figure 19-6 • Health Expenditures and Average Yearly Growth by Government Policy. (Source: CMS.gov, Centers for Medicare and Medicaid Services. "Table 23 National Health Expenditures; Nominal Dollars, Real Dollars, Price Indexes, and Annual Percent Change." National Health Expenditure Accounts; https://www.cms.gov/Research-Statistics-Data-and-Systems/Statistics-Trends-and-Reports/NationalHealthExpendData/NationalHealthAccountsHistorical.html, accessed on July 2019.)

clinics, and growing employment in the labor market. Montana reportedly saved $25 million by moving people off state-funded programs onto Medicaid.[9] Michigan reportedly created 30,000 new jobs as a result of the state's expansion, along with $2.3 billion in new economic activity.[10] The cost of expansion in 2019 was $128 billion, less than the $172 billion originally forecasted. By contrast, states that have not expanded Medicaid found that residents were much more likely to report financial barriers to getting healthcare.

The overall answer as to the impact of PPACA on total spending is, as my colleague Marty Gaynor once wrote, "definitely maybe, but that's not final."[11] The reason is that hoped-for efficiencies depend on how VBP initiatives play out over the long run.[12] So, after nearly 10 years, we do not know. We do know that the anticipated savings of $200 billion a year has not yet been achieved. Moreover, inflation-adjusted healthcare spending per capita has accelerated from 1.7% annually (2003-2010) to 2.8% annually (2010-2018).[13] Stay tuned.

shifted the focus and balance between the 2 groups by federalizing the SSI program and reducing state flexibility and discretion in running their programs. SSI benefits were now available for all individuals who were aged, blind, or disabled; moreover, these groups became automatically eligible for Medicaid. In the absence of any insurance mechanism for long-term care, Medicaid became the primary funder of SNFs. By contrast, the AFDC portion of Medicaid was allowed to vary from state to state.

The expansion of SSI eligibility, along with the growth in the elderly population, caused a shift in financing. In 1972, 18% of Medicaid spending went to AFDC children under 21 years old; by 1984, this had fallen to 11.7%. The SSI population's consumption of Medicaid funds grew from 52.8% in 1972 to 73% by 1987—even though they constituted only 28% of Medicaid recipients (vs 66% in AFDC). In 1987, Medicaid recipients who resided in nursing homes accounted for only 7% of total recipients but 42% of program costs. Medicaid now paid for almost half of all nursing home expenditures in this country.

## MEDICAID ISSUES: BALANCING ACTS

Since its inception, Medicaid has had to deal with the different needs of the 2 categorical groups originally entitled to benefits: recipients of AFDC and SSI. The former are primarily poor women and children in need of primary care; the latter are primarily elderly people needing long-term care in skilled nursing facilities (SNFs). The 1972 Social Security Amendments

## MEDICAID TODAY[14]

This balancing act remains today. Medicaid is the principal source of care for the low-income population and the principal source of coverage for long-term care. Children account for 39% of all Medicaid enrollees (fiscal year 2016), while the elderly and disabled account for 23%; in terms of expenditures, the figures are reversed, with children accounting for 19% and the elderly/disabled accounting for 53% (Figure 19-7).

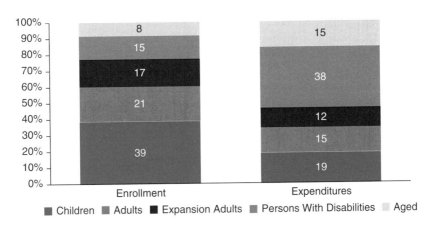

**Figure 19-7** • Estimated Medicaid Enrollment and Expenditures for Benefits, by Enrollment Category as a Share of Total, Fiscal Year 2017. (Source: US Department of Health and Human Services. "2018 Actuarial Report on the Financial Outlook for Medicaid." Available online: https://www.cms.gov/files/document/2018-report.pdf.)

Medicaid covers several vulnerable populations and thus serves as a major "safety net" for the following populations:

- 21% of the US population
- 39% of all US children
- 83% of poor children
- Approximately 50% of all births
- 48% of children with special healthcare needs
- 45% of nonelderly adults with disabilities
- 60%+ of nursing home residents
- 44% of national spending on LTSS
- 61% of all nonelderly individuals with income below 100% of the FPL
- 21% of adults with mental health services
- 17% of adults with substance abuse disorders

As of fiscal year 2018, Medicaid covered over 75 million people at an estimated total cost of $616 billion, with the federal government paying $386 billion of that amount. By contrast, the Medicare program provided healthcare benefits to nearly 59 million individuals at a cost of roughly $711 billion. Medicaid is the third-largest domestic program in the federal budget, after Social Security and Medicare, accounting for 9.5% of federal spending in fiscal year 2017.

## Beneficiary Cost Sharing

Beneficiary cost sharing is limited under the Medicaid program. States can require certain beneficiaries to share in the cost of Medicaid services, but there are limits on (1) the amounts that states can impose, (2) the beneficiary groups that can be required to pay, and (3) the services for which cost sharing can be charged.

In general, premiums and enrollment fees often are prohibited. However, premiums may be imposed on certain enrollees, such as individuals with incomes above 150% of FPL, certain working individuals with disabilities, and certain children with disabilities. States can impose cost sharing at the point of service, such as copayments, coinsurance, deductibles, and other similar charges, on most Medicaid-covered benefits, up to federal limits that vary by income. Some subgroups of beneficiaries are exempt from cost sharing (eg, children under 18 years of age and pregnant women). The aggregate cap on participation-related cost sharing (eg, monthly premiums) and point-of-service cost sharing

(eg, copayments) is generally up to 5% of monthly or quarterly household income. In addition, beneficiaries receiving certain Medicaid-covered LTSSs are required to apply their income exceeding specified amounts toward the cost of their care. These reductions from a beneficiary's income are referred to as posteligibility treatment of income and are not subject to the 5% aggregate cost-sharing cap described earlier. The amounts a beneficiary may retain for their personal use vary by care setting (ie, nursing facility vs home and community based).

## MEDICAID ELIGIBILITY

In general, individuals qualify for Medicaid coverage by meeting the requirements of a specific eligibility pathway offered by their state. Some eligibility pathways are mandatory, meaning all states with a Medicaid program must cover them; others are optional. Within this framework, states are afforded discretion in determining certain eligibility criteria for both mandatory and optional eligibility groups. In addition, states may apply to CMS for a waiver of federal law to expand health coverage beyond the mandatory and optional eligibility groups specified in federal statute.

An eligibility pathway is the federal statutory track referenced under Title XIX of the SSA that extends Medicaid coverage to one or more groups of individuals. Each pathway specifies the group of individuals covered by the pathway (ie, "categorical criteria"), the financial requirements applicable to the group (ie, "financial criteria"), whether the pathway is mandatory or optional, and the extent of the state's discretion over the pathway's requirements.[15]

All Medicaid applicants, regardless of their eligibility pathway, must meet federal and state requirements regarding residency, immigration status, and documentation of US citizenship. Often an applicant's eligibility pathway dictates the Medicaid state plan services that a given program enrollee is entitled to (eg, women eligible due to their pregnancy status are entitled to Medicaid pregnancy-related services). When applying to Medicaid, an individual may be eligible for the program through more than one pathway. In that situation, an individual is generally permitted to choose the pathway that would be most beneficial in terms of the treatment of income and sometimes assets for determining eligibility, but also in terms of the available benefits associated with each eligibility pathway. The subsections that follow describe Medicaid's categorical and financial eligibility criteria.

## Categorical Eligibility

Medicaid's categorical eligibility criteria are the nonfinancial requirements for a population to qualify for Medicaid coverage under a particular eligibility pathway offered by the state. If a state participates in Medicaid, the following eligibility groups *must* be provided coverage:

- Certain low-income families, including parents, that meet the financial requirements of the former AFDC cash assistance program
- Pregnant women with annual income at or below 133% of FPL
- Children with family income at or below 133% of FPL
- Aged, blind, or disabled individuals who receive cash assistance under the SSI program
- Children receiving foster care, adoption assistance, or kinship guardianship assistance under SSA Title IV–E
- Certain former foster care youth
- Individuals eligible for the Qualified Medicare Beneficiary program
- Certain groups of legal permanent resident immigrants

Examples of eligibility groups to which states *may* provide Medicaid include the following:

- Pregnant women with annual income between 133% and 185% of FPL
- Infants with family income between 133% and 185% of FPL
- Certain individuals who require institutional care and have incomes up to 300% of the SSI federal benefit rate
- Certain *medically needy* individuals (eg, children, pregnant women, aged, blind, or disabled) who are otherwise eligible for Medicaid but who have incomes too high to qualify and spend down their income on medical care
- Nonelderly adults with income at or below 133% of FPL (ie, the PPACA Medicaid expansion)

## Financial Eligibility

Medicaid is also a means-tested program that is limited to those with financial need. However, the criteria used to determine financial eligibility—income and sometimes asset tests—vary by eligibility group. For most eligibility groups, the criteria used to determine eligibility are based on modified adjusted gross income (MAGI); there is no resource or asset test used to determine Medicaid financial eligibility for MAGI-eligible individuals.

## SERVICES COVERED

Medicaid coverage includes a broad range of primary and acute-care services as well as LTSSs. Not all Medicaid enrollees have access to the same set of services. An enrollee's eligibility pathway determines the available services within a benefit package. Federal law provides 2 primary benefit packages for state Medicaid programs (Figure 19-8): (1) traditional benefits and (2) alternative benefit plans (ABPs; ie, plans that cover the 10 essential health benefits offered under PPACA).

The services that Medicaid offers cover diverse constituents:

### Low-Income Families

- Pregnant women: Prenatal care and delivery costs
- Children: Routine and specialized care for childhood development (immunizations, dental, vision, speech therapy)
- Families: Affordable coverage to prepare for the unexpected (emergency dental, hospitalizations, antibiotics)

### Individuals With Disabilities

- Children with autism: In-home therapy, speech/occupational therapy
- Cerebral palsy: Assistance to gain independence (personal care, case management, and assistive technology)
- HIV/AIDS: Physician services, prescription drugs
- Mental illness: Prescription drugs, physician services

### Elderly Individuals

- Medicare beneficiaries: Help paying for Medicare premiums and cost sharing
- Community waiver participants: Community-based care and personal care

| Type of Benefit | Traditional Benefits | ABPs |
|---|---|---|
| Mandatory | • Inpatient hospital services<br>• EPSDT (< the age of 21)<br>• Nursing facility care (aged 21+)<br>• Physician services<br>• FQHC services<br>• Family planning services<br>• Pregnancy-related services<br>• Home health | • Hospitalization services<br>• EPSDT (< the age of 21)<br>• Preventive services<br>• Prescription drugs<br>• FQHC services<br>• Family planning services<br>• Maternity and newborn care<br>• Rehabilitative services<br>• Mental health and substance use disorder services |
| Optional | • Clinic services<br>• Prescription drugs<br>• Physical, occupational, and speech therapy services<br>• Dental services for adults<br>• Personal care | For special needs subgroups, option to receive traditional benefits or enroll in an ABP plan |

Notes: ABP – Alternative Benefit Plan
EPSDT – Early and periodic screening, diagnostic, and treatment services
FQHC – Federal qualified health center

**Figure 19-8 •** Examples of Medicaid Mandatory and Optional Benefits for Traditional Benefits and Alternative Benefit Plans (ABPs). (Source: Title XIX of the Social Security Act and Related Federal Guidance.)

• Nursing home residents: Care paid by Medicaid since Medicare does not cover institutional care

Medicaid covers a continuum of LTSSs ranging from HCBSs that allow persons to live independently in their own homes or in other community settings to institutional care provided in SNFs and intermediate care facilities. In fiscal year 2016, HCBSs represented 57% of total Medicaid expenditures on LTSSs, whereas institutional LTSSs represented 43%. This is a dramatic shift from 1995 (2 decades earlier) when institutional settings accounted for 82% of national Medicaid LTSS expenditures.

## STATE INITIATIVES TO CONTROL MEDICAID SPENDING VIA MANAGED CARE

In 2017, Medicaid was the second-largest item in state budgets, after elementary and secondary education. Federal Medicaid matching funds are the largest source of federal revenue (55.1%) in state budgets. Accounting for state and federal funds, Medicaid accounts for 26.5% of total state spending (Figure 19-9).

Medicaid enrollees generally receive benefits via 1 of 2 service delivery systems: FFS

or managed care (Figure 19-10). Under FFS, healthcare providers are paid by the state Medicaid program for each service provided to a Medicaid enrollee. As noted in earlier chapters, FFS payment is inherently inflationary and contributes to higher state outlays on Medicaid. Under managed care, by contrast, Medicaid enrollees get most or all of their services through an MCO that contracts with the state on a capitated basis. Most states use a combination of FFS and managed care approaches across their diverse population groups based on the services used.

Because Medicaid plays a large role in state budgets, states have an interest in containing the costs of the program. This helps to explain why over two-thirds of all Medicaid beneficiaries receive their care in comprehensive, risk-based MCOs offered by private sector health plans. Initially, states used managed care to deliver healthcare services to the healthier Medicaid populations, including children and parents. Recently, more states are turning to managed care for their aged, disabled, and other populations: (1) long-term care support services (eg, nursing facilities, community-based home health), (2) behavioral health carved into an integrated Medicaid managed care benefits package, (3) dental services, and (4) prescription drugs.

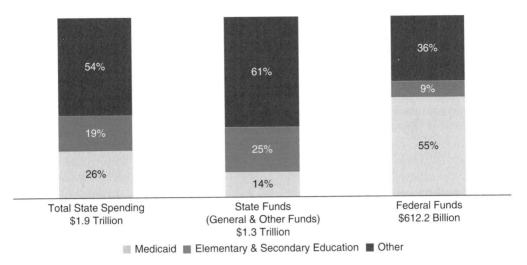

**Figure 19-9** • Medicaid Is a Budget Item and a Revenue Item in State Budgets. (Source: Kaiser Family Foundation. Estimates Based on the National Association of State Budget Officers [NASBO] 2018 State Expenditure Report: Fiscal Years 2016-2018 [Data for Actual FY 2017]. See Also Rudowitz, Ordera, and Hinton, Medicaid Financing: The Basics, Kaiser Family Foundation, 2019. https://www.kff.org/medicaid/issue-brief/medicaid-financing-the-basics/view/print/.)

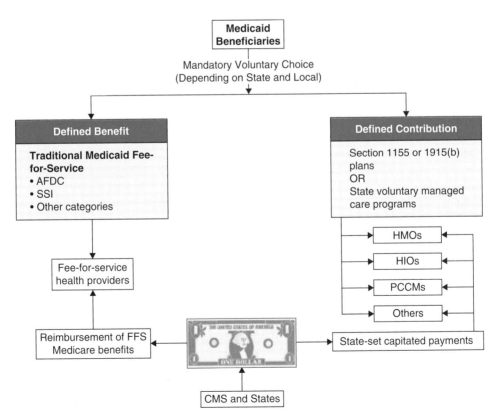

**Figure 19-10** • Medicaid Fee-for-Service (FFS) and Managed Care Programs. AFDC, Aid to Families with Dependent Children; CMS, Centers for Medicare and Medicaid Services; HIOs, Health Insuring Organizations; HMOs, Health Maintenance Organizations; PCCM, Primary Care Case Management; SSI, Supplemental Security Income. (Source: Steve Wood, Clear View Solutions LLC. Presentation to Wharton School, Spring 2017.)

There are 3 main types of Medicaid managed care[16]:

- **Comprehensive risk-based managed care**—States contract with MCOs to provide a comprehensive package of benefits to certain Medicaid enrollees. States usually pay the MCOs on a capitated basis, which means the states prospectively pay the MCOs a fixed monthly rate per enrollee to provide or arrange for most healthcare services. MCOs then pay providers for services rendered to enrollees.
- **Primary care case management (PCCM)**—States contract with primary care providers to provide case management services to Medicaid enrollees. Typically, under PCCM, the primary care provider receives a monthly case management fee per enrollee for coordination of care, but the provider continues to receive fee-for-service payments for the medical care services used by Medicaid enrollees.
- **Limited benefit plans**—These plans look like MCOs in that states usually contract with a plan and pay it on a capitated basis. The difference is that limited benefit plans provide only 1 or 2 Medicaid services (eg, behavioral health or dental services).

The most prevalent type is the comprehensive, risk-based managed care provided through MCOs (69% of beneficiaries as of July 1, 2018). Overall, payments to MCOs accounted for nearly half (46%) of total Medicaid spending; 25 states with such MCOs covered more than 75% of Medicaid beneficiaries in these plans.

Capitated managed care more heavily penetrates the 2 lowest-cost categories of enrollees (the non-elderly nondisabled and children) where the bulk of enrollment lies; FFS Medicaid payments more heavily penetrate 2 other categories with a smaller number of enrollees (the elderly disabled and the dual eligibles). The past two administrations have sought to coordinate the Medicare and Medicaid benefits of the dual eligibles, who are enrolled in managed care plans.

## IMPACT OF MEDICAID MANAGED CARE ON THE IRON TRIANGLE

It is difficult to draw conclusions about the impact of Medicaid managed care on the iron triangle. This is because managed care networks and organizations can be configured, staffed, and funded in many different ways. Studies examining this issue have arrived at different and sometimes conflicting conclusions. As a result, the evidence is mixed.

### Access

There is some evidence that Medicaid managed care improves access to care, but the scope of the improvements is state specific and depends on how access is measured. In general, there is evidence that Medicaid managed care sometimes improves access to a usual source of primary care, while also reducing emergency department (ED) utilization and ambulatory-sensitive hospitalization. At the same time, studies that focus on pregnant beneficiaries' access to prenatal care show mixed results. Overall, according to an earlier literature review, 2 studies showed improvement, 2 studies showed some improvement, 5 studies reported mixed evidence, and 6 studies reported no improvement.

### Quality and Health Outcomes

The literature on Medicaid managed care and quality has often examined whether pregnant beneficiaries have healthier babies than those covered under FFS: They do not. Little research focuses on care management programs for high-need, high-cost beneficiaries. Health plans, like the Medicaid agencies themselves, have only a limited ability to change traditional delivery systems and an equally limited ability to respond to the social determinants of health that play a large role in the fragmented care Medicaid enrollees receive. Overall, according to an earlier literature review, 4 studies reported mixed evidence, 7 studies reported no impact, and 1 study reported a negative impact.

### Cost

The findings with regard to cost, finally, are slightly more encouraging: 6 studies reported savings, 2 reported modest or projected savings, 4 reported no savings, and 2 reported no clear evidence.[17] The literature finds little savings at the national level but some success by states with relatively high provider reimbursement rates in their FFS programs. The cost savings are due primarily to reductions in provider reimbursement rates rather than managed care techniques, although reductions in ED utilization and inpatient hospital care also contribute. The trend to add high-need, high-cost beneficiaries into managed care increases the cost savings potential, most likely via overuse of ED and inpatient care services. However, the extent of such savings is still uncertain.

---

### Critical Thinking Exercise: CareMore

CareMore Health System has received a lot of "kudos" from healthcare observers and a lot of "ink" from the media.[18] It has also been the subject of a Harvard Business School case for its innovative managed care approach to delivering care to the Medicaid population in the states of Tennessee and Iowa.[19] CareMore's managed care infrastructure includes a narrow network of PCPs (not all employed), "extensivist physicians" to deal with medically complex patients and attack the social determinants of health, neighborhood care centers for the chronically ill, and case managers to coordinate care. CareMore developed these managed care elements to treat Medicare enrollees in managed care plans in California. After having been sold to Anthem, CareMore is now trying to use this model for Medicaid enrollees in managed care plans. What issues might CareMore face in attempting to migrate the model to a new patient population?

---

## INNOVATIVE STATE-MANAGED CARE APPROACHES

Several states have undertaken innovative approaches to manage their Medicaid programs. In addition to Medicaid managed care, states have deployed primary care programs targeting managed care beneficiaries, Medicaid ACOs, health homes for Medicaid beneficiaries with chronic illnesses, and delivery system reform incentive payments. Some of the efforts undertaken in Massachusetts and North Carolina are briefly summarized in the following sections.

### MassHealth

The Commonwealth of Massachusetts has historically operated a generous Medicaid program that covers roughly one-quarter of its residents and accounts for 40%+ of the state's budget. To contain this spending (and try to "bend the trend"), the Commonwealth obtained a waiver to migrate its Medicaid program away from open-access, FFS provider networks to offer 3 types of ACOs. The most popular ACO, financed through capitation arrangements, required the ACO to offer comprehensive services; among the 2 other models, one employed the shared savings model used in Medicare ACOs, while the other administered the ACO through an MCO. ACO-eligible beneficiaries (ie, nonelderly, those without other coverage) were auto-assigned to an ACO, with the ability to switch during an open-enrollment period.

The program faced challenges during the first year of operation (calendar year 2018): low base rates, high rate of "patient churn" among ACO models, and poor financial performance among safety-net providers participating in the program (perhaps due to faulty risk adjustment). For the following year, participating providers will be involved in P4P models.

### North Carolina

North Carolina's Medicaid program covers one-fifth of the state's population. In 2015, the state's General Assembly mandated a transition from FFS to managed care. The state is now busily engaged in a multitasking effort to contract with 5 "prepaid health plans" (PHPs) in 2019, expand Medicaid (as one of the 14 states that did not adopt PPACA), and pilot programs in the social determinants of health. Enrollment is mandatory for some Medicaid populations (family and children, pregnant women), whereas others are temporarily excluded (dual eligibles) or totally excluded (medically needy). In all, about 1.6 million beneficiaries will enroll in a "standard plan" that provides integrated physical health, behavioral health, and pharmaceutical services. In October 2018, the federal government approved the state's Section 1115 waiver to develop a "healthy opportunities pilot" to cover evidence-based nonmedical services that address specific social needs linked to health status and outcomes. The pilot will address housing instability, transportation insecurity, food insecurity, and interpersonal violence and toxic stress for a limited number of high-need enrollees. Political turmoil in the state—due to divided state government, court challenges to the drawing of the state's congressional districts, and budget stalemates, among others—threatened to delay the rollout, however. In mid-2020, the legislature put off expansion of Medicaid for a year, partly due to COVID-19; in July 2020, the legislature and governor agreed on the rollout of the transformation to privatize Medicaid.

## SUMMARY

It is not easy to succinctly characterize or summarize the Medicaid program. Medicaid varies considerably across states and over time. Its highest-cost beneficiaries are those that are also covered by Medicare (the dual eligibles). Unlike the federal Medicare program, states bear part of the fiscal responsibility for Medicaid. Also unlike the Medicare program, states cannot "print money" (borrow) to finance their Medicaid programs, but must balance Medicaid expenditures with other state outlays (such as education). State Medicaid programs received an enormous boost from the PPACA but have still relied heavily on managed care to keep their books balanced. To date, the results here are mixed.

### QUESTIONS TO PONDER

1. What are the most important differences between Medicare and Medicaid?
2. Why are the Medicaid "waiver programs" of such interest? Why do several states make use of them?
3. Why are private MCOs so interested in entering the Medicaid market?
4. Overall, how successful have states been in using MCOs to address the iron triangle?
5. Overall, how successful was the PPACA in addressing the iron triangle?

## REFERENCES

1. Social Security is a cash benefit program run by the federal government. It is important to distinguish 3 programs under Social Security: Supplemental Security Income (SSI), Social Security Disability (SSD), and Social Security Retirement. To qualify for SSI and SSD, you have to meet the Social Security definition for disability. The SSI program is for low-income people who have little or no work history. There is a standard monthly benefit amount that people on SSI get. SSD is based on one's work history. The amount of your monthly benefit is based on your work history and varies from person to person. The more you have worked and paid Social Security taxes in the past, the higher your SSD benefit will be. Social Security Retirement is a monthly cash benefit you can receive after you turn 62. However, if you wait until regular retirement age, your monthly benefits will be higher. Regular retirement age is between the ages of 65 and 67. The monthly benefit amount depends on how much you have worked during your lifetime. If you have not worked much in your lifetime, you can get SSI when you turn 65.
2. David Blumenthal and Melinda Abrams. "The Affordable Care Act at 10 Years: Payment and Delivery System Reforms," *N Engl J Med.* 382 (March 12, 2020): 1057-1063.
3. Deborah Peikes, Erin Taylor, Ann O'Malley, et al. "The Changing Landscape of Primary Care: Effects of the ACA and Other Efforts Over the Past Decade." *Health Aff.* 39 (3) (2020): 421-428.
4. This review is based on several recent reviews. Charles Courtemanche, James Marton, Benjamin Ukert, et al. "Effects of the Affordable Care Act on Health Care Access and Self-Assessed Health After 3 Years," *Inquiry.* 55 (2018). See also: Madeline Guth, Rachel Garfield, and Robin Rudowitz. *The Effects of Medicaid Expansion Under the ACA: Updated Findings from a Literature Review* (KFF, March 17, 2020). Available online: https://www.kff.org/medicaid/report/the-effects-of-medicaid-expansion-under-the-aca-updated-findings-from-a-literature-review/. Accessed on April 8, 2020. See also: David F. Perkis and Audrey Rich. *The Affordable Care Act: More Health Care Services at Lower Cost?* (Federal Reserve Bank of St. Louis, September 2019). Available online: https://research.stlouisfed.org/publications/page1-econ/2019/09/12/the-affordable-care-act-more-health-care-services-at-lower-cost. Accessed on April 10, 2020.
5. David Blumenthal, Sara Collins, and Elizabeth Fowler. "The Affordable Care Act at 10 Years: Its Coverage and Access Provisions," *N Engl J Med.* 382 (March 12, 2020): 1057-1063. "The increase in new coverage is not easily reconciled with the decrease in the uninsured. Some of the newly enrolled on the HIEs had other coverage previously."
6. Josh Bivens and Ben Zipperer. *Health Insurance and the COVID-19 Shock* (Washington, DC: Economic Policy Institute, August 26, 2020).
7. The Commonwealth Fund. *What Is Medicaid's Value* (December 13, 2019). Available online: https://www.commonwealthfund.org/publications/

explainer/2019/dec/medicaids-value. Accessed on April 8, 2020.

8. David Blumenthal, Sara Collins, and Elizabeth Fowler. "The Affordable Care Act at 10 Years: Its Coverage and Access Provisions," *N Engl J Med.* 382 (March 12, 2020): 1057-1063.

9. Susan L. Hayes, Akeiisa Coleman, Sara R. Collins, and Rachel Nuzum. *The Fiscal Case for Medicaid Expansion* (The Commonwealth Fund, February 15, 2019). Available online at: https://www.common wealthfund.org/blog/2019/fiscal-case-medicaid-expansion. Accessed on April 10, 2020.

10. Susan L. Hayes, Akeiisa Coleman, Sara R. Collins, and Rachel Nuzum. *The Fiscal Case for Medicaid Expansion* (The Commonwealth Fund, February 15, 2019). Available online: https://www .commonwealthfund.org/blog/2019/fiscal-case-medicaid-expansion. Accessed on April 10, 2020.

11. Martin Gaynor. "Is Vertical Integration Anti-Competitive? Definitely Maybe (But That's Not Final)," *J Health Econ.* 25 (1) (2006): 175-180.

12. Melinda Buntin and John Graves. "How the ACA Dented the Cost Curve," *Health Aff.* 39 (3) (2020): 403-412.

13. Joseph Antos and James Capretta. "The ACA: Trillions? Yes. A Revolution? No," *Health Affairs Blog* (April 10, 2020).

14. This section draws on: Robin Rudowitz, Rachel Garfield, and Elizabeth Hinton. *10 Things to Know About Medicaid: Setting the Facts Straight.* Issue Brief (Kaiser Family Foundation, March 2019).

15. Individuals in need of Medicaid-covered LTSS must demonstrate the need for long-term care by meeting state-based eligibility criteria for services, and they also may be subject to a separate set of Medicaid financial eligibility rules in order to receive LTSS coverage.

16. Congressional Research Service. *Medicaid: An Overview* (June 24, 2019). Available online: https://fas.org/sgp/crs/misc/R43357.pdf. Accessed on April 8, 2020.

17. Michael Sparer. *Medicaid Managed Care: Costs, Access, and Quality of* Care (Princeton, NJ: The Synthesis Project. Robert Wood Johnson Foundation, September 2012). Also see: MACPAC. *Managed Care's Effect on Outcomes.* Available online: https://www.macpac.gov/subtopic/managed-cares-effect-on-outcomes/. Accessed on April 12, 2020. Tiffany Fan, Natalie Miller, Chris Ragsdale, et al. *Medicaid Expansion and Medicaid Managed Care.* Presentation to the Wharton School, November 2019.

18. Vivek Garg, Amberly Molosky, Sandeep Palokodeti, et al. "Rethinking How Medicaid Patients Receive Care," *Harvard Business Review* (October 5, 2018). Available online: https://hbr.org/2018/10/rethinking-how-medicaid-patients-receive-care. Accessed on August 9, 2020.

19. Robert Huckman and Brian Powers. *CareMore Health System.* HBS Case # 9-618-008 (revised August 2, 2017). (Boston, MA: Harvard Business School, 2017).

# SECTION IV

## Technology Sectors in the Ecosystem

# The Healthcare Technology Sectors

20

## THE HUNT FOR BIOMEDICAL INNOVATION

Perhaps as never before, countries around the world are looking at biomedical innovation as a source of (1) *knowledge creation* by their scientific communities, (2) *value creation* for their populations, and (3) *wealth creation* by fostering industries and expansion of employment. In the United States, for example, bipartisan passage of the 21st Century Cures Act (2016) seeks to accelerate new product development and faster patient access to new treatments and therapies. It also elevates the role of biomedical research through an additional $6.3 billion in funding for the National Institutes of Health (NIH) and other agencies. China's Twelfth and Thirteenth Five-Year Plans (FYP 2011-2015, 2016-2020) emphasize a shift away from manufacturing to higher-end technology sectors such as biotechnology, biomedical and advanced medical equipment, and information technology. China is also on pace to surpass the United States in terms of research funding levels, indicating biomedical innovation is a national priority.[1]

At the same time, countries around the world are looking at the price tag for these new biomedical innovations. Not only is healthcare a rising percentage of every country's gross domestic product (GDP), but inflation in the prices of biomedical innovation often outstrips the rate of increase in spending on healthcare services. Newspaper headlines now commonly display the annual cost of new biotechnology treatments to patients and their insurers. Recently, Novartis announced that its new gene therapy (AVXS-101) to treat spinal muscular atrophy in newborns could be valued as much as $4 million per patient (although it did not say it would charge this price). This follows on the heels of Novartis pricing its drug Kymriah (based on CAR-T technology) to treat acute lymphoblastic leukemia in children at $475,000, and Spark Therapeutics's decision to price its new drug for blindness, Luxturna, at $850,000 for a one-time treatment.

These 2 observations underlie the tension every country faces between the benefits of technological innovation and the affordability of such innovation (similar to the iron triangle). There are now multiple calls for "an effective innovation agenda" that calls for, among other things, greater coordination among government agencies responsible for funding and paying for this innovation.[2] This chapter (and the next 4) seek to inform this discussion by focusing on the sources of that innovation and the industrial context in which it occurs.

## INNOVATION IN THE HEALTHCARE VALUE CHAIN

Innovation occurs in the context of industrial value chains. A value chain is defined as the string of firms and industries (sellers) whose outputs serve as the inputs of other firm and industries downstream (buyers). Thus, in a traditional production model, a value chain links together raw material suppliers, manufacturers, distributors, and end customers. Using raw materials from their own suppliers, product manufacturers design and make innovative products and then market them to downstream end-users. This chapter examines the producers of innovative products found in the right-hand box of Figure 3-9. The following chapters cover 4

| Pharma/Biotech | HC Providers/Services |
|---|---|
| High margins | Low margins |
| Low capital invested | High capital invested |
| High return on invested capital | Low return on invested capital |

**Figure 20-1** • Value Creation in Healthcare (HC).

specific sectors: pharmaceuticals, biotechnology, medical devices, and information technology.

## SIMILARITIES AMONG THE TECHNOLOGY SECTORS

The technology sectors share several important similarities. They are the only truly global sectors in the healthcare industry. The adage that "all healthcare is local" (see Chapter 2) clearly applies to providers and insurers but not to the suppliers. The pharmaceutical, medical device, and (increasingly) biotechnology sectors clearly sell their products to global markets. The technology sectors are also the key source of research and development (R&D) spending—at least in the United States—and thus the source of most innovation (hospital innovation centers notwithstanding). Not surprisingly, they earn much higher returns and margins compared to providers of healthcare services (Figure 20-1) and

other industrial sectors (Figure 20-2). A recent analysis suggests that the large, fully integrated pharmaceutical firms also earn higher gross margins, pretax margins, and net incomes compared to other public firms in the Standard & Poors 500.[3]

This chapter and the next 4 chapters emphasize several themes that cut across these sectors. One is innovation and the value and benefits conferred by innovative products; such benefits can accrue to both patients and their providers. Another recurring theme is the level of R&D investment, the mix of public versus private R&D investment, and the productivity of these investments (see box titled "What Is R&D?"). R&D investments in the pharmaceutical and biotechnology sectors greatly exceed those in other technology sectors (Figure 20-3). A third recurring theme is the importance of market structure and competition among firms in each of these sectors, as well as the growing overlap between the pharmaceutical and biotechnology sectors (now increasingly referred to as "biopharmaceuticals" or, more generally, life sciences). A fourth recurring theme is the set of strategies that firms in these sectors engage in to manage R&D productivity and deal with competitive pressures. These strategies include mergers and acquisitions (M&As), occupation of niche markets (or "focus"), diversification, and strategic alliances. A fifth

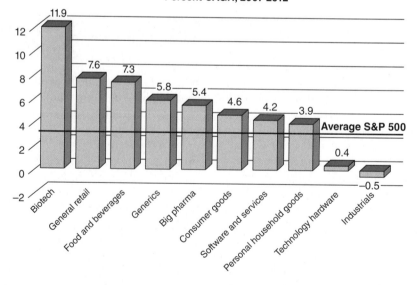

**Figure 20-2** • Attractive Returns. CAGR, Compound Annual Growth Rate. (Source: Figure 1.3, in Lawton R. Burns [Ed.], *The Business of Healthcare Innovation*, 3rd ed. Cambridge, United Kingdom: Cambridge University Press; 2020.)

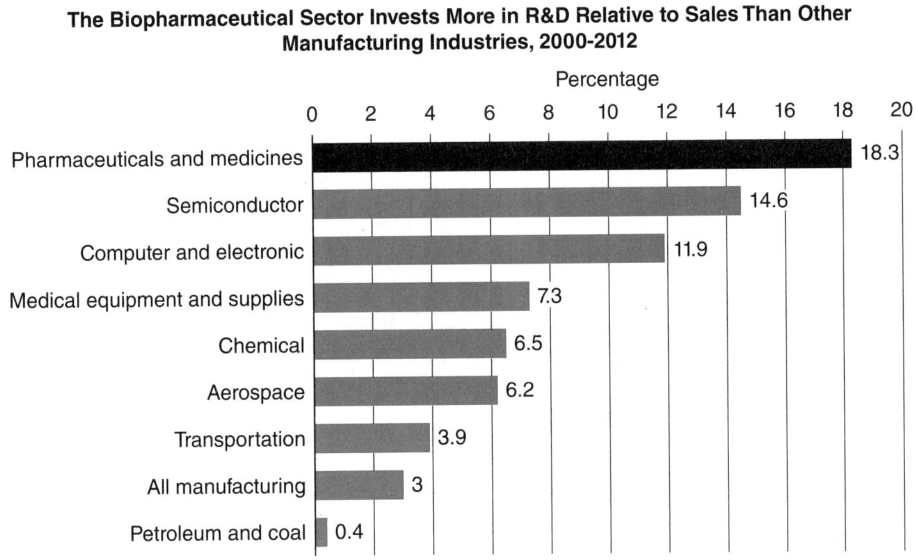

**The Biopharmaceutical Sector Invests More in R&D Relative to Sales Than Other Manufacturing Industries, 2000-2012**

Percentage

| Industry | Percentage |
|---|---|
| Pharmaceuticals and medicines | 18.3 |
| Semiconductor | 14.6 |
| Computer and electronic | 11.9 |
| Medical equipment and supplies | 7.3 |
| Chemical | 6.5 |
| Aerospace | 6.2 |
| Transportation | 3.9 |
| All manufacturing | 3 |
| Petroleum and coal | 0.4 |

**Figure 20-3** • Investment in Research and Development (R&D) Among Different Industries. (Source: Figure 1.4, in Lawton R. Burns [Ed.], *The Business of Healthcare Innovation*, 3rd ed. Cambridge, United Kingdom: Cambridge University Press; 2020.)

recurring theme is the growing demand for the products developed in these sectors by patients and providers located downstream from them, a theme also known as "the technological imperative" (described later).

### What Is R&D?

R&D is planned, creative work aimed at discovering new knowledge or developing new or significantly improved goods and services. This includes (1) activities aimed at acquiring new knowledge or understanding without specific immediate commercial applications or uses (*basic research*); (2) activities aimed at solving a specific problem or meeting a specific commercial objective (*applied research*); and (3) systematic use of research and practical experience to produce new or significantly improved goods, services, or processes (*development*). Roughly two-thirds of this effort—$102 billion of the total of $159 billion (2015)— is financed by the private sector in the United States (Figure 20-4). There is a clear division of labor in the R&D effort: The public sector funds basic research, largely through the NIH, whereas the private sector funds applied R&D (Figure 20-5).

### DIFFERENCES AMONG THE TECHNOLOGY SECTORS

There are, nevertheless, important differences among the technology sectors, which subsequent chapters document in great detail. Some of the major differences are summarized here. Although they all earn high margins, these margins do differ, as well as their expense components (Figure 20-6). Pharmaceutical firms earn higher margins and have lower cost of goods sold compared to medical device firms; both earn higher returns than makers of medical supplies. Both have high sales, general, and administrative (SG&A) costs due to heavy reliance on sales representatives.

In addition, the pharmaceutical, biotechnology, and medical device sectors differ in terms of their product cycles, capital intensity, and entry barriers (Figure 20-7). There are a host of other differences between pharmaceuticals and medical devices (see Figure 20-8).

### COMMONALITIES IN THE INNOVATION PROCESS

Five commonalities in the innovation process cut across the producer sectors studied here: risk, capital, time, space, and scale. Most of

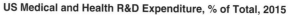
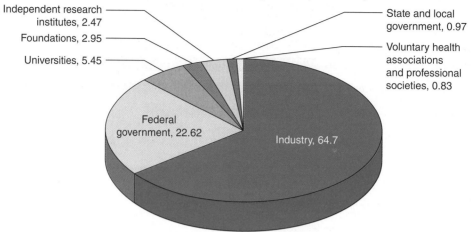

## US Medical and Health R&D Expenditure, % of Total, 2015

Independent research institutes, 2.47
Foundations, 2.95
Universities, 5.45
Federal government, 22.62
Industry, 64.7
State and local government, 0.97
Voluntary health associations and professional societies, 0.83

### Estimated US Medical and Health Research ($ in millions)

| Research Segment | 2013 | 2014 | 13-'14 change | 2015 | 14-'15 change |
|---|---|---|---|---|---|
| Industry (US Operations) | $89,666 | $98,097 | 9.40% | $102,679 | 4.56% |
| Federal Government | 33,634 | 35,435 | 5.36% | 35,924 | 1.38% |
| Other Sources | 16,807 | 18,260 | 8.65% | 20,113 | 10.15% |
| Total US Medical and Health R&D Spending | $140,107 | $151,792 | 8.34% | $158,716 | 4.56% |

**Figure 20-4** • US Medical and Health Research and Development (R&D) Expenditure and Research. (Source: Figure 1.5, in Lawton R. Burns [Ed.], *The Business of Healthcare Innovation*, 3rd ed. Cambridge, United Kingdom: Cambridge University Press; 2020.)

the healthcare sectors examined here are characterized by high risk. Failure rates in the life sciences are especially high, as are the failure rates of new ventures in all of the sectors studied here. Indeed, small firms account for much of the innovation across these sectors, and firm survival rates here are notoriously low. Firms in these sectors require success

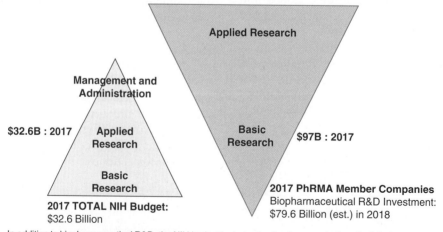

Biopharmaceutical Companies Do the Vast Majority of Research to Translate Basic Science Into New Medicines

Applied Research

Management and Administration

Applied Research

Basic Research

$32.6B : 2017

Basic Research

$97B : 2017

**2017 TOTAL NIH Budget:**
$32.6 Billion

**2017 PhRMA Member Companies**
Biopharmaceutical R&D Investment:
$79.6 Billion (est.) in 2018

In addition to biopharmaceutical R&D, the NIH budget includes funding in support of medical devices, diagnostics, prevention, training, and other activities.

**Figure 20-5** • Biopharmaceutical Research. NIH, National Institutes of Health; R&D, Research and Development. (Source: Figure 1.6, in Lawton R. Burns [Ed.], *The Business of Healthcare Innovation*, 3rd ed. Cambridge, United Kingdom: Cambridge University Press; 2020.)

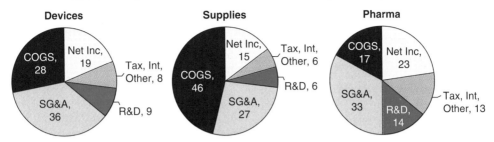

Figure 20-6 • Expense Components of Producer Sectors. COGS, cost of goods sold; R&D, Research and Development; SG&A, selling, general, and administrative costs. (Source: Figure 1.7, in Lawton R. Burns [Ed.], *The Business of Healthcare Innovation*, 3rd ed. Cambridge, United Kingdom: Cambridge University Press; 2020.)

| | Product Cycles | Growth | Capital Intensity | Profitability | Self-Sufficiency | Barriers |
|---|---|---|---|---|---|---|
| Devices | Short | Moderate to High | Low | High | High | High |
| Pharma | Long | Moderate | High | Moderate to High | High | High |
| Biotech | Medium | High | Low | Low to Moderate | Moderate | Low |

Figure 20-7 • Pharma, Biotech, and Devices: Some Dissimilarities. (Source: Figure 1.9, in Lawton R. Burns [Ed.], *The Business of Healthcare Innovation*, 3rd ed. Cambridge, United Kingdom: Cambridge University Press; 2020.)

| Pharma | Devices |
|---|---|
| $1.4T Sales WW (2017) | $405B Sales WW (2017) |
| Prices well understood | Prices not understood |
| Expenditures easily discerned | Expenditures buried |
| Heavy policy pressure | Lighter policy pressure |
| Brands more comparable | Brands less comparable |
| Products are featureless | Products bristle with features |
| More consumerism | Less consumerism |
| Buyers & consumers not separate | Buyers & consumers separate |
| Unconcentrated customers | Concentrated customers |
| Channel inefficiencies | Channel efficiencies |
| Payer formularies & tiers | No payer formularies & tiers |
| Price elastic demand | Price inelastic demand |

Figure 20-8 • Pharmaceuticals Versus Medical Devices. WW, Worldwide. (Source: Figure 1.10, in Lawton R. Burns [Ed.], *The Business of Healthcare Innovation*, 3rd ed. Cambridge, United Kingdom: Cambridge University Press; 2020.)

with the technologies they develop and early market success in order to survive. They also require heavy injections of capital from venture capitalists and the public (in the form of initial public offerings [IPOs], secondary offerings, and so on) in order to sustain themselves through the innovation process, especially as this process may take years. Capital and time often interact in the form of "boom and bust" cycles in some of these sectors (eg, biotechnology), as a sector goes in and out of fashion with venture capitalists or as the window for IPOs periodically opens and closes.

Time is important in studying these sectors for 3 other reasons. First, the products developed in these sectors have development cycles that can be either long in duration (eg, pharmaceuticals and biologicals) or short in duration (eg, medical devices, information technology). Second, the sector itself may be either youthful (eg, biotechnology, information technology) or older (eg, pharmaceuticals). These time dimensions dictate much of the strategic behavior of firms within these sectors and also their capabilities to innovate. Third, there is a tendency for analysts and observers (as well as investors) to overestimate the impact of new technology on these sectors in the short term and to underestimate the impact of new technology in the long term. Thus, the technological innovations mentioned in this volume may take longer to play out but may have a more profound impact than was originally anticipated.

Another important commonality is space. As noted earlier, some sectors (eg, pharmaceuticals) are truly global businesses, whereas others, such as biotechnology, are largely domestic businesses found in many nations with a common aim to become global businesses. Still other sectors, such as medical devices and information technology, are largely domestic (medical devices are heavily based in the United States), although they, too, are trying to penetrate foreign markets. Lastly, firm scale and scope are important dimensions. All of the sectors are growing. They all face issues of managing large size and diversity of operations and thus face the need to coordinate their complex operations. They also all pursue strategies of M&As, whereas some simultaneously pursue strategies of vertical integration and diversification. Due to the common avenues of growth pursued, these firms are ripe for strategic analysis.

## THE TECHNOLOGICAL IMPERATIVE IN HEALTHCARE

The technology sectors listed earlier are responsible for supplying a majority of the innovative products that are used by physicians and hospitals and that are increasingly demanded by consumers. This supply and demand logic has exerted both positive and negative effects.

On the one hand, technology is commonly cited as being the major driver of rising healthcare expenditures worldwide. Scholars have characterized this driver as the technological imperative[4]—that is, innovative treatments and equipment are demanded by patients and their (physician) agents on the grounds of quality and are reimbursed by payers and their fiscal intermediaries. Indeed, empirical evidence from the United States documents that the cost of new technology and the intensity with which it is used consistently account for anywhere from 20% to 40% of the rise in health expenditures over the past 40 years (Figure 20-9).

Particularly disturbing to many, given this level of spending, is evidence that high levels of spending on technology, particularly in the United States, do not always translate into added "value" (outcomes divided by costs).[5] The problem here is manifold: the utilization of technology without weighing the commensurate benefits, the overutilization of technology in the United States (which increases spending without added benefit), the price of new innovations, and market-based competition among provider organizations to have the latest equipment—the "technology wars"—which increases the diffusion and utilization of expensive technology at the expense of older, less expensive alternatives.[6]

US governmental efforts to contain spending on medical technology (eg, certificate of need laws enacted in the 1970s, the Inpatient Prospective Payment System enacted in 1983, the threat of presidential-led health reforms in 1993/1994) exerted only short-term effects, followed by a resumption in spending. Governmental restrictions on access to this technology, on the prices charged for the technology made available, and on the wages paid to labor who apply this technology have been favored methods of controlling healthcare costs in other countries.[7] Other regulatory initiatives underway in the United States as part of healthcare reform seek to redesign both provider organization

**Relative Contribution to Healthcare Inflation**
**Academic Studies Covering Period 1960-2007 and 1940-1990**

| | Smith, Newhouse & Freeland (2009) | Smith, Heffler and Freeland (2000) | Cutler (1995) | Newhouse (1992) |
|---|---|---|---|---|
| Aging of Population | 7 | 2 | 2 | 2 |
| Changes in Third-Party Payment | 11 | 10 | 13 | 10 |
| Personal Income Growth | 28-43 | 11-18 | 5 | <23 |
| Prices in the Healthcare Sector | 5-19 | 11-22 | 19 | NA |
| Administrative Costs | NA | 3-10 | 13 | NA |
| Defensive Medicine and Supplier-Induced Demand | NA | 0 | NA | 0 |
| Technology-Related Changes in Medical Practice | 27-48 | 38-62 | 49 | >65 |

**Figure 20-9** • Technology and Service Intensity as Drivers of Rising US Healthcare Costs. (Source: Sheila Smith, Joseph P. Newhouse, Mark S. Freeland. "Income, Insurance, and Technology: Why Does Health Spending Outpace Economic Growth?" *Health Aff.* 28 [2009]: 1276-1284.)

and provider payment incentives in an effort to "bend the curve"[8] or "transform" the healthcare system and move it from volume to value.[9]

On the other hand, there is growing public recognition, based on continuing scholarly evidence, that new technology has a definite "value proposition"—that it confers benefits to stakeholders downstream such as patients, the companies that employ them, the health plans that cover them, and the physicians and hospitals who treat them. Technological innovation

contributes to increases in longevity and mobility, reductions in disease and pain, improvements in worker productivity, and improvements in quality of life, especially for patients with particular conditions.[10] Some technologies such as the drug cocktails for patients with HIV/AIDS have reduced actual mortality rates since the mid-1990s and avoided over three-quarters of a million premature deaths (Figure 20-10). Other drug therapies for patients suffering from hypertension have likewise served to avoid hospitalizations

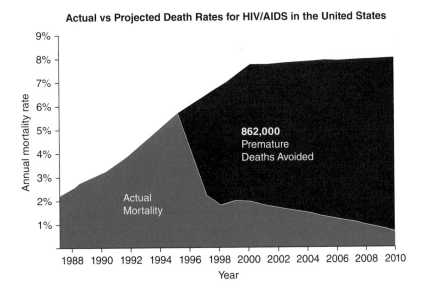

**Figure 20-10** • Health Impact of New Technology. (Source: PhRMA.)

**Annual Hospitalizations and Deaths Avoided Through the Use of Recommended Hypertensive Medications**

|  | Annual Hospitalizations Avoided | Annual Premature Births Avoided |
|---|---|---|
| Prevention Achieved: Based on Current Treatment Rates | 833,000 | 86,000 |
| Potential Additional Prevention: If Untreated Patients Receive Recommended Medicines | 420,000 | 89,000 |

**Figure 20-11** • Recommended Medicines Can Save Lives and Dramatically Improve Health. (Source: David M. Cutler, Genia Long, Ernst R. Berndt, et al. The Value of Antihypertensive Drugs: A Perspective on Medical Innovation. *Health Aff.* 26 [2007]: 97-110.)

and reduce premature deaths (Figure 20-11).[11] Overall, evidence suggests that increased health spending is "worth it": Over the past 20 years, each additional dollar spent on healthcare services in the United States produced health gains valued at $2.40 to $3.00 (eg, in terms of increased life expectancy, reduced disability, improved overall health).[12] Moreover, there is considerable evidence that increased spending on new technologies such as drug therapies is more than off-set by the savings from avoided hospitalizations and physician office visits (Figure 20-12).[13] That is, spending on technology may "substitute" for

spending on hospitals and physicians, although not all economists are convinced of this.[14] Based on this recognition, there continues to be public pressure for more healthcare spending and access to new technology worldwide.

This chapter does not seek to attack or defend the technological imperative in healthcare. It takes the position that technology does not increase costs by itself, but rather must be viewed as part of the healthcare ecosystems in which it is used. What is critical are the payment structures and incentives established within a given country that promote or retard the use

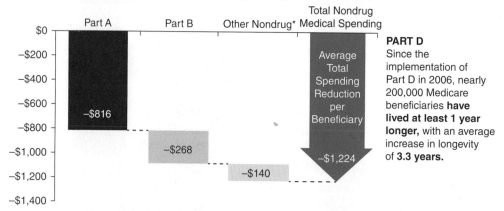

*Average Reduction in Medical Spending in 2006 and 2007 for Beneficiaries Who Gained Drug Coverage Through Medicare Part D*

**PART D** Since the implementation of Part D in 2006, nearly 200,000 Medicare beneficiaries **have lived at least 1 year longer,** with an average increase in longevity of **3.3 years.**

*Home health, durable medical equipment, hospice, and outpatient institutional services

The Medicare drug benefit increased access to medicines for those previously without drug coverage, resulting in reduced medical spending and an overall saving of $13.4 billion in 2007, the first full year of the benefit.

**Figure 20-12** • Gaining Drug Coverage Reduced Other Medical Spending. (Source: http://phrma-docs.phrma .org/files/dmfile/chart-pack-biopharmaceuticals-in-perspective4.pdf.)

of technologies for given patients (and their diffusion to other patients). This chapter also takes the position that any analysis of increased spending on technology must be combined with an analysis of the benefits achieved by using these technological resources.[15] Finally, this chapter takes it as a given that technological innovation will continue to drive the dynamics of the healthcare industry into the future, as it did during the past century.[16]

## THE INNOVATION CHALLENGE

All of the healthcare sectors examined here are considered "high technology."[17] Like other high-tech industries, innovation is the key driver of competitive advantage and commercial success. R&D investments can account for up to one-third of a medical technology firm's stock price and are correlated with the firm's gross margins 4 to 5 years down the road.[18] At the same time, innovation is also the continuing challenge facing firms in these sectors. The high price-to-revenue multiples for many of these firms suggest that financial markets expect these firms to grow revenues and sustain gross margins above and beyond other investment sectors, all of which necessitate continued innovation.[19]

Successful innovation hinges on many factors, including serendipity of discovery, wise paths taken in the past, wise investment decisions in the present, wise options taken out on the future, and access to new technologies via M&As and strategic alliances. A recent monograph illustrates the critical interplay between uncertain scientific endeavors and support from management above in abetting this innovation.[20] These factors occur in the context of favorable market structures, the possession of key resources and capabilities, and fruitful ties with other organizations upstream and downstream in the value chain.

This chapter (and the following 4 chapters) examine the source of technological innovation in the healthcare system. Specifically, for the firms in each of the innovative sectors listed earlier, these chapters address the following set of questions:

- What products do these companies make, and what is so innovative about them?
- What are the different business models of innovation pursued by firms in this sector, and how do they finance them?

- What are the strategies pursued by firms in this sector?
- What are the key success factors for innovative firms in this sector?
- How have firms in this sector, and the sector itself, grown over time?
- What are the important competitive and regulatory forces shaping this sector?

## WHY STUDY THE PRODUCERS OF HEALTHCARE TECHNOLOGY?

### Importance in Health Administration Curricula

Historically, the manufacturers of innovative products in the healthcare ecosystem were ignored in most graduate-level courses in health administration taught in schools of business and public health. Into the early 2000s, introductory texts included few, if any, chapters dedicated to the technology sectors. This situation has fortunately changed. Texts now include at least one chapter on "technology," the pharmaceutical sector, or both, as well as a discussion of some of the regulatory bodies governing these sectors (eg, Food and Drug Administration).[21] Few texts, however, discuss industry dynamics or company business models; few discuss new start-ups; and none take a global perspective.

The limited understanding of these sectors can foster a narrow view of the overall healthcare ecosystem on the part of academic researchers and executives of health provider organizations. Graduate curriculums of health administration devote considerable attention to the provider and purchaser sectors in the ecosystem, along with the fiscal intermediaries that separate them (ie, the first 3 boxes in the healthcare value chain; see Figure 3-9). Why might this be of concern?

As an illustration, one cannot fully understand the technological imperative in the US healthcare ecosystem unless one understands the relationship that manufacturers of new products have with individual physicians.[22] The failure to understand this relationship can undermine efforts by health provider organizations to control their own costs. Executives of provider organizations may not fully appreciate that their physicians often develop closer alliances and attachments to the manufacturing firms than to their own organizations. These attachments have as much to do with the innovative features of the products made as with the intense sales and marketing support that goes with them. Indeed, manufacturers and physicians have developed a 2-way exchange of mutual benefits that executives and purchasers may have trouble altering. For their part, manufacturers offer clinicians access to the latest technology, information about the product, assistance and training in its use, involvement in clinical trials, training of the clinician's residents and nursing team, donations and honoraria, and opportunities for "naming" rights on new equipment. For their part, clinicians can serve as "thought leaders" and thereby provide avenues for influencing colleagues to use the product, feedback on the product to assist with next-generation product development, leaders for clinical trials, and access to patients.

This entire set of exchanges—discussed in detail in Chapter 23 on medical devices—is poorly understood. They are also now under scrutiny by the federal and state governments in the United States as part of a larger inquiry into "conflicts of interest." Indeed, the United States enacted a congressionally mandated transparency program called the Open Payments Act—also known as the Sunshine Act—as part of the Patient Protection and Affordable Care Act to increase awareness of financial relationships by collecting and reporting any payments or transfers of value product manufacturers make to physicians or teaching hospitals. What is not clearly known at this point is what effect such transparency will have on the process of interactions between producers and providers and the ultimate impact on innovation.

## Importance of Providers Focusing on Upstream Supply Costs

To aggravate this problem, many provider organizations historically concerned themselves primarily with the "downstream" portions of the value chain—that is, public purchasers in the government (Medicare and Medicaid), private purchasers (employers), and the fiscal intermediaries (private insurers) who reimburse them. They largely ignored the "upstream" players in the value chain, such as the manufacturers and the distributors of their products. Fortunately, this deemphasis on the supply chain has also been corrected. Supply chain management now plays a more critical role in hospital systems, embodied in the chief resource officer (CRO).

This attention to the supply chain is important for several reasons. Healthcare supplies (eg, drugs, medical devices, medical-surgical supplies) account for 19% of a hospital's total expenditures, according to US government figures. If one includes the costs of handling and distributing these supplies internally, as well as the cost of all services contracted from the outside, the percentage of hospital expenditures may reach as high as 30% (see Figure 11-26). These are portions of the hospital's cost structure that now represent a major area for cost containment and improved supply utilization. With appropriate training at the level of the chief executive officer (CEO), chief operating officer (COO), chief financial officer (CFO), chief medical officer (CMO), chief nursing officer (CNO), and the newly emergent CRO—the "O-zone layer"—provider organizations may be able to achieve improvements.

Not only are supply chain costs the second largest cost bucket for hospitals, but they are also fragmented among lots of expense areas in the hospital, each with its own manager who may not have been trained in managing supply expense.[23] Hospitals have made great strides to focus on "supply chain management" and managing the cost and utilization of "physician preference items" (PPIs)—the products for which their physicians have specific vendor and/or model preferences.[24]

Within the large bucket of supply expense, the 2 biggest categories of spending are drugs and medical-surgical supplies, including medical devices (see Figure 11-27). Costs for these supplies have been rising quite rapidly. Retail pharmaceutical costs as a percentage of national health expenditures have doubled in the United States over the past 4 decades from 5% (1980) to 10% (2019). These cost figures do not include pharmaceutical products shipped to hospitals, which are embedded in hospital cost figures and which may account for 10% to 15% of total prescription drugs costs.[25] Although there are no precise national statistics on the percentage of hospital costs devoted to drugs, we might estimate them by multiplying the percentage of hospital market basket spending devoted to products (19.5%) by the percentage of products that are drugs (18%), which yields roughly 3.5% of hospital costs. Research on hospital finance suggests the amount may be as high as 7.9% of hospital costs.[26] Combining both retail and institutional sales, trend data suggest that pharmaceutical costs are approaching shares of total spending by hospital and physician services—areas that historically have accounted for the majority of health spending (see Figure 6-17).[27]

Medical device costs have also been rising. Device spending in the United States reached $55 to $65 billion at the turn of the millennium and now amounts to $162 billion. Much of this rise is due to the technological imperative noted earlier. As an illustration, executives at one group purchasing organization (GPO) reported that despite their successful efforts to secure a lower contract price with a device manufacturer for its products, the overall costs of the contract rose 25% in 1 year due to increases in new product introductions (primary reason) and utilization (secondary reason).[28]

There is no precise estimate of what percentage of hospital costs are accounted for by medical devices. The Centers for Medicare and Medicaid Services (CMS) in the United States does not break these costs out in their annual tabulations of national healthcare expenditures. As a result, medical device costs are not separately depicted in Figure 6-17, but rather are buried inside the trend line for hospital spending. This is because most devices are implanted in hospitals and thus are purchased by hospitals on behalf of their physicians. Extrapolating again from the figures provided earlier, however, we might estimate the amount by multiplying the percentage of hospital market basket spending devoted to products (19.5%) by the percentage of products that are medical-surgical (27%), which yields roughly 5% of hospital costs. This figure is close to the 6.2% suggested by research on hospital finance and the device industry itself.[29]

This identification of drug and device costs buried in the hospital spending bucket is important. We might take the 3.5% to 7.9% and 5.0% to 6.2% of hospital spending on drugs and devices, respectively, and reallocate them to retail pharmaceutical spending (thus yielding a more robust measure of technology spending). We would then find the 3 trend lines in Figure 6-17 converging more closely together. Stated differently, the United States is beginning to spend as much on the products as it does on the providers who use them.

## Growing Prominence of the Technology Sectors in the Economy

Finally, these technology sectors are important in their own right, composing a major part of

| Medical Device Firms | Biopharmaceutical Firms |
| --- | --- |
| Cardinal Health | J&J |
| Abbott Labs | Pfizer |
| Stryker | Merck |
| Becton Dickinson | Abbvie |
| Baxter | Eli Lilly |
| Boston Scientific | Bristol-Myers |
| Zimmer | Celgene |
| | Biogen |
| | Regeneron |

**Figure 20-13** • Medical Device and Biopharmaceutical Firms on the 2017 Fortune 500 List. (Source: Advisory Board, "The 42 Health Care Companies that Made This Year's Fortune 500 (May 24, 2018). Available at https://www.advisory.com/daily-briefing/2018/05/24/fortune-500. Accessed on February 21, 2019.)

the US corporate world. Nine biopharmaceutical firms and 8 medical device firms are listed among the US Fortune 500, based on 2017 revenues (Figure 20-13). This list does not include the large foreign-based pharmaceutical firms that do a lot of business in the United States. On a worldwide basis, firms in the pharmaceutical, biotechnology, and medical device industries generated over $1,440 billion in revenues in 2015.

## Technology Sector Margins Support Other Parts of the Value Chain

The profit margins earned within these sectors are the envy of other parts of the healthcare ecosystem, which frequently look to the producers for help with their own margins. Thus, for example, GPOs have earned the bulk of their revenues from contract administration fees paid by the manufacturers in order to do contracted business with the GPOs' hospital members. Insurers have begun negotiating value-based contracts with drug and device manufacturers to reimburse the latter based on the clinical outcomes derived from their expensive, innovative products. In the past, pharmaceutical wholesalers relied more on upstream drug manufacturers than on downstream hospital customers for the bulk of their ever-shrinking margins. Hospital efforts to partner with manufacturers (described earlier) represent another example of less profitable portions of the healthcare industry seeking assistance and relief from the more profitable sectors. Indeed, the middle 3 blocks of the healthcare value chain (see Figure 3-9)—providers and the 2 sets of intermediaries—enjoy much lower returns than do the technology sectors. Faced with governmental pressures to restrain increases in provider reimbursement and employer concerns over rising healthcare outlays for their employees, providers and their intermediaries will increasingly (be forced to) look to the manufacturing sectors for financial assistance.

## Growing Importance of the Healthcare Supply Chain in Public Policy and Public Health

Events in early 2020 highlighted the importance of personal protective equipment (PPE), ventilators, and active pharmaceutical ingredients (APIs)—topics that never received much attention. They were incredibly important, however, for managing the initial onslaught of patients infected with COVID-19. The country learned that it sourced its PPEs from China. The country also learned that over 70% of the manufacturing sites that produce the APIs for medicines dispensed in the United States are overseas, with almost a third coming from India and China. China was singled out in particular, given that it makes roughly 80% of the world's antibiotics; the United States, by contrast, has witnessed the number of its antibiotic manufacturers decline from more than 30 (in the late 1980s) to zero— in large part due to aggressive investments made by state-backed enterprises in China, which offered to make antibiotics at lower cost.[30]

Title III of the 2020 Coronavirus Aid, Relief, and Economic Security (CARES) Act helped to shine the light on logistical issues such as the security of the medical product supply chain, the strategic national stockpile of medical supplies, and preventing interruptions in medical device production. In other words, the healthcare supply chain has become an issue of national security. The Trump administration responded by awarding a 4-year, $354 million contract to Phlow Corp to manufacture APIs and generic medicines domestically. The administration also announced it was making a $765 million loan to Eastman Kodak as part of the Defense Production Act to make the APIs used in generic drugs. These efforts followed on the heels of the administration's invocation of the 1950 act to award a $489 million contract to General Motors to manufacture 30,000 ventilators.

## IMPACT OF TECHNOLOGY SECTORS ON LOCAL AND NATIONAL ECONOMIES

Technology sectors are also playing increasingly important roles in national and local economies. One report provides empirical evidence for the substantial economic impact of several technology sectors (pharmaceuticals, biotechnology, devices) during the decade from 1996 to 2006. The sectors' impact has been both broad and deep. They have contributed to the nation's job growth (via direct, indirect, and induced means) at a faster rate than the rest of the economy and impacted the nation's GDP at a rate triple that of other sectors in the economy. These sectors supported the largest number of jobs in the local economies of several states (California, New York, New Jersey, Pennsylvania, and Illinois). Moreover, investment levels per employee in the biopharmaceutical sectors are approximately 8 times the R&D spend per employee in all manufacturing industries.[31]

At a national level, governments are protecting their pharmaceutical industries against foreign competition and the threat of foreign takeover (eg, France's defense of Sanofi and support of its merger with Aventis in the early 2000s to prevent a takeover by Swiss-based Novartis). Such moves are undertaken for reasons of national pride as well as the desire to maintain highly skilled labor (eg, R&D scientists). National governments (eg, China) are also actively developing biotechnology sectors in order to attract skilled workers, develop an R&D base in a growing industry, and become a regional hub for such activity. Countries such as the United Kingdom are making major investments in information technology in order to improve the efficiency of their national health systems and their levels of customer service.

Similar developments are occurring at the local government level. Cities in the United States, such as San Diego, San Jose, Boston, Philadelphia, and Raleigh-Durham, are seeking to develop technology clusters in pharmaceuticals and biotechnology in order to foster economic development and investment.[32] Other cities (eg, Warsaw, Indiana) have developed clusters of medical device firms. These areas are leveraging the advantages that physical proximity affords scientists in the life and medical sciences to generate, transmit, and share knowledge.

Such clustering also serves to attract and retain scientific talent and companies in search of this talent and also permits other businesses and the local economy to reap the benefits of the innovation that is locally grown. In this manner, cities develop crucial interactions among scientists, entrepreneurs, and venture capitalists.

Michael Porter has argued that proximity of specialized companies leads to unusual competitive success. This is partly based on increased productivity by ensuring better access to employees and suppliers. It is also partly based on superior access to new and specialized information. Finally, it is partly the fact that proximity generates both competition and cooperation (eg, value chain linkages between manufacturers and the suppliers of needed inputs and specialized infrastructure). Such clustering serves to increase local firms' ability to innovate and compete both nationally and globally.[33]

Not surprisingly, the current strategy of many countries is to emulate the local clusters found in the United States, particularly in biotechnology.[34] Due to global competition and national investments in innovation, US-based companies find their historical leadership position now seriously challenged. PricewaterhouseCoopers has developed a Medical Technologies Innovation Scorecard that evaluates the innovative capacity and capabilities of 9 Western and Asian countries.[35] The scorecard suggests the emergence of new national leaders in medical technology over the next decade who can develop smaller, faster, and more affordable devices that deliver healthcare to "the bottom of the pyramid" (the poor), that enable the delivery of healthcare anywhere, and that help to "bend the trend" in rising healthcare costs.

## SUMMARY

This chapter "kicks off" an analysis of another little-known portion of the healthcare ecosystem—the companies that make innovative technologies. The technology sectors are quite important to providers who rely on them to treat their patients. These sectors are also important to insurers who have to pay for them. Finally, they are important to governments at all levels that wish to build engines for economic growth and job creation. They deserve consideration in healthcare administration curricula and warrant your understanding.

## QUESTIONS TO PONDER

1. What prevents US healthcare providers from being global players (ie, operating in other countries) the way that technology firms do?
2. What is the "technological imperative" in healthcare? Is this a good thing or a bad thing?
3. According to this chapter, why do students of healthcare management need to understand the technology sectors?
4. Do we have to manage the technology costs of healthcare in the same way that we manage the costs of hospitals and physicians?
5. Do we finance healthcare technology differently than we finance the services of hospitals and physicians?

## REFERENCES

1. Ben Guarino, Emily Rauhala, and William Wan. "China Increasingly Challenges American Dominance of Science," *Washington Post* (June 3, 2018).
2. Tanisha Carino. "To Get More Bang for Your Health-Care Buck, Invest in Innovation," *Health Affairs Blog* (January 24, 2019). Kevin Schulman and Barak Richman. "Toward an Effective Innovation Agenda," *N Engl J Med.* 380 (2019): 900-990.
3. Fred Ledley, Sarah McCoy, Gregory Vaughn, et al. "Profitability of Large Pharmaceutical Companies Compared With Other Large Public Companies," *JAMA.* 323 (9) (2020): 834-843.
4. Victor Fuchs. *The Health Economy* (Cambridge, MA: Harvard University Press, 1986). Annetine Gelijns and Nathan Rosenberg. "The Dynamics of Technological Change in Medicine," *Health Aff.* 13 (3) (1994): 28-46.
5. Laurence Baker, Scott Atlas, and Christopher Afendulis. "Expanded Use of Imaging Technology and the Challenge of Measuring Value," *Health Aff.* 27 (6) (2008): 1467-1478. Lawton Burns, Elizabeth Bradley, and Bryan Weiner. "The Management Challenge of Delivering Value in Health Care: Global and U.S. Perspectives," in Lawton Burns, Elizabeth Bradley, and Bryan Weiner (Eds.), *Health Care Management: Organization Design and Behavior*, 6th ed. (Clifton Park, NY: Cengage Learning, 2011):

2-32. Peter S. Hussey, Gerard F. Anderson, Robin Osborn, et al. "How Does the Quality of Care Compare in Five Countries?" *Health Aff.* 23 (3) (2004): 89-99.

6. Congressional Budget Office. *Technological Change and the Growth of Health Care Spending* (Washington, DC: Congressional Budget Office, 2008). Cinda Becker. "The Best Care Money Can Buy?" *Mod Healthc.* 34 (2004): 26-29.

7. Organisation for Economic Co-operation and Development. *Value for Money in Health Spending* (Paris France: OECD, 2010).

8. Commonwealth Fund. *Bending the Curve: Options for Achieving Savings and Improving Value in U.S. Health Spending* (New York, NY: Commonwealth Fund, 2007).

9. Lawton R. Burns and Mark V. Pauly. "Transformation of the Healthcare Industry: Curb Your Enthusiasm?" *Milbank Q.* 96 (1) (2018): 57-109.

10. Paul Wallace. "The Health of Nations: A Survey of Health-Care Finance," *Economist* (July 17, 2004): 3-19. David Cutler and Mark McClelland. "Is Technological Change in Medicine Worth It?" *Health Aff.* 20 (5) (2001): 11-29. David Cutler, Allison Rosen, and Sandeep Vijan. "The Value of Medical Spending in the United States, 1960-2000," *N Engl J Med.* 355 (2006): 920-927.

11. David Cutler, Genia Long, Ernst R. Berndt, et al. "The Value of Antihypertensive Drugs: A Perspective on Medical Innovation," *Health Aff.* 26 (1) (2007): 97-110.

12. Value Group. *The Value of Investment in Health Care: Better Care, Better Lives.* Available online: https://www.aha.org/2006-03-10-value-investment-health-care-better-care-better-lives. Accessed on August 7, 2020.

13. J. Michael McWilliams, Alan Zaslavsky, and Haiden Huskamp. "Implementation of Medicare Part D and Nondrug Medical Spending for Elderly Adults With Limited Prior Drug Coverage," *JAMA.* 36 (4) (2011): 402-409.

14. Craig Garthwaite and Mark Duggan. "Empirical Evidence on the Value of Pharmaceuticals," Chapter 15 in Patricia Danzon and Sean Nicholson (Eds.), *Oxford Handbook of the Economics of the BioPharmaceutical Industry* (Oxford, United Kingdom: University Press, 2011). J. Michael McWilliams, Alan Zaslavsky, and Haiden Huskamp. "Implementation of Medicare Part D and Nondrug Medical Spending for Elderly Adults With Limited Prior Drug Coverage," *JAMA.* 36 (4) (2011): 402-409. M. Christopher Roebuck, Joshua Liberman, Marin Gemmill-Toyama, et al. "Medication Adherence Leads to Lower Health Care Use and Costs Despite Increased Drug Spending," *Health Aff.* 30 (1) (2011): 90-91. Martin Gaynor, Jian Li, and William Vogt. *Is Drug Coverage a Free Lunch? Cross-Price Elasticities and the Design of Prescription Drug Benefits*

(Cambridge, MA: National Bureau of Economic Research, NBER Working Paper Series, Working Paper No. 12758, 2006). Frank Lichtenberg. *The Effect of Pharmaceutical Use and Innovation on Hospitalization and Mortality* (Cambridge, MA: National Bureau of Economic Research, NBER Working Paper Series, Working Paper No. 5418, 1996). Terry McInnis. *Pharmacist—The Most Transformative Force in Healthcare or the Demise of a Profession?* (American College of Clinical Pharmacy, October 2011). Available online: https://www.accp.com/report/index.aspx?iss=1011&art=5. Accessed on August 7, 2020.

15. Penny E. Mohr, Curt Mueller, Peter Neumann, et al. *The Impact of Medical Technology on Future Healthcare Costs* (Bethesda, MD: Project Hope, 2001).

16. Rosemary Stevens. *In Sickness and in Wealth* (New York, NY: Basic Books, 1989). Paul Starr. *The Social Transformation of American Medicine* (New York, NY: Basic Books, 1982).

17. "High-technology" firms are those engaged in the design, development, and introduction of new products and innovative manufacturing processes, or both, through the systematic application of scientific and technical knowledge. They also typically use state-of-the-art techniques, devote a high proportion of expenditures to R&D, and employ a high proportion of scientific, technical, and engineering personnel. Compare Daniel Hecker. "High-Technology Employment: A Broader View," *Monthly Labor Rev.* (June 1999): 18-28.

18. Peter Lawyer, Alexander Kerstein, Hirotaka Yabuki, et al. "High Science: A Best-Practice Formula for Driving Innovation," *In Vivo* (April 2004): 70-82.

19. Peter Lawyer, Alexander Kerstein, Hirotaka Yabuki, et al. "High Science: A Best-Practice Formula for Driving Innovation," *In Vivo* (April 2004): 70-82.

20. Philip Rea, Mark V. Pauly, and Lawton R. Burns (Eds.). *Managing Discovery: Harnessing Creativity to Drive Biomedical Innovation* (Cambridge, United Kingdom: Cambridge University Press, 2018).

21. Stephen Williams and Paul Torrens. *Introduction to Health Services,* 7th ed. (Albany, NY: Delmar Publishers, 2008). Phoebe Barton. *Understanding the US Health Services System,* 4th ed. (Chicago, IL: Health Administration Press, 2010). Anthony Kovner and Steven Jonas (Eds.). *Health Care Delivery in the United States,* 9th ed. (New York, NY: Springer Publishing, 2008). Leiyu Shi and Douglas Singh. *Delivering Health Care in America: A Systems Approach,* 4th ed. (Boston, MA: Jones & Bartlett, 2008).

22. Lawton Burns, Michael Housman, Robert Booth, et al. "Implant Vendors and Hospitals: Competing

Influences Over Product Choice by Orthopedic Surgeons," *Health Care Manag Rev.* 34 (1) (2009): 2-18. Mark Pauly and Lawton R. Burns. "Price Transparency for Medical Devices," *Health Aff.* 27 (6) (2008): 1544-1553.

23. Lawton R. Burns. *The Health Care Value Chain* (San Francisco, CA: Jossey-Bass, 2002).

24. Lawton R. Burns, Michael Housman, Robert Booth, and Aaron Koenig. "Physician Preference Items: What Factors Matter to Surgeons? Does the Vendor Matter?" *Med Devices.* 11 (2018): 39-49.

25. Lawton R. Burns. *The Health Care Value Chain* (San Francisco, CA: Jossey-Bass, 2002). Pembroke Consulting. *Pharmaceutical Purchases by Channel* (2009). IMS data provided courtesy of Adam Fein.

26. Nancy Kane and Richard Siegrist. *Understanding Rising Hospital Inpatient Costs: Key Components of Cost and the Impact on Poor Quality* (Unpublished Report, August 12, 2002). Available online: www.heartland.org/custom/semod_policybot/pdf/14629.pdf. Accessed on March 3, 2011.

27. This trend was noted in the 1990s by Patricia Danzon and Mark Pauly. "Insurance and New Technology: From Hospital to Drugstore," *Health Aff.* 20 (5) (2001): 86-100.

28. David Ricker, personal communication.

29. Nancy Kane and Richard Siegrist. "Understanding Rising Hospital Inpatient Costs: Key Components of Cost and The Impact on Poor Quality" (Unpublished Report, August 12, 2002). Available online: www.heartland.org/custom/semod_policybot/pdf/14629.pdf. Accessed on March 3, 2011.

30. Gardiner Harris and Alex Palmer. "China Has Near-Total Control of the World's Antibiotic Supply. Is America at Risk as a Result?" *Stat+* (April 28, 2020).

31. Data are for the years 2000 to 2004. Archstone Consulting and Lawton R. Burns. *The Biopharmaceutical Sector's Impact on the U.S. Economy: Analysis at the National, State, and Local Levels* (Stamford, CT: PhRMA, 2009).

32. Ross DeVol. *America's Biotech and Life Science Clusters* (Washington, DC: Milken Institute, 2004). Kerry Dolan. "San DNAgo," *Forbes Magazine* (May 26, 2003): 122-126.

33. Michael Porter. "Clusters and the New Economics of Competition," *Harvard Business Review* (November-December 1998): 77-90.

34. Des Dearlove. "The Cluster Effect: Can Europe Clone Silicon Valley?" *Strategy + Business* 24 (Fall 2001): 67-75.

35. Christopher Wasden and Douglas Mowen. "The Changing Face of Medical Technology Innovation," *In Vivo* (September 2010): 88-98. PricewaterhouseCoopers. *Medical Technology Innovation Scorecard: The Race for Global Leadership* (Florham Park, NJ: PricewaterhouseCoopers, January 2011).

# 21

# The Pharmaceutical Sector

This chapter and the next examine the sectors that manufacture pharmaceuticals and biologics. By way of definition, a *pharmaceutical* is a product made through chemical synthesis (ie, the preparation of a compound using plant- and chemical-based substances that use chemical reactions to derive a pill or capsule). By contrast, a *biologic* is manufactured in or extracted from living biological sources (eg, bacteria, yeast, and mammalian cells) and can include vaccines, allergenics, somatic cells, gene therapies, tissues, recombinant therapeutic proteins (including monoclonal antibodies), peptides (protein fragments), and living cells. An easier way to distinguish these 2 products is that pharmaceuticals are small molecules (<700 daltons) that allow them to be taken orally; biologics are large molecules (>700 daltons) that are usually administered by a physician via an injection, but can sometimes be patient-administered via an auto-injector.

The 2 sectors are nevertheless lumped together as biopharmaceuticals (or, "biopharma" for short). Why now use this convention? Over the past decade or two, pharmaceutical companies have diversified into making large-molecule biologics, whereas biotechnology companies have diversified into making small molecules. It is no longer possible to distinguish the 2 sectors by the companies that make these 2 types of products.

## WHY THE PHARMACEUTICAL SECTOR IS SO INTERESTING

The pharmaceutical sector is large, profitable, and contentious. There are a lot of companies, several big companies, companies that earn some healthy profit margins (see Chapter 20), and companies that are frequently in the headlines—and not always for good reasons. Look at some news stories between 2007 and 2016:

- 2007: Eli Lilly was fined $1.42 billion to resolve a government investigation into the off-label promotion of the antipsychotic Zyprexa.
- September 2009: Pfizer was fined $2.3 billion for misbranding the painkiller Bextra with "the intent to defraud or mislead," promoting the drug to treat acute pain at dosages the US Food and Drug Administration (FDA) had previously deemed dangerously high.
- November 2011: Merck agreed to pay a fine of $950 million related to the illegal promotion of the painkiller Vioxx, which was withdrawn from the market in 2004 after studies found the drug increased the risk of heart attacks.
- July 2012: GlaxoSmithKline agreed to pay a fine of $3 billion to resolve civil and criminal liabilities regarding its promotion of drugs (eg, misbranding the drug Paxil for treating depression in patients under 18), as well as its failure to report safety data.

- November 2013: Johnson & Johnson agreed to pay a $2.2 billion fine to resolve criminal and civil allegations relating to its promotion of the prescription drugs Risperdal, Invega, and Natrecor for uses not approved as safe and effective by the FDA, as well as targeting elderly dementia patients in nursing homes and paying kickbacks to physicians.
- September 2014: GlaxoSmithKline apologized to China for bribing healthcare workers to use its drugs and agreed to pay a fine of nearly half a billion US dollars to the Chinese government.
- December 2016: Mylan CEO Heather Bresch admitted publicly that her firm had raised the prices on its EpiPen by 500% over the prior 9 years.

As noted in Chapter 20, the pharma sector carries great risk, but can also lead to attractive returns. It can also bring great therapeutic benefits to patients, but excesses and mistakes are frequent. The sector is highly regulated (eg, by the FDA) and features a very complex value chain, both internally and externally. The sector faces many current challenges but is also likely to have an interesting future. If you are unsure about this last point, just consider the role played by the biopharma sector

in helping the country manage its way through the COVID-19 crisis in the spring of 2020, including rapid diagnostic testing, the hunt for therapies, and the hunt for vaccines. The sector went from "whipping boy" to "wunderkind" almost overnight.

## OVERVIEW OF PHARMA: THE BIG PICTURE

### Market Overview

The global biopharma sector generated revenues just over $1.2 trillion in 2018 (Figure 21-1). The top 10 companies accounted for nearly 40% of sales in 2018 (Figure 21-2), and the top 10 therapeutic classes accounted for roughly 50% of sales and 70% of all prescriptions written in the United States (Figure 21-3). The therapeutic areas with the highest projected growth rates are immunosuppressants, dermatologicals, and anticoagulants. The top 15 drug products for 2018 are presented in Figure 21-4. Generics make up roughly 28% of total sales revenues and nearly 90% of prescription volume. In terms of global sales, North America and Europe account for 40% and 25%, respectively, of the global market; however, the fastest growth is in the emerging markets (Figure 21-5).

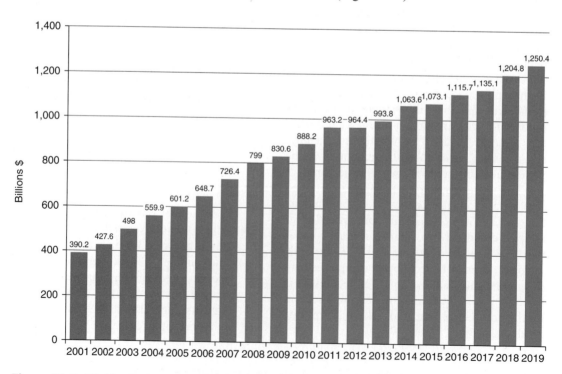

**Figure 21-1** • Worldwide Pharma Revenues (2001-2019). (Source: IQVIA, Statista.)

**Pharmaceutical Industry—Evolution of Global Ranking 2003-2018**

| # | 2003 Company | Share | 2008 Company | Share | 2013 Company | Share | 2018 Company | Share |
|---|---|---|---|---|---|---|---|---|
| 1 | Pfizer | 8.95% | Pfizer | 6.36% | Novartis | 6.02% | Pfizer | 5.25% |
| 2 | GlaxoSmithKline | 6.88% | Sanofi | 5.85% | Pfizer | 5.81% | Roche | 5.19% |
| 3 | Merck & Co | 4.76% | GlaxoSmithKline | 5.74% | Roche | 5.03% | Novartis | 5.17% |
| 4 | Johnson & Johnson | 4.52% | Novartis | 5.28% | Merck & Co | 4.81% | Johnson & Johnson | 4.71% |
| 5 | Aventis | 4.39% | Roche | 5.04% | Sanofi | 4.77% | Merck & Co | 4.32% |
| 6 | Novartis | 4.38% | AstraZeneca | 4.66% | GlaxoSmithKline | 4.28% | Sanofi | 4.06% |
| 7 | AstraZeneca | 4.24% | Johnson & Johnson | 3.73% | Johnson & Johnson | 3.61% | Abbvie | 3.71% |
| 8 | Roche | 3.41% | Merck & Co | 3.35% | AstraZeneca | 3.30% | GlaxoSmithKline | 3.51% |
| 9 | Bristol-Myers Squibb | 3.23% | Eli Lilly | 2.86% | Eli Lilly | 2.64% | Amgen | 2.60% |
| 10 | Eli Lilly | 2.77% | Bristol-Myers Squibb | 2.69% | AbbVie | 2.41% | Gilead Sciences | 2.51% |
| 11 | Wyeth | 2.77% | Abbott Labs | 2.60% | Teva | 2.35% | Bristol-Myers Squibb | 2.49% |
| 12 | Abbott Labs | 2.45% | Schering-Plough | 2.50% | Amgen | 2.34% | Eli Lilly | 2.48% |
| 13 | Takeda | 2.21% | Wyeth | 2.46% | Novo Nordisk | 1.91% | AstraZeneca | 2.43% |
| 14 | Sanofi | 2.04% | Amgen | 2.23% | Bayer | 1.91% | Bayer | 2.21% |
| 15 | Amgen | 1.82% | Bayer | 2.23% | Takeda | 1.90% | Novo Nordisk | 2.05% |
| | | 58.80% | | 57.60% | | 53.10% | | 52.70% |

**Figure 21-2** • Top 15 Pharma Companies by Global Sales. (Source: Hardman & Co. "Global Pharmaceuticals: 2018 Industry Statistics." Available Online: https://www.hardmanandco.com/research/corporate-research/global-pharmaceuticals-2018-industry-statistics/.)

**Worldwide (WW) Sales ($bn)**

| Rank | Therapy Area | 2018 WW Sales | 2024 Projected WW Sales |
|---|---|---|---|
| 1 | Oncology | 123.8 | 236.6 |
| 2 | Antidiabetics | 48.5 | 57.6 |
| 3 | Antirheumatics | 58.1 | 54.6 |
| 4 | Vaccines | 30.5 | 44.8 |
| 5 | Antivirals | 38.9 | 42.2 |
| 6 | Immunosuppressants | 14.2 | 36.1 |
| 7 | Dermatologicals | 15.8 | 32.1 |
| 8 | Bronchodilators | 28 | 30.7 |
| 9 | Sensory organs | 22.3 | 30.5 |
| 10 | Anticoagulants | 19.3 | 24.6 |
| 11 | Antihypertensives | 22.9 | 24.1 |
| 12 | MS therapies | 22.7 | 21.1 |
| 13 | Antifibrinolytics | 13.8 | 18.2 |
| 14 | Antihyperlipidaemics | 9.6 | 17.7 |
| 15 | Sera & gammaglobulins | 10.5 | 15.1 |
| | Top 15 | 479 | 686 |
| | Other | 385 | 536 |
| | **Total WW Prescription & OTC Sales** | **864** | **1,222** |

**Figure 21-3** • Top 15 Global Therapeutic Classes. bn, Billion; MS, Multiple Sclerosis; OTC, Over the Counter; WW, Worldwide. (Source: Evaluate Pharma. "World Preview 2019, Outlook to 2024." https://info.evaluate.com/rs/607-YGS-364/images/EvaluatePharma_World_Preview_2019.pdf.)

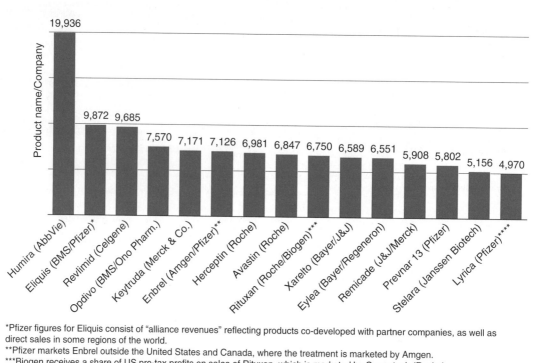

**Figure 21-4 •** Top 15 Pharmaceutical Products in 2018 ($ Billions). (Source: Statista, Genetic Engineering & Biotechnology News.)

*Pfizer figures for Eliquis consist of "alliance revenues" reflecting products co-developed with partner companies, as well as direct sales in some regions of the world.
**Pfizer markets Enbrel outside the United States and Canada, where the treatment is marketed by Amgen.
***Biogen receives a share of US pre-tax profits on sales of Rituxan, which is marketed by Genentech (Roche).
Sales figures do not include US pre-tax profits generated by Biogen, since the company only discloses those profits combined with profits from Gazyva® (obinutuzumab), and does not break out each product separately. Biogen reported combined Rituxan-Gazyva pre-tax profits of $1.432 billion for 2018, and $1.316 billion for 2017.
****Pfizer lists separately the Lyrica revenues generated in all of Europe, Russia, Turkey, Israel, and Central Asian countries ($347 million in 2018, $553 million in 2017). Those revenues are listed by Pfizer's "Essential Health" operating segment, while its "Innovative Health" segment records Lyrica revenues generated elsewhere in the world, including the United States ($4.622 billion in 2018, $4.511 billion in 2017).

### World Pharmaceutical Sales 2017-2019 by Region in Billion US$*

* All values are based at constant exchange rates (CER). 2018 figures are estimates.
** ROW = rest of world.

**Figure 21-5 •** World Sales by Region. (Source: Statista, AstraZeneca, IQVIA.)

**Nominal and Inflation-Adjusted per Capita Spending on Retail Prescription Drugs, 1960-2017**

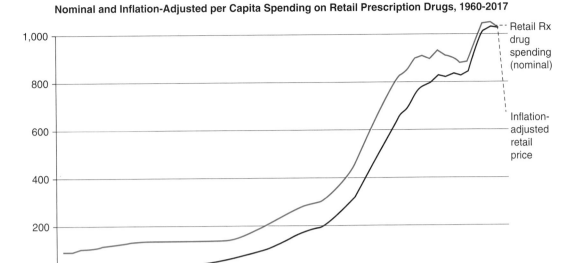

**Figure 21-6** • US Spending on Retail Prescription Drugs, 1960 to 2017. (Source: Kaiser Family Foundation Analysis of National Health Expenditures Account.)

## Trends in the US Market

The cost of prescription drugs has become a hot-button issue with consumers and policy makers. For example, in September 2019, Speaker of the House Nancy Pelosi unveiled plans to impose price controls on US pharmaceutical manufacturers.

Figure 21-6 shows the steady historical growth in US spending on pharmaceuticals. On a per-capita basis, inflation-adjusted retail prescription drug spending in the United States increased from $90 in 1960 to $1,025 in 2017. Despite the absolute growth, the percentage of national health expenditures devoted to retail pharmaceuticals has remained fairly steady at 11% to 12% during the past decade. Prescription drugs represented a shrinking share of total health spending through 2013, but increased in 2014 and 2015 with the introduction of some high-cost specialty drugs (Figure 21-7). The Altarum Institute projects that this percentage will remain stable going forward through 2027. Indeed, if any one sector of healthcare has exhibited particularly outsized spending, it is hospital care (Figure 21-8).

Likewise, out-of-pocket per-capita spending on prescription drugs has been relatively flat ($145 in 2016, $144 in 2017) compared to out-of-pocket per-capita costs for physician services, which rose from $182 to $185, and hospital services, which rose from $99 to $104.

Out-of-pocket costs for prescription drugs are expected to increase but will likely represent a smaller portion of overall prescription drug spending. Prices for common generic drugs have dropped by 37% since 2014, while branded drug prices have increased by over 60% (Figure 21-9). However, as noted in Chapter 16, the net prices paid are much lower than the list prices.

## MARKET STRUCTURE OF PHARMA

The pharmaceutical sector has undergone significant consolidation over the past 30 years, beginning in the late 1980s. Figure 21-10 illustrates how the pharma firm with the largest global sales (Pfizer) achieved its status: It was a "mass-mergerer." Only one-third of the 38 large-cap pharma companies that existed in 1988 remained in 2009 (total number of 13), but with more than 5 times the market value ($188 billion in 1988 vs $1,109 billion in 2009). The top 15 global pharma companies as of 2018 are listed in Figure 21-2; the top 10 accounted for roughly 40% of sales.

However, despite the consolidation, the pharma market is quite competitive. It is perhaps more accurate to state that pharma is a consolida*ting* but *not* a consolida*ted* industry. There are roughly 5,000 pharma firms, and the

**Percent Growth in Per Capita Spending by Drug Type, 2009-2017**

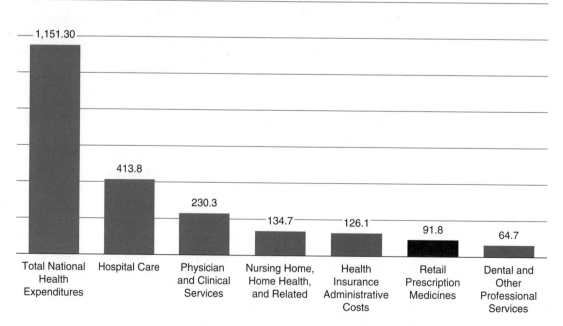

**Figure 21-7** • Growth in Specialty Drug Spending. (Source: IQVIA, Medicine Use and Spending in the U.S., April 2018; IQVIA Institute of Human Data Science.)

top 10 firms commanded a smaller share of total sales in 2016 (41%) than they did 10 years earlier (45% in 2006). This is despite the fact that there were 500 mergers and acquisitions (M&A) and 2,500 collaborations and licensing deals in the prior year (2015). The result is, thus, not a consolidated industry but a clustered, networked industry in which strategic partnerships are very important. According to Deloitte, the number of new research and development (R&D) partnerships increased from 4,000 to 9,000 between 2005 and 2014; the number of

**Prescription Medicine Spending Contributed Less Than One-Tenth of Total Healthcare Spending Growth in the Past Decade**

**Cumulative spending growth over 10 years in billions (2009-2018)**

**Figure 21-8** • Spending Growth. (Source: PhRMA, Centers for Medicare and Medicaid Services.)

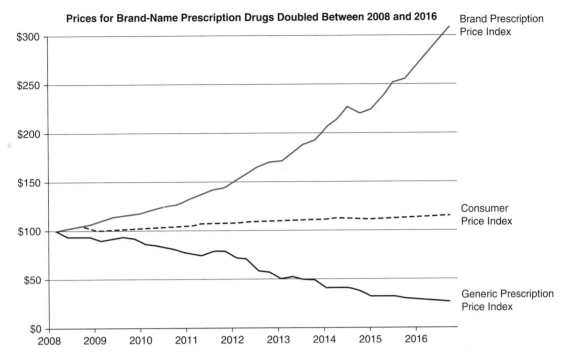

**Figure 21-9** • Prices for Brand Name Prescription Drugs. (Source: Kaiser Family Foundation Analysis of Data from Express Scripts 2015 Prescription Price Index.)

R&D consortia increased from 34 to 334; and the number of early-stage partnerships rose from 256 to 578.[1]

## RESEARCH AND DEVELOPMENT

As noted in Chapter 20, the pharmaceutical sector spends heavily on R&D. R&D is the key to the value of all biopharma firms; their stock prices reflect the prospects of the drugs in their clinical pipelines. It should thus come as no surprise that the internal value chain of a biopharma firm centers heavily on R&D. R&D spending as a percentage of sales by the largest pharma firms has more than doubled in the past 30 years, from 7.8% in 1987 to 16.1% in 2017. In absolute dollar terms, spending over this period grew by more than 300% (after adjusting for inflation).[2] There is some debate regarding the

**The Building of Pfizer**

| Date | Event | Market Share |
|------|-------|--------------|
| 1994 | Pfizer (ranked #22) | 2.7% |
| 1995 | Acquisition of American Cyanamid | 1.3% |
| 1995 | Upjohn merged with Pharmacia | |
| 2000 | Pharmacia acquires Searle (Monsanto) | |
| 2000 | Acquisition of Warner-Lambert | 2.6% |
| 2002 | Acquisition of Pharmacia | 3.3% |
| 2010 | Acquisition of Wyeth/American Home Products | 2.0% |
| | Pfizer accumulated market share | 11.9% |
| 2016 | Pfizer ranked #1 | 5.6% |

**Figure 21-10** • History of a Global Sales Leader at Pfizer.

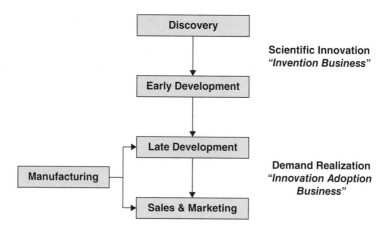

**Figure 21-11** • The Pharmaceutical Value Chain.

actual average cost to develop a new drug, however, with estimates ranging from $985 million to $2.8 billion.[3]

Chapter 20 defined R&D; this section illustrates what R&D looks like in a pharmaceutical firm. Simply stated, R&D defines the "twin towers" of these science-based firms: discover a new drug and then develop and commercialize it (Figure 21-11). The first stage is rooted in discovering an innovative product; the second stage is rooted in commercializing it. The latter includes creating the clinical information needed to bring it to the FDA for approval and

then bring it to the market and get clinicians to adopt it. The various stages in this "twin tower" process are depicted in Figure 21-12. They are briefly summarized in the following sections.

## Discovery

As noted in Chapter 20, discovery is not the same as basic science, which is largely funded by the National Institutes of Health (NIH) and largely conducted in university and research institute settings. Discovery in biopharma is applied research. Everything that is conducted has an

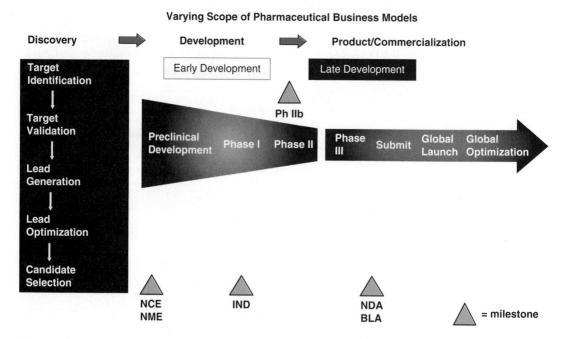

**Figure 21-12** • Varying Scope of Pharmaceutical Business Models. BLA, Biologics License Application; IND, Investigational New Drug; NCE, New Chemical Entity; NDA, New Drug Application; NME, New Molecular Entity.

end goal of (1) developing a new molecule and (2) creating the knowledge and processes around that molecule to prove that it has its intended effects and activity that make it a useful therapeutic for patients. Discovery involves 5 phases[4]:

- **Target Identification:** The discovery scientist picks a target that is hypothesized to have an important therapeutic effect on a human disease state. This is often done using in vivo testing and assay development.
- **Target Validation:** The scientist generates evidence that blocking or triggering the target will have the desired beneficial effect. The approach should potentially be preferred over rivals using predictive "disease models." Scientists also screen libraries of compounds for desired target impact.
- **Lead Generation:** The scientist works with others to use assay development, screening, and early medicinal chemistry to create the molecule. This is conducted iteratively with "structure-activity relationship" (SAR) models.
- **Lead Optimization:** Scientists use additional chemistry to study how the promising molecule behaves and then optimize it into something that can be potent, orally active, soluble, and ideally once-a-day. The goal is to select the most promising "hits" for further design, engineering, and biologic testing (using both in vitro and animal models of disease). One important goal here is to use specific animal models to predict activity and toxicity of the drug candidate and also provide data to justify initial human dosing and clinical trial design.
- **Candidate Selection:** The scientific team picks the most promising candidate (ie, meets acceptance criteria for development) to take forward into clinical testing, as well as perhaps 1 or 2 more as backups. After selection, scientists issue a "declaration" of their drug as a "new chemical entity" (NCE) or "new molecular entity" (NME).[5]

The discovery process begins with identifying diseases and associated "targets." These targets might be complex biological processes or systems or very specific molecules. Companies then seek drug candidates that have desirable effects on disease targets. This search can take many different forms, including broad, brute-force approaches that screen thousands of compounds for interaction with the target ("high-throughput screening"), or delicate and highly specific approaches that essentially handcraft drug candidates designed to interact with the unique 3-dimensional structure of the target. Once drug candidates with desirable on-target effects are identified, these are further evaluated in increasingly complex disease models.

## Patents and Patent Expirations

Pharma companies file for a patent soon after the discovery of a drug and its novel mechanism of action. From that point, the company has a 20-year patent for the product, but R&D can take up to 15 years; thus, by the time the product is approved and available on the market, the patent can be close to running out. Once the 20-year exclusivity period is up, generic competitors can enter the market and compete with the branded drug on price (covered later). To further protect their investment, companies often seek to extend their exclusivity period for a drug by filing secondary patents.

There can be patents around the biology of the disease process, around the structure of the human proteins involved, around the disease models used to try to find molecules, and around the chemical classes and structures that may have utility as a therapeutic. Additionally, there can be patents around product/process development and manufacturing processes. As a general point, patents around the composition of matter of the NCE and related compounds are considered the most valuable.

It is important to understand that it takes typically at least 2 years to receive a patent from an application. During those 2 years that the patent is under review, it is confidentially held and not a matter of public record. Additionally, a patent is not a right to proceed with the development of the NCE. It is a right to exclude others from the scope defined and granted. The reason this is important is that several patents may be required to protect an exclusive position for an NCE. For example, one company may have a patent around the compound and its ability to modulate the biological target. Another company might have a patent on the biological target and its role in human disease. Both may be required to develop the compound for that disease. None of these may be sufficient to protect the company from a competitive compound that works through different chemistry at a different site of action in the body to treat the same disease.

## Development

Drug development starts when the biopharma firm finds the molecule it wants to take into testing and ultimately into the physician's clinic. Many of the activities conducted during discovery (eg, pharmacology and toxicology) become *preclinical development* activities to satisfy FDA regulators and provide documentation needed to complete an investigational new drug (IND) application. The IND is needed to do clinical trials in humans. The IND tells the story of the investigational drug product, shows that a new experimental drug is worthy of human testing, and shows that every precaution has been taken to identify toxicity in humans. The IND is not "approved" by the FDA; the company is permitted to proceed after 30 days if no objection comes from the FDA.

Preclinical development also requires scaling up "good manufacturing practices" (GMPs): develop the process to produce larger quantities of drug, assess the product's physical characteristics and formulation requirements, develop a plan for further process scale-up and optimization (cost reductions), work with suppliers and contract manufacturers to make the drug for clinical supply, and develop assays for product release testing (critical quality attributes).

Preclinical development is followed by 4 stages of *clinical development*:

- **Phase I:** Safety studies with a small number of healthy volunteers (20-100), usually in a single center, usually short in duration, and involving no placebo or randomization of subjects. The goal here is to document safety and tolerability (eg, assess side effects associated with higher doses). Studies here try to gather data on ADME (absorption, distribution, metabolism, and excretion of the drug), which covers the drug's pharmacodynamics (PD; what the drug does to the body) and the drug's pharmacokinetics (PK; what the body does to the drug), as well as data on the half-life of the drug.

- **Phase II:** Efficacy studies with a larger number of patients (eg, 50-200) with the disease in a multicenter trial of longer duration and involving randomization of subjects with a comparator (eg, placebo, active comparator, or competing drug). Phase IIa seeks to demonstrate "proof-of-concept" regarding the compound's therapeutic potential in humans, the drug's PKs in the target population, and the drug's preliminary dose range. PK and PD studies may indicate dosing for different subpopulations. These are followed by phase IIb trials that have more subjects and longer duration and are intended to determine safety, efficacy, dosing, and other design elements in a large study.

- **Phase III:** "Pivotal" trials negotiated with regulatory authorities that are designed to support product registration. These entail large populations of patients (500-1,000+) with the disease who are treated in multicenter trials conducted on a global basis for longer durations (can be 1+ years) using placebos or active comparators in randomized testing. The goal here is to demonstrate safety and efficacy in more typical patients, determine the drug's risk/benefit profile, assess the drug's long-term safety, and finalize the remaining data required for FDA label and market access (reimbursement). These data are needed to convince the FDA to approve the drug and convince physicians to prescribe it for their patients.

- **Phase IV:** Subsequent clinical trials conducted after the drug's approval designed to answer questions of clinicians and insurers regarding subsets of patients, combination therapies, or treatment strategies using the new drug. They are often conducted to demonstrate the drug's superiority in an attribute important to stakeholders—whether clinical or economic. These studies may also be used to obtain pharmacoeconomic data, evidence regarding new formulations, dose regimens, or routes of administration, as well as new indications.

All of the information collected during clinical development is then submitted to the FDA in the form of a new drug application (NDA) for a small molecule, or a new biologic application

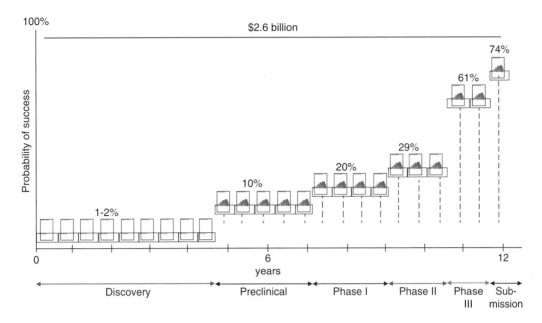

**Figure 21-13 •** Pharmaceutical Business Model: Long Cycle Time and High Risk.

(BLA) for a large-molecule biologic product. The FDA pulls together an advisory committee of physician scientists prominent in the relevant disease area who then vote on whether or not to approve the new drug. The FDA also conducts an inspection at the biopharma firm's plants that will manufacture the drug.

## Target Product Profile

Over the time of the drug's development, the biopharma firm needs to develop the drug's target product profile (TPP). The TPP defines the "go/no go" criteria for proceeding to the next phase as well as the drug's "must have" product characteristics. Referring back to Chapter 5, the TPP represents biopharma's attempt to answer the drug's impact on "the iron triangle." Thus, it answers the key questions about the drug's (1) efficacy (including key claims and clinical endpoints); (2) safety attributes; (3) dosing (including frequency and packaging); and (4) economic value (including cost-effectiveness, quality of life, and so on). All of this is designed to increase the "willingness to pay" for the drug in the marketplace.

## Managing Uncertainty and Clinical Trial Failure

All biopharma activities undertaken through phase IIb (including discovery and early development) can be considered as "managing uncertainty." Everything conducted from phase III on (late-stage development and commercialization) can be considered as "large-scale execution." Why is this so? Figure 21-13 shows the odds of success during each of the stages and phases described earlier. They slowly increase from the discovery stage (1%-2%) to preclinical development (10%) and then to phase I (20%) and phase II (29%) before they skyrocket to phase III (61%). The figure also shows the huge cost incurred and the long time taken (12 years). The average cost of drug development has risen from $179 million (1970s) to $413 million (1980s) to $1.0 billion (1990s and early 2000s) to $2.6 billion (early 2010s). These costs cover the investment in both successful and unsuccessful projects. Reasons for rising R&D costs include the requirement by regulators to run larger clinical trials, the increased complexity of those trials (clinical trial testing protocols), the longer duration of those trials, the higher cost of the drugs used, the larger number of testing procedures conducted during those trials, and the growing number of eligibility criteria needed to recruit subjects into those trials.

Of particular interest, however, is the high failure rate of potential new drugs in phase II trials. Data presented in Figure 21-14 show that phase II trials not only have lower success rates compared to phase I and phase III, but they

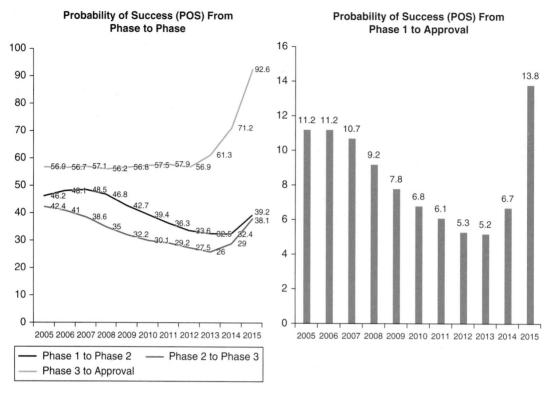

**Figure 21-14 •** Probability of Trial Success. (Source: Chi Heem Wong, Kien Wei Siah, and Andrew W. Lo. "Estimation of Clinical Trial Success Rates and Related Parameters," *Biostatistics.* 20 [2] [2019]: 273-286.)

have fallen more over time. The major type of failure incurred here concerns the molecule's "efficacy": It did not work or work safely. There are no hard data on what contributes to these failures. However, experts in translational medicine argue that the quality of the drug candidates advanced from phase I to phase II is quite (too) variable and that biopharma firms are sending too many molecules into phase II that are based on shaky science.[6]

Most of what's placed in human testing by the large biopharmaceutical companies comes from their own laboratories—about 78% of phase I projects, 69% of phase II projects, and 47% of phase III projects.[7] The fact that in-house discoveries as a percentage of products in human testing falls as human testing progresses suggests that companies may be in-licensing later-stage projects to offset the attrition that occurs as in-house discoveries fail—an expensive and inefficient approach to filling out an insufficient pipeline.

Ensuring that in-house discovery operations, which consume 25% of R&D spending, are focused on projects where the company has a reasonable chance of producing a competitive

drug candidate is an obvious start. Improving the quality of drug candidates placed in human testing is perhaps the most important step companies can take toward improving their economic returns to R&D spending. And because even the largest of biopharmaceutical companies generate no more than 2% to 3% of global biomedical innovation, this implies that in addition to optimizing their internal discovery operations, companies should be systematically and aggressively looking outside their own laboratories for drug candidates to place into human testing.

## R&D PIPELINE PRODUCTIVITY

The high failure rate of phase II clinical trials leads naturally to a consideration of the "productivity" of the biopharma R&D pipeline. Figure 21-15 shows the long-term trend in new drug approvals by the FDA from 1975 to 2019. For the most part, it reflects a remarkable, steady-state process. On average, there have been roughly 20 to 30 new drugs approved every year for the past 40 years. If one takes an even

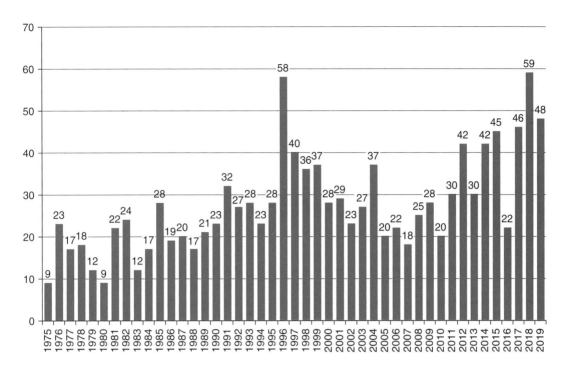

**Figure 21-15** • New Drug Approvals, 1975 to 2019. (Source: US Food and Drug Administration.)

longer time series analysis (say going back to 1950), the chart looks exactly the same.[8] More importantly, since 1950, the productivity of that constant R&D output in the face of rising R&D costs has obviously fallen. This is now known as "eRoom's law" (the reverse spelling and obverse

of "Moore's Law"), which argues that the efficiency of pharma R&D has been cut in half roughly every 9 years (Figure 21-16).

What explains this falling productivity? One set of explanations deals with the science: The low-hanging fruit in drug development—blockbuster

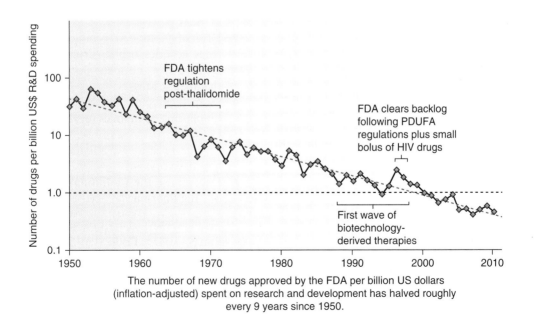

The number of new drugs approved by the FDA per billion US dollars (inflation-adjusted) spent on research and development has halved roughly every 9 years since 1950.

**Figure 21-16** • eRoom's Law. FDA, US Food and Drug Administration; PDUFA, Prescription Drug User Fee Act; R&D, Research and Development. (Source: Scannell et al., Nature Reviews Drug Discovery 11:191, 2012.)

drugs to treat common chronic conditions in the late 1980s and 1990s—has already been picked.[9] This creates 2 problems. First, there has been a "crowding" of biopharma R&D programs in existing drug classes. Second, what remains to be picked to treat unmet patient needs are the less favorable prospects for finding new drugs that are based on more complex science that is not well understood. The emerging areas of genomics and biomarkers are still not well understood, making harvesting discovery based on such technologies more elusive.

A second set of explanations, rooted more in economics, is that the rise of generic drugs since the 1990s, which are not only efficacious but also cheap, has "raised the bar" with downstream customers (patients, employers, insurers) regarding their willingness to pay for expensive new drugs. A third set of explanations rests with the risk aversion of regulators, such as the FDA in the United States and the National Institute for Health and Care Excellence (NICE) in the United Kingdom, that heightened after the Vioxx scandal that surfaced in 2004. Regulators learned that Merck obscured cardiovascular health risks to patients in reporting its clinical trial results. Such events raised the safety hurdles and the cost-effectiveness hurdles that new drugs must meet in order to receive approval for marketing.

A fourth set of explanations lies in supply and demand factors that foster more drugs going into phase II trials. On the supply side, there has been a steady supply of new ideas for drug firms funded by NIH research, with changes over time in both its volume and character. On the demand side has been the rise in national income and insurance coverage for drugs covered in Chapter 16, both of which stimulate and justify biopharma funding of ever-more-costly research. It is hard to disentangle the drivers of this change. The falling productivity observed in biopharma R&D is likely due to a changing marketplace for new drugs that has rewarded higher R&D spending per discovery.

Meanwhile, the "clock is ticking" for biopharma firms in terms of loss of exclusivity (LOE) due to patent expirations (otherwise known as "expiries" or "patent cliffs"). The percentage of industry revenues at risk for expirations grew from 8% (1999-2002) to 16% (2009-2012) and then abated a bit to 8%

(2019-2023). The last figure may not seem high, but it represents roughly $40 billion in sales.

Replacing this lost revenue is often challenging. Biopharma firms have engaged in a multitude of strategies to try to "raise the bar" on their constant level of R&D productivity. Since the late 1980s, the favorite go-to strategy was M&A. Unfortunately, research shows that M&A does not improve R&D productivity or increase R&D expenditures. More generally, large scale has no relationship with R&D intensity (investment) and at best a weak impact on R&D productivity, which are the 2 drivers of firm value. Large scale may, in fact, make it harder to develop new drugs (due to bureaucratic complexity and other factors). Indeed, the large scale of biopharma firms may have likewise rendered big drug companies less efficient.[10]

More recently, biopharma firms have engaged in several additional strategies beyond M&A to improve their R&D output. These include efforts to:

- Develop the research capabilities of small biotechnology firms by shifting emphasis away from small molecules to embrace developments in gene therapy, protein therapy, monoclonal antibodies, peptides, and cell therapy
- Reorganize internally to resemble small biotech firms
- Diversify geographically into emerging markets
- Diversify into new product lines (vaccines, generics, orphan drugs, and so on)
- De-diversify and focus on a handful of therapeutic areas
- Swap therapeutic franchises with other biopharma companies (eg, Novartis and Glaxo)
- Engage in strategic alliances and business development
- Decompose the traditional value chain of "Big Pharma"

Strategic alliances have proven to be more beneficial to R&D productivity than have M&A efforts. This is evident from the 24% decline in early-stage programs being conducted in "Big Pharma" from 2011 to 2017. McKinsey data show that the success of drugs developed "in house" had a 14% success rate in making it from phase I to launch; conversely, drugs in-licensed from other companies as part of business development activity had a much higher success rate of 26%. The same relative advantage appears later during the 2012 to 2014 period: 11% versus 20%.[11] Similar data on the comparative advantage of strategic alliances over in-house development have been presented by academic researchers.[12] Research shows that in-licensed drugs have a much greater likelihood of moving from phase I to launch. This means a growing deemphasis on in-house R&D (both the number of programs and their size) and increasing time spent on monitoring external research, such as that taking place in academia and other research institutes.

Another possible remedy is to reverse the long tradition of fully integrated pharmaceutical companies (FIPCOs), concentrate on specific stages in the value chain of drug development and commercialization, and outsource activities of lesser value. For example, outsourcing of biopharma manufacturing to "contract manufacturing organizations" (CMOs) would allow for fuller asset utilization since facility owners could aggregate demand from more than one biopharma company into any given plant. Similarly, outsourcing of sales activities to "contract sales organizations" (CSOs) could reduce head counts in their field forces. Finally, outsourcing R&D to biotech firms that serve as "contract research organizations" (CROs) could allow Big Pharma to focus on what they excel at—the commercialization of products.

Finally, there are signs that the R&D productivity stasis depicted in Figure 21-15 may be improving. Some suggest that, since 2010, the downward trajectory in "eRoom's Law" has been arrested and has slightly improved (addressed more fully in Chapter 22)[13]; others suggest that the downward slide has continued.[14] Nevertheless, one needs to curb their enthusiasm and exuberance here, since the timelines (number of years) for both discovery and development have barely changed over the past 2 decades: The duration for discovery (from screening to development candidate) is still 4 years, while the duration for development (from preclinical to approval) is still 10 years (and maybe even more). Moreover, the phase II failure rates still remain high, around 85% (2012-2017), suggesting that failure may remain an inescapable feature of biopharma R&D.[15]

> ### Critical Thinking Exercise: Merck's Acquisition of Schering-Plough
>
> A Harvard Business School case chronicles Merck's acquisition of Schering-Plough in 2008 for $41 billion.[16] Some Merck officials justify the merger based on the rationales espoused in the case (eg, scale economies, diversification, deal with imminent patent expiries, annex Schering's "formidable R&D pipeline"). Others justify it by the eventual discovery of Merck's current blockbuster drug, Keytruda, which came with the Schering-Plough deal. What do you think of these rationales? What else could Merck have done with the $41 billion?

## COMMERCIALIZATION

### Registration and FDA Approval

Prior to marketing and product launch, the biopharma firm requires regulatory approval that the product is safe and effective for its intended use (a decision that almost never considers economic factors); this is known as "market authorization." The key stakeholders here are the FDA in the United States and the European Medicines Agency (EMA) in the European Union. The biopharma firm submits an NDA that provides all the relevant data and information collected during R&D. Much of the information is contained in the packaging insert that comes with each drug prescription (in very small print). The NDA must provide sufficient data to determine (1) the drug's safety and efficacy, (2) an acceptable risk-benefit profile, and (3) adequate manufacturing methods and controls to preserve identity, strength, and purity of the product. There are 3 types of NDAs[17]:

1. 505(b)(1) (NDA)
   - Used for an NCE.
   - Contains full reports of investigations of safety and effectiveness.
2. 505(b)(2) (abbreviated NDA [ANDA])
   - Used for a combination of 2 approved products, new use for an approved active pharmaceutical ingredient (API), new dosage form, or new route of administration.

- Contains full reports of investigations of safety and effectiveness but where at least some of the information required for approval comes from studies not conducted by or for the applicant and for which the applicant has not obtained a right of reference. These include:
  - Published literature
  - FDA's previous findings of safety and efficacy (ie, an approved product)
3. 505(j) (Generic)
   - Used for a generic product.
   - Contains information to show that the proposed product is identical in active ingredient, dosage form, strength, route of administration, labeling, quality, performance characteristics, and intended use, among other things, to a previously approved product.

The FDA has developed 4 distinct approaches to speed the availability of drugs intended to treat serious diseases and/or address unmet medical needs. These include the following:

- Fast track—to fulfill an unmet need
- Breakthrough therapy—significant improvement over current therapy
- Accelerated approval—use of surrogate endpoints (eg, laboratory measurements) or intermediate endpoints likely to predict a clinical benefit; confirmatory trials required
- Priority review—6 months (vs 10-12 months) with same requirements for approval

## Market Access

After regulatory approval, the biopharma firm needs to make pricing and market access decisions. These include (1) country-specific clinical and economic evaluations; (2) coverage, funding, reimbursement decisions, and price negotiations with payers; and (3) local purchase decisions (eg, gain access to pharmacy benefit manager [PBM] and hospital formularies). The key stakeholders here are public and private payers (insurers). When payers determine whether or not to cover a product, decisions are driven by both clinical and economic factors. These include the product's TPP but also budgetary considerations, cost-effectiveness analyses, and the clinical and economic benefit relative to comparator therapies.

To obtain market access, manufacturers generally have to consider a trade-off between price, volume, and time. A low list price or high rebates/discounts will generally increase payers' willingness to cover the product. Payers can place restrictions on the product beyond the regulatory label to reduce the number of patients eligible for the product. Some payers will use time as a negotiation tool to slow the manufacturer's time to market (and thereby lower the associated costs for the payer). For drugs that go to the retail channel, PBMs and insurers are the major stakeholders; for drugs that go to the institutional channel, the hospital pharmacy and therapeutics committee and the hospital's group purchasing organization are the major stakeholders. In other countries, the stakeholder is often a national regulatory authority such as NICE in the United Kingdom.

In recent years, pharma firms have entered into their own version of value-based contracts (VBCs) or "risk-sharing agreements" with public payers and private insurers to gain market access. The "value" can be defined in both financial and clinical terms. Financial terms can include capitated agreements whereby the insurer pays only so much per patient per month (PMPM), the insurer pays for only a certain number of scripts per month, the insurer pays nothing or a discounted price if the patient stops taking the medication, or the insurer's total cost liability is capped. Clinical terms can include the patient's adherence and persistence with the prescribed medication, the percentage of the insurer's patients reaching a target level (eg, blood pressure levels), the lack of patient response to the medication, or the occurrence of adverse events.

## Sales and Marketing

Finally, the firm needs to target potential physician prescribers, position the drug in the physician's current treatment paradigm, and influence patient utilization decisions. Drugs are no longer sold and marketed primarily through large, in-house sales forces. Between 2005 and 2016, the size of pharma's sales force shrunk from 101,000 to about 71,000 representatives. Much of this shrinkage was driven by patent expiry of blockbuster drugs (eg, statins) developed during the 1990s that were marketed to primary care physicians treating large patient populations with chronic disease. After such drugs went generic, they did not require such heavy sales support.

Another driver shrinking the sales force has been the rise of specialty care drugs that have supplanted the primary care drugs. Such specialty drugs required pharma to find a new business model. Unlike high cholesterol and its treatment with statins, cancer was not a single disease with a massive patient population treated by primary care physicians that could be blanketed by thousands of sales reps. Rather, cancer included thousands of rare diseases, all under the umbrella of oncology, but perhaps treated by different specialties.[18] Each of these diseases had smaller patient pools and smaller populations of prescribing physicians. Moreover, there was much less crowding of drugs in these specialty therapeutic categories (see Chapter 22). Instead, there was often just one drug available to treat a certain patient population, which put sales reps in a very different position. Reps now served as account managers, providing the service of liaison between physicians and companies, with responsibility for demonstrating new modes of administration and explaining reimbursement.

Smaller patient markets also meant that physicians and patients occupied a different place when the sales rep entered the picture. Physicians now needed help to identify which patients should be screened for rare diseases or might be eligible for a certain drug; patients sometimes needed help paying for these expensive drugs with coupons available from the manufacturer.

The size of the pharma sales force also shrank due to reduced market access to physicians. Part of the reduced market access was driven by the development of drug formularies on the part of managed care organizations and the PBMs they contracted with (see Chapter 16). Part of the reduced access was driven by providers themselves. In an effort to curb sales reps' influence over doctors' prescribing habits, many hospitals and physician networks limited their access to physicians. A report in *JAMA* showed that reducing "detailing" (ie, the time that reps spent with physicians) reduced the prescribing of drugs promoted by the reps, while increasing the prescribing of the nondetailed drugs. The number of physicians deemed "accessible" fell to 44%, down from 80% in 2008.[19] Not only did reps get to see fewer physicians and see them less frequently, but when they did see them, they got less time with them—down from 6 minutes in 2012 to 3 minutes by 2016.

Even though doctors spend less time with sales reps, they are still interested in the information the reps present. Many doctors now elect to get the information through different media or ways that accommodate their very busy schedule. Doctors spend an average of 84 hours a year reading digital marketing material. According to Accenture,[20] 1 in 4 sales force interactions have been replaced by digital interactions. Sales reps complement the digital approach, using iPads to answer doctors' questions about drugs or show research. They also use video chats after typical business hours to engage with physicians during convenient times.

With regard to marketing, the FDA restricts what pharma firms can tell physicians about which indications their drug is authorized for. Every prescription drug marketed in the United States carries an individual, FDA-approved label. This label ("the insert") is a written report that provides detailed instructions regarding the approved uses and doses, which are based on the results of clinical studies that the drug maker submitted to the FDA. Physicians are free, however, to prescribe a drug "off label" for other indications they think are suitable. This practice is legal and common: 1 in 5 prescriptions written today are for off-label use.

Marketing efforts involve patients as well as physicians. In 2016, medical marketing to physicians comprised $20.3 billion, nearly 68% of total marketing spend. Medical marketing included an additional $9.6 billion (32%) spent on direct-to-consumer (DTC) advertising, mostly on prescription drugs but also on disease awareness, health services, and laboratory (e.g., genetic) tests. DTC advertising is legal in only two countries—the US and New Zealand. Such advertising has been legal in the US since 1985, but accelerated after 1997 when the FDA eased up on a rule obliging companies to offer a detailed list of side-effects in their long format television commercials. What is notable here is that, between 1997-2016, the greatest increase in marketing spend was on DTC ($7.5 billion, a 357% rise) compared to an increase of only $4.7 billion (30% rise) on physician marketing. Such increased DTC marketing is associated with an increase in patient requests, prescription volumes, patient visits, and higher costs.[21]

Marketing activities also include lobbying and campaign contributions. Such activities are often designed to counter proposed regulations and governmental efforts to control drug spending. Between 1999 and 2018, compared to all industrial sectors, the pharmaceutical and health product sector accounted for the single largest share (7.3%) of spend on lobbying Congress and federal agencies. Biopharmaceutical companies or their trade associations comprised 17 of the top 20 biggest spenders in such lobbying; they also comprised 15 of the top 20 contributors to presidential and congressional campaigns. Twice as much money was spent by the sector on elections at the state level ($877 million vs $414 million), usually to blunt cost containment measures.[22]

## GENERIC DRUG COMPANIES

There is a major imbalance between branded drugs that are still on patent and generic drugs (branded drugs that have lost their patent protection). The United States had a total prescription volume in 2017 of 4.5 billion "scripts," worth a total of $475 billion in sales. Branded drugs account for just 10% of prescriptions in the United States but 76% of the revenues; generics account for 90% of prescriptions but only 24% of revenues.

Generic drugs provide a major benefit to consumers. A generic is the same as the branded drug in terms of its strength, dosage form, route of administration, quality, active ingredient, and therapeutic effect. It also resembles the brand drug in terms of chemistry, manufacturing, controls, labeling, and testing. Once a

product's patent protection lapses, any specialty chemical producer is able to make the product with access to all the published patent data and the know-how that have been created. Minimal clinical work past the establishment of bioequivalence is required in order to register and sell a generic product. And as multiple generic companies enter the market, prices may eventually drop to 10% to 15% over the cost of manufacture. Generic products represent a delayed, but major benefit for consumers in the technology for advancing healthcare at affordable pricing. Without the initial patented innovation, this would never be possible.

All of this was made possible by the 1984 Hatch-Waxman Amendments to the Federal Food Drug and Cosmetic Act. Generic drugs no longer needed to prove their safety and efficacy. Under the bill, generic drug manufacturers needed only to submit an ANDA to prove their product's bioequivalence to the original branded drug. This was a cheaper process for generic drug manufacturers, as the cost of conducting clinical and nonclinical studies or risking liability for patent infringement damages was no longer part of the equation. Manufacturers filing ANDAs could only do so (1) for drugs that had not been patented or (2) when a branded drug's patent had expired. Because branded drugs lose so much of their revenue when generic drugs are introduced, the act provided them with patent extension options, which now average about 3 years.

There has been a steady increase in the number of ANDAs (Figure 21-17). This has led to increased competition among generic firms and their products and lower and lower

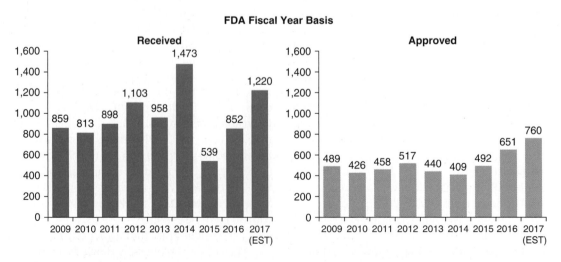

**Figure 21-17 •** Trend in Abbreviated New Drug Application Approvals. FDA, US Food and Drug Administration. (Source: GDUFA Approvals, May 2017.)

generic drug prices. The generic drug manufacturer market is fragmented, with lots of players having small market shares. Among the market leaders are Teva, Mylan, and Sandoz. The top 10 competitors combined control a stable share of 60% of prescriptions; the top 5 competitors' shares have continued to decline with more competitors (200+) and more new products.

Unlike brand companies that depend on the discovery and commercialization of new molecules and biologics, generic drug companies must successfully challenge patents and file for approval for generic versions of branded products. This represents the generic drug company's pipeline. First-to-file ANDAs or patent challenges are of particular importance in the US market because the filer is granted 180 days of exclusivity. During this period, the FDA is statutorily precluded from approving other applications, thereby ensuring some price stability.

## DRUG PRODUCT MANUFACTURING

There are 2 major phases in manufacturing a drug: drug substance manufacturing and drug product manufacturing. The former includes manufacturing the API in bulk through a series of chemical or biological reactions. In this phase, the operation is typically technology driven. Different companies take quite different approaches. Some companies outsource almost their entire drug substance operation to take advantage of avoiding capital investment and keep a lean workforce; however, this approach can adversely impact cost of goods sold, overall profit margins (there are tax benefits linked to drug substance operations), and API availability. API availability garnered little notice until the COVID-19 crisis in the spring of 2020. It came to the public's attention that the supply chain for these base ingredients stretched back into China, were difficult to obtain from China, were not made in the United States, and were essential for the drug treatments required to deal with the virus. Other firms engage in internal manufacturing operations only to the last few steps of bulk drug synthesis in order to capture the tax benefit.

Drug product manufacturing encompasses the further processing of the drug product at form/fill/finish (F/F/F) sites. For tablets, excipients such as starches and lactose are added to the bulk chemical and coated, compressed, and dispensed in pills, which will be subsequently packaged in bottles (the most common form in the United States) or blisters (each tablet individually sealed) for world markets. Excipients help to process APIs more efficiently (through lubrication, manageable sizes, and so on) and also can enhance the drugs' pharmacokinetics—particularly for absorption and distribution. In the F/F/F phase of the operation, complexity rather than technology is the major concern (eg, when a single product is made in 3 different strengths and supplied to 100 countries with different packages).

Manufacturing is governed by the FDA's enforcement of current GMPs (cGMPs) on drug manufacturing and testing. These standards are designed to provide patients with a product that has equivalent identity, safety, strength, quality, and purity to the one used to establish the clinical database. The FDA establishes cGMPs through regulations and guidance. It is the pharmaceutical companies' responsibility to set up and maintain quality systems to assure product quality.

## RISING DRUG PRICES

Rising drug prices have been a hot issue in recent years. Turing Pharmaceuticals, under its notorious CEO, Martin Shkreli (a former hedge manager), bought the US manufacturer of Daraprim—a drug developed in the 1960s to treat toxoplasmosis—in 2015. Shkreli immediately raised the price of this generic medicine from $13.50 per pill to $750 per pill, an increase of over 5,000%. This brought the annual cost of treatment for some patients to hundreds of thousands of dollars. Shkreli was not alone. Heather Bresch, CEO of Mylan Pharmaceuticals, purchased the marketing rights to the EpiPen (used to prevent anaphylactic shock in children) in 2007 and then proceeded, over the next 9 years, to raise its price by 461% from $100 to $600. Zaltrap was approved in 2012 for the treatment of metastatic colorectal cancer. Its initial price tag of $11,000 per month was seen as too high by oncologists, given that the drug improved survival time by just 1.4 months. This led Memorial Sloan Kettering Cancer Center to ban prescribing of the drug.

Some new product launches come with some astronomical prices. Kymriah (to treat acute lymphoblastic leukemia) cost $475,000; Luxturna (to treat retinal dystrophy due to biallelic RPE65 mutation) cost $850,000; and

Soliris (to treat paroxysmal nocturnal hemoglobinuria) cost $440,000.

Pricing is a complex issue due to (1) differences across countries in their willingness to pay (WTP) the high prices charged by pharma firms and (2) differences across countries in their national incomes (wealth), which likely drive their WTP. In most major developed markets, healthcare costs are heavily borne by the public sector. They can nevertheless vary in terms of who the key stakeholders are (national vs regional vs local governments, public employers, social insurance funds) and the mechanisms they use to decide whether or not to cover a drug (eg, cost-utility/effectiveness analysis, budget impact assessment, or clinical value assessment). Outside the United States, manufacturers are not free to set the price of a drug in many public systems; in such cases, pricing may be dictated by health technology assessments (HTAs), price negotiations with manufacturers, and international reference pricing.

An understanding of the producer sectors is needed to interpret charges historically and currently laid against them. Pharmaceutical companies are often (and increasingly) viewed as charging high prices for their products and earning unseemly high levels of return.

Figure 21-9 shows that prices for branded drugs doubled between 2008 and 2016, rising faster than the consumer price index. This issue now dominates US policy discussions and congressional hearings as this book is prepared.

Why do drug prices continue to rise over time? The previous discussion hints at some answers, but the real story is much more complex and multifactorial (Figure 21-18).[23] The industry's critics focus on distribution chain intermediaries such as the PBMs (see Chapter 16) and the lack of aligned incentives among these parties. Any explanation must discern differences between specialty drugs versus branded drugs, between branded drugs versus generic drugs, between new product introductions versus existing drug price inflation, and between the actions of drug manufacturers versus their pharmaceutical distribution channel partners. Several conclusions can be reached. First, not only have drug costs risen faster than inflation, but they have also risen faster for specialty drugs. Second, rising costs of branded drugs were driven more by price inflation of existing products than by entry of new innovative products. Third, rising costs of specialty drugs were driven more by new product entry than by inflation of existing prices.[23]

| | |
|---|---|
| High launch prices and high annual price increases for branded drugs | Slow development of biosimilar drugs |
| High launch prices and increases for orphan drugs | Anticompetitive practices by some manufacturers (eg, pay-for-delay, product hopping) |
| Lack of competition and natural monopolies for drugs | Manufacturers use current patent protection to extend monopoly pricing |
| Lack of robust competition among generic firms until recently | Insurance that makes patients price-insensitive |
| Structure of cost sharing:<br>  1. High copays may reduce utilization<br>  2. High copays do not control prices<br>  3. Coupons induce use of high-cost drugs | Coinsurance that steepens the slope of demand curve → higher price charged |
| | US payers focus on demand side controls (not supply side) |
| PPACA stipulation that all plans must have stop-loss limit geared to person's income → if patient expects to hit the limit, price is irrelevant | Medicare's loose annual budget |
| Exchange plans cannot cap spending on "covered benefits" or control price | Greater prevalence of discounts for PCP-prescribed drugs that makes physicians more willing to switch and promotes substitutability |
| Medicare ACOs focus on Parts A and B (not Part D) | Lower prevalence of discounts for specialist-prescribed drugs for chronic illness that makes physicians reluctant to switch |
| Lack of comparative effectiveness information | |
| Complexity of pharma distribution channel | |

**Figure 21-18 •** Causes of Rising Drug Prices. ACO, Accountable Care Organization; PCP, Primary Care Physician; PPACA, Patient Protection and Affordable Care Act.

| **Critical Thinking Exercise: Consumer Relief From Rising Drug Prices** |
|---|

On July 24, 2020, President Trump signed 4 executive orders relating to drug pricing that direct the secretary of the Department of Health and Human Services (DHHS) to take several steps. Some of these steps include the following:

- End "the system of kickbacks by middlemen" (eg, the PBM rebates covered in Chapter 16) that lies behind the high out-of-pocket costs many Americans face at the pharmacy counter. Under this action, American seniors would directly receive these kickbacks as discounts in Medicare Part D. In 2018, these Part D discounts totaled more than $30 billion, representing an average discount of 26% to 30%.
- Require federally qualified health centers (FQHCs, see Chapter 13) who purchase insulins and epinephrine in the 340B program to pass the savings from discounted drug prices directly on to medically underserved patients. This would increase access to life-saving drugs for the patients who face especially high costs among the 28 million patients who visit FQHCs every year, over 6 million of whom are uninsured.
- Finalize a rule allowing states to develop safe importation plans for certain prescription drugs. Also, authorize the reimportation of insulin products made in the United States if the DHHS secretary finds reimportation is required for emergency medical care pursuant to section 801(d) of the Food, Drug, and Cosmetic Act.
- Create a pathway for safe personal importation through the use of individual waivers

to purchase drugs at lower cost from preauthorized US pharmacies.

- Take action to ensure that the Medicare program and seniors pay no more for the most costly Medicare Part B drugs than any economically comparable Organisation of Economic Co-operation and Development (OECD) country, ending foreign countries' "free-loading" off the backs of American taxpayers and pharmaceutical investments.

However, Wilkinson and colleagues state that "Although these executive orders could be viewed as far-reaching proposals that may attract attention during this presidential election year, they have no immediate legal effect. The executive orders direct Alex Azar, the Secretary of the U.S. Department of Health & Human Services ('HHS'), to implement the four policies through federal rulemaking procedures; however, these executive orders do not address some of the underlying barriers that hindered progress on similar proposals."[25]

At the time of this text going to press, the pharmaceutical sector was considering 2 drug pricing policies to replace President Trump's plan. Its alternative included (1) discounts for high-cost drugs injected in physicians' offices with patient copays set at that amount, and (2) a 5% cap on what Medicare Part D patients would pay for pharmacy-administered drugs. How much financial relief will these steps provide US consumers? How big of an impact on the US national health expenditures will this likely have?

## SUMMARY

The overriding business model that defines the pharmaceutical sector is the interplay of high risk, long timelines for development, and the financial returns required to motivate stakeholders to invest. It is quite typical for a pharma's bench-to-bed program to span at least a dozen years before the first sale is earned. In addition to a time to sales of 11 to 17 years, the chance of

having a registered product is roughly 2 out of 100 projects that are conceived. This translates to an R&D model where the fully loaded cost of "dry wells" (projects that die) is greater than the cost of "wet wells." Of the roughly $2.6 billion in R&D spend to bring a drug to market, two-thirds of the cost may be attributable to dry-well efforts that have to be funded by the successful few. After accounting for dry wells, the second largest expense is the cost of capital over this long timeline; only then does the actual cost of the "wet-well" program push on the economics of the pharmaceutical business.

The innovation business model is fundamentally a race on a treadmill. It requires companies to invest in discovery and development of innovations that matter to physicians and patients by providing benefit greater than status quo treatments. There are strong rewards to being first and to being "best in class," with very mediocre rewards to anything else. Innovation is not judged by the amount of new science or the number of Nobel laureates whose path-breaking work is harnessed. Rather it is judged by what the innovation does for patients relative to what they had before.

### QUESTIONS TO PONDER

1. Several novel drugs have entered the market with sky-high price tags. And yet, the percentage of national health expenditures spent on retail drugs and the level of out-of-pocket spend on those drugs have remained quite stable. How do you reconcile these 2 factual observations?
2. The "twin towers" of drug innovation encompasses the discovery of a new drug and then its commercialization. Which of these 2 factors do you think is more important? Why?
3. Many critics of the pharmaceutical sector lay the blame for high drug prices and spending at the feet of patent protection, which awards market exclusivity to the innovator drug. Advocates for the pharma sector counter by arguing their companies will not invest in drug development without the promise (and reward) of patent protection. Do you see any resolution to these opposing views?
4. What might explain the stability (or stagnancy) in R&D productivity over so many decades?
5. Of the various, alternative strategies to try to improve R&D productivity, which one(s) do you think is or are most promising?
6. Why has "market access" become such a major issue and problem for pharma?

## REFERENCES

1. Deloitte.com. "How Biopharmaceutical Collaborations Are Fueling Biomedical Innovation." Available online: https://www2.deloitte.com/us/en/pages/life-sciences-and-health-care/articles/how-biopharma-collaborations-are-fueling-biomedical-innovation.html. Accessed on April 21, 2020.
2. Richard Evans and Scott Hinds. "The Pharmaceutical Sector," in Lawton R. Burns (Ed.), *The Business of Healthcare Innovation*, 3rd ed. (Cambridge, United Kingdom: Cambridge University Press, 2020): Chapter 2.
3. Olivier Wouters, Martin McKee, and Jeroen Luyten. "Estimated Research and Development Investment Needed to Bring a New Medicine to Market, 2009-2018," *JAMA.* 323 (9) (2020): 844-853.
4. This section summarizes a section from the following source: Jonathan Northurp, Marina Tarasova, and Lee Kalowski. "The Pharmaceutical Sector: Rebooted and Reinvigorated," in Lawton R. Burns (Ed.), *The Business of Healthcare Innovation,* 2nd ed. (Cambridge, UK: Cambridge University Press, 2012): Chapter 2.
5. NCEs are small molecules that do not have active ingredients that typically bind to a target and cause a biological process to stop or start; NMEs are large-molecule, biological products that have active ingredients. For this declaration, the biopharma must be able to answer the following questions: Can we make it? Can we evaluate it? Is there a market for it? And can we patent it? These answers are developed by a multidisciplinary team that includes not only scientists but also marketing staff, patent attorneys, business leaders, experts in biomarkers, and clinicians.
6. Garret Fitzgerald, personal communication.
7. Richard Evans and Scott Hinds. "The Pharmaceutical Sector," in Lawton R. Burns (Ed.), *The Business of Healthcare Innovation,* 3rd ed. (Cambridge, United Kingdom: Cambridge University Press, 2020): Chapter 2.
8. Bernard Munos. "Lessons From 60 Years of Pharmaceutical Innovation," *Nat Rev Drug Discov.* 8 (December 2009): 959-968. Available online: https://www.nature.com/articles/nrd2961. Accessed on August 10, 2020.
9. Jack Scannell, Alex Blanckley, Helen Boldon, et al. "Diagnosing the Decline in Pharmaceutical R&D Efficiency," *Nat Rev Drug Discov.* 11 (3) (2012): 191-200.
10. Lawton R. Burns, Sean Nicholson, and Joanna Wolkowski. "Pharmaceutical Strategy and the Evolving Role of Mergers and Acquisitions (M&A)," in Lawton R. Burns (Ed.), *The Business of Healthcare Innovation*, 2nd ed. (Cambridge,

United Kingdom: Cambridge University Press, 2012): Chapter 3.

11. McKinsey Quarterly. "Improving the Pharma Research Pipeline," 2004 (#4) and June 2016.

12. Patricia Danzon, Sean Nicholson, and Nuno Pereira. "Productivity in Pharmaceutical Biotechnology R&D: The Role of Experience and Alliances," *J Health Econ.* 24 (2) (March 2005): 317-339.

13. Jason Rhodes. "Presentation to the Vagelos Life Sciences and Management Program (LSMP)," Wharton School (November 2019).

14. Richard Evans and Scott Hinds. "The Pharmaceutical Sector," in Lawton R. Burns (Ed.), *The Business of Healthcare Innovation,* 3rd ed. (Cambridge, United Kingdom: Cambridge University Press, 2020): Chapter 2.

15. Jason Rhodes. "Presentation to the Vagelos Life Sciences and Management Program (LSMP)," Wharton School (November 2019).

16. Frank Rothaermal and Michael McKay. *Merck and Co. Inc.* HBS Case # MH0035 (Revised January 2, 2015) (Boston, MA: Harvard Business School, 2015).

17. These NDA descriptions are courtesy of Monica Ferrante. "Presentation to the Vagelos Life Sciences and Management Program (LSMP)," Wharton School (October 2019).

18. Lisa LaMotta. "5 Trends Shaping the Pharma Sales Force," *BioPharma Dive* (September 18, 2017). Available online: https://www.biopharmadive.com/news/spotlight-trends-pharma-sales-force-digital-marketing/504949/. Accessed on April 20, 2020.

19. ZS Associates. *Want Better Access to Physicians? Understand What's Top of Mind.* 2016 Access-Monitor report. Available online: http://mmedical.com/docs/default-source/footnotes-references/zs-want-better-access-to-physicians-nderstand-what%27s-top-of-mind.pdf. Accessed on August 11, 2020.

20. Accenture. *The Rebirth of the Pharmaceutical Sales Force.* (2015). Available online: https://www.accenture.com/t20161128T001132Z__w__/us-en/_acnmedia/Accenture/Conversion-Assets/DotCom/Documents/Global/PDF/Dualpub_13/Accenture-Rebirth-Pharmaceutical-Salesforce.pdf. Accessed on August 11, 2020.

21. Lisa Schwartz and Steven Woloshin. "Medical Marketing in the United States, 1997-2016," *Journal of American Medical Association* 321 (1) (2019):80-96.

22. Olivier Wouters. "Lobbying Expenditures and Campaign Contributions by the Pharmaceutical and Health Product Industry in the United States, 1999-2018," *JAMA Int Med.* 180 (5) (2020): 688-697.

23. Henry Waxman, Bill Corr, Kristi Martin, and Sophia Duong. *Getting to the Root of High Prescription Drug Prices: Drivers and Potential Solutions.* The Commonwealth Fund (July 10, 2017). Available online: https://www.commonwealthfund.org/publications/fund-reports/2017/jul/getting-root-high-prescription-drug-prices-drivers-and-potential. Accessed on August 10, 2020.

24. Immaculada Hernandez, Chester Good, David Cutler, et al. "The Contribution of New Product Entry Versus Existing Product Inflation in the Rising Costs of Drugs," *Health Aff.* 38 (1) (2019): 76-83.

25. Constance A. Wilkinson, Alan J. Arville, John S. Linehan, Jennifer E. Michael, Christopher R. Smith, Alexis Boaz. "President Trump Signs Executive Orders on Drug Pricing and Domestic Supply Chain Reform." Available online: https://www.ebglaw.com/news/president-trump-signs-executive-orders-on-drug-pricing-and-domestic-supply-chain-reform/. Accessed on December 14, 2020.

# The Biotechnology Sector

22

## THE GROWING ROLE OF BIOLOGICS AND BIOTECHNOLOGY

### Biological Products

Section 351 of the Public Health Service (PHS) Act defines a biological product as a "virus, therapeutic serum, toxin, antitoxin, vaccine, blood, blood component or derivative, allergenic product, or analogous product, applicable to the prevention, treatment, or cure of a disease or condition of human beings." Some examples of biologics include vaccine immunoglobulin products (antibodies), products containing cells or microorganisms, most protein products, gene/cell/tissue therapy products (including viruses), in vivo diagnostic allergenic products, and tests to screen potential blood donors for infectious agents (eg, HIV). Some specific, well-known illustrations are Herceptin for breast cancer, Enbrel for rheumatoid arthritis, and Botox for both dermatologic and neurologic use.

The pharmaceutical and biotechnology sectors undertake many of the same research and development (R&D) processes.[1] However, the 2 sectors differ markedly in their scientific foundation (chemistry vs biology), historical origins (19th vs 20th centuries), financing (internal vs external), and profitability (Figure 22-1). The biotech sector originated with the founding of Genentech in 1976 by university scientists working with a venture capitalist. Scientists genetically engineered colonies of *Escherichia coli* bacteria, making them express a foreign gene that let them resist an antibiotic. To achieve this, the researchers used a process called recombination. They used proteins ("restriction enzymes") to cut bacterial DNA; the enzymes left uneven cuts on the molecule ends called "sticky ends" where foreign DNA could be inserted; the bacteria could then start expressing the new DNA as if it were its own. This new technology revolutionized the production of biological molecules: Instead of inefficient traditional methods such as deriving them from animals, they could be mass produced more inexpensively in fermentation vats of microbes.

This discovery paved the way for the field of genetic engineering. Five years after its founding, there were an additional 155 biotech start-ups, founded by entrepreneurs with venture capital (VC) financing of their university research programs. In contrast to Big Pharma, which has witnessed no significant new industry entrants over time, biotech is characterized by high entry and exit rates. Figure 22-2 depicts the increase in the number of biotech companies.[2] Today, there are over 2,500 firms.

There is another important contrast between pharmaceutical and biotechnology companies. A pharmaceutical company is a drug development company that makes money; a biotechnology company is a drug development company that loses money initially and maybe for a long time. Substantial financing is required to successfully execute any business model in biotechnology because of the large amount of capital and time required for a relatively high-risk chance at building a successful company and obtaining a financial return. The need for

| Pharmaceuticals | Biotechnology |
|---|---|
| • Founded in 1800s | • Founded in 1976 |
| • Large industrial enterprises | • Entrepreneurial start-ups |
| • Historically relied on in-house R&D efforts | • Often linked to university research programs |
| • Vertically integrated: research and commercialization | • Focus on discovery primarily with little development |
| • Blockbuster products | • Niche products, orphan drugs |
| • Internal capital financing | • External capital financing PE/VC |
| • No new firm creation | • Lots of firm creation |
| • Few firm failures | • Lots of failures |
| • High threat of generic competition | • Low threat of generic competition |

**Figure 22-1** • Pharmaceuticals Versus Biotechnology. PE, Private Equity; R&D, Research and Development; VC, Venture Capital.

capital is incessant. In 2017, about 30% of biotechnology companies had less than 12 months of cash on hand, and on average, all but the large-cap public biotechnology companies (at least $5 billion market cap) posted net annual losses (Figure 22-3).[3]

This distinction between pharma and biotech success is now breaking down. The biotechnology side of biopharma has been outperforming the pharma side for much of the past decade (Figure 22-4) due to their discovery of orphan drugs that carry high prices (see later discussion). The larger, established biotech firms are now quite profitable; the remainder are still struggling. Still, overall, it takes the top 500 biotech companies to parallel the stature of the top 5 pharma companies (Figure 22-5).

## Biotech Sector Maturation

The biotechnology portion of biopharma is enjoying its "heyday." The sector now features multiple technology-based modalities that support rapid, low-cost commercialization; it enjoys high demand but limited supply of VC-backed startups; it is supported by a stable community of financiers (venture capitalists); it is a maturing sector that now contributes significantly to the market for initial public offerings (IPOs); it is increasingly engaged in creative partnerships and deals with Big Pharma; it enjoys a strong talent flow of R&D personnel; it has had an enormous impact on human health across many diseases; and it is a sector that many US cities and other countries wish to cultivate.

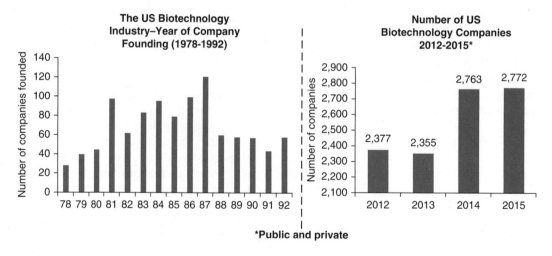

**Figure 22-2** • Historical Formation of Biotechnology Companies. (Source: Figure 3.3, in Lawton R. Burns [Ed.], *The Business of Healthcare Innovation*, 3rd ed. Cambridge, United Kingdom: Cambridge University Press; 2020.)

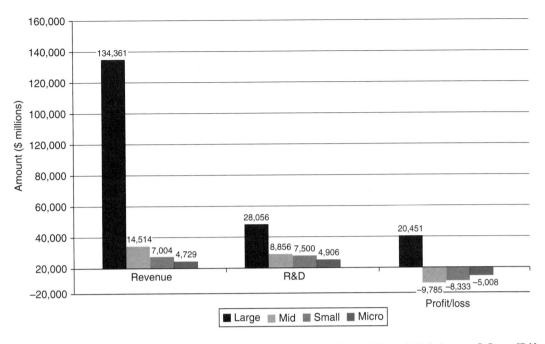

**Figure 22-3** • Public Biotechnology Company Financial Status 2017. (Source: Figure 3.29, in Lawton R. Burns [Ed.], *The Business of Healthcare Innovation*, 3rd ed. Cambridge, United Kingdom: Cambridge University Press; 2020.)

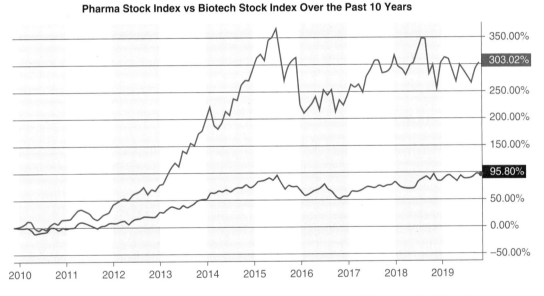

**Figure 22-4** • Pharma Versus Biotech Stock Performance. (Source: Yahoo! Finance; Eric Schmidt, Presentation to the Wharton School, 2019.)

| | US Biotech (~500 public companies) | US Pharma (Top 5 companies) |
|---|---|---|
| Market Value (billion) | ~$900 | ~$800 |
| Revenues (billion) | $150 | $175 |
| R&D Investment (billion) | $46 | $25 |
| Net Income (billion) | $8 | $45 |
| Marketed Products | ~100 | ~200 |
| Products in Development | 750+ | 245 |

**Figure 22-5** • Snapshot Comparison of US Biotech and Pharma Sectors. R&D, Research and Development. (Source: Ernst & Young, Cowen & Company; Eric Schmidt, Presentation to the Wharton School, 2019.)

## INSIDE BIOTECH

### Boost to R&D

The promise and performance of biotech is to translate and "productize" early-stage science into real research programs at a faster speed, lower cost, and a greater rate of success than has historically been the case. Why might this be happening? One possible explanation is innovation in the technological base that underlies biopharma's R&D model. Under the traditional R&D model based on chemistry that focused on small molecules (new chemical entities [NCEs]), the following success rates were observed: For every 1 million compounds that were screened, 10,000 compounds were made, 1,000 were tested in cells, 100 were tested in vivo, 10 were taken into preclinical development, and only 1 was taken into clinical trials (see Figure 21-13).

Evidence suggests the odds have improved with more biology-based research modalities being thrown at the R&D pipeline than in prior decades. These modalities are sometimes referred to as research "platforms." The 1970s and 1980s marked the revolution in recombinant DNA and protein biologics (at biotech firms such as Genentech, Amgen, Biogen, and Genzyme). From there, biotech evolved from making simple secreted proteins (insulin) to more complex products (antibodies). While in the early 2000s antibodies were not really established, today their total sales are enormous. Humira, AbbVie's anti-inflammatory drug for arthritis, is the number one seller (see Figure 21-4). More recently, other modalities, such as antisense molecules (short, synthetic nucleic acids whose sequence complements the gene of a disease-causing gene thus altering its expression); RNA interference (RNAi; whereby RNA molecules inhibit gene expression by catalytic destruction of targeted mRNA molecules); and messenger RNA (mRNA) (longer nucleic acid polymers that code for protein of desired expression), have come to the fore, joined by cell therapy and gene therapy. Some of these technologies are briefly described in the following list[4]:

- **Monoclonal antibodies (mAbs):** mAbs are the basis of many approved biotechnology drugs. Antibodies are a key component of the immune system capable of binding proteins and molecules with unique specificity, thereby blocking specific molecular interactions. Cells that produce mAbs are special in that they produce identical antibodies that all bind to the same specific part of a protein termed an "antigen." This highly specific binding is valuable therapeutically to block naturally occurring molecular interactions that cause a disease or unwanted symptom. Most chemically synthesized pharmaceuticals act similarly to block specific molecular interactions, but mAbs have certain advantages: (1) They can be more specific and bind their target more tightly, (2) they may have lower risk of toxicity, and (3) they can be used to block interactions that cannot be blocked with small molecules. By 2016, mAb therapeutics reached about $89 billion in global sales. As of 2017, there were 71 mAb-based human therapeutic products available in the United States.

- **Genomics:** Genomics is the study of the structure and function of genes. Genomics technologies enable scientists to quickly decipher DNA sequences that code for genes. During the 1990s and early 2000s, genomics led to the discovery of many new molecular targets. However, scientists soon recognized that determining the function of genes and their proteins was a significant rate-limiting step in finding new molecular targets for drug discovery. Additional technologies like gene expression analysis and proteomics served to elucidate gene function and validate targets for intervention. Today, next-generation DNA sequencing capabilities—with their faster speed and higher computing power—have opened the doors further toward personalized medicine by lowering the cost of gene sequencing. Within this world of genomic medicine, several types of companies have emerged: tool companies with sequencing capabilities, companies that focus on direct-to-consumer personal genetic tests (eg, 23andMe), and personal genomics companies that analyze the genes of paying customers. The utility of genomic analysis today remains a question, since most diseases are multifactorial and typically involve many genes.

- **Cell therapy:** Cell therapy is defined as the administration of living whole cells to the patient for the treatment of diseases. The origin of the cells can be from the same individual (autologous source) or from another individual (allogeneic source). Cell therapy has greatly expanded its potential through new technologies such as genetic modification and cell engineering. The first commercially successful example of engineered cell therapy is the chimeric antigen receptor T-cell therapy (CAR-T), developed to treat cancer. In 2017, 2 products received approval by the US Food and Drug Administration (FDA) for treating refractory blood cancers: Novartis's Kymriah and Gilead/Kite's Yescarta. These are regarded as historic breakthroughs for the era of cancer cell therapy.

- **Genome editing (CRISPR/Cas9):** Genome editing is a method of making specific changes to the DNA of a cell or organism. Most often, genome editing refers to the specific alteration of DNA sequences that code for proteins; however, it can also include modifying other parts of the genetic system that regulate DNA in various different ways. During recent years, genome editing has become one of the fastest advancing areas in biotechnology. CRISPR/Cas9 is an enzyme system that is able to change or edit the DNA code of cells in a very quick and accurate way. Although there are other gene editing tools that had previously been discovered, the CRISPR/Cas9 system is the easiest to deploy in order to edit DNA in the desired way and is, therefore, the most widely used today. With the CRISPR/Cas9 system, scientists are able to create new animal model systems, as well as new assays and screens, more easily than before. In addition, since the discovery of CRISPR/Cas9 technology in 2012, several biotechnology companies have formed to focus on developing new therapeutics using DNA editing to treat genetic diseases.

- **Gene therapy:** Gene therapy is the process of inserting a new gene into human cells to have a therapeutic effect. Since many diseases have some genetic basis, gene therapy has the potential to allow scientists to correct the fundamental defect that is causing a diseased state, provided there is sufficient understanding of which gene is defective in a given disease. As is also the case with gene editing, gene therapy has far-reaching implications for safety, because it can irreversibly alter the genetic structure of cells and often requires the use of viral delivery technologies that bring additional risk.

- **Single-cell sequencing:** Cancer cell genomes often differ from the genomes of normal cells by harboring rapidly evolving mutations. Because of these variations, it may be important to analyze the genome of single cells to better understand the biology of a disease and how best to treat it. Single-cell genome sequencing involves isolating a single cell, performing whole-genome amplification (WGA), and then sequencing the DNA using a next-generation sequencer. Today, the major applications for single-cell genomics are cancer sequencing and microbiome sequencing. Scientists are also learning more about the mechanism of different diseases by studying single-cell genomes.

Two observations about these modalities are worth mentioning. First, there is an acceleration in these therapies. Biotech firms invest as much or more in R&D (as a percentage of sales) as do their pharma counterparts and enjoy higher operating margins (Figure 22-6). Second, over time, biotechnology may slowly assume some characteristics of engineering, including lower costs and faster R&D cycles. Indeed, data show that biotech firms allocate lower R&D costs per FDA-approved priority review for new molecular entities ($1.63 billion in R&D expense) compared to pharma ($6.3 billion in R&D expense).[5]

The new modalities have led to increased success in developing new drugs. One example of such success is Regeneron Pharmaceuticals, one of the largest biotechnology companies by market capitalization ($50 billion in 2016). After struggling for 22 years, Regeneron finally achieved commercial success in late 2011 with the launch of its first major drug, Eylea (aflibercept), to treat one version of age-related macular degeneration that leads to rapid loss of vision. Eylea earned sales revenues of $24.8 million in 2011, enabling the company to achieve its first year of net profitability. Eylea then earned $838 million

| Industry | Cost of Goods Sold | R&D as a % of Sales | SG&A as a % of Sales | Operating Margins |
|---|---|---|---|---|
| Large Pharma | ~20% | 13%-17% | 25%-30% | 35%-40% |
| Top 5 Biotech | ~10% | 15%-25% | 20%-25% | ~50% |

**Figure 22-6** • Relative Profitability of Pharma and Biotech. R&D, Research and Development; SG&A, Selling, General, and Administrative Expenses.

in 2012 and $1.3 billion in 2013, at a time when some analysts wondered if the era of multi-billion-dollar drugs was over. In 2011, the company also demonstrated the strength of its pipeline by submitting 3 biologics license applications (BLAs) to the FDA for approval. In 2015, Regeneron received FDA approval for a potential new bestseller (Praluent, alirocumab) to lower cholesterol in patients resistant to statins. The box titled "Case Study: Regeneron" provides a "deep dive" into Regeneron's remarkable history.

## Biotech Success Rates

Taking a *long-term perspective*, data reveal that biotech firms outperformed pharma during the period from 1998 to 2012 in terms of originating new molecular entities (NMEs) receiving "priority review" by the FDA. A total of 162 products received such review. Of the 26 new biological entities (NBEs) receiving such review, biotechs were responsible for 92% of them; of the 136 NCEs receiving such reviews, biotechs were responsible

for nearly half (48%). Among the "commercializing companies" (ie, those with principal rights to market in North America at time of FDA approval) behind these products, 44% were biotechs. Taking a *short-term perspective*, the number of active commercial investigational new drugs (INDs, see Chapter 21) has steadily increased since 2013 from 6,115 to 7,211 in 2017. The odds of success from phase I to approval have increased slightly between 2013 and 2015.[7]

There are several specific explanations for biotech's relatively high degree of R&D success compared to pharma. These include the following:

- Due to their larger mass (large molecules), biologics have greater "specificity" (ie, they bind to the target and wrap themselves around it). This means they have lower potential for off-target toxicity and side effects. This also means they have greater success in clinical trials in terms of product safety.

---

### Case Study: Regeneron[6]

Similar to large, established biotech firms (Biogen, Amgen, Genentech), Regeneron has built a greenfield, fully integrated biotechnology company (FIBCO) over the past 25 years with a robust pipeline of 13 drugs and $2.1 billion in revenues (as of 2013). However, unlike all other major biopharma companies, which in-license a significant percentage of their research projects from outside using business development strategies, Regeneron's entire pipeline has been homegrown and based on its own in-house technologies. This has allowed the company to retain the value and revenues generated by its own discoveries.

According to its chief science officer, Regeneron created a "discovery and development

wheel" of technologies, which it keeps "turning" to generate more drug opportunities. Its target discovery and validation technologies are deeply rooted in biological and genetic platform innovations such as "VelociGene" (ie, the testing of genes as potential drug targets by the high-throughput generation of mice missing each gene) that, in turn, allowed the company to develop "turnkey therapeutics" (fully humanized antibodies/traps) such as "VelocImmune" (ie, the creation of a mouse with a humanized immune system that can efficiently produce human antibodies that can be used as drugs against these targets). The technology platforms have allowed parallel processing of multiple candidates and thus "multiple shots on goal." In-house processing and manufacturing capabilities at the company's Tarrytown and Rensselaer sites support both clinical testing of the firm's pipeline and subsequent market development for its products. Unlike most other biopharma companies that often have a specialized manufacturing plant for each of their products, Regeneron uses a very similar process for each of its drug candidates, allowing it to build interchangeable, multiuse manufacturing suites and facilities, greatly decreasing its costs and time to production while increasing flexibility. Essentially, Regeneron has "McDonaldized" its manufacturing processes.

Regeneron took more than 2 decades and a series of failures to develop its end-to-end capability (repeatedly developing products from start to finish)—and did so in a learning and adaptive fashion. It did not bet on 1 big idea and did not rely on 1 drug. Instead, the company assembled a lot of smart people in the same room to think and work together to develop homegrown platform technologies that allowed the firm to innovate constantly and generate numerous drug candidates.

How did Regeneron accomplish this over such a long period of unprofitability? Regeneron monetized its assets to absorb a series of failures and support the development of its technological capabilities. It sold minority stakes to large pharma firms (Sanofi, Bayer) and used their monies to finance R&D over the long term but without giving up control. On its way to becoming a FIBCO in 2013, Regeneron increased its workforce size 2.5-fold between 2008 and 2012, mostly by adding scientists and retaining a research-centered culture. The heavy research focus had some possible downsides, however. The company's R&D spending as a percentage of total revenues was high (35%-42%) compared to its peers (19%-30%), contributing to a lower operating margin (30%+) and a relatively high price-earnings multiple of 20 to 21. The company's large size also posed an ongoing threat to its cultural cohesion, a problem that plagued Biogen and IDEC after their merger.

Regeneron's achievements have all come under the same top management team and the same core of scientists with which it began. Research by Bain & Company on the top 35

biotechnology companies (based on market or acquisition values of $3+ billion) suggests that firms replace up to 50% of their C-suite executives during the 4-year period surrounding their first product launch. This suggests the enormous challenge facing start-ups that wish to become FIBCOs. The shareholders of these start-ups often fare no better: Among the 21 biotechnology firms launching their first drug between January 2000 and June 2011, half destroyed shareholder value, ranging from 8% to 82% relative to the S&P 500. Of the 35 companies, only 30 achieved FIBCO status.

Regeneron is not a case study of the discovery of a particular novel product, but of a company built to make—and keep making—novel product discoveries. Regeneron is the antithesis of Big Pharma in that de facto control of the company is in the hands of its scientists, who plan strategy and new ventures, while management's main job is to make sure that high-quality employees and adequate financing are always at hand. Regeneron is not unique in this regard; many of the newer and smaller biotech companies were started by scientists with an idea, although in some of them, management seized control when the science did not pan out. Ironically, one of the companies closest to Regeneron in history and orientation is Genentech, also founded by scientists, which was successful in developing products (Avastin and Lucentis) very similar in many ways to 2 of Regeneron's current mainstays (Zaltrap and Eylea).

The most surprising thing about Regeneron has been its ability to stay on and even grow in the face of the repeated failures of its initial products—products based on the original ideas upon which its scientist-owner managers founded the company. Genentech also had an initial dry period when it operated at a significant loss, as did many similar companies, but the determining characteristic of Regeneron was that it had the perseverance to survive long enough to eventually deliver. One part of that perseverance lay in the persistence and loyalty of its scientists, who resisted the temptation to seek academic asylum when the going got tough. Another part was the willingness of the company's investors to stay the course and hang in there a lot longer than is typical of most investors.

- Biotech firms have been smart (or lucky) in going after rare (eg, orphan) diseases with high unmet need, which leads to rapid adoption by patients and physicians.
- Orphan diseases involve clinical trials with smaller patient sizes and may not require large, expensive phase III trials. This reduces the amount of capital needed to develop them. Orphan products also have no competitors, which allows companies to charge a higher price for their products.
- The complexity of biologics minimizes the threat of generics, which makes them more immune to patent cliffs.
- Biotech firms have also been smart (or lucky) in going after diseases in high-cost areas that require specialty therapeutics. Such drugs have lower risk and higher returns than drugs for chronic conditions that are mass marketed to primary care physicians.
- Biotechs have avoided the "diseconomies of scope" that plague pharma firms. Companies that specialize in just a few therapeutic categories may be more efficient, leaving them with smaller scale and product scope. Biotechnology firms began as small start-up operations focused on discovery and then development of one or a small number of drugs.
- Biotechs have had to operate more efficiently than pharma. They are perpetually raising money and need to move products forward as quickly and inexpensively as possible at every stage of development. By contrast, big pharma enjoys financial slack that can be used to conduct additional testing at each stage of clinical development. Their financial slack has also been deployed to acquire biotechnology companies and their products, which may be reflected in their R&D costs.
- Biotechs may be spending proportionately more on R&D, thus helping them to maintain higher organic growth.

Biological products have thus emerged as the R&D engine and the top sellers of biopharma products. In 1999, biologics accounted for only 10% of sales of the top 15 products; the percentage rose to 27% by 2009 and then to 68% by 2018! Between 2011 and 2016, small-midsize biopharma firms served as the originators for roughly two-thirds of all new drug applications (NDAs; see Chapter 21), whereas the larger biopharma firms served as the marketers of those drugs.

The biotech sector now serves as the "farm system" for Big Pharma: Biotechs have taken the lead in terms of discovery, while Big Pharma takes the lead in terms of development and commercialization. Strategic alliances thus represent a major strategy for both biotech and pharmaceutical firms. Among the major alliances in recent years are Kymera with Vertex, Goldfinch Bio with Gilead, and Voyager with AbbVie. Total licensing deals in the biopharma industry from 2013 to 2017 ranged from over 1,000 to over 1,600 deals annually, with average deal size ranging from $250 to $340 million per deal, continuing to trend higher over time. Taking the long view, deal activity has grown vastly since the early days of the biotechnology sector and remains strong today.[8] Moreover, since 2013, the number of merger and acquisition (M&A) deals involving the US biotechnology sector ranged from 350 to 550 transactions annually, while the aggregate deal value ranged from $132 to $350+ billion.

## ORPHAN DRUGS

Much of biotech's success lies in entering the "orphan drug" space. In 1995, only 23% of new drugs approved by the FDA were orphan drugs; by 2015, the percentage had skyrocketed to 58%. An orphan drug is a pharmaceutical product aimed at populations with rare diseases or disorders—defined in the United States as less than 200,000 patients (or a disease that affects more than 200,000 persons but is not expected to recover the cost of developing and marketing a treatment drug). The development of orphan drugs was financially incentivized by the Orphan Drug Act of 1983. The act provided 7 years of marketing exclusivity from approval, reduced R&D costs via a 50% tax credit as well as R&D grants for phase I to phase III, and waived "user fees" (payments to the FDA to review their product applications). The National Organization for Rare Disorders (NORD), which was instrumental in establishing the act, currently estimates 30 million Americans suffer from 7,000 rare diseases.

Since 1983, more than 400 drugs and biologic products for rare diseases have been developed and marketed. By contrast, during the decade prior to 1983, fewer than 10 such products supported by industry came to market. The Orphan Grants Program has brought more than 45 products to marketing approval.

Orphan drugs have "remarkable" price points. The average orphan drug cost to patients was $111,820 in 2014 (vs $23,331 for a nonorphan drug); the median orphan drug cost was $66,057 (vs $4,775 for a nonorphan drug). While the average and median drug prices have increased year-on-year for both orphan and nonorphan drugs since 2010, the median price increase was higher for orphan than for nonorphan drugs (1.8 times vs 1.7 times).[9]

Figure 22-7 illustrates the pricing power of biologicals that enjoy orphan drug status. The example presented here from Avonex (interferon beta-1a) shows persistent price increases over a long period of time (2005-2018). The story is similar for other biotech drugs that, despite many going off patent, still enjoy strong

### US Avonex Price Hikes

| Date | % Increase | Approximate Price |
|---|---|---|
| May 2005 | 5% | $15,500 |
| December 2005 | 9% | $16,900 |
| June 2006 | 9% | $18,400 |
| February 2007 | 5% | $19,400 |
| August 2007 | 6% | $20,500 |
| November 2007 | 12% | $23,000 |
| June 2008 | 9% | $25,050 |
| November 2008 | 9% | $27,300 |
| March 2009 | 9.5% | $29,900 |
| December 2009 | 7.5% | $32,100 |
| February 2010 | 5.5% | $33,900 |
| July 2010 | 4.5% | $35,400 |
| December 2010 | 6% | $37,500 |
| May 2011 | 6% | $39,800 |
| December 2011 | 6.5% | $42,350 |
| March 2012 | 8.5% | $45,950 |
| August 2012 | 6% | $48,600 |
| November 2012 | 4.5% | $50,900 |
| June 2013 | 7.5% | $54,700 |
| November 2013 | 8% | $59,100 |
| September 2014 | 4% | $62,000 |
| March 2015 | 5.5% | $65,700 |
| August 2015 | 6% | $69,600 |
| December 2015 | 4% | $72,300 |
| May 2016 | 5% | $75,900 |
| January 2017 | 8% | $82,000 |
| January 2018 | 8% | $88,500 |

**Figure 22-7 •** Avonex Drug Price Hikes Over Time. (Source: PriceRx.)

intellectual property (IP) rights and, thus, continue to earn high revenues (Figure 22-8).[10]

The higher prices of orphan drugs may not be matched by their higher effectiveness, however. Researchers have reported that although orphan drugs were 5 times more likely to offer a health benefit compared to other FDA-approved drugs, their median cost was substantially higher ($47,650 vs $2,870) and entailed a 2.7 multiple in cost to gain the same extra year of health.[11]

## BIOSIMILARS AND THE THREAT OF GENERICS

The rising price of biologics has created considerable interest in generic versions—known as "biosimilars." Generic versions of small-molecule drugs (NCEs) have saved consumers almost $2 trillion in the past decade, with increasing savings year-over-year (Figure 22-9). The United States leads the rest of the world in adoption of generics (Figure 22-10). Generic drugs exert positive impacts on the iron triangle:

- **Cost:** Generic drugs save approximately $300 billion per year, with that amount growing every year. Generic competition reduces prices of branded drugs by approximately 40%.
- **Quality:** Generics are identical in effectiveness to branded counterparts (ie, bioequivalence); improved access may result in higher-quality health outcomes for patients.
- **Access:** Patients pay less out of pocket for generics. There is a 7-fold difference in copays: average generic copay of less than $6 versus average brand name copay of more than $40. This improves access to patients with high-deductible health plan coverage.

Policy makers would like to see the same consumer benefits for expensive biologic products.

A biosimilar uses the same mechanism(s) of action for the proposed condition(s) of use as the reference product and the same condition(s) of use proposed in labeling previously approved for the reference product. The biosimilar also has the same route of administration and dosage form and strength as the reference product and has no clinically meaningful differences with regard to safety, purity, and potency

| Rank | Drug | 2018 Sales ($B) | Patent Expiry |
|------|------|-----------------|---------------|
| 1 | Gilead's HIV franchise | 14.9 | 2018-2030 |
| 2 | Celgene's Revlimid | 9.7 | 2027 |
| 3 | Amgen's Enbrel | 4.9 | Biologic |
| 4 | Amgen's G-CSF franchise | 4.7 | Biologic |
| 5 | Biogen's Rituxan (US only) | 4.5 | Biologic |
| 6 | Biogen's Tecfidera | 4.3 | 2028 |
| 7 | Amgen's denosumab | 4.2 | Biologic |
| 8 | Regeneron's Eylea | 4.0 | Biologic |
| 9 | Gilead's HCV franchise | 3.9 | 2029 |
| 10 | Alexion's Soliris | 3.4 | Biologic |

**Figure 22-8** • Intellectual Property Rights Are Strong. B, Billions; G-CSF, Granulocyte Colony-Stimulating Factor; HCV, Hepatitis C Virus. (Source: Cowen & Company; Eric Schmidt, Presentation to the Wharton School, 2019.)

vis-à-vis the reference product. Based on this, it is called "bioequivalent" and can be substituted for the brand without patient knowledge; without such equivalence and substitutability, the drug is known as a "biogeneric."

However, there are major differences between generic chemical drugs and biosimilars (Figure 22-11). These have enormous implications for the development of biosimilars. Rather than the cost of $3 to $5 million for making a generic drug, a biosimilar can cost $100 to $200

million and require the full range of clinical trials. The abbreviated NDA route for generic drugs only requires scientific demonstration of bioequivalence; biosimilars must take a different route to approval [351(k)] that requires animal, clinical, and analytical studies.

As of 2019, 60 biosimilars had been approved in Europe, but only 25 had been approved in the United States; of those, only 9 were commercially available. Moreover, 17 of the largest commercial health insurers in the United States

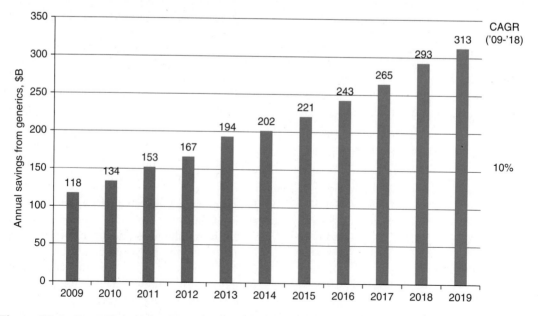

**Figure 22-9** • Two Trillion Dollars in Savings From Generics in the Last Decade. B, Billion. (Source: Association for Accessible Medicines. "AAM 2019 Generic Biosimilars Access and Savings US Report." Available Online: https://accessiblemeds.org/2020-Access-Savings-Report.)

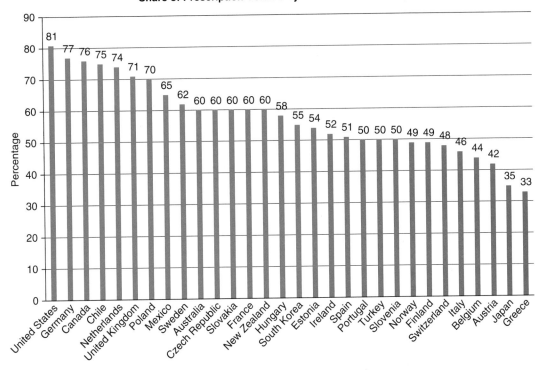

**Share of Prescription Volume by Unbranded Generics, 2018**

**Figure 22-10** • United States Has High Rates of Generic Adoption. (Source: Statista, Organisation of Economic Co-operation and Development, IQVIA, Patented Medicine Prices Review Board.)

(covering 60% of commercial enrollees) rarely preferred biosimilar versions over brand name biologics when making their coverage decisions; insurers required patients to try the biosimilar first only 14% of the time.[12] If biosimilars had 50% market share, the United States could save $4.8 billion per year (a conservative estimate based on historical sales); yet, over the past 4 years, the country has saved only $1 billion. Why is this the case? Both the adoption and the price discounting for biosimilars have been limited. For all but one of the biosimilars presented in Figure 22-12, the market penetration is 5% or less, and the price discount is 30% or less.

This begs the question: Why is adoption so limited?[13] One reason is the higher manufacturing cost and thus the lower margins available for manufacturers of biosimilars. The manufacturing cost per patient per year for a small-molecule drug is $10; for a large molecule (eg, hormone), it is $200; and for a complex biologic (eg, mAb), it is $3,000. Overall, branded biologics may have average gross margins approximately 10% lower than small

| Characteristics | Generics | Biosimilars |
|---|---|---|
| Size | ~500 daltons | >150k daltons |
| Chemical structure | Simple, well defined, and chemically identical to reference product | Complex, heterogeneous with differences in protein folding and glycosylation |
| Analytical characteristics | Active drug identical to that of the reference product | Similar but not identical to reference product; hard to characterize |
| Manufacturing process | Relatively simple; uses medicinal chemical reactions | Complex; produced in living cells with several stages of purification and production |
| Impact of process change | Likely to be negligible | Small changes can alter final protein structure and function |

**Figure 22-11** • Comparison of Biosimilars and Generics.

| Biosimilar | Biosimilar Market Share | Price Discount |
|---|---|---|
| Inflectra | 5.3% | −25.8% |
| Renflexis | 1.0% | −18.5% |
| Fulphila | 2.2% | −10.3% |
| Udencya | 2.3% | −8.1% |
| Zarxio | 54.9% | −38.3% |
| Nivestym | 0.3% | −28.0% |
| Retacrit | 1.5% | −3.4% |

**Figure 22-12** • Limited Adoption and Price Discounts for Biosimilars: the Bigger the Price Discount, the Bigger the Market Share. (Source: IQVIA and CMMS. See Also: "Incenting Competition to Reduce Drug Spending: The Biosimilar Opportunity." https://www.pacificresearch.org/wp-content/uploads/2019/07/BiosimilarsCompetition_F.pdf.)

molecules, leaving (slightly) less headroom for price discounts from biosimilar competition.

A second reason is the high entry barrier for biosimilars. Branded biologics may have 75 or more patents compared to 1 to 3 for small molecules, leading to claims of "patent abuse." The requirement for clinical trials significantly increases the costs that must be incurred to achieve approval relative to small-molecule generics. Finally, the trade secrets regarding the manufacture of complex biologicals remain barriers even after patent expiry, conferring strong IP protection.

A third reason is the lack of (perceived) interchangeability of biosimilars for the branded biological product. Physicians are reportedly risk averse and unwilling to switch their patients away from the latter to use the former. This is despite the fact that a 2018 study comparing 20 years of global data showed no meaningful differences in safety or efficacy when patients switched. For their part, insurers may also be unwilling to switch, given they may lose the rebates paid to them by the pharmacy benefit managers (PBMs) who contract with the manufacturers of the branded product. This is known in the industry as "the rebate trap."

To be sure, the FDA has been trying to accelerate the adoption of biosimilars. The first effort was the Biologics Price Competition and Innovation Act (BPCI, 2009), which created an abbreviated approval pathway for biological products. The next effort was the Biosimilars Action Plan (July 2018) to implement the BPCI regulations. This ambitious yet vague plan includes streamlining the review process and clarifying what performance data are needed to demonstrate biosimilarity.

So, what does the future likely hold? The accumulation of more evidence and growing clinical experience with biosimilars will shift the United States toward interchangeable use with branded biologics. This shift could come quickly, with one analysis suggesting a tripling of biosimilar sales in the United States by 2024 to $2.5 billion[14]; at the same time, however, the shift may take 10 or more years to produce significant changes in physician prescribing behavior. As obstacles to biosimilar adoption are reduced, major biologics will face significant biosimilar competition, leading to price discounts; however, these discounts are likely not going to be as steep as the discounts of small-molecule generics. Finally, branded biologics with sufficiently low levels of sales may never face biosimilar competition; however, their ability to raise prices without tempting biosimilar competition may be limited.

## BIOTECH ORGANIZATION AND MANAGEMENT

As intimated earlier, part of biotech's promise rests on small size and low bureaucracy. Research suggests that such organizational characteristics may be associated with innovation.[15] The large pharmaceutical companies began as chemical companies in Europe more than 100 years ago, which forward-integrated into fine chemicals and then again into synthetic (medicinal) chemistry. This is where the drug industry really began. These large and fully integrated pharmaceutical companies (FIPCOs) spanned the entire value chain of activity—from discovery and chemistry capabilities through development into commercialization. With the stagnation in R&D productivity and the patent cliffs following the first decade of the new millennium, large pharma firms were forced to reexamine the nature of their vertically integrated business model. Although they didn't entirely gut their research programs, many shrank their in-house research footprint, which was a high fixed-cost portion of their business. They began to outsource much of their innovation to biotechs in the form of R&D partnerships and in-licensing of biotech science.

By contrast, biotechs are small companies with small top management teams and flat (rather than hierarchical) organizational structures. They are also reputed for their innovative cultures, which are "technically oriented" throughout the organization, less commercially focused (except in the large companies), less process heavy and less bureaucratic, more entrepreneurial and fast paced, with rapid decision making and mixing of expertise across multiple organizational levels. The firms are also more focused, with fewer than 10 clinical programs underway and little to no infrastructure for purposes of commercialization (eg, sales reps). Biotechs tend to focus on select portions of the pharma value chain where they can add value, while outsourcing the rest. According to researchers, this culture can be described in terms of the following 5 major attributes[16]:

- Tolerance for failure but no tolerance for incompetence
- Willingness to experiment but highly disciplined
- Psychologically safe but brutally candid
- Collaboration but with individual accountability
- Flat but strong leadership

### Critical Thinking Exercise: Amgen

A Harvard Business School case extols the virtues of strategic planning and the role of management in the early success of Amgen—one of the biotech pioneers.[17] A book by Amgen's former CEO repeats some of the same lessons as the case.[18] These managerial lessons include the following:

- Detailed, long-range plans
- Using plans as a communication channel between executives and scientists
- Use of product development teams
- Use of business plans that include timing, probabilities of success, the availability of financing, collaboration and partnerships, facilities requirements, and staffing opportunities
- Maintaining a large cash cushion
- Building up technological capabilities as infrastructure for the future

Executives strongly believed that these management lessons separated Amgen from its competitors and were the key cause of its success. What do you think?

## BIOTECH INVESTMENT: THE BIG PICTURE

There has been a proliferation of new product technologies, novel therapies, and externalization of R&D via strategic alliances. Biotechs have enjoyed a ramp-up in VC funding since 2013, along with new public company formations (almost 250 IPOs over the past 5 years) and rising drug prices. There is thus clearly a high demand. On the other hand, however, there has been a relatively flat supply of new biotech products and start-ups, especially when compared to the software industry. VCs launch only 100 to 125 new companies annually.[19] The complexity of the science underlying the biotech sector has served as a serious barrier to entry and constrained the supply of products and firms.

Biotech only represents about 11% of all venture investments across sectors. While it is a small piece of the pie on a relative basis, it is large on an absolute basis in terms of funding. Moreover, over half of the IPO exits are biotech companies, which have enjoyed increases in their public market valuations. These IPOs tend to be for companies in preclinical development or phase I stages. One explanation for this is that large private tech companies that are valued at more than a billion dollars are making deliberate strategic decisions to stay private and build before they exit. They can do this given the availability of capital for the tech space. Another reason may be that they cannot exit and thus keep raising money given the huge inflows of money. Conversely, biotech investors are very wary of having private companies with public market valuations, since falling values make it harder to raise money. For those companies that are going to go public, VCs wait for open windows as long as the company is sufficiently mature in terms of its product platform, its product pipeline, and the readiness of its management team. VCs kill off roughly one-third of the biotech ventures in their portfolios.

Biopharma as a share of global VC funding has also been fairly constant, suggesting the sector has kept pace. Nevertheless, funding for VC-backed biotechs continues to increase, translating into increased investment per company. This suggests there is no longer a technology funding chasm with underfunded biotechs. There are more and more companies that are very well capitalized, and perhaps not overcapitalized as in a bubble. Rather, there now seems to be a very logical transition of the capital markets from early-stage ventures through going public following release of early clinical results. IPO valuations continue upward in the face of strong demand for biotech products. The segment now features early clinical companies, mid-stage biotechs, and mature biotechs that have fully integrated their value chain activities all the way through to commercialization. Capital markets are now able to see a single company move along the entire lifestyle spectrum and are willing to fund it. This translates into more access to capital across all stages, including the venture stage.

## BIOTECH BUSINESS MODELS

Selecting a business model for a new biotech firm is an important and consequential decision that affects financing and business development strategy, exit, and value realization. Biotech business models can be described as falling on a spectrum from platforms to products (Figure 22-13). Platform companies typically have a "horizontal" capability that can be applied to multiple products. This could be a novel therapeutic modality such as gain-of-function gene therapy

using a viral vector like adeno-associated virus (AAV) or gene editing using CRISPR/Cas9. In these cases, the underlying technology often may be applied across many therapeutic areas. Platforms may also be based around specific areas of biology, such as modulating the tumor microenvironment in immuno-oncology or preventing axonal degeneration in central nervous system diseases like multiple sclerosis (limiting, by definition, the possible product portfolio to a specific therapeutic area). By contrast, product companies focus on a single product or on a limited set of products within a particular disease.

Although these 2 models blend in the middle of the spectrum, they are fundamentally quite different in terms of the scope of their underlying technology, the breadth of expertise required to lead and staff them, their operational complexity, their capital requirements, and their partnering options. They are described in more detail in the following sections.

### Platform Companies

Platform companies must access and manage the expertise required to build their "horizontal" technology platform (eg, antibodies, RNA interference, viral gene therapy) as well as the

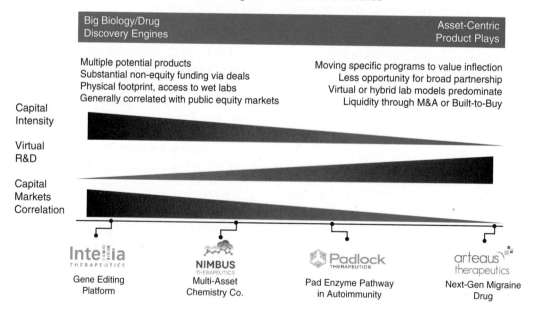

Figure 22-13 • Biotechnology Business Models. M&A, Mergers and Acquisitions; R&D, Research and Development. (Source: Figure 4.1, in Lawton R. Burns [Ed.], *The Business of Healthcare Innovation*, 3rd ed. Cambridge, United Kingdom: Cambridge University Press; 2020.)

expertise needed to pursue diverse "vertical" therapeutic areas (eg, rare hematologic diseases, ophthalmology). This is a practical challenge that requires management to set strategy for, operationalize, and integrate multiple research streams in parallel. With their necessary early focus on developing the core platform, these new companies often falter due to a lack of specific disease-area expertise. Successful platform companies recognize the need for disease-specific expertise and bring it on board early in their development.

Platform companies also typically have high capital requirements—to first build their technology platform and to then apply it across multiple programs to develop a product pipeline. As a result, in comparison to narrower product companies, they are likely to (1) create broader investor syndicates, (2) enter in strategic partnerships with large pharma and biotech companies to access expertise and nondilutive capital (albeit at the cost of product rights), and (3) go public to access additional capital at a lower cost of capital than is available in the private capital markets (vs exiting through M&A).

New platform technologies, such as antibodies or RNAi, can take a decade or more to be reduced to practice, generate clinical data and achieve their first product approval. Notably, once those new modalities are introduced into practice, the venture can leverage its "off-the-shelf toolkit" and transition from (1) an open-ended, fixed-cost investment to get from platform-to-practice that may cost a billion dollars and take many years to (2) a more direct marginal cost, product-by-product economic model.

## Product Companies

At the other end of the spectrum are more asset-centric or product-specific companies. These are less capital intensive because the entire investment is directed to specific products rather than building a horizontal platform. They may be built in a virtual or semivirtual fashion, with small, expert internal teams (eg, medicinal chemists that design new molecules) that manage networks of external contract research organizations (CROs) that conduct the synthetic chemistry, pharmacokinetics/pharmacodynamics testing, and the animal testing, and manage the wet labs. As a result, they are able to engage in research on a direct and largely variable cost basis from the start. With few product programs (often only

1 or 2), they are less likely to enter into strategic partnerships and also less likely to finance and exit via the public markets. Instead, they typically exit through M&A, often through structured acquisitions that may occur during preclinical stages, ahead of any human clinical data. Structured acquisitions typically have an upfront payment and near- and longer-term milestones based on clinical and commercial objectives. In these structured acquisitions, liquidity is realized for investors, management, and other shareholders (eg, scientific founders), while shifting financing costs and risks onto the acquirer.

## NEW BIOTECH VENTURE CREATION

Geographically, successful biotechnology rests on a supportive ecosystem, sometimes known as "economic clusters." Such clusters foster key transfers and exchanges of knowledge, assets, and cooperative efforts that not only occur among scientists within organizations but also among scientists and other professionals across organizations. Beyond the immediate geographic cluster, new biotechs also rest on connectivity with larger pharmaceutical and biotechnology companies. Such connectivity includes 2-way flows: talent from the larger companies that inhabit the start-ups as executives-in-residence (EIRs), and product out-licensing from the start-ups to the larger firms.

### Economic Clusters

The near majority of VC funding of biotechs is being funneled into start-ups located in a handful of "clusters." Between 2012 and 2016, the percentage of VC funding going to such areas as Cambridge (Massachusetts) and San Francisco rose 128%, accounting for 48% of biotech VC funding (up from 31%). These geographic clusters have also enjoyed a large ramp-up in R&D employment.

### How Economic Clusters Work[20]

Economic clusters in the biomedical sciences originated in the United States with the founding of the first biotech firms in the 1970s and 1980s, largely through the efforts of academic scientists with some help from local VCs. The biotech pioneers included (1) Genentech, cofounded by

University of California, San Francisco biochemist Herbert Boyer and geneticist Stanley Cohen at Stanford; (2) Biogen, cofounded by MIT biologist Phillip Allen Sharp and Harvard biochemist Walter Gilbert; and (3) Genzyme, cofounded by Henry Blair at Tufts Medical School. These entrepreneurial efforts spurred other academic researchers to follow suit and establish their own biomedical sciences start-up firms. These efforts, in turn, encouraged large pharmaceutical firms to relocate their R&D facilities to within easy striking distance of the biotech firms with whom they could establish partnerships and more easily gain information on and licensing rights to the new technologies being developed—largely as a strategy to offset the slumping efficiency and lagging productivity of their own in-house R&D programs.

Geographic regions that host a concentration of knowledge-intensive firms incite innovation by breaking down boundaries in several ways. First, they increase the likelihood of serendipitous encounters and personal interactions that spawn new ideas that foster innovation. Second, they allow firms to closely monitor the activities of their competitors, which in turn intensifies rivalry, the diffusion of ideas, and the recognition of the need to keep abreast of (and copy) some of the most recent technological developments. Third, they stimulate and accelerate knowledge spillovers and access to knowledge and capital stocks that are crucial inputs to innovation. Fourth, they diminish costs (eg, those associated with transportation and communication) incurred in gaining access to needed resources.[21] Fifth, they enable greater exposure to a wider variety of new (and disparate) ideas and materials that can be usefully recombined to generate new innovations. According to Michael Porter, an economic cluster can be thought of as a "geographically proximate group of interconnected companies and associated institutions in a particular field, linked by commonalities and complementarities."[22] The competitive advantage of such co-location equates with access to key complementary resources that nonproximate competitors lack.

To be sure, co-location alone is not a guarantee of innovation and competitive advantage. The characteristics of the local geographic network of firms also play a role. These include the structure of the local network: the density and redundancy of ties among local firms, the cohesion (eg,

levels of knowledge, trust, coordination) in the network, and the presence of knowledge brokers that serve to connect firms that might benefit mutually from such connections.[23] Of course, it almost goes without saying that if a co-located firm is to benefit, it must have sought-after capabilities of its own to be in a position to leverage the innovation advantage of proximity. Such capabilities include intraorganizational network cohesion and an ability to process and utilize the information to which they are exposed.

## Cluster Location

Why do clusters of life sciences firms locate where they do? One model, the "county manager" view, emphasizes the efforts undertaken by local governments that use various policy instruments to attract such companies to serve as engines for job creation. These instruments can include property tax forgiveness, relaxation of planning or environmental regulations, construction of transportation and communication infrastructure, and construction subsidies. A second model, the "entrepreneurial" view, focuses on the decisions made by founding scientists to undertake a start-up and to do so in that region. These can include favorable university policies, attractive levels of internal and external research funding, the ready availability of high-caliber researchers and graduates from the universities in the region, high R&D spending levels, the availability of capital (eg, VC and private equity firms), low local property taxes, high total county income, easy highway access, and an abundance of county amenities. The 2 models are complementary, analogous to forces of demand ("pull") and supply ("push"),[24] and amply supported by empirical evidence.[25]

A more elaborate treatment of these push-pull forces posits the importance of "the triple helix": the joint (but not necessarily coordinated) efforts of government, academia, and industry to create high-tech clusters.[26] According to this argument, academia and industry are more tightly linked to one another but less tightly linked to government. The 3 strands of the helix can be briefly summarized as follows:

- *Academia* supplies an abundance of extraordinarily creative scientists, many of whom serve as the scientific cofounders of start-ups. The universities they come from house the offices of technology transfer that facilitate the establishment of companies based on the technologies developed by their researchers. The universities also provide students as interns and graduates as employees, as well as land and/or space for start-ups.

- *Industry* provides entrepreneurial scientists with business partners. These include VCs, larger firms that license or acquire the technologies developed by the start-ups, the managerial cadre of these firms that can help lead the start-ups, legal firms that can help with IP protection, and research institutes in which the scientists can conduct their research and entrepreneurial effort.

- *Government* bodies at state and local levels can aid the formation of start-ups by codifying the rules for new and controversial activities (eg, recombinant DNA research and application), offering tax concessions to build plants and other facilities, and approving the construction of manufacturing facilities (eg, through public offices of economic development). At a higher level, governmental actions at the federal level can help inculcate a start-up culture, particularly in the life sciences. Examples include (1) the 1974 Employee Retirement Income and Security Act (ERISA), which fueled investment in VC funds; (2) cuts in the capital gains tax rate in 1978 and 1982, which stimulated long-term investment; (3) the 1980 Bayh-Dole Act, which granted universities IP rights to federally funded inventions and the means to license them to industry; (4) the 1982 Supreme Court decision (*Diamond v. Chakrabarty*) that allowed the patentability of genetically modified bacteria, facilitating the rise of the biotechnology sector; and (5) federal funding of basic scientific research in the life sciences through the National Institutes of Health (NIH), National Science Foundation, Department of Energy, and Department of Agriculture.

## The Life Sciences Cluster in Cambridge, Massachusetts

The Cambridge cluster developed as a geographic focal point in tandem with MIT's heavy investment in the development of Kendall Square (an area alternatively defined as the MIT campus or everything within a 10-minute walk of the Kendall/MIT subway station). The Boston Consulting Group proclaimed the area to be "the most innovative square mile on earth."[27] Figure 22-14 describes the industrial sectors that compose the Cambridge cluster; Figure 22-15 provides a geographic view of the co-location for many of the life sciences firms in Kendall Square.

The Cambridge economic cluster amply illustrates the triple helix. First, the 2 major universities (Harvard and MIT) feature several creative scientists (many Nobel Prize winners) on their faculties, establishing their leadership in key research areas and serving as a hub for attracting especially able and committed students. Their institutions were among the first to establish offices of technology transfer (MIT in 1940, Harvard in 1977), as well as partnerships with large corporations working in the life sciences (Hoechst AG, Monsanto).

Second, local business leaders organized early VC funds (eg, the American Research and Development Corporation) to invest in new companies (eg, Digital Equipment) that spawned other sources of capital that fueled the start-ups. Major pharmaceutical firms developed a research presence in the Boston metropolitan area, starting with Johnson & Johnson in 1982, American Home Products in 1992, and Abbott Laboratories (now AbbVie) in 2000. Novartis set up its research lab in Cambridge, Massachusetts, in 2003. Other pharmaceutical firms were soon to follow suit: Pfizer in 2014, Amgen in 2014, and AstraZeneca in 2016.[28] The Dutch medical device firm Philips recently announced plans to move its US research hub to Kendall. Former executives of these companies (particularly Abbott and Baxter) served as the chief executive officers for Biogen and Genzyme.

Third, the Commonwealth of Massachusetts Department of Economic Development simplified the permit process to outcompete other cities in attracting biotechnology companies to locate their manufacturing plants in the area. Synergy between the complex biotechnology manufacturing process and preexisting R&D activity served to strengthen and amplify cross-investments and geographical lock-in.

The Cambridge area developed as local scientist-inventors reclaimed factory space ("abandoned wasteland") that had closed down

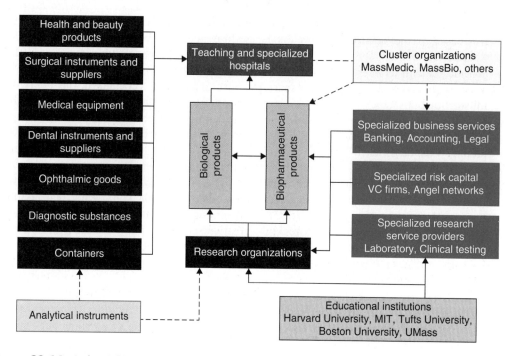

**Figure 22-14 •** Industrial Sectors in Cambridge Cluster. VC, Venture Capital. (Source: Figure 4.2, in Lawton R. Burns [Ed.], *The Business of Healthcare Innovation*, 3rd ed. Cambridge, United Kingdom: Cambridge University Press; 2020.)

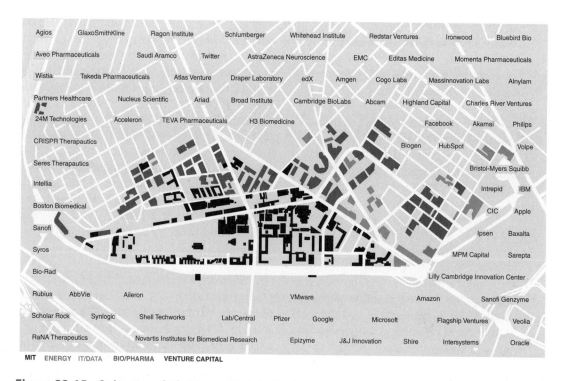

**Figure 22-15 •** Co-location of Life Sciences Firms in Cambridge Cluster. (Source: Figure 4.3, in Lawton R. Burns [Ed.], *The Business of Healthcare Innovation*, 3rd ed. Cambridge, United Kingdom: Cambridge University Press; 2020.)

in the 1940s and 1950s to house their companies. Phillip Sharp (a co-recipient of the 1993 Nobel Prize for his work on gene structure and function) chose the area for his start-up Biogen due to its proximity to his laboratory in the university and future employees of his company.[29] Biogen's move was shortly followed by Genzyme, creating a nascent biotechnology hub. Cambridge also benefited from the start of the Internet era in the 1990s given that MIT was home to web inventor Tim Berners-Lee. The university leased space to entrepreneurs who developed the Cambridge Innovation Center in 1999, which attracted and hosted many small tech start-ups in affordable and adjacent space. Start-up entrepreneurs reported that they could count on running into their counterparts on the way to and from lunch. Add to this the "Sloanies," named after the University's Sloan School of Management: a captive pool from which interns and employees might be recruited (and their former faculty advisors) and angel investors solicited. Unlike the Bay Area, start-ups in the Cambridge area faced less competition for these sources of support, which in turn attracted VC investment and larger tech firms such as Google and Amazon.[30]

## Cluster Advantage

The role of geography in innovation has long been recognized.[31] The US biotechnology sector is largely concentrated in 9 geographic regions.[32] Collectively, these regions account for three-quarters of all biotechnology companies, more than 60% of NIH research funding, and two-thirds of all biotechnology-related patents. Empirical analyses suggest that tighter clustering of biotechnology firms in a given state enhances regional industry efficiency, measured by the value of shipments and receipts and the number of patents.[33]

Data suggest that VC funding in recent years has disproportionately flowed to the Cambridge and San Francisco clusters, suggesting a geographic consolidation of financial investment. A parallel consolidation of R&D and managerial employment in biopharma has also occurred. Such concentrations may well be associated with shorter times to exit (number of years since founding) and higher exit valuations. The value of the Cambridge location is greater

for companies outside of the cluster, suggesting a positive selection bias that occurs for those companies that come there. This may reflect a self-fulfilling prophecy by virtue of having better companies enter the market, which can then hire better talent and recruit better leadership.

Some confirmatory evidence comes from the Commonwealth's own report on its life sciences efforts.[34] The report asserts the state is the number one life sciences cluster worldwide, garnering the highest level of NIH funding per capita and 10% of NIH funds overall. Thirty-seven percent of biopharma VC funding went to Massachusetts in 2017, and US-based investors outside of the state led 60% of investment in Massachusetts-based biopharma companies in 2017. Cambridge-based companies received 62% of all biotech venture investment in the state, and 50% of all Massachusetts biotechs that went public in 2017 were located in Cambridge. The commonwealth also sports the following impressive growth statistics: 28% job growth and 35% R&D growth (2008-2017) and 71% lab space growth (2009-2018).

## Cluster Envy

Based on these impressive achievements and statistics, it is little wonder that other US cities and other countries want to emulate the Cambridge example. New York City's mayor and New York State's governor announced in December 2016 they planned to invest $500 million to build up life science firms in Manhattan and statewide. Never mind that the city lacks both a Harvard and an MIT, as well as a host of pharmaceutical firms and biotech start-ups. Despite such shortcomings, the governor offered an additional $650 million in tax incentives, innovation space, and tax-free land at college campuses around the state.[35]

Other countries have also taken notice and begun to set up shop in Cambridge. Canada, the Netherlands, Denmark, and others have opened up biotech incubators and accelerators in the area. It is estimated that as many as 65 countries are members of the Science and Technology Diplomatic Circle to foster interactions on scientific and technology programs.[36]

Finally, other countries like China are attempting to establish their own indigenous life sciences clusters. China's version of Kendall

Square is called "Pharma Valley," located within the Zhangjiang Hi-Tech Park.[37] Pharma Valley has 500 biotech companies clustered in a 10-square-kilometer area, representing as much as 70% to 80% of China's innovative biopharma activity. Foreign pharmaceutical firms have been attracted to the area to work with the local CROs and start-ups. Unlike Kendall Square, nearly all funding for China's cluster comes from the Chinese Central Government ($254 billion) rather than VC and private equity ($45 billion, 2017). The government has also pursued reforms in its pharmaceutical sector to speed up the drug approval process and the regulatory apparatus to abet the cluster's development. But like other US cities, China lacks some of the key Kendall Square infrastructure, such as top-tier universities, academic medical centers, and VC—for now.

## SUMMARY

There are a few "hot areas" in healthcare; biotechnology is clearly one of them. Biotech science is cutting edge; biotech organization and management are unconventional; and biotech funding is robust. All of these developments are manifestly evident in the Biotech clusters located on both coasts of the United States. Perhaps more so than in pharmaceuticals, managing creativity and discovery in biotech is on the agenda of entrepreneurs, financiers, and governments everywhere.

## QUESTIONS TO PONDER

1. Why are biotech firms more successful in drug discovery than "Big Pharma"?
2. If biotech firms are better than pharma in drug discovery, why do so many of them fail and/or lose lots of money?
3. In terms of their relative success in R&D, have biotech firms been smart or just lucky?
4. Why hasn't the threat of generics penetrated biotech the way it has penetrated pharma?
5. How likely are US cities or other countries to successfully emulate the economic cluster of Cambridge, Massachusetts?

## REFERENCES

1. These include preclinical studies, in vitro studies in animal and human systems, and in vivo animal studies (to determine systemic uptake and exposure, metabolism, pharmacological effect, potential toxicities, and target organs of a drug), in vitro physiochemical and ADME (absorption, distribution, metabolism, and excretion) properties, selectivity and safety screens, in vivo studies, pharmacokinetics and ADME-efficacy models, and toxicological/safety assessments.
2. Figure courtesy of Cary Pfeffer. "The Biotechnology Sector," in Lawton R. Burns (Ed.), *The Business of Healthcare Innovation.* 3rd ed. (Cambridge, United Kingdom: Cambridge University Press, 2020): Chapter 3.
3. Figure courtesy of Cary Pfeffer. "The Biotechnology Sector," in Lawton R. Burns (Ed.), *The Business of Healthcare Innovation.* 3rd ed. (Cambridge, United Kingdom: Cambridge University Press, 2020): Chapter 3.
4. Definitions are taken from Cary Pfeffer. "The Biotechnology Sector," in Lawton R. Burns (Ed.), *The Business of Healthcare Innovation.* 3rd ed. (Cambridge, United Kingdom: Cambridge University Press, 2020): Chapter 3.
5. Donald L. Drakeman. "Benchmarking Biotech and Pharmaceutical Product Development," *Nat Biotechnol.* 32 (7) (July 2014): 621-625.
6. This section is adapted from the following source: Alex Rosen, Lawton R. Burns, Philip A. Rea, et al. "Regeneron: Agility, Resilience, and Balance," in Philip A. Rea, Mark V. Pauly, and Lawton R. Burns (Eds.), *Managing Discovery in the Life Sciences* (Cambridge, United Kingdom: Cambridge University Press, 2018): Chapter 12.
7. Chi Heem Wong and Kien Wei Shah. "Estimation of Clinical Trial Success Rates and Related Parameters," *Biostatistics.* 20 (2) (2019): 273-286.
8. Cary Pfeffer. "The Biotechnology Sector," in Lawton R. Burns (Ed.), *The Business of Healthcare Innovation*, 3rd ed. (Cambridge, United Kingdom: Cambridge University Press, 2020): Chapter 3.
9. EvaluatePharma. *Orphan Drug Report 2015*, 3rd ed. (October 2015). Available online: http://info.evaluategroup.com/rs/607-YGS-364/images/EPOD15.pdf. Accessed on November 16, 2020.
10. Figures from presentation by Eric Schmidt, PhD, to the Vagelos Life Sciences and Management Program (LSMP) at the Wharton School (November 2019).
11. James Chambers, Madison Silver, Flora Berklein, et al. "Orphan Drugs Offer Larger Health Gains but Less Favorable Cost-Effectiveness Than Non-orphan Drugs," *J Gen Intern Med.* 35 (2020): 2629-2636.

12. Ed Silverman. "Biosimilars Got the Cold Shoulder From Health Plans When It Came to Preferred Coverage," *Stat* (May 20, 2020).

13. This section on barriers to development of biosimilars is based on a presentation to HCMG 841 at The Wharton School in Fall 2019 by Michele Dragoescu, Sneha Hariharan, Kenneth Kasper, and Michael Kim.

14. Ed Silverman. "Debates Over Biosimilar Uptake Notwithstanding, Sales Growth Should Accelerate by 2024," *Stat* (March 9, 2020).

15. Lawton R. Burns, Sean Nicholson, and Joanna Wolkowski. "Pharmaceutical Strategy and the Evolving Role of Mergers and Acquisitions (M&A)," in Lawton R. Burns (Ed.), *The Business of Healthcare Innovation,* 2nd ed. (Cambridge, United Kingdom: Cambridge University Press, 2012): Chapter 3.

16. Gary Pisano. "The Hard Truth About Innovative Cultures," *Harvard Business Review* (January-February, 2019).

17. Nitin Nohria. *Amgen: Planning the Unplannable.* HBS Case # 9-492-052 (Boston, MA: Harvard Business School, 1992).

18. Gordon Binder and Philip Bashe. *Science Lessons: What the Business of Biotech Taught Me About Management* (Boston, MA: Harvard Business School, 2008).

19. Jason Rhodes. "Presentation to the Vagelos Life Science and Management Program (LSMP)," the Wharton School (November 2019).

20. This section is adapted from Lawton R. Burns and Philip A. Rea. "Organization of the Discovery Process," in Philip A. Rea, Mark V. Pauly, and Lawton R. Burns (Eds.), *Managing Discovery in the Life Sciences* (Cambridge, United Kingdom: Cambridge University Press, 2018): Chapter 15.

21. Such friction was likely more important in earlier periods when manufacturers co-located around physical resources (eg, steel companies located near sources of coal and iron ore).

22. Michael Porter. "Clusters and the New Economics of Competition," *Harvard Business Review* (November-December 1998): 77-90. Michael Porter. "Location, Competition, and Economic Development: Local Clusters in a Global Economy," *Econ Dev Q.* 14 (1) (2000): 15-34.

23. Ronald Stuart Burt. *Structural Holes* (Cambridge, MA: Harvard University Press, 1992). Ronald Stuart Burt. "Structural Holes and Good Ideas," *Am J Sociol.* 110 (2004): 349-399. David Obstfeld. "Social Networks, the Tertius Iungens Orientation, and Involvement in Innovation," *Admin Sci Q.* 50 (2005): 100-130.

24. Stuart Schweitzer, Judith Connell, and Fredric Schoenberg. "Clustering in the Biotechnology Industry," *Int J Healthc Technol Manag.* 7 (6) (2006): 554-566.

25. Man-Keun Kim, Thomas Harris, and Slavica Vusovic. "Efficiency Analysis of the US Biotechnology Industry: Clustering Enhances Productivity." Available online: https://agbioforum.org/v12n34/v12n34a17-kim.htm. Accessed on November 16, 2020. Stephan Goetz and R. Shannon Morgan. "State-level Locational Determinants of Biotechnology Firms," *Econ Dev Q.* 9 (2) (1995): 174-184. Linda Hall and Sharmistha Bagchi-Sen. "An Analysis of R&D, Innovation, and Business Performance in the US Biotechnology Industry," *Int J Biotechnol.* 3 (3) (2001): 1-10. Stephan Goetz and Anil Rupasingha. "High-Tech Industry Clustering: Implications for Rural Areas," *Am J Agricultural Econ.* 84 (5) (2002): 1229-1236. Joseph Cortright and Heike Mayer. *Signs of Life: The Growth of Biotechnology Centers in the United States* (Washington, DC: The Brookings Institution Center on Urban and Metropolitan Policy, 2002). Tapan Munroe, Gary Craft, and David Hutton. *A Critical Analysis of the Local Biotechnology Industry Cluster in Alameda, Contra Costa and Solano Counties* (Oakland, CA: East Bay Bioscience Study, 2002). Available online: http://eastbayeda.org/research_facts_figures/archived_studies.htm. Accessed on November 16, 2020. Slavica Vusovic. *State Level Location Determinants for Biotechnology Firms.* Unpublished Master's Thesis. (Reno, NV: Department of Resource Economics, University of Nevada, 2006).

26. Henry Etzkowitz and Loet Leydesdorff. "The Triple Helix: University-Industry-Government Relations: A Laboratory for Knowledge Based Economic Development," *EASST Rev.* 14 (1) (1995): 14-19. Ashley Stevens. "The Biopharmaceutical Industry in Massachusetts—The Triple Helix in Action," *J Biolaw Bus.* 10 (3) (2007): 3-10.

27. Michael Blanding. "The Past and Future of Kendall Square," *MIT Technology Review* (August 18, 2015). Available online: https://www.technologyreview.com/s/540206/the-past-and-future-of-kendall-square/. Accessed on May 30, 2016.

28. "The Biotechnology Industry: Clusterluck," *The Economist* (January 16, 2016). Available online: http://www.economist.com/node/21688385/print. Accessed on May 30, 2016.

29. Sharp's co-founder, Walter Gilbert, himself received the 1980 Nobel Prize for his work on DNA sequencing.

30. Michael Blanding. "The Past and Future of Kendall Square," *MIT Technology Review* (August 18, 2015). Available online: https://www.technologyreview.com/s/540206/the-past-and-future-of-kendall-square/. Accessed on May 30, 2016.

31. Thomas J. Allen. *Managing the Flow of Technology* (Cambridge, MA: MIT Press, 1977). Richard Pouder and Caron H. St. John. "Hot Spots and Blind Spots: Geographical Clusters of Firms and Innovation," *Acad Manag Rev.* 21 (1996): 1192-1225. Kiersten Bunker Whittington, Jason Owen-Smith, and Walter W. Powell. "Networks, Propinquity, and Innovation in Knowledge-Intensive Industries," *Admin Sci Q.* 54 (2009): 90-122.

32. The 9 regions are Boston-Worcester-Lawrence (MA-NH-ME-CT), San Francisco-Oakland-San Jose (CA), San Diego (CA), Raleigh-Durham-Chapel Hill (NC), Seattle-Tacoma-Bremerton (WA), New York-Northern New Jersey-Long Island (NY-NJ-CT-PA), Philadelphia-Wilmington, Atlantic City (PA-NJ-DE-MD), Los Angeles-Riverside-Orange County (CA), and Washington DC-Baltimore (DC-MD-VA-WV). Man-Keun Kim, Thomas Harris, and Slavica Vusovic. "Efficiency Analysis of the US Biotechnology Industry: Clustering Enhances Productivity," *AgBioForum.* 12 (3&4) (2009): 422-436.

33. Man-Keun Kim, Thomas Harris, and Slavica Vusovic. "Efficiency Analysis of the US Biotechnology Industry: Clustering Enhances Productivity," *AgBioForum.* 12 (3&4) (2009): 422-436.

34. Massachusetts Biotechnology Council. *2018 Industry Snapshot* (Cambridge, MA: MassBio, 2018).

35. Lev Facher. "Can New York's Biotech Scene Grab Some of that Kendall Square Magic?" *Stat* (December 13, 2016).

36. Kate Sheridan. "Foreign Governments Want to Boost their Biotech Industries—So They're Setting Up Shop in Boston," *Stat* (February 22, 2019).

37. Yi-Ling Liu. "Pharma Valley, China's Equivalent of Kendall Square, Is Expanding Rapidly," *Stat* (December 3, 2018).

# 23

# The MedTech Sector

## WHAT IS MEDTECH?

The label "MedTech," shorthand for medical technology, subsumes lots of disparate, technology-heavy sectors in healthcare. These include the following:

- Vascular intervention (VI): coronary stents
- Cardiac rhythm management (CRM): pacemakers, defibrillators
- Transcatheter heart valves
- Orthopedic implants (for hip and knee replacements)
- Surgical instruments
- Diagnostics
- Imaging equipment: x-ray machines, computed tomography (CT) scanners
- Robotics
- Nanomedicine

While imaging equipment has been used in hospitals since the early 20th century, the majority of medical products used through the mid-20th century were fairly primitive (eg, bandages, sutures).

This chapter focuses on "medical devices," which compose the bulk of revenues generated from MedTech sales. Figure 23-1 shows the upward trajectory in medical device innovation in the latter half of the 20th century, which parallels the rise in healthcare spending in the United States. The US Food and Drug Administration (FDA) defines a medical device as:

an instrument, apparatus, implement, machine, contrivance, implant, in vitro reagent, or other similar or related article . . . intended for use in the diagnosis

of disease or other conditions, or in the cure, mitigation, treatment, or prevention of disease, in man or other animals, or intended to affect the structure or any function of the body of man or other animals, and which does not achieve its primary intended purposes through chemical action within or on the body of man or other animals and which is not dependent upon being metabolized for the achievement of any of its primary intended purposes.

Medical devices became prominent with the development of the pacemaker in the 1950s by an engineer, Earl Bakken, who founded Medtronic, the largest MedTech firm today. Medtronic has since diversified to operate in 4 major medical device segments (Figure 23-2). Among these 4 segments, the largest in terms of 2017 revenues is cardiovascular ($10.5 billion), followed closely by minimally invasive therapies ($9.9 billion), restorative therapies ($7.5 billion), and diabetes ($1.8 billion).

## MEDTECH VERSUS PHARMA

Figures 20-6, 20-7, and 20-8 draw some sharp contrasts between the pharmaceutical and medical device sectors. There are several other important differences. Medical device innovation is "bedside to bench": Discoveries typically originate at the patient's bedside in the form of clinician recognition of unmet needs that device therapy might address. Such recognition subsequently gets communicated to engineers (once independent but now employed at MedTech

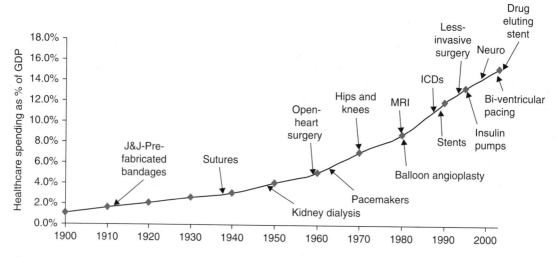

**Figure 23-1** • Medical Devices: A Relatively New Industry. GDP, Gross Domestic Product; ICD, Implantable Cardioverter-Defibrillator; MRI, Magnetic Resonance Imaging. (Source: Kurt Kruger, Presentation to the Wharton School, Fall 2006.)

firms) who conduct the "bench research" that translates this into product discoveries. By contrast, pharma is based on "bench to bed-side" research. Clinicians are thus more heavily involved in research and development (R&D) in MedTech discovery—a role evident across many of the MedTech product segments.[1] This observation highlights the "premise" of MedTech: to make a difference at the point of care in the hospital and solve the patients' clinical needs.

As a result, MedTech firms devote more effort to commercialization efforts to stay close to their physician customers and physician inventors (covered later). The clinician is also the major customer of the medical device firm and a key influencer in the decision on which product to use; by contrast, there is much less direct-to-consumer (DTC) advertising in Med-Tech. This makes marketing and sales channels much more efficient in MedTech since companies appeal to a much smaller number of clinicians at a handful of medical centers performing such procedures. This also makes marketing and sales relatively more important

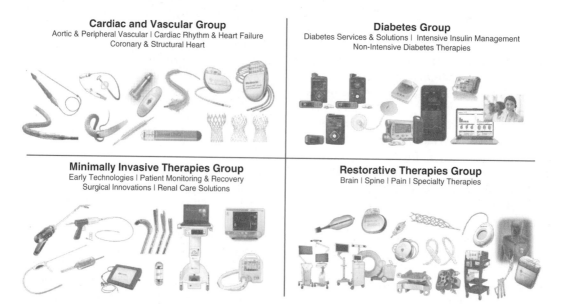

**Figure 23-2** • Four Technologies to Address Multiple Disease States and Conditions at Medtronic. (Source: Medtronic. Used with permission from Medtronic.)

for competitive success. Although the products of MedTech competitors are differentiated in terms of their features, they are perhaps less differentiated than the firms would like.[2] As a result, the firms also compete on differentiating their clinician sales and service functions.

Medical device innovation is much less costly than pharma innovation ($50-$100 million vs $1-$2.6 billion), partly due to the shorter product development cycle time (4-8 years vs 10-12 years) and partly due to the heavier reliance of MedTech firms on iteration and "incrementalism" in product development. Figure 23-3 illustrates the continual iterations of a core, mature technology such as pacemakers. Moreover, devices are subject to quality defects, while drugs are subject to side effects. Finally, the prices paid for MedTech products are typically borne by the hospital (the "institutional channel") rather than by the patient (the "retail channel"); this diminishes the role of consumerism and any understanding of the prices paid for medical devices. Such costs are buried in the hospital portion of the patient's bill and paid by Blue Cross or Medicare Part A.

## THE MEDTECH SECTOR TODAY

Figure 23-4 lists the largest MedTech sectors by 2017 global revenues: Orthopedics and cardiovascular are the largest 2 categories. Figure 23-5 lists some of the largest MedTech firms (2017 revenues). On average, sales in the United States compose half of their revenues, although there is a lot of variation across specific firms.[3] US-based firms derive the majority of their sales at home; conversely, non–US-based firms derive most of their sales outside of the United States. Firms prefer to sell to the United States because the consumption of medical devices per capita is much higher in the United States ($497) versus the rest of the world ($23). Similarly, the number of implanted devices and rates of implantation per million people are often much higher in the United States.

The general drivers of MedTech resemble the drivers of many of the other provider and technology sectors covered in this book. These include the aging of the population, the rise in chronic illness (which includes heart disease), growing obesity (which puts stress on the joints), and the explosive growth of the middle class in developing economies who can afford device therapy.

## TECHNOLOGICAL INNOVATION

A specific driver of the MedTech sector is the continual development (what Medtronic calls a "strong cadence") of new technologies and therapies to address unmet patient needs. Medtronic focuses on 3 core product areas that have historically served as the foundation of its cardiovascular segment: aortic and peripheral vascular (APV), cardiac rhythm and heart failure (CRHF), and coronary and structural heart (CSH). The future drivers of growth in these mature, core product areas, as well as in other product areas, are continuous innovation in existing products, invention of new products, and development of disruptive therapies (Figure 23-6). Other drivers include clinical research evidence that supports new patient indications warranting device therapies.

The "technological imperative" (covered in Chapter 20) characterizes this sector as well as the sectors covered in the prior 2 chapters. Over time, the basis of innovation has shifted from surgical tools *to* surgical implants *to* less invasive (ie, nonsurgical) therapies *to* robotics (eg, robotic surgery), implantable diagnostics (eg, sensors to measure blood pressure deep within the heart), implantable circuitry (to monitor and treat epilepsy), 3-dimensional printing, biomaterials, advanced energy, and nanomedicine (defined as the highly specific medical intervention at the nano-scale for screening, diagnosis, and treatment, such as improved cancer detection; see Figure 23-7 for some examples). Over time, the mix of scientific disciplines involved in such innovation has changed and diversified—from engineers and polymer scientists and computer scientists to now also include physical chemists, nanomolecular engineers, molecular biologists, and experts in bioinformatics. Some researchers have labeled this as "technological convergence."[4]

## BUSINESS MODEL INNOVATION

MedTechs have been forced to tweak their business models over time to satisfy new types of customers. The clinician is no longer the *sole* customer and, according to some observers, may be more of a *primus inter pares* (first among equals) in decision making. New influencers have emerged, including the hospital's vice-president for materials management (VPMM)

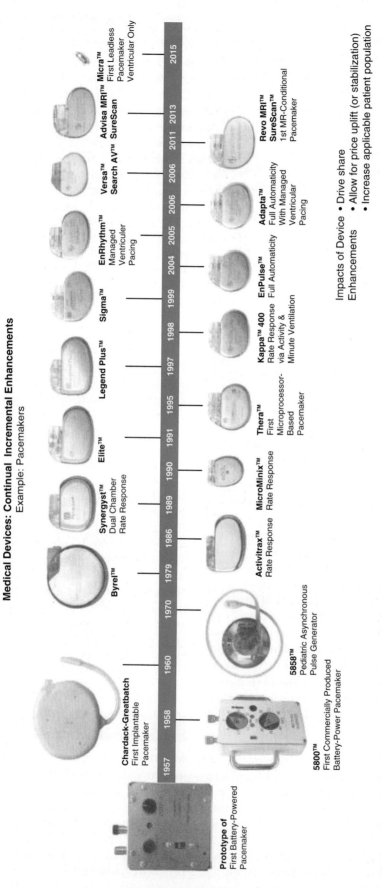

**Medical Devices: Continual Incremental Enhancements**
Example: Pacemakers

**Figure 23-3** • Continual Incremental Enhancements in Medical Devices: Pacemakers. (Source: Medtronic. Used with permission from Medtronic.)

| | Revenues ($billion) | Growth rate (%) |
|---|---|---|
| Orthopedics | 42.4 | 3.0 |
| Cardiovascular | 36.3 | 4.9 |
| General surgery | 18.5 | 5.0 |
| Ophthalmology | 16.5 | 3.3 |
| Urology, ENT, and respiratory | 9.9 | 8.2 |
| Diabetes Care | 9.5 | 9.6 |
| Neurological products (stim & vascular) | 4.6 | 12.9 |
| Robotic surgery | 3.9 | 16.6 |
| subtotal | 141.4 | 5.2 |
| Diagnostics | 41.4 | 5.0 |
| Imaging | 30.3 | 3.0 |
| subtotal | 71.6 | 4.1 |
| Total Medical Devices | 213.0 | 4.8 |
| Commodities/supplies | 116.8 | 3.5 |
| Grand total devices and supplies | 329.8 | 4.4 |

**Figure 23-4** • Major Categories of Medical Devices, 2017 Worldwide Revenues ($ Billion). ENT, Ear, Nose, and Throat. (Source: Figure 5.2, in Lawton R. Burns [Ed.], *The Business of Healthcare Innovation*, 3rd ed. Cambridge, United Kingdom: Cambridge University Press; 2020.)

who procures the technologies, the director of the cardiac cath lab or the administrator of the hospital's cardiovascular product line, and the hospital's chief financial officer (CFO), who pays the bills for the expensive technologies. These parties often seek to persuade clinicians to (1) consider both price and quality in their choice of medical devices, (2) switch from one device manufacturer to another manufacturer who offers a better deal, (3) choose the device they want as long as it fits under a price cap, or (4) choose a device from a hospital formulary.

| Company | Products | Revenues ($ billion) | Growth rate (%) |
|---|---|---|---|
| Medtronic Plc | Diversified | 29.6 | 0.8 |
| Abbott Laboratories | Diversified | 27.2 | 30.2 |
| Johnson & Johnson | Diversified | 26.6 | 5.9 |
| Danaher Corporation | Hospital Products | 18.2 | 8.2 |
| Stryker Corporation | Orthopedics | 12.4 | 9.6 |
| Becton, Dickinson and Company | Diversified | 12.2 | −1.1 |
| Baxter International Inc. | Diversified | 10.6 | 3.8 |
| Boston Scientific Corporation | Diversified | 9.0 | 8.1 |
| Zimmer Biomet Holdings, Inc. | Orthopedics | 7.8 | 1.2 |
| Terumo Corporation | Cardiovascular | 5.0 | 16.0 |
| Smith & Nephew Plc | Orthopedics | 4.8 | 1.9 |
| Edwards Lifesciences Corporation | Cardiovascular | 3.4 | 14.8 |
| Hologic, Inc. | Diversified | 3.1 | 8.7 |
| Intuitive Surgical, Inc. | Robotics | 3.1 | 14.7 |
| Varian Medical Systems, Inc. | Oncology | 2.6 | 0.0 |
| **Total** | | **175.6** | **8.2** |

Notes: J&J and Danaher are diversified, we show revenues for only medical devices/life sciences; J&J's revenues in 2017 include the acquisition of AMO; Abbott's revenues in 2017 include the acquisition of St. Jude Medical.

**Figure 23-5** • Large Medical Device Companies, 2017. (Source: Figure 5.6, in Lawton R. Burns [Ed.], *The Business of Healthcare Innovation*, 3rd ed. Cambridge, United Kingdom: Cambridge University Press; 2020.)

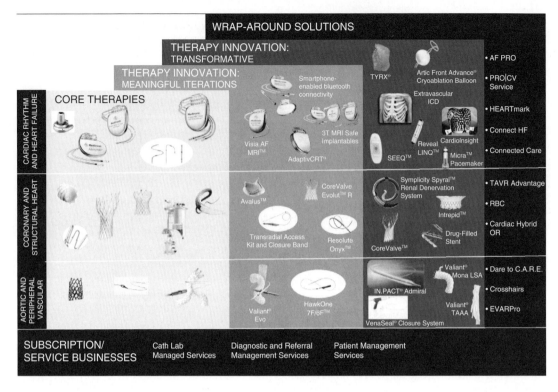

**Figure 23-6** • Technology Approach at Medtronic. (Source: Medtronic. Used with permission from Medtronic.)

In addition, value-based purchasing (VBP) has entered the MedTech space. The focus is now shifting from a clinician's preference for specific inputs used in a procedure (device, instruments) to many stakeholders' interest in improved patient outcomes, the cost of achieving those outcomes with a given technology, and other factors that can influence the effectiveness of any device (eg, product utilization levels, patient compliance, patient self-care behaviors). Large MedTech firms are responding to these dictates by offering not only new products but also new services (wrap-around programs and innovative solutions) to help hospitals manage their way

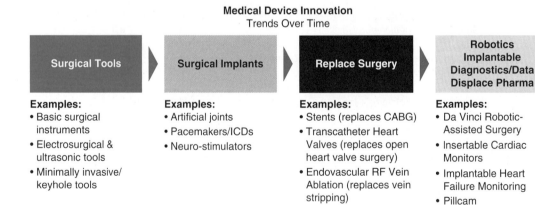

**Figure 23-7** • Medical Device Innovation Trends Over Time. CABG, Coronary Artery Bypass Graft; ICD, Implantable Cardioverter-Defibrillator; RF, Radiofrequency. (Source: Medtronic. Used with permission from Medtronic.)

through VBP. These include new products to "optimize therapy" to deal with risk-based payments, new services to help hospitals manage under bundled payments (which are typically targeted at cardiovascular and orthopedic patients), and new programs to help hospitals manage their chronically ill patients (eg, diabetics).

As one example, Medtronic developed its TYRX Absorbable Antibacterial Envelope to reduce the incidence of infections (and the extra cost of managing them) following implantation of electronic cardiac devices; Medtronic shares (with the payer or the hospital) in both the risk (rewards) of higher (lower) patient utilization.[5] Other examples include MedTech's management of a hospital's cardiac catheterization lab or heart failure clinic. In making this transition, MedTech is taking on several new roles beyond technology leader. These include the following:

- Become a value-based healthcare provider with the hospital
- Help hospitals to improve quality and reduce costs of care
- Manage risk sharing as a partner with providers
- Bundle technology products with consulting and management services
- Develop informatics systems
- Become disease specialists
- Manage hospital logistics
- Serve as a capital partner to cash-strapped providers

The "jury is out" regarding the ability of MedTechs to make such transitions and earn service-based revenues comparable to product-based sales. Researchers have noted several headwinds to the transformation to "value," including the limited spread of risk-based and value-based payment, the mixed evidence on the performance of bundled payment, the enormous "hype" surrounding VBP without commensurate supporting evidence, the "quality tower of babble" (see Chapter 1), and providers' difficulty in measuring and managing quality.[6] Other likely problems include difficulties in (1) generating scale economies and efficiencies providing services (which rest on using MedTech personnel to work with providers); (2) working with hospitals' physicians who may not want to learn from MedTech; and (3) cross-selling of products and services (ie, being a "one-stop shop"). MedTechs have

attempted risk contracting in prior decades without much success and do not see much current success with the types of contracts that pharma has entered. VBP represents a long-term strategic bet for MedTech in an area that is a huge departure from their base in product innovation. Finally, the proliferation of stakeholders inside a given hospital means more "points of call" for the MedTech sales representative and more loci of contention in reaching any agreement.

## THE TWIN PILLARS IN ACTION

Like the technological sectors covered in Chapters 21 and 22, MedTech rests on 2 pillars: *product* development and *market* development (commercialization). The former entails the development of innovative technological features, the ability of these technologies and features to meet unmet clinical needs, R&D activities, clinical trials of new products, development of intellectual property, and management of regulatory and reimbursement processes. The latter entails product launch, the sales force to support the product launch and promote the technology's adoption (eg, by informing physicians about new device products to treat new patients indicated for such products by the clinical trials), product training and feedback, and cultivation of relationships with physician customers.

Each pillar is necessary but insufficient; both pillars are synergistic and reinforcing. However, in terms of timelines, tackling the first pillar absorbs many more years; Figure 23-8 illustrates the total development time for a particular VI device, the drug-eluting stent. Moreover, these 2 pillars are supported by a host of corporate strategies, internal management capabilities, and risk management efforts to mitigate threats against them. These activities are illustrated in an extended description of VI products in the following sections.

### Value Drivers in Vascular Intervention

Several large MedTechs have historically developed, manufactured, and sold 4 categories of products used in VI: coronary stents, balloon dilatation catheters, guidewires, and guiding catheters. Such products grew in prominence with the introduction of 3 major advances in treating coronary artery disease (CAD) between the late 1970s and early 2000s:

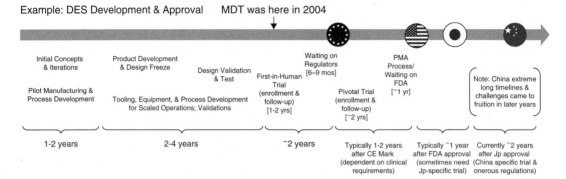

**How Quickly Can You Develop & Release a New Product?**
Cycle Time Depends on Complexity

Example: DES Development & Approval      MDT was here in 2004

| | | |
|---|---|---|
| Initial Concepts & Iterations | Product Development & Design Freeze | |
| Pilot Manufacturing & Process Development | Tooling, Equipment, & Process Development for Scaled Operations; Validations | Design Validation & Test |

First-in-Human Trial (enrollment & follow-up) [1-2 yrs]

Waiting on Regulators [6–9 mos]

Pivotal Trial (enrollment & follow-up) [~2 yrs]

PMA Process/ Waiting on FDA [~1 yr]

Note: China extreme long timelines & challenges came to fruition in later years

| 1-2 years | 2-4 years | ~2 years | Typically 1-2 years after CE Mark (dependent on clinical requirements) | Typically ~1 year after FDA approval (sometimes need Jp-specific trial) | Currently ~2 years after Jp approval (China specific trial & onerous regulations) |
|---|---|---|---|---|---|

• Higher risk medical devices ("Class III") have a more onerous approval path than lower risk ("Class II" and "Class I").

• Traditionally, European regulatory approval (CE Mark) is first path to market.

• Note: new European regulation changes (in process) making this much more difficult; simultaneously FDA is trying to ease the process, at least for early feasibility of new technology.

**Figure 23-8** • How Quickly Can You Develop and Release a New Product? DES, Drug-Eluting Stent; FDA, US Food and Drug Administration; PMA, Premarket Approval. (Source: Medtronic. Used with permission from Medtronic.)

angioplasty, bare metal stents (BMS), and drug-eluting stents (DES).

CAD results from atherosclerosis, which is the development of plaque on the inside surface of coronary artery walls that prevents oxygen transport to the myocardium and results in damage to the myocardial tissue (myocardial infarction, or heart attack). Prior to 1977, the gold standard of treatment for CAD was coronary artery bypass with graft (CABG) surgery.[7]

In 1977, Dr. Andreas Gruentzig introduced balloon angioplasty, also known as percutaneous transluminal coronary angioplasty (PTCA) or percutaneous coronary interventions (PCI).[8] During PTCA, the physician inserted a guiding catheter into the femoral artery in the thigh and then advanced it to the sclerotic coronary artery. The physician next advanced a stainless steel guidewire through the guiding catheter to the aorta aided by fluoroscopy and then delivered a balloon dilatation catheter over the guidewire through the inside of the guiding catheter. The balloon was inflated and deflated several times to crack the plaque and compress it against the wall, thereby restoring blood flow.

Angioplasty was much less invasive and expensive than CABG and involved less procedural time. As a result, by the 1990s, PTCA procedures supplanted CABGs and fueled the growth of products used in PTCA procedures (stents, dilatation catheters, guidewires, and guiding catheters). By the early 2000s, PTCA procedures

(1 million in the United States, 2.2 million globally) dwarfed the number of CABG procedures (300,000 in the United States, 500,000 globally).[9]

Julio Palmaz developed a BMS that (1) improved upon PTCA by inserting a tubular metal scaffold inside the artery wall to prevent restenosis (the re-narrowing of the vessel cavity due to elastic recoil) and (2) improved upon an earlier stent design by adding a heparin coating that reduced subacute thrombosis. BMS sales rose dramatically with the reduction in restenosis rates from 25% to 35% (under PTCA) to 20% to 25%. By 1999, 84% of PCIs involved stenting.[10] The 2003 introduction of the DES—a BMS covered with a polymer that transported a drug and regulated its release kinetics—dramatically reduced restenosis rates down to the single digits.

## Company Value

Wall Street analysts, investors, and consultants place a premium on growth in earnings in evaluating the attractiveness of a sector.[11] MedTech's strategy can be expressed in straightforward language: increase the quantity of *newly* developed devices sold at a premium price (high average selling price [ASP]). An estimated 50% to 60% of MedTech's revenues historically come from products less than 12 months old.[12] MedTechs maintain premium pricing, resist price discounting, and avoid or delay commoditization pursuing the twin pillars of *product* and *market* development. This requires a continual stream of new products and/or new features that physicians want, that are differentiated from the product features found in competitors' devices, and that are supported by customer service from sales representatives.

## Pillar I: New Technology/ Product Development

### Technology and Technical Features

Cardiovascular medical devices constituted a large share of Class III products approved by the FDA between 1992 and 2007 (see box titled "FDA Classification of Medical Devices"). Such advances are covered by premarket approvals (PMAs) and PMA supplements. PMAs comprise approvals of first-time market entry by innovative medical devices on a product level; supplements cover changes to them. Of the 456 Class III approvals, 145 were for cardiovascular devices. Of these 145 approvals, the highest number (65 of 145) was awarded to VI products such as stents and catheter systems (eg, BMS and DES).

---

### FDA Classification of Medical Devices

Low-risk medical devices (Class I) are usually exempt from regulatory review. Class II medical devices that have substantial equivalence to an already existing device require a premarket notification [known as 510(k)]. The 510(k) pathway promotes evolutionary enhancements by providing a quicker pathway to market for newer versions of legally marketed lower-risk devices. Class III devices, involving higher risk, are approved using a PMA process. According to the FDA, Class III products are defined as those that support or sustain human life, are of substantial importance in preventing impairment of human health, or present a potential, unreasonable risk of illness or injury. The review process for such products requires a demonstration of clinical safety and efficacy based on clinical trials. In contrast to 510(k) approvals for lower-risk (Class II) devices, the approval times for Class III devices are longer and more costly but may yield higher market returns.

---

### BMS Products

BMS are mesh-like metal tubes that serve to prop open arteries. They vary in their length, diameter/profile, metal composition, architecture (eg, slotted vs coiled/modular configuration), scaffolding (ie, number and thickness of struts), and manufacturing technique. Such differences affect their deliverability, flexibility, steerability in navigating blood vessels, and radiopacity (ie, visibility under fluoroscopy imaging).

Early stents were limited in their radiopacity and suffered from trade-offs in their strength versus flexibility. The *Palmaz-Schatz* stent was strong and stable enough to function as a scaffold within the vessel and resist its natural tendency to recoil. However, it was not flexible enough to easily wind its way through the patient's vasculature to reach the target lesion.[13] These features—a by-product of its manufacturing technique—made it difficult for the average physician to use and required lots of skill. Subsequent BMS products engineered a better combination of flexibility (strut thickness) and strength that physicians preferred, even though they were higher in price.[14] Later-generation stents made out of cobalt chromium had a potentially superior stent platform compared to earlier-generation stainless steel stents due to improved deliverability (eg, via thinner struts, a lower profile, and continued radiopacity), which required smaller incisions and enjoyed easier navigation to the aorta.

Some stents reportedly had high ease of use due to their more flexible slotted tube, a rapid exchange system for the balloon catheter (described later), and multiple lengths.[15] Nevertheless, despite these improvements, BMS stent technology slowly converged in the early 2000s, leading to greater competition and pricing pressures. For MedTech firms with a VI franchise, the objectives shifted to building capabilities in commercialization such as product launch, sales representative coverage, and training sales managers.

### DES Products

DES products applied a polymer coating to the BMS platform that bonded with, transported, and released a drug to prevent restenosis. Competing DES products used different drugs to coat their stent—sirolimus (used by J&J), paclitaxel (Boston Scientific), and everolimus (Guidant)—as well as different drug dosages, drug kinetics (ie, rate of drug elution), and thicknesses in the polymer coating.[16] Other differentiators included greater radiopacity and thinner struts, which reduced stent size, increased stent deliverability, and reduced late-stage thrombosis.[17] According to physicians, DES success depended on all 3 DES components (stent platform, polymer, and agent) as well as on the interactions among them.[18]

### Balloon Dilatation Catheters

Balloon materials varied in their ability to maintain their shape, available sizes, push-ability, and track-ability. More importantly, balloon catheters varied in their delivery systems. The 2 major alternative systems were balloons delivered (1) "over the wire" and (2) via "rapid exchange."[19] These systems are described next.

### Guidewires and Guiding Catheters

Guidewires were very important during the early days of balloon angioplasty. Gruentzig's initial angioplasty product required a 4-hour procedure due to the lack of a steerable guidewire. In 1982, John Simpson developed the over-the-wire (OTW) delivery system using a steerable guidewire to help place the angioplasty catheter.[20] The OTW delivery system required a guidewire roughly 10 feet long and 2 people to handle it. In 1991, while working with John Simpson, Paul Yock developed the rapid exchange system, which shortened the guidewire and required only a single person to operate both the catheter and the guidewire. It was preferred due to ease of use, ability to quickly exchange catheters during the procedure, and improved deliverability. Rapid exchange subsequently became the state-of-the-art delivery system for PTCAs by the mid-2000s.

### Component Strength

According to analysts, companies making VI products differed in their relative strength across these components. One firm was strong in balloons; another was strong in stents (BMS initially, DES later on) and guide catheters; a third was strong in BMS, balloons, and wires.[21] MedTech firms often lacked a rapid exchange delivery system, which roughly 50% of the market used.[22] The development of DES products thus heavily relied on intercompany alliances to access the needed technology, share the costs of development, and reduce risk.

## Ability to Address Unmet Clinical Needs

The introduction of PTCA marked a radical improvement in the treatment of CAD over medication therapy by keeping open blocked arteries and eliminating the need for invasive surgery, its attendant costs, and patient trauma. The subsequent introduction of stent products further reduced the incidence of angiographic restenosis (ie, >50% narrowing of a previously treated site), the need for subsequent follow-up procedures (eg, PTCA), and the patient's level of chest pain. DES's ability to lower restenosis rates conferred significant value to patients, including lower risk of repeat procedures, reduced need to take a daily medication, and reduced chest pain.[23] There was also a significant value advantage to the implanting physician, including better patient outcomes (see later discussion), greater durability of the procedure's results, and potentially greater patient referrals.[24]

## R&D and Product Development

### R&D Spending

R&D spending composes one-third of the medical device firm's stock price.[25] Such spending serves as a leading indicator of the product pipeline, future sales and earnings, and future market share. R&D spending supports basic and applied research, product development, clinical trials, and regulatory affairs, which in turn exert a major impact on customer demand, product sales, and revenue growth. R&D investment is critical for MedTechs, especially as the cost of acquiring external innovation via acquisition rises.

### Product Platform Strategy

Devices are systems of components packaged together into product "platforms" or "families." Device companies crafted the product platform strategy by the early 1990s to overcome their historical "disabilities in development": ad hoc product development, incongruous development cycles, and excessive customization of components (and its high costs) across product models.[26] By contrast, the platform serves as the common "hardware" for multiple product generations that can leverage the product line and reduce development costs.

Platforms serve as a foundation for technological advancement in the longer term (3-5 years) and a springboard for iterative change in platform features in the shorter term (1-3 years).[27] Platforms serve as the major source of product differentiation; iterative innovation within the platform can serve as a second source of differentiation, an effort to maintain market leadership, or an effort to gain parity with rivals that pioneer incremental changes.

A MedTech's platform strategy is its key to product leadership and competitive success. Platforms are introduced every 2 to 3 years to alter the playing field; in between, the company needs to deliver meaningful new product iterations in a predictable fashion. In this manner, the device firm pursues "rhythm" (periodicity) in its product launches that is rapid and predictable.[28] This provides the sales representatives with a continual flow of "new toys in the bag" to show and interest physician customers, as well as reinforce the firm's image as an innovator in the eyes of the physicians who adopt the technology.[29] It also helps to increase market share.[30]

The medical device firm's value is thus the sum of R&D investments in new technological platforms, the accumulation of smaller technical advances in product iterations between platform redesigns, and the resulting increase in revenues from the continual sale of new products. Analysts refer to this as "cumulative innovation with differentiation."[31] The cumulative effect of this continued innovation is manifold: image as an innovator, product differentiation, growth, increased revenues, and the ability to offer flexible pricing (higher prices on new models and lower prices on slightly older models). Due to the pace of innovation, product portfolio development may be more important than patent protection.[32] Product portfolio development also trumps marketing; in fact, "marketing" is referred to as "what you do when you have no real innovation."[33] As noted earlier, a large percentage of a MedTech's sales derive from new products introduced in the past year or two.

### Intellectual Property

Innovation is a major contributor to the creation of intangible assets of MedTechs. Firms protect intangible assets through the generation of intellectual property (IP) such as patents. Nevertheless, the value conferred by IP is bounded by several factors. These include the shorter product life cycles, common platform technologies, the product iteration strategies used by most major companies, the infrequent use of randomized controlled trials (RCTs), the lack of "data exclusivity" periods, and weaker market exclusivity protection.

### Clinical Trials

Investments in RCTs, expertise in trial design and execution, and favorable trial results are important drivers of new approvals, product flow, and earnings.[34] Favorable results—presented at professional meetings and published in peer-reviewed journals—constitute important clinical milestones that serve to motivate physician adoption. Physicians who treat CAD are used to large-scale RCTs of drugs and may need to see comparable trial results of medical devices in order to recommend device therapies. RCTs also provide patient outcome data needed to persuade the FDA to approve new products, the Centers for Medicare and Medicaid Services (CMS) to reimburse them, and CMS to possibly expand device coverage to new patient populations.

Results from the RCTs not only increase the volume of devices sold but also support premium pricing. Compelling clinical outcomes, economic outcomes, and the ability to substitute for a more costly inpatient episode support high device prices.

## Management of the Regulatory and Reimbursement Processes

Management of the FDA review process is a related capability.[35] Because the FDA has limited resources and staffing, device firms need to dialogue with FDA reviewers about their products on an ongoing basis to reduce cycle times and accelerate the time-to-market process. This dialogue can include the most appropriate classification of the medical device, the regulatory pathway to pursue [510(k) vs PMA], the appropriate clinical studies to conduct (if needed), subject selection, clinical endpoints to be achieved, the necessary types of studies and documentation to include in the regulatory submission, and postapproval reporting guidelines.

Medical device companies and inventors also need to focus on securing reimbursement in tandem with regulatory approval. This involves determining the clinical setting in which the device will be used, analyzing coverage for prior products and related procedures, and identifying the appropriate procedure codes and reimbursement rates. This information assists them in establishing prices for their devices. MedTech firms also conduct coding and reimbursement seminars to train hospital personnel on proper coding for the DES procedure to minimize errors and increase hospital revenues. Finally, like pharmaceutical manufacturers, MedTech firms are seeking value-based contracts with hospital providers to try to ensure continued adoption of their products (see the following Critical Thinking Exercise box).

Like other MedTechs and many pharmaceutical companies, Medtronic has pushed to develop value-based contracts (VBCs) with hospital providers. Medtronic's efforts are chronicled in a recent Harvard Business School case.[36] Medtronic believed that if hospitals were increasingly subjected to demonstrating "value" (eg, higher quality and/or lower cost), then Medtronic would thrive to the extent it helped its hospital customers, which meant that both parties would need to be accountable for the value of the products and services used in patient care.

For its part, Medtronic believed it needed to engage in risk-sharing contracts with providers (where it would share its clinical expertise and ability to improve patient outcomes) as well as participate in providers' bundled payment programs and chronic care management programs. A signature Medtronic VBC effort was its TYRX Antibacterial Envelope, an implantable mesh that was designed to wrap around and stabilize the placement of a cardiac implantable electronic device and thereby reduce the risk of infections. The product would not only reduce the cost of treating postsurgical infections but also lower patient mortality rates. Medtronic believed that such products would help hospitals to improve their quality, reduce their costs, and earn shared savings from public and private insurers, which then could be shared with Medtronic.

What "tailwinds" does Medtronic enjoy to help them with this strategic move? What "headwinds" does it face? Is VBC a product or a service? How successful have product manufacturers been at selling products and services together in bundles? Do such bundles mark a significant change in the type of customer that Medtronic now needs to deal with?

## Pillar II: Commercialization and Market Development

Commercialization and market development include product launch and execution, the key role of the sales force, product training and feedback, and cultivation of relationships with physician customers. The importance of these activities is evident in the VI market.

### Product Launch and Execution

Product launch efficiency translates into earlier and higher sales by virtue of penetrating the market ahead of a competitor or eating into an incumbent's existing market share. Launch execution is very important in the VI segment due to some of the shortest product development life cycles in the device market.[37] Successful launch depends on 2 specific activities: create awareness and anticipation ahead of product launch, and cultivate key opinion leaders in the medical community and on Wall Street.[38] These activities are described in the following sections.

#### Build Awareness

To build awareness and anticipation, MedTechs painted restenosis as the biggest problem in cardiovascular medicine at cardiology conferences, education seminars, and public relations efforts.

They offered continuing medical education to interventional cardiologists and their nurses on their DES products, explained the method of action in their DES and the science behind the technology, and presented evidence drawn from 40 clinical studies. The database supporting the superiority of DES encompassed 6 years of worldwide safety and efficacy data, making it perhaps the most extensively studied stent. Over a 2-year period, they issued 42 major media announcements beginning with phase II data, the announcement of the brand name, completion of enrollment in its RCTs, and announcement of the RCT results. MedTech's efforts left the impression that using any other product would be tantamount to medical malpractice.

#### Cultivate Key Opinion Leaders

Medical device companies seek to cultivate "key opinion leaders" (KOLs; eg, high-volume implanters, physicians who give frequent clinical presentations, and/or physicians who are highly influential among their peers). KOLs play an important role in building the market for VI products. They can help design and conduct the RCTs to have a higher probability of success; they can provide credibility and visibility to the RCT results; they can highlight the product's superiority; and they can influence their colleagues to adopt the device. MedTechs also seek to demonstrate the market potential of their products to another set of KOLs—Wall Street analysts that follow MedTechs—via presentations at investment banking conferences and participation in earnings calls.

## Key Role of the Sales Force

The sales force is a key component of market development by virtue of their ability to (1) stimulate demand for devices among physicians to treat the anticipated influx of new patients and patient conditions indicated in RCT results, and (2) sell the competitive advantages of the company's technologies and components to physicians (eg, using educational materials based on RCT results) and thereby grow the business.[39]

Competitive advantage in commercialization is largely based on having accessible and knowledgeable sales representatives, strong training programs for physicians and their staff, customer service, and customer loyalty. Indeed, loyalty to the sales representative can sometimes outweigh loyalty to the company.[40] Strategies focus on increasing customer intimacy, key account management, increasing the number of sales representatives, clinical efficacy messaging, and promotion. Sales force efforts to cultivate physician preference can also serve to blunt the efforts of centralized purchasers (eg, group purchasing organizations [GPOs], hospital systems) that seek to discount pricing on less differentiated CRM products.[41]

In general, if firms maintain technological parity with their competitors, they may gain competitive advantage through sales and service.[42] Similarly, during periods of innovation slowdown, sales representatives' efforts can help the device firm to maintain or gain market share by converting physicians to their product line.

## Product Training and Feedback

### Product Training and Fellowship Programs
Medical devices and their electronics are complex technologies. Both referring physicians (demand side) and implanting physicians (supply side) require education and training to increase their awareness, understanding, and selection of devices. On the demand side, sales representatives may need to educate primary care physicians about the new capabilities of devices that allow doctors to manage their patients and thus increase the likelihood of referring their patients

to cardiologists who implant the devices. On the supply side, sales representatives offer training to implanting clinicians on new technologies along with continued education on product launches and addition of new features.

MedTechs may complement physician training with a "Fellows Program"—that is, a dedicated field organization that targets fellows (postresidency trainees) as a central customer and funds fellowship programs to increase the supply of specialists who could implant their products. MedTechs also use "institute programs" to train practicing physicians on their device therapy.

### Product Feedback
MedTechs sometimes tie new product launches to gathering physician feedback on their devices via physician surveys and evaluations. Such surveys provide "key learnings" to help with subsequent product development and training. It can also be used to publish case studies and abstracts that drive adoption among other physicians.

Sales representatives serve as a conduit of information to the clinician, as well as an information channel back to the device company on how well the launch is working and what product design and performance features might be changed. They can also convey information from clinicians on unmet clinical needs that new devices might be able to address, along with the clinician's suggestions for technologies that might address those unmet needs.

Physician input and feedback can provide a lot of good ideas for product development and form a large part of a MedTech's R&D effort. Some analysts estimate that the majority (up to 80%) of the initial ideas for new and important medical device advances come from the physician end-user, not from the internal R&D of the MedTech.[43] This requires that the company's sales force and engineers have not only *good* relationships with the outside clinician community but also *extensive* relationships with them that require a high "coverage ratio" by the firm's sales representatives. Market development thus spans the thousands of linkages that the sales representatives and product engineers have with practicing cardiologists.

## Physician Customer Relationships

### Array of Physician Customers
For VI procedures such as stent implantations, the main customer is the interventional cardiologist; cardiac surgeons, by contrast, are more

heavily involved in CABG and valve procedures. Interventional cardiologists are some of the fastest adopters of innovative devices and among the clinicians who work most closely with MedTechs. They are also part of a clinical specialty that heavily relies on evidence-based medicine (EBM) and RCT data to assess new technology. EBM has increasingly become an important consideration in the physician's decision to use a device and thus in the market penetration achieved by that device. Med-Techs frequently distinguish their physician core customer from the patients treated by the physician. This is because most patients have little brand awareness and no brand preference and thus leave the decision regarding choice of implant to their physicians.

Although the main VI customer is the interventional cardiologist, a secondary customer is the director of the cardiac cath lab or cardiovascular product line. The cardiologist exercises discretion over the choice of technology, whereas the cath lab or product line director focuses more on pricing and negotiation. VI technology vendors were historically selected on the basis of having the best products (technology). Cath lab directors may place importance on the device company having a broad line of interventional cardiology products, which allows for simpler contracting, improved tracking and management of inventory, opportunities to standardize and save money, the possibility of vendor partnerships, and greater bargaining power.

### Physician Customer Segments

MedTechs can segment their physician customers in several ways. One method is to categorize physicians as "service-oriented spenders" (ie, price-insensitive implanters who value the services of knowledgeable sales representatives), "price-sensitive technologists" (ie, want the latest technology, don't want to pay for it, and do not value sales representative relationships), or "traditionalists" (ie, value relationships with sales representatives). Another method is to cross-classify physicians by their practice size (eg, solo practice, 2-5 physicians) and setting (open, closed, or academic). Some MedTechs also segment physicians in terms of their implant experience and customer loyalty or the strength of the MedTech's relationship with the executives of the hospitals in which they perform their procedures.

## Pillar Supports: Corporate Strategy, Internal Management, and Risk Management

### Corporate Strategy

Supporting their twin pillar efforts, MedTechs use several corporate strategies to increase firm value. These include mergers and acquisitions (M&A) and diversification.

#### Mergers and Acquisitions

M&A allows the firm to acquire new products from the outside (inorganic growth) to bolster R&D if the firm cannot develop new products internally (organic growth). Much of the new innovation in device technology comes from smaller start-up firms that serve as feeders to the technology pipelines of the larger firms. Larger firms compete with one another to buy the start-up firms. Figure 23-9 illustrates how Medtronic grew "inorganically" via M&A, joint ventures, and partnerships; Figure 23-10 shows that M&A continues as a steady trend in the medical device sector. In terms of the number of M&A transactions, the most active "mass mergerers" have been Stryker and Medtronic. In terms of transaction values, the most active players have been Medtronic, Abbott Labs, and Becton Dickinson.[44]

M&A can confer other benefits. An acquisition increases the size of the firm's sales force, increases the scope of its "face to the customer," and increases product breadth that puts "more toys in the bag" of the sales representative. That is, acquisitions can increase the firm's market access to clinician and hospital customers, as well as help with potential cross-selling synergies. More sales representatives allow the firm to enter new geographic territories, gain or retain market share, and conduct market development by seeking to stimulate demand.

M&A plays a major role in the development of VI franchises, particularly as larger firms acquire smaller firms with innovative technology. Competition in stents from the outset has been defined by acquiring, rather than developing, new technology. As one illustration, Medtronic pursued 2 acquisitions during the 1998 to 2000 period to build its VI franchise: AVE (BMS stents) and PercuSurge (guidewires). Abbott acquired Guidant's VI business from Boston Scientific to enter the DES market.

| Company | Business Unit | Fiscal Year | Type |
|---|---|---|---|
| HeartWare | CVG | 2017 | Purchase |
| Intact Medical | RTG | 2017 | Purchase |
| NOK (Nederlandse Obesitas Kliniek) | MTG | 2017 | Acquire majority ownership (51%) |
| Smith & Nephew Plc | MITG | 2017 | Purchase SNN Gynecology Business |
| Mazor Robotics | RTG | 2017 | Partnership |
| Qualcomm Life | Diabetes | 2017 | Partnership |
| Team Spine MN | RTG | 2017 | |
| Renova Group (Stentex JV) | CVG | 2017 | Joint Venture |
| Responsive Orthopedics, LLC | RTG | 2017 | Purchase |
| Bellco | MITG | 2016 | Purchase |
| IOOS | CVG | 2016 | |
| Baylis Medical | RTG | 2016 | Acquire OsteoCool Device Technology |
| Aircraft Medical | MITG | 2016 | Purchase |
| Cardiored S.A. | CVG | 2016 | |
| Twelve | CVG | 2016 | Purchase |
| Lazarus Effect | RTG | 2016 | Purchase |
| Agentek | Diabetes | 2016 | |
| Medina Medical | RTG | 2016 | Purchase |
| Saudi JV | CVG | 2016 | |
| RF Surgical | MITG | 2016 | Purchase |
| CardioInsight | CVG | 2016 | Purchase |
| Intruventional Inc | MITG | 2016 | |
| Aptus Endosystems | CVG | 2016 | Purchase |
| Arsenal Investments | CVG | 2015 | Debt Investment |
| BDX | Diabetes | 2015 | Partnership |
| Glooko | Diabetes | 2015 | Partnership |
| IBM Watson Health | Diabetes | 2015 | Partnership |
| Diabeter | Diabetes | 2015 | Purchase |
| Sophono | RTG | 2015 | Purchase |
| Advanced Uro-Solutions | Neuro | 2015 | Purchase |
| Covidien | Corp | 2015 | Purchase |

**Figure 23-9 •** Inorganic Mergers and Acquisitions Growth at Medtronic. (Source: Medtronic company documents.)

| | 2013 | 2014 | 2015 | 2016 | 2017 |
|---|---|---|---|---|---|
| Total number of transactions | 166 | 191 | 225 | 251 | 240 |
| Number of transactions over $50m | 37 | 41 | 64 | 50 | 44 |
| Number of transactions over $250m | 15 | 15 | 21 | 19 | 16 |
| Total value of transactions over $250m | 11.6 | 85.5 | 22.7 | 59.9 | 42.0 |

**Figure 23-10 •** Mergers and Acquisitions (M&A) in Medical Devices (Actual Numbers and Transaction Value, $ Billions). (Source: Figure 5.22, in Lawton R. Burns [Ed.], *The Business of Healthcare Innovation*, 3rd ed. Cambridge, United Kingdom: Cambridge University Press; 2020.)

To be sure, M&A strategies are often supplemented by internal R&D efforts. Many large MedTechs acquired the first-generation product externally and then innovated subsequent iterations via internal R&D programs.[45] Ironically, competition for external acquisitions increases their transaction prices, thereby increasing the value of internal R&D investments.

*Diversification*

A second popular strategy—*diversification*—is often used by MedTech firms to span a wider number of anatomical areas in their product portfolios (Figure 23-11). Diversification can confer technological and commercial advantages that support the twin pillars.[46] On the technological side, diversification may confer scope economies in the manufacturing and product development process and increase the firm's attractiveness to entrepreneurs that have developed new technologies that fit well with the firm's broad product portfolio. On the commercial side, a diversified portfolio may appeal to clinical customers. It also helps the firm to address patient comorbidities and develop an integrated approach to tackling patient diseases. Finally, diversification can foster growth when antitrust laws limit further horizontal mergers within industry segments.[47]

Diversification played an important role in the development of DES products. J&J's lead in DES was partly based on its ability to screen 600+ drug compounds in house before it settled on sirolimus.[48] In a similar fashion, Abbott's success in DES rested on combining its pharmaceutical capability with the Guidant vascular business (acquired from Boston Scientific) to enter the DES market. J&J and Abbott had in-house expertise and experience with drugs, whereas competitors had to rely on time-consuming alliances to source the drug components and expend effort to handle the complex science (analytical chemistry, pharmacology, pharmacokinetics), the higher clinical hurdles, and higher regulatory hurdles.[49]

Finally, diversification and the ability to offer a broad product portfolio may reduce the transaction costs with large hospital systems and GPOs. That is, it can simplify contracting, improve convenience in procurement, enhance efficiency in inventory management, allow for standardization in stocking and product training, and offer the possibility of both cross-selling synergies (for the seller) and discounts across a bundle of products (for the buyer). It can thus help MedTechs to combat consolidation on the buyer side, to blunt efforts by GPOs and hospital systems to "rationalize" (ie, reduce)

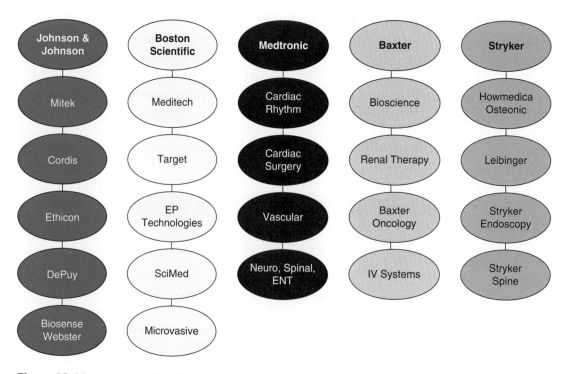

**Figure 23-11** • Anatomical Diversification via Mergers and Acquisitions. ENT, Ear, Nose, and Throat; IV, Intravenous.

the number of product vendors for contracting, and to appeal to economic customers looking for a product bundling capability.[50]

## Internal Management

The history of many successful MedTechs demonstrates the importance of internal management processes for product innovation, sales execution, and firm performance. Guidant maintained a "start-up mentality"[51] that featured a willingness to invest in long-term product development, relentless pursuit of new technology, a product family (ie, platform) approach to product innovation, efficient low-cost management, lean manufacturing, and development of organizational systems to measure performance, incentivize employees, and mitigate risks (covered later).[52]

Given the other value drivers discussed earlier, successful device firms must be able to develop strong internal managerial processes in the face of large company size, diversified product portfolios, and large sales forces.[53] Growing size multiplies the amount of complexity to be managed and the risks to the enterprise (covered next). There is some evidence that large medical device firms enjoy scale economies that confer competitive advantage over their smaller rivals,[54] scope economies by operating across multiple clinical areas (VI, CRM, cardiac surgery), and larger free cash flows that enable investment in R&D and M&A deals.[55]

## Enterprise Risk Management

### Overview of Risks

Wall Street analysts commonly assess several risks facing MedTechs: technology risk (vulnerability to new products/platforms or alternative therapeutic approaches), regulatory risk (product approval), reimbursement risk (product coverage), liability risk (eg, recalls), and currency risk (currency fluctuations outside the United States).[56] Large MedTechs have developed a comprehensive view of all of the risks that need to be managed.[57] This comprehensive view spans the following functional areas and competitive strategies:

- Innovation/technology: pipeline, transformation of product portfolio to deliver value, peripheral vision of emerging and disruptive technologies

- Customer relationships: physician collaborations, emergence of economic customers, managing conflicts of interest
- Business transformation: change in the healthcare delivery ecosystem (eg, accountable care organizations), employment of physician customers
- Geographic portfolio: opportunities in developed and developing markets, geopolitical and economic stability in emerging markets
- M&A: investments, strategic fit, integration success
- Clinical evidence: RCT design, selection of clinical endpoints
- Economic evidence: health technology assessment (HTA), willingness-to-pay (WTP), comparative effectiveness research (CER)
- Competition: local competitors in emerging markets
- Pricing and reimbursement: global economic pressures, national health budgets, the National Institute for Clinical Excellence (NICE) in the United Kingdom, managing price pressures
- Image and brand reputation: industry image, firm reputation, customer communications
- Operations: supply chain management, component excellence, resilience
- Information technology/cybersecurity: data storage, enterprise resource planning (ERP) systems
- Quality: quality assurance processes, performance metrics (field actions)
- Talent and organization: attraction and retention of talent, top management cohesion, talent acquisition in emerging markets
- Regulatory environment: changing regulations, government scrutiny and enforcement
- Product liability and recalls: class action lawsuits, product recall management, manufacturing quality systems, record-keeping
- Anticorruption: standards of business conduct, Foreign Corrupt Practices Act (FCPA) and other laws, anti-kickback statutes
- IP: IP protection in an expanding global market

### Quality Management
Manufacturing, product testing, and product quality are all important elements of quality

management and, thus, enterprise risk management. There are entire texts devoted to the importance of engineering standards in medical devices.[58] In order to continue marketing products that clinicians want, medical device companies need to invest in quality management systems to implement quality assurance and quality control, maintain good manufacturing practices (GMPs), and avoid production interruptions and product recalls.

The historical record suggests that although recalls of devices have a negative impact on a company's sales and market share, they are not fatal to its survival.[59] First, adverse events with medical devices are quite common but rarely lead to patient deaths.[60] Second, product recalls—a subset of adverse events—are also frequent in number, but involve only a small percentage of devices on the market.[61] Third, survey results suggest that product recalls may not necessarily exert a long-lasting influence on physicians' purchasing decisions or affect their willingness to use the same product again.[62]

## DES Postscript

Over the past decade, there have been no breakthrough innovations in stents (beyond smaller sizes, greater radiopacity, and easier deliverability). Instead, the stent market has matured, resulting in a state of "clinical equipoise"— when a clinician has no good basis for a choice between 2 or more product options. With newer-generation stents, clinical results are very strong with few adverse events. Large-scale RCTs only show "noninferiority." The result for MedTech firms has been a significant erosion in ASP from $2,500 in 2005 to $1,000 in 2015.

With falling profits, MedTechs have considered their options: reduce their cost of goods sold to prop up sagging margins, look for market adjacencies (eg, focus on the tools used in PCI procedures), try to market different therapies to existing customers, or find new customer markets for growth. They have turned to the last strategy and increased their sales and marketing efforts in emerging markets (eg, China). Sales in China have increased by double digits between 2007 and 2017; the country is expected to do more PCI procedures than any other market within the coming few years. However, MedTechs face obstacles capturing a share of this growth market. These include the emergence of local domestic competitors using "copied technology," government regulations that favor the local competitors, and the bifurcation of the market in which multinational corporations (like Western MedTechs) heavily penetrate the Tier 1 large cities, while domestic competitors heavily penetrate the Tier 2 and 3 cities.[63] The MedTechs must also tackle the same issues addressed earlier: train and educate Chinese physicians, lobby for adequate reimbursement, and develop local sales infrastructure.

## SUMMARY

The value of a medical device and its MedTech manufacturer rests on the twin pillars of technology and commercialization. Simply put, you have to have a good product and then convince physicians to use it.

The first pillar encompasses the technology and its development. This includes the device, its constituent components, the technology's ability to address unmet clinical needs, the iterative innovation of the technology and its components, the iterative development of new platforms that combine those components, the R&D effort invested in this continued innovation, the RCTs that test and document the quality-enhancing benefits associated with the innovation, and the management of the regulatory and reimbursement processes. In this manner, new technological products forestall commoditization and resist price discounting.

The second pillar, commercialization, encompasses all activities to market the device to physician customers and facilitate their acceptance. This includes the product launch, development of large sales forces to promote the product and assist physicians, dissemination of RCT results to persuade physicians to adopt the product, physician training and feedback on the device, and cultivation of relationships with physician customers.

The twin pillars drive sales volume and support premium pricing; they are thus the major revenue drivers. Both pillars are supported by corporate strategies to broaden the company's product line and sales force, as well as by risk management efforts to mitigate threats against them.

---

### QUESTIONS TO PONDER

1. One could argue that, in contrast to pharma and biotech, success in MedTech rests more on the second of the twin pillars (ie, commercialization). Why might this argument be valid? Do you agree with it?
2. How does technological innovation in MedTech differ from technological innovation in pharma and biotech?
3. How do the business models of biotech and MedTech differ?
4. How do the customers of pharma, biotech, and MedTech differ?

## REFERENCES

1. Lawton R. Burns, Eduardo Cisneros, William Ferniany, and Harbir Singh. "Strategic Alliances Between Buyers and Suppliers: Lessons from the Medical Imaging Industry," in Christine Harland, Guido Nassimbeni, and Eugene Schneller (Eds.), *The SAGE Handbook of Strategic Supply Management* (New York, NY: Sage Publications, 2012).
2. Lawton R. Burns, Michael Housman, Robert Booth, and Aaron Koenig. "Physician Preference Items: What Factors Matter to Surgeons? Does the Vendor Matter?" *Med Devices.* 11 (2018): 39-49.
3. Kurt Kruger and Max Kruger. "The Medical Device Sector," in Lawton R. Burns (Ed.), *The Business of Healthcare Innovation*, 3rd ed. (Cambridge, United Kingdom: Cambridge University Press, 2020): Chapter 6.
4. Lawton R. Burns, Stephen Sammut, and David Lawrence. "Healthcare Innovation Across Sectors: Convergences and Divergences," in Lawton R. Burns (Ed.), *The Business of Healthcare Innovation*, 2nd ed. (Cambridge, United Kingdom: Cambridge University Press, 2012): Chapter 8.
5. Jason Weidman. Presentation to the Wharton School (December 2019).
6. Lawton R. Burns and Mark V. Pauly. "Transformation of the Healthcare Industry: Curb Your Enthusiasm?" *Milbank Q.* 96 (1) (March 2018): 57-109.
7. CABG is an invasive surgical procedure that involved cracking open the patient's chest and bypassing the clogged coronary artery with a blood vessel harvested from the leg and grafted around the narrowed section of the coronary artery.
8. Simon Basseyn, Sourav Bose, Lawton R. Burns, and Chris Groskaufmanis. "Angioplasty: Catheters, Guidewires, and Balloons," in Philip Rea, Mark V. Pauly, and Lawton R. Burns (Eds.), *Managing Discovery in the Life Sciences* (Cambridge, United Kingdom: Cambridge University Press, 2018): Chapter 6.
9. Glenn Reicin, Matt Miksic, Steven Harr, et al. *Hospital Supplies and Medical Technology: The 2005 Investors' Guide to Interventional Cardiology* (February 23, 2005).
10. Patrick Serruys, Michael Kutryk, and Andrew Ong. "Coronary Artery Stents," *N Engl J Med.* 354 (February 2, 2006): 483-495.
11. Lawrence Keusch, Paul Matsui, and Alan Kessler. *Medical Devices: Year 2000 Outlook* (New York, NY: Goldman Sachs, January 12, 2000). Hans Bostrom, Mark Tracey, Lawrence Keusch, et al. *Healthcare: Medical Devices—Europe* (New York, NY: Goldman Sachs, July 20, 2001). Kurt Kruger and Max Kruger. "The Medical Device Sector," in Lawton R. Burns (Ed.), *The Business of Healthcare Innovation*, 3rd ed. (Cambridge, United Kingdom: Cambridge University Press, 2020): Chapter 6. Dave Powell, Oliver Scheel, and Bill Tribe. *Medical Devices: Equipped for the Future?* (Chicago, IL: AT Kearney, 2014).
12. David Cassak. "Guidant's Start-Up Mentality," *In Vivo* (September 1998): 42-56. David Cassak. Presentation to the Wharton School (November 2006).
13. Stephen Levin. "Medinol: Can Technology Still Win in Stents?" *In Vivo* (October 2002): 44-52.
14. David Cassak. "Building Billion-Dollar Businesses: An Interview with Robert Croce," *In Vivo* (December 2005): 27-36.
15. Sean Salmon. "Marketing in the Stent Wars." Presentation to the Wharton School (n.d.).
16. Glenn Reicin, Matt Miksic, Steven Harr, et al. *Hospital Supplies and Medical Technology: The 2005 Investors' Guide to Interventional Cardiology* (February 23, 2005).
17. Stephen Levin. "Turning Around Medtronic Vascular: An Interview with Scott Ward," *In Vivo* (October 1, 2006).
18. Patrick W. Serruys, Michael J.B. Kutryk, and Andrew T.L. Ong. "Coronary Artery Stents," *N Engl J Med.* 354 (5) (February 2, 2006): 483-495.
19. Guidant's over-the-wire catheter was called Opensail; the rapid exchange platform was called Cross-sail.
20. David Cassak. "Richard Stack, MD: Filling the Cath Lab Pipeline," *In Vivo* (June 2006): 37-41.
21. Glenn Reicin and Jason Wittes. *Hospital Supplies and Medical Technology: Our Annual Trip Through Europe* (New York, NY: Morgan Stanley, March 15, 2002).

22. Stephen Levin. "Renewed DES Safety Debate Creates Second-Generation Mover Advantage," *In Vivo* (October 1, 2006).

23. Plavix (clopidogrel) helped to prevent platelets in the blood from sticking together and forming a blood clot.

24. Sean Salmon. "Marketing in the Stent Wars." Presentation to the Wharton School (n.d.).

25. Jeffrey Englander and Phillip Seligman. *Industry Surveys—Healthcare: Products and Supplies* (New York, NY: Standard & Poors, 2009). Frost & Sullivan. *U.S. Medical Devices Market Outlook* (2008). Peter Lawyer. "Payback: Making Innovation Count in Uncertain Times," *In Vivo* (January 1, 2007). Peter Lawyer, Alexander Kirstein, Hirotaka Yabuki, et al. "High Science: A Best-Practice Formula for Driving Innovation," *In Vivo* (April 2004): 70-82. Peter Lawyer, James Andrew, Marin Gjaja, and Christoph Schweizer. "Payback II: Medical Devices Ride the Cash Curve," *In Vivo* (March 2007): 47-53.

26. Clayton Christensen. *We've Got Rhythm! Medtronic Corporation's Cardiac Pacemaker Business.* Harvard Business School Case 9-698-004 (Boston, MA: Harvard Business School Publishing, July 8, 1997).

27. Clayton Christensen. *We've Got Rhythm! Medtronic Corporation's Cardiac Pacemaker Business.* Harvard Business School Case 9-698-004 (Boston, MA: Harvard Business School Publishing, July 8, 1997). Mikelle Eastley and Steven Wheelwright. *Cardiac Pacemakers, Inc. (A).* Harvard Business School Case 9-698-021 (Boston, MA: Harvard Business School Publishing, March 23, 1998).

28. With respect to VI products, Guidant's Multi-Link stent introduced in 1997 went through several product iterations: Duet (launched 1998), TriStar (1999), Tetra (2000), Penta (2001), Pixel (2001), Zeta (2002), and Vision (2003). Sheryl Zimmer, Bruce Jacobs, Tao Levy, et al. *Med-Tech 101: The Medical Device Handbook* (New York, NY: Deutsche Bank Securities, September 2002).

29. Mikelle Eastley and Steven Wheelwright. *Cardiac Pacemakers, Inc. (A). Harvard Business School Case 9-698-021* (Boston, MA: Harvard Business School Publishing, March 23, 1998).

30. Lawrence Keusch, Paul Matsui, and Kenneth Lin. *Healthcare: Medical Devices—United States* (January 30, 2002).

31. Jeffrey W. Englander and Phillip M. Seligman. *Industry Surveys–Healthcare: Products and Supplies* (August 27, 2009). Kurt Kruger and Max Kruger. "The Medical Device Sector," in Lawton R. Burns (Ed.), *The Business of Healthcare Innovation*, 3rd ed. (Cambridge, United Kingdom: Cambridge University Press, 2020): Chapter 6. Alexander Pryde. *The Medical Technology Market: Commercial Information Sharing and Its Effects on Market Competitiveness and Efficiency* (Edinburgh, United Kingdom: Management School, University of Edinburgh, 2009).

32. Greg Freiherr. "Sustaining Corporate Growth in a Rapidly Changing Industry," *Medical Device Link* (September 1999). Philip Aspden. *Medical Innovation in the Changing Healthcare Marketplace: Conference Summary* (Washington, DC: National Academies Press, 2002). Gold and Diller. *Industry Surveys: Healthcare Products and Supplies* (February 23, 2006; August 31, 2006).

33. David Cassak. "It's the Technology. End of Story," *In Vivo* (November 2001): 31-41.

34. David Cassak. "Medtronic: The Beat Goes On," *In Vivo* (1999). David Cassak. "Guidant's Loss of Innocence," *In Vivo* (June 1, 2003). Kurt Kruger and Max Kruger. "The Medical Device Sector," in Lawton R. Burns (Ed.), *The Business of Healthcare Innovation*, 3rd ed. (Cambridge, United Kingdom: Cambridge University Press, 2020): Chapter 6. Zimbalist. *Medtronic Equity Research* (2003). Guidant. *Fiscal Year 2002: 10-K Report.* Lawrence Keusch, Paul Matsui, and Kenneth Lin. *Healthcare: Medical Devices—United States* (April 2, 2002). Lynn Pieper, Kimberly Weeks, and Whit Kincaid. *Guidant Corporation–Market Perform* (San Francisco, CA: Thomas Weisel Partners, February 14, 2003).

35. Kurt Kruger and Max Kruger. "The Medical Device Sector," in Lawton R. Burns (Ed.), *The Business of Healthcare Innovation*, 3rd ed. (Cambridge, United Kingdom: Cambridge University Press, 2020): Chapter 6. Stefanos Zenios, Josh Makower, and Paul Yock. *Biodesign: The Process of Innovating Medical Technologies* (Cambridge, United Kingdom: Cambridge University Press, 2010): Chapter 4.2. MaRS Entrepreneur Guides. *Navigating the Regulatory Landscape for Healthcare Product Development: Key Principles and Best Practices* (Ontario, Canada: MaRS Discovery District, October 2012).

36. Robert Kaplan, Michael Porter, Thomas Feeley, et al. *Medtronic: Navigating a Shifting Healthcare Landscape.* HBS Case # 9-718-471 (Revised June 28, 2018) (Boston, MA: Harvard Business School Publishing, 2018).

37. Stephen Levin. "Labcoat: Less Is More in Next Generation Drug-Eluting Stents," *In Vivo* (December 2005): 43-49.

38. Sean Salmon. "Marketing in the Stent Wars." Presentation to the Wharton School (n.d.).

39. David Cassak. "Guidant's Loss of Innocence," *In Vivo* (June 1, 2003).

40. Kurt Kruger and Max Kruger. "The Medical Device Sector," in Lawton R. Burns (Ed.), *The Business of Healthcare Innovation*, 3rd ed. (Cambridge, United Kingdom: Cambridge University Press, 2020). Chapter 6. Lawton R. Burns, Michael Housman, Robert Booth, and

Aaron Koenig. "Implant Vendors and Hospitals: Competing Influences Over Product Choice by Orthopedic Surgeons," *Health Care Manag Rev.* 34 (1) (2009): 2-18.

41. Lawrence Keusch, J.C. Davies, and Kenneth Lin. *Healthcare: Medical Devices—United States* (New York, NY: Goldman Sachs, April 11, 2001).

42. David Cassak. "Medtronic: The Beat Goes On," *In Vivo* (1999).

43. Jeffrey W. Englander and Phillip M. Seligman. *Industry Surveys—Healthcare: Products and Supplies* (August 27, 2009).

44. Kurt Kruger and Max Kruger. "The Medical Device Sector," in Lawton R. Burns (Ed.), *The Business of Healthcare Innovation*, 3rd ed. (Cambridge, United Kingdom: Cambridge University Press, 2020): Chapter 6.

45. Stephen Levin. "Abbott: Cracking the Cardiology Cartel," *In Vivo* (May 1, 2001).

46. Mikelle Eastley and Steven Wheelwright. *Cardiac Pacemakers, Inc. (A)*. Harvard Business School Case 9-698-021 (Boston, MA: Harvard Business School Publishing, March 23, 1998).

47. David Cassak. "Guidant: The New Rules of the Device Game," *In Vivo* (July 1, 2003).

48. Stephen Levin. "Abbott: Cracking the Cardiology Cartel," *In Vivo* (May 1, 2001).

49. David Cassak. "XTENT and the Next DES Boom," *In Vivo* (February 2008): 42-52. David Cassak. "From Guidant to Abbott: An Interview with John Capek," *In Vivo* (May 1, 2008).

50. Sheila Marcelo and Lynda M. Applegate. *Medtronic Vision 2010 (A): Transforming for the 21st Century.* Harvard Business School Case 9-800-357 (Boston, MA: Harvard Business School Publishing, March 29, 2000). Greg Freiherr. "Sustaining Corporate Growth in a Rapidly Changing Industry," *MDDI* (September 1, 1999).

51. Guidant's "start-up mentality" had nothing to do with being a real start-up, however. Guidant was not formed via an initial public offering (IPO) or via entrepreneurs setting up a new company, but rather via the 1994 spin-off of 5 device companies that Eli Lilly had acquired. Rather than entering the market as a newborn, Guidant entered as a good-sized, "developed teenager" valued at close to $1 billion.

52. David Cassak. "Medtronic: The Beat Goes On," *In Vivo* (1999). David Cassak. "The Guidant Legacy: An Interview with Ron Dollens," *In Vivo* (January 1, 2007). Other internal management capabilities include good corporate governance, cohesion among the top management team, team structures and cross-functional organization around the customer that combine product lines with sales, and the emergence of project managers who can manage these matrix relationships. MedTechs also mention culture, leadership development, employee growth and development, quality and reliability processes, communications strategy, sales and marketing execution, continuous improvement, operating efficiencies, and employee retention and engagement.

53. Robert L. Simons and Antonio Davila. *Guidant Corporation: Shaping Culture Through Systems.* Harvard Business School Case 198-076 (Boston, MA: Harvard Business School Publishing, April 1998, Revised May 2000.) Catherine M. Dalton. "Leadership, Alignment, and Performance at Guidant Corporation: An Interview with Ronald W. Dollens," *Harvard Business Review* (March 15, 2005).

54. Robert A. DeGraaff. Personal communication. Based on his doctoral thesis, *Analysis of Corporate Acquisitions by Medical Device Manufacturers.* Ph.D. Thesis (Philadelphia, PA: The Wharton School, University of Pennsylvania, 2006).

55. Peter Lawyer. "Payback: Making Innovation Count in Uncertain Times," *In Vivo* (January 1, 2007). Peter Lawyer, Alexander Kirstein, Hirotaka Yabuki, et al. "High Science: A Best-Practice Formula for Driving Innovation," *In Vivo* (April 2004): 70-82. Peter Lawyer, James Andrew, Marin Gjaja, and Christoph Schweizer. "Payback II: Medical Devices Ride the Cash Curve," *In Vivo* (March 2007): 47-53.

56. Hans Bostrom, Mark Tracey, Lawrence Keusch, et al. *Healthcare: Medical Devices—Europe* (New York, NY: Goldman Sachs, July 20, 2001).

57. Stephen Oesterle. Presentation to the Wharton School (November 2014).

58. Gail Babura. *Medical Device Technologies: A System Based Overview Using Engineering Standards* (Waltham, MA: Academic Press, 2012): Chapters 3, 5, 8, and 19.

59. Indeed, pacemaker and implantable cardioverter defibrillator (ICD) recalls occur frequently: From 1990 to 2000, 52 advisories were issued affecting 408,500 pacemakers and 114,645 ICDs. Moreover, the total number of devices affected by advisories increased steadily during this period. William Maisel, Michael Sweeney, William Stevenson, et al. "Recalls and Safety Alerts Involving Pacemakers and Implantable Cardioverter-Defibrillator Generators," *JAMA.* 286 (7) (2001): 793-799. William Maisel, Megan Moynahan, Bram Zuckerman, et al. "Pacemaker and ICD Generator Malfunctions: Analysis of Food and Drug Administration Annual Reports," *JAMA.* 295 (16) (2001): 1901-1906. William Maisel. "Safety Issues Involving Medical Devices: Implications of Recent Implantable Cardioverter-Defibrillator Malfunctions," *JAMA.* 294 (8) (2005): 955-958.

60. The FDA and Center for Devices and Radiological Health receive adverse events as medical device reports (MDRs) for both 510(k) and PMA devices. A manufacturer or provider is required

to submit an MDR if its medical device may have caused or contributed to a death or a serious injury or, in the case of a device malfunction, if the malfunction were to recur and could likely result in a death or serious injury. MDRs are housed in a large database, the Manufacturer and User Facility Device Experience (MAUDE). Between 1996 and 2009, manufacturers filed 182,394 MDRs associated with 7,823 510(k)s. Nearly two-thirds of the reports (66.4%) were associated with a device malfunction; 29.5% of the reports were associated with a patient injury, but less than 2% involved a patient death. Theresa Wizemann. *Public Health Effectiveness of the FDA 510(k) Clearance Process* (Washington, DC: National Academies Press, Institute of Medicine, 2011).

61. On an annual basis, the percentage of devices on the market approved via the 510(k) pathway that are recalled is between 1% and 2%. For 510(k) devices, 99.8% did not experience a recall over a 5-year study period. Nearly three-quarters of individual recalled 510(k) devices are recalled only once; another 16% are recalled twice. The analysis of recall-free 510(k) "survival" of devices showed that 98.4% of the devices cleared in 2003 to 2009 remained on the market, free of recall, 1 year after the 510(k) decision. Similar results hold for medical devices approved under the PMA track: A high percentage of PMA devices (99.7%) did not experience a recall. Roughly 1% of approvals are PMAs. Due to their higher product complexity, they are represented disproportionately (14%) among Class I device recalls, defined by the FDA as situations "where there is a reasonable probability that the use of, or exposure to, a violative product will cause serious adverse health consequences or death".

62. The experience of Zimmer's hip implant, the Durom Cup hip, offers one illustration. The Durom Cup was first sold in the United States in 2006. In July 2008, Zimmer Holdings initiated a voluntary recall following patients' complaints about premature device failures resulting from loosened components. A few months after halting the sales of the device, Zimmer returned it to the market and resumed sales. There was a 6% sales increase attributable to the product's introduction, followed by a sales reduction in 2009, and then a sales rebound in 2010. Zimmer Holdings Annual Reports. Available online: http://investor.zimmer.com/annuals.cfm?id=8. Accessed on November 20, 2020.

63. James Deng and Lawton R. Burns. "China's Medical Technology Sector," In Lawton R. Burns and Gordon Liu (Eds.), *China's Healthcare System and Reform* (Cambridge, United Kingdom: Cambridge University Press, 2017): Chapter 15.

# Healthcare Information Technology

# 24

## THE INFORMATION TECHNOLOGY IMPERATIVE

The healthcare ecosystem is "awash in data." It is one of the most data-intensive sectors in the US economy, with more information generated with each patient encounter. Such encounters mushroomed following enactment of Medicare and Medicaid in 1965, spurring payer and provider efforts to get their arms around the costs and utilization patterns of these patient populations. Hospitals and physician offices adopted desktop computers and information software to bill insurers. Hospitals also began to apply healthcare information technology (HCIT) to specialized areas like pharmacy, radiology, and clinical laboratories to gather and analyze clinical information. The enactment of the Inpatient Prospective Payment System (IPPS) in 1983 increased the need for HCIT to manage costs under budgeted payments. During the 1990s, changes in physician payment under Medicare and pressures from managed care payers likewise required physician practices to more widely implement software systems to manage their practice finances.

Capturing this information has been challenging. As noted in Figure 3-12, there are 2 major flows in the healthcare ecosystem: money and products. The first includes the flow of reimbursement; the second concerns the flow of products through the supply chain. Conspicuous in its absence from Figure 3-12 is the flow of information. This has long been regarded as the "Achilles heel" of the healthcare ecosystem that undermines the efficiency of the other flows. For example, pay-for-performance (P4P) and value-based purchasing (VBP) programs used by insurers rely on the electronic collection and transmittal of clinical data (and then their utilization by providers).

Not surprisingly, correcting the problem of information flow has been central to US healthcare policy for nearly 2 decades. To wit:

- In 2004, President Bush created the position of the "National Coordinator" to lead the Office of the National Coordinator (ONC) for Health Information Technology whose responsibilities included ensuring that every American had access to his or her electronic health information and establishing connectivity of health information technology.
- In 2009, the American Recovery and Reinvestment Act (ARRA) implemented the Health Information Technology for Economic and Clinical Health (HITECH) Act (passed in 2008), which spent $36 billion to incentivize physicians (up to $64,000 in subsidies) to adopt electronic medical records (EMRs) and demonstrate "meaningful use" (MU) of the technology—or penalize them financially if they did not do so.[1] HITECH foresaw three MU stages in the evolution of the EMR, spanning from (1) data capture and sharing to (2) transmission and exchange of clinical information to (3) clinical decision support and access to all relevant data. HITECH also included funding of health information exchanges (HIEs) to grease the flow of information across provider organizations.
- In 2015, the Medicare Access and CHIP Reauthorization Act (MACRA)

shuttered the meaningful use program and shifted incentives to P4P and VBP models. MACRA also signaled the government would move away from standard regulations of EMR use, and focus instead on use of certified EMR technology and HCIT interoperability to allow data exchange among providers and coordination of care via its Advancing Care Information initiative. Having ready access to both clinical and financial information became even more important for physicians to get reimbursed under Medicare.

## SMALL SECTOR, GROWTH SECTOR[2]

The HCIT sector is much smaller than pharma (roughly 11%-15% of national health expenditures [NHEs]) and MedTech (roughly 6%). Leerink currently estimates that HCIT accounts for approximately $50 billion of the country's $4.4 trillion in annual spending accounts, or just over 1% of NHE. This suggests a significant growth opportunity for HCIT. Assuming healthcare reaches the cross-industry information technology penetration average of 3.3%, HCIT firms may generate $100 billion in near-term revenue, approximately double today's market size (Figure 24-1).

Figure 24-2 shows the growth in the market capitalization of selected HCIT firms and the recent surge in initial public offerings (IPOs). Mergers and acquisitions (M&A) still outpaced IPOs by a 9:1 ratio in 2019 (Figure 24-3). Compared to 2015, 2019 saw almost 10 times the number of deals, representing a 75% compound average growth rate (CAGR).

One of the major promises of HCIT is that it might help all players to improve efficiency and reduce wasteful spending. The Institute of Medicine (IOM) estimated that wasteful spending amounted to roughly $1 trillion, or nearly a third of all healthcare spending. Of this total amount, the largest portion was attributable to $285 billion in administrative spending, or nearly one-third of total wasted spending. Such spending is most amenable to reduction using HCIT, particularly in the provider sector, which accounts for roughly two-thirds of NHE. A major potential source of provider savings from HCIT may lie in EMRs (covered later), population health management, clinical decision support systems (CDSS), care coordination, telehealth and telemedicine, remote monitoring, and revenue cycle management.

Providers are not the only market for HCIT solutions. Payers and patients are also growing customer markets for many of the same applications (Figure 24-4). Payer solutions include membership management, wellness management, and underwriting quotes. Patient solutions include connected devices (wearables), mobile applications, personal health, and wellness management. Other applications include business intelligence and analytics, patient engagement, and consumer health information.

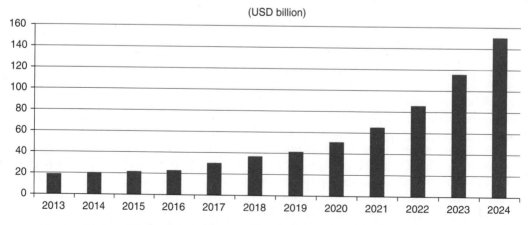

**Figure 24-1** • US Digital Health Market Size, 2012-2024. (Source: Figure 7.4, in Lawton R. Burns [Ed.], *The Business of Healthcare Innovation*, 3rd ed. Cambridge, United Kingdom: Cambridge University Press; 2020.)

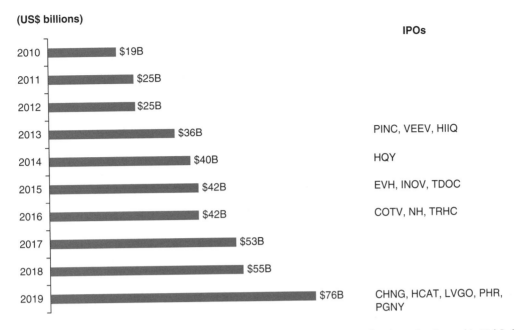

**(US$ billions)**

**IPOs**

- 2010 — $19B
- 2011 — $25B
- 2012 — $25B
- 2013 — $36B — PINC, VEEV, HIIQ
- 2014 — $40B — HQY
- 2015 — $42B — EVH, INOV, TDOC
- 2016 — $42B — COTV, NH, TRHC
- 2017 — $53B
- 2018 — $55B
- 2019 — $76B — CHNG, HCAT, LVGO, PHR, PGNY

**Figure 24-2** • Market Capitalization of Selected Healthcare Information Technology Stocks and Initial Public Offerings (IPOs). (Source: FactSet, SVB Leerink Estimates.)

There are multiple ways to classify companies that work in the HCIT space. Analysts often divide the industry into 4 subsectors: (1) EMRs, alternatively known as the clinical systems players; (2) the niche provider-facing solutions; (3) niche payer-facing solutions; and (4) niche pharma-facing solutions. EMRs provide an electronic health record platform and related software/services to providers, including revenue cycle management, practice management, patient portals, and hosting solutions. Provider-facing firms encompass niche software

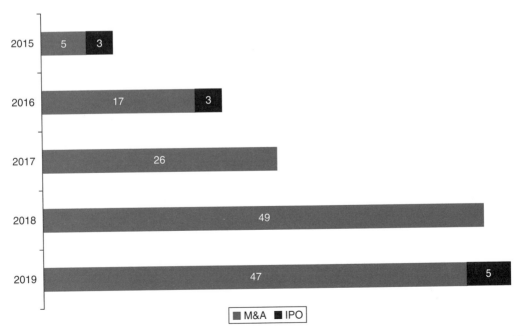

- 2015 — M&A: 5, IPO: 3
- 2016 — M&A: 17, IPO: 3
- 2017 — M&A: 26
- 2018 — M&A: 49
- 2019 — M&A: 47, IPO: 5

■ M&A  ■ IPO

**Figure 24-3** • Healthcare Information Technology Private Mergers and Acquisitions (M&A) and Initial Public Offerings (IPOs) (Both United States and Europe). (Source: SVB Leerink.)

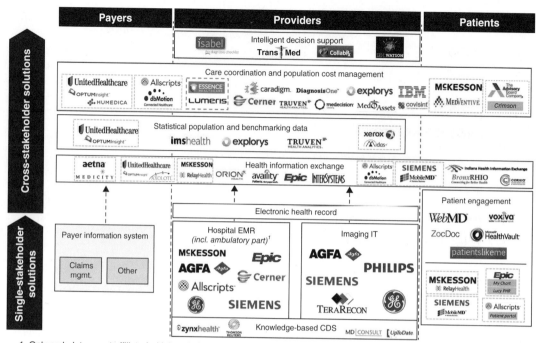

1. Only ambulatory part affiliated with hospitals; excluding practice management
Note: CDS = Clinical Decision Support

**Figure 24-4** • Healthcare Information Technology Market Segments. (Source: John Glaser, Presentation to the Wharton School, November 2017.)

and services solutions that are sold to healthcare providers such as hospitals, health systems, and ambulatory practices. Solutions generally focus on cost management, outsourcing, and efficiency enhancements. Payer-facing firms similarly sell niche HCIT platform solutions to insurers. While this originally encompassed solely large payers (eg, Aetna, United) and government contracts, these firms have begun to expand into the employee benefits manager sector as companies take on a greater share of health insurance cost. Solutions can include telehealth, consumer-directed benefits, payments accuracy, and broader analytics. Finally, the pharma-facing firms sell niche HCIT platform and data solutions to the life sciences industry, including pharmaceutical companies and clinical research organizations (CROs). Solutions within this subsector include clinical trials management, big data and artificial intelligence (AI) solutions to streamline processes, quality/regulatory solutions, and consulting.

Figure 24-5 provides an alternative way to classify firms in the HCIT market, using 4 categories: clinical solutions, nonclinical solutions, payer solutions, and outsourcing services. The size of the markets for the products that

contribute to the categories are shown. The largest market, nonclinical solutions, was projected to grow at a 13% CAGR from $15 billion to $28 billion between 2015 and 2020. The second largest market, clinical solutions, was projected to grow at a faster rate, 20%, from $13 billion to $33 billion (2015-2020). The payer solutions and outsourcing services markets are both smaller in size and more modest in growth. Such growth has naturally attracted venture capital (VC) investment (Figure 24-6). The biggest targets of VC funding have been telemedicine, analytics, and wearables (discussed later). Indeed, perhaps due to the COVID-19 crisis in the spring of 2020, such digital health businesses received a record $6.3 billion in venture investment during the first half of that year.[3]

## ELECTRONIC MEDICAL RECORDS AND THEIR CONTROVERSIES

EMRs are among the most notable entrants into the HCIT sector. EMR vendors have an aggregate 111 years of public company experience across the group. Combined with government subsidies during the MU era (2011-2016), this

| | 2015 Market Size | 2020 Market Size | CAGR (2015-2020) |
|---|---|---|---|
| **Clinical Solutions** | 13,049 | 32,685 | 20% |
| –Electronic Health/Medical Records | 3,269 | 5,644 | 12% |
| –m Health Solutions and Apps | 3,763 | 13,859 | 30% |
| –PACS and VNA | 1,510 | 2,533 | 11% |
| –Healthcare IT Integration Systems | 983 | 1,922 | 14% |
| –Medical Image Analysis Software | 686 | 1,292 | 14% |
| –Telehealth Solutions | 781 | 2,921 | 30% |
| –Specialty Management Information Systems | 631 | 1,418 | 18% |
| –Computerized Physician Order Entry | 408 | 798 | 14% |
| –Laboratory Information Systems | 363 | 681 | 13% |
| –Clinical Decision Support Systems | 204 | 428 | 16% |
| –Radiology Information Systems | 175 | 397 | 18% |
| –Digital Pathology | 152 | 323 | 16% |
| –Practice Management Systems | 90 | 159 | 12% |
| –Radiation Dose Management | 34 | 310 | 56% |
| **Nonclinical Solutions** | 15,103 | 27,641 | 13% |
| –Supply Chain Management | 2,713 | 4,168 | 9% |
| –Revenue Cycle Management | 2,511 | 4,371 | 12% |
| –Population Health Management | 2,466 | 4,309 | 12% |
| –Healthcare Asset Management | 2,449 | 5,118 | 16% |
| –Healthcare Analytics | 2,891 | 6,431 | 17% |
| –Pharmacy Information Systems | 1,003 | 1,343 | 6% |
| –Workforce Management Systems | 367 | 507 | 7% |
| –Healthcare Information Exchanges | 260 | 394 | 9% |
| –Financial Management Systems | 222 | 334 | 9% |
| –Medical Document Management Systems | 140 | 450 | 26% |
| –Medication Management Systems | 32 | 50 | 9% |
| –Customer Relationship Management | 49 | 168 | 28% |
| **Payer Solutions** | 5,513 | 8,588 | 9% |
| –Claims Management | 1,324 | 2,059 | 9% |
| –Customer Relationship Management | 970 | 1,559 | 10% |
| –Pharmacy Analysis and Audit | 805 | 1,178 | 8% |
| –Fraud Management | 714 | 1,191 | 11% |
| –Payment Management | 611 | 930 | 9% |
| –Member Eligibility Management | 319 | 478 | 9% |
| –Provider Network Management | 209 | 317 | 9% |
| –Computer Assisted Coding Systems | 99 | 160 | 10% |
| –Medical Document Management | 18 | 33 | 13% |
| –Other (General Ledger, Payroll Management) | 446 | 684 | 9% |
| **Outsourcing Services** | 12,822 | 18,150 | 7% |
| –IT Infrastructure Management Services | 6,029 | 8,598 | 7% |
| –Payer HCIT Outsourcing Market | 3,446 | 4,700 | 6% |
| –Provider HCIT Outsourcing Market | 2,114 | 3,112 | 8% |
| –Operational HCIT Outsourcing Market | 1,233 | 1,740 | 7% |
| **Total** | 46,488 | 87,064 | 13% |

Size of US health IT submarkets: projected (2015 and 2020; in US$ million)

**Figure 24-5** • Size of Healthcare Information Technology Submarkets in United States, 2015 and 2020 ($ Millions). (Source: Figure 7.5, in Lawton R. Burns [Ed.], *The Business of Healthcare Innovation*, 3rd ed. Cambridge, United Kingdom: Cambridge University Press; 2020.)

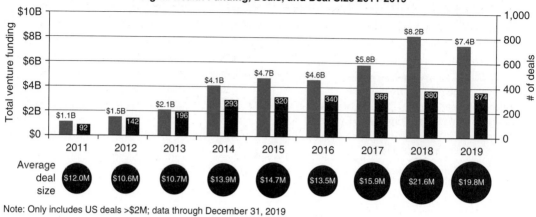

Figure 24-6 • Digital Health Funding. B, Billion. (Source: Rock Health Funding Database.)

puts the EMRs furthest along the maturity curve within the HCIT sector. It is therefore instructive to look at the historical experience of the EMR to gauge the promise of the entire HCIT sector.

## History of EMRs

Historically, the medical record constituted the notes of private encounters of physicians with their patients. Each patient's medical record was kept in a file folder and catalogued in alphabetical order in large filing cabinets or filing shelves. Before the 1960s, such charting was primarily "narrative" (ie, here is what happened). During the 1960s, the problem-oriented medical record, which included the patient's history, symptoms, test results, treatment plans, progress notes, discharge summary, and any follow-up steps, was developed as a comprehensive approach to recording and accessing patient medical data gathered from all care team members. Moreover, physicians "communicated" with one another by virtue of adding their notes to the record and reading the notes of colleagues already in the record (assuming they practiced in the same clinic or hospital and could find the file).

The early EMRs were developed at academic medical centers in the early 1970s, although they still remain to this day a hybrid collection of computerized and paper data.[4] Some EMRs were added to hospital billing and scheduling systems, while others were developed as clinical systems to help improve medical care and medical research. Early EMRs also included data interchange for claims processing and image scanning as a method for document capture. Most were developed on large mainframe computers, with limited storage and wired terminals.

As inadequacies of the paper record became more evident, the IOM advocated an EMR.[5] EMR adoption was delayed by high costs, data entry errors, poor physician acceptance, and lack of incentives. Clinical use nevertheless increased with the rise of the Internet, the development of physician workstations, and the integration of personal computers with EMRs that allowed access to physician notes, orders, consults, laboratory results, radiological studies, direct patient measurements, nursing assessments and notes, and patient care procedures. The field of "medical informatics" arose as providers recognized that the medical information in the EMR could be used for CDSS. CDSS was often a component of computerized physician order entry (CPOE), which required physicians to respond to computer-generated reminders to improve their compliance with preventive care protocols.

EMRs are increasingly used in patient exam rooms to document and access patients' records, access online medical information and decision-making tools, and prescribe medications. They have changed the dynamics of the doctor-patient interaction in good ways (eg, clinician-patient e-mail, virtual consults, and telemedicine) and in bad ways (eg, distracted physicians). EMRs now include lab results, imaging results, and medication histories. Physicians can use mobile devices with high-resolution cameras to capture images from the bedside and insert them into the EMR. EMRs also include e-prescribing interfaces to local pharmacies. Patients have likewise voiced their interest in accessing their healthcare data, which has led to more personal use of EMR information in the form of a personal health record (PHR; covered later).

Family health histories can be entered into the EMRs and used to assess disease risk and identify the role of genetic and social factors in one's health status. Biobanks are now linked to personal and family health information in EMRs to accurately identify subjects with specific diseases and phenotypes and to identify genotype-phenotype associations. Public health agencies have also found value in EMRs as part of biosurveillance systems and the new National Institutes of Health (NIH) initiative, "All of Us."

Between 2000 and 2010, different vendors developed "best-of-breed" EMRs for specialty settings (ambulatory care, anesthesia, emergency department, etc). Over the past decade, providers have migrated away from multivendor, "best-of-breed," focused EMRs to a single-vendor, end-to-end EMR suite (Figure 24-7). EMRs have thus become comprehensive solutions that span clinical, billing, reporting, and administrative functions that permit a more coherent view of the patient. Major vendors here are Cerner and EPIC, who had 26-29% and 25-26% market share, respectively, in 2014 and 2019. Providers have increasingly rigorous expectations from these systems, not only because they pay a lot of money to install them but also because of the new demands placed on them by public and private payers to support P4P and VBP initiatives.

## Diffusion of EMRs

The diffusion of EMRs has been tracked most closely for the 2 sets of providers accounting for the largest share of NHE: hospitals and physicians (see Figure 24-8). The data show that adoption has increased substantially among both groups over time, due to financial penalties for nonadoption imposed by the HITECH Act and the need to respond to the P4P and VBP initiatives in MACRA.

## Controversies Regarding EMRs and HCIT

There are many contentious issues surrounding HCIT in general and EMRs in particular.

First, many practitioners and researchers assume that EMR adoption facilitates physician efforts to engage in clinical integration, care management, and population health management. Second, they assume that EMR adoption reduces healthcare costs and improves healthcare quality. Third, many analysts have characterized EMRs as disruptive innovations that will transform healthcare. Fourth, many argue that "big data" contained in the EMR are **the** way forward for the healthcare industry. These claims are assessed in the following sections.

## Interoperability

The biggest and most serious complaint about EMRs is their inability to talk with one another. This problem is known as "interoperability"— that is, the lack of data standards, common interfaces, or common architecture (eg, software capabilities) that allow different EMR systems to exchange information among providers. This problem complicates clinician communication, workflows, and quality of care by hindering the availability of the right data at the right time in the hands of the right provider. This problem also inhibits continuity of care by preventing each successive clinician from knowing what the prior clinician did.

Given the large number of EMR vendors and the fragmentation of their market shares, there is no dominant vendor and thus no dominant EMR platform. EPIC has been likened to a "closed system" vendor that makes it hard to communicate with other vendors' EMRs. To address this issue, the ONC issued a final rule in March 2020 to establish policies to hold accountable those who restrict the exchange, access, or use of electronic health information ("information blocking"). This is partly designed to protect patients or providers from becoming "locked in" to a particular technology or healthcare network because their electronic health information is not portable. Even among hospital systems that have purchased EMRs from the same vendor (eg, EPIC), their EMRs may be unable to talk to one another. Some observers claim the vendors do not want to share their data. The problem gets worse. Even for a given hospital system that has affiliated with community physicians (see Chapter 12), there are on average 16 disparate EMR vendors in these practices; only 2% of hospitals have a single vendor supporting their practices.[6]

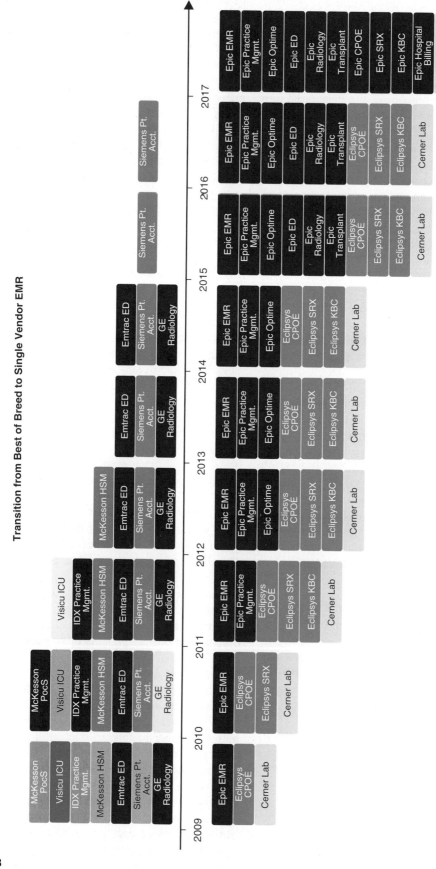

**Figure 24-7** • Transition From Best of Breed to Single Vendor Emergency Medical Record (EMR). (Source: Michael Restuccia. Presentation by Bill Hanson to the Wharton School, Fall 2019.)

**Adoption of EHRs at Physician Practices and Hospitals**

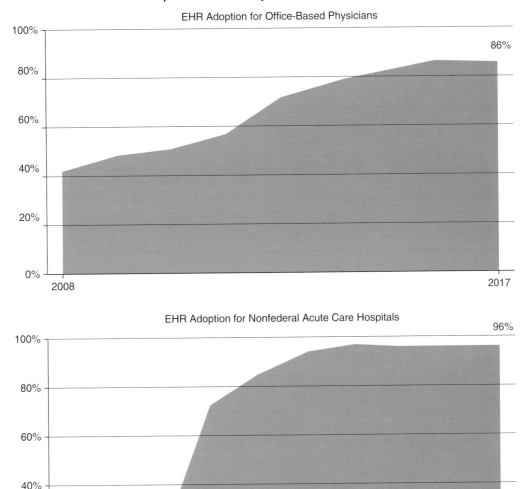

Figure 24-8 • Emergency Medical Record Adoption. EHR, Electronic Health Record. (Source: Fred Schulte and Erika Fry. Death by 1,000 Clicks: Where Electronic Health Records Went Wrong. Kaiser Family Foundation, March 18, 2019, https://khn.org/news/Death-by-a-Thousand-Clicks/.)

## EMR Impact on Clinical Integration, Care Management, and Population Health Management

Patient mortality and morbidity are driven heavily by patient behaviors and then secondarily by genetics and the physical and social environment. EMR adoption can at best impact providers in their efforts to access, collect, and transmit information on the health of the populations they care for (eg, by compiling disease registries). However, there is no logical reason why adoption of an EMR should impact the mortality and morbidity patterns in the local population. Why might this be so?

First, there is inconsistent evidence that EMR adoption facilitates physician efforts to engage in clinical integration, chronic care management, and population health management.[7] A major field investigation of physician groups found that the number of HCIT components used was not associated with the use of care management practices.[8] That is, care management was not dependent on information technology. Another found that EMR capabilities were not associated with diabetes management, asthma maintenance, or other processes of care (preventive services).[9] A third study found that changes in EMR capability were not associated with changes in a medical group's index of care management activity.[10]

Second, studies report that HCIT usage is not associated with care coordination.[11] What explains these surprising findings? Physicians require several pieces of patient information to coordinate care, including results from patient referrals for consultation, the patient's history and reasons for referral, and hospital discharge information. One study reported that hospital-employed physicians were slightly less likely to routinely receive all 3 types of information compared to nonemployed physicians. Moreover, there were only small differences in the receipt of such information when comparing physicians not using information technology with physicians using information technology. The researchers concluded that EMR adoption and electronic sharing of patient data among physicians may not be enough to ensure care coordination.[12] Another study reported that EMR usage did not improve care coordination across sites of care such as inpatient, outpatient, and emergency department areas.[13] EMR adoption may require other factors to be present in order to coordinate care, including the presence of a cohesive provider team, dense social networks of interaction among team members, and use of a care coordinator who acts as a communications hub between the care team providers and patient.[14]

In general, research shows that HCIT is infrequently used to coordinate care[15]; instead, EMRs may play primarily the role of data storage and access. Barriers to a coordinative role include the need for interpersonal sharing of information to coordinate care, the need to reengineer internal workflows in tandem with installations of HCIT, and the lack of reimbursement for care coordination. Existing incentive programs to promote MU of HCIT have resulted in only limited adoption of optional care coordination objectives.[16] Recent data suggest that only 16% of clinicians reported they sent a summary of care record for the majority of their patient transitions and referrals. The care coordination activities with the greatest HCIT support are not the care coordination activities that clinicians value most and are most routinely implemented.[17]

## Impact of EMRs on Cost and Quality

HCIT has long been heralded as the "silver bullet" solution that will cure the healthcare ecosystem's many problems. Policy makers and researchers have long anticipated cost and quality benefits from the adoption and diffusion of HCIT among providers. In 2005, for example, RAND researchers estimated potential savings of $142 to $271 billion based on the experience of other economic sectors' investment in information technology. Such optimistic projections may have prompted the US government to offer subsidies to physicians to make these investments as part of HITECH.[18]

Research has subsequently proven that such assumptions and projections were incorrect. Researchers now recognize that HCIT is exceedingly complex with varying results depending on the context in which it is implemented (eg, the business practices of the adopter, the type of provider).[19]

There have been multiple reviews of the literature on EMRs over the past decade. Overall, these reviews suggest no effect on cost and only mixed effects on quality.[20] Data from the Medicare Coordinated Care Demonstration found that extensive use of HCIT and EMRs had no effect on either cost or quality.[21] A national study of physician groups found that EMR use was not associated with the quality of care rendered to chronically ill patients, a finding replicated in other studies.[22] One review examined some of the functionalities required under the MU regulations, including CDSS alerts and physician reminders.[23] Most studies reported positive effects of alerts and reminders on quality measures, such as medication management, screening, and preventive care. One study, however, found no impact on patient mortality, adverse drug events, and readmission rates[24]; another found no evidence of improved safety in terms of detecting adverse drug events.[25]

Studies conducted in ambulatory settings likewise found mixed or weak effects of HCIT on quality.[26] A literature review found some benefits regarding quality but no evidence on cost-effectiveness, mortality, or hospital lengths of stay. The authors concluded that EMRs may improve clinical process measures of quality, but cost savings are not anticipated, at least in the short term, due to the high cost of implementation, although medium- and long-term positive results were expected.[27] The evidence for the benefits of CDSS was also mixed.[28]

Why the mixed results? One reason is that HCIT helps physicians to comply with clinical guidelines but not to deliver higher quality of care.[29] Another reason is that the evidence varies depending on the type of HCIT (eg, EMRs), the different components of EMRs (eg, CPOE, CDSS), and the different functionalities of EMRs (eg, physician reminders, physician alerts).

Moreover, research suggests that provider organizations implementing EMRs and HCIT need to make a series of concomitant changes to realize the benefits of the records and avoid undesired consequences. These include implementation of CDSS, alignment of HCIT with care delivery, workflow mapping and redesign, the HCIT implementation process, provider training and learning, simulation, ongoing support, the provider organization's commitment to change (including time and money invested), and choice between bedside versus central station desktop EMRs. Achieving this involves a heavy emphasis on the implementation of parallel changes in people and work processes and on interfaces linking information systems across care settings. The Agency for Healthcare Research and Quality concluded it is unlikely that there will be any major improvements in the quality and cost of care from the use of HCIT without use of computerized decision support, which itself is a challenge.[30] Another set of researchers concluded that it was difficult to draw any clear conclusions regarding the financial effects of HCIT across patient care settings (inpatient, outpatient, emergency department) and across information technology tools.[31]

National data show no impact of EMR adoption on hospital efficiency (eg, patient cost per day).[32] Among physicians, EMR adoption fostered revenue gains for some, but revenue losses for many due to increased practice and staffing costs.[33] One review examined some of the functionalities required under MU regulations, including CDSS alerts and physician reminders.[34] Most studies reported mixed impacts on cost that ranged from a 75% decrease to a 69% increase in targeted costs. One study found no cost savings in hospitals even 5 years after adoption.[35]

## Failure to Disrupt

### EMRs

Despite the high adoption levels and funding of HIEs, compatibility and interoperability among HCIT systems used by different providers have lagged. Hospitals have lacked a financial incentive to share their patients' data with other competitors. HCIT vendors, for their part, have tried to lock in their customers, have not invested heavily in data transfer, and have made it difficult for local hospitals using the same vendor to share information from their EMRs.

There are other barriers to EMR adoption that limit its potential to disrupt healthcare.[36] These include:

- A fundamental misalignment of incentives, with healthcare providers spending capital and time on implementing systems and health insurers reaping the financial benefits of the investments. Investments in HCIT reduce duplicative testing and generate savings that accrue to the insurer but lead to lost revenues among providers.
- The need to tightly integrate with care processes and uncertainty regarding software vendors. Healthcare providers must decide between (1) changing their own processes to match those of off-the-shelf software and (2) spending money to configure software to align with preexisting processes. Either pathway causes strain.
- Physician dissatisfaction with EMRs that disrupt their workflow, detract from face-to-face time with patients, and lead to both frustration and burnout.
- Initial cost, maintenance costs, training costs, and lack of capital.
- Technical support, technical infrastructure.
- Productivity loss, change to existing work habits, and workflow challenges.
- Errors in the EMR, including unreliable patient medication lists, data on the wrong patient, and unreliable lab results.

## Personal Health Records (PHRs)

Beyond EMRs, there have been several other entrants to the "let's disrupt healthcare using HCIT" derby. At the turn of the millennium, there were several efforts to develop PHRs. A PHR includes electronic copies of information that patients have received from their providers, as well as information that patients themselves enter. PHRs must be distinguished from patient portals, which are typically offered by a hospital or large health system to provide patients with a window into their lab results, histories, and other data. PHRs are intended to increase the patient's engagement in and awareness of their own health status, as well as allow them to transmit their clinical data across all the providers they see (even if the latter are not exchanging that information themselves).

The initial efforts to roll such products out to consumers—by Microsoft's "Health Vault" and Google's "Google Health"—totally failed. One problem can be summarized as the combination of customer ignorance and apathy: "I don't know and I don't care." Consumers were either not aware of the product or were not interested in it. Another reason is that patients could just as easily use hospital portals or those maintained by health plans instead of the PHR. As a related issue, many users stated that although the PHRs were "user friendly," they did not add value, did not meet an unmet need, and were time consuming (data entry).[37] A third barrier was the lack of partnerships with large provider systems that would work with firms like Google and Microsoft to transmit their data to populate the PHR. PHRs need connections to providers and an open platform that permits the importation of data from multiple sources and applications.[38] Finally, people may have been reluctant to share their private health information with Microsoft and Google.

After the debacle of Health Vault and Google Health, a firm called Dossia—owned by 10 self-insured employers—tried to resurrect the PHR strategy to provide their employees with lifelong, portable, comprehensive, patient-controlled EMRs. According to Dossia's chief executive officer (CEO), "this was a truly disruptive, transformative innovation designed to put the power of health and healthcare management firmly in the patient's hands."[39] The firm survived 8 years (2008-2016) and then failed. One major reason was that the individuals responsible for managing health benefits at the employers did not buy into the idea of PHRs; instead, they believed that benefits consultants, health plan administrators, pharmacy benefit managers, and healthcare providers were better experts in making decisions.

## HITECH

The HITECH Act similarly failed. According to a Kaiser analysis, rather than creating an electronic ecosystem of information, the United States has hundreds, if not thousands of EMRs that operate as a sprawling, disconnected patchwork.[40] This is reminiscent of the description of the US healthcare ecosystem in Chapter 1. Moreover, it has "handcuffed" providers to technology they dislike (eg, switching back and forth between focusing on the patient and the computer) and created patient safety risks of death or injury (due to software glitches, design flaws, and user errors), while enriching and empowering the HCIT sector that sells it. The HITECH Act did not enforce interoperability standards; EMRs also failed to use standard drug, laboratory, and diagnosis codes. Unlike the global network of automated teller machines (ATMs), proprietary EMRs made by 700+ vendors did not talk to one another, resulting in physicians transferring patient information via telephone, fax, and CD-ROM.

What went wrong? In a hurry to stimulate the US economy, HITECH and ARRA pushed providers to adopt the EMRs quickly and do a lot of things with them—before they were ready and before the software was ready for them. In a 2017 interview, even President Obama admitted the shortcomings: "there are still just mountains of paperwork . . . and the doctors still have to input stuff, and the nurses are spending all their time on all this administrative work. We put a big slug of money into trying to encourage everyone to digitalize, to catch up with the rest of the world . . . that's been harder than we expected." Finally, HITECH required such documentation by US physicians that their clinical notes were 4 times longer than those of their non-US counterparts.

## Big Data: The Way Forward?

Despite these many problems and limitations, many believe (perhaps rightly) that the "big data" captured in part by EMRs is the way forward for the healthcare ecosystem. Big data encompasses data digitization, data consolidation, data science (eg, identifying patients at risk), data visualization, and data-enabled treatment automation. Healthcare is behind other industrial sectors in these activities and should hopefully benefit by catching up. But there is more. The EMR has become a "meta-document" that is used for many purposes, such as feeding a knowledge engine that can make clinical recommendations, fueling research, improving operating efficiency, and converting data into assets that can serve new drug development and start-up creations in both information technology and biotechnology. Thus, the benefits of big data may extend far beyond patient care.

<h2>OTHER INFORMATION TECHNOLOGY SUBSECTORS</h2>

### Cloud Computing

In 2018, Eric Schmidt (Google's former CEO) gave a keynote address to an HCIT industry conference that urged healthcare providers to move their data to the cloud instead of the locally hosted sites. In retrospect, many unwisely failed to heed his advice: The following year (2019) saw a record number of ransomware attacks on healthcare organizations and breach of health records. At the same time that we moved to share data and make them more accessible, we now also had to protect that data to preserve patient privacy. Cloud computing might accelerate in the future with cybersecurity risks. Surprisingly, however, despite a heightened level of awareness around cybersecurity risk, there is no groundswell in commercial demand for healthcare-centric security solutions. The cloud's penetration of healthcare was only 15% as of early 2020. The large tech vendors that have helped healthcare to shift to the cloud have been Microsoft Azure and Amazon Web services, followed by Google Cloud as a distant third.

Market forecasts going forward are quite bullish. The global healthcare data storage market is expected to grow at a CAGR of 16.4% between 2019 and 2026 and reach $8.11 billion. Growth will be driven by a greater volume of digital data generated not only by healthcare providers but also by telemedicine, chronic disease management, and the applications developed by "big tech" (profiled later). At a minimum, the cloud will serve as data storage (much like the EMR, but on a grander scale); at a maximum, it may serve the goals of artificial intelligence (AI, covered below).

### Wearables

One interesting market segment is consumer wearables. Figure 24-9 shows some of the possible applications according to function and body part; Figure 24-10 shows the anticipated

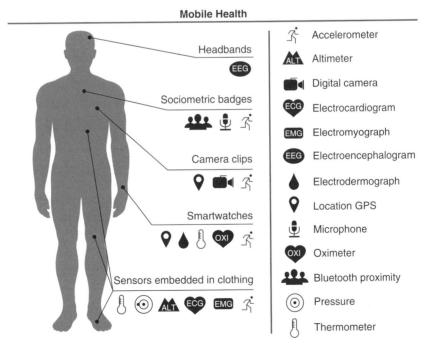

**Figure 24-9 •** Mobile Health Applications. (Source: Figure 7.6, in Lawton R. Burns [Ed.], *The Business of Healthcare Innovation*, 3rd ed. Cambridge, United Kingdom: Cambridge University Press; 2020.)

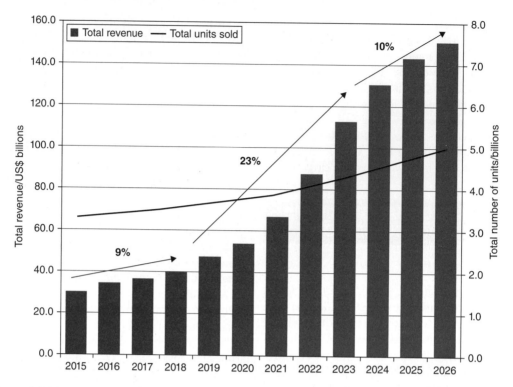

**Figure 24-10 •** Growth of Smart Wearable Devices. (Source: IDTechEx - Wearables Forecast 2017.)

growth in revenues for this segment (eg, 23% CAGR between 2019 and 2023). Gartner has made a more optimistic forecast, suggesting the wearables device market may reach $87 billion by 2023; other firms have offered much less optimistic forecasts.[41] There is a broad spectrum of devices, which spans from low-acuity, fitness-oriented products to high-acuity, chronic disease–oriented products. As of October 2016, there were more than 259,000 mobile health applications ("apps") available for download. When combined with an EMR, these devices can provide real-time, continuous data that offer a comprehensive view of the patient's health that can improve clinician decision making and thus patient outcomes. They may also improve the patient's engagement in their own health.

Nevertheless, consumer use has been modest. Between 2015 and 2017, consumer adoption of digital health tools has been highest in online health information (79% by 2017), followed by online reviews of providers (58%). There has been much lower adoption of mobile tracking devices (24%), wearables (24%), and live video telemedicine (19%).[42] Moreover, evidence about the impact of such digital tools on clinical diagnosis, treatment adherence, and patient outcomes has been mixed.[43]

## Analytics[44]

Another interesting HCIT segment is analytics. Analytics includes several tools described in the following list. Figure 24-11 highlights some of the emerging areas of application for analytics.

- *Business analytics:* Tools to explore past data to gain insight into future business decisions
- *Business intelligence:* Tools and techniques to turn data into meaningful information and knowledge, including data digitization
- *Big data:* Data sets that are so large or complex that traditional data processing applications are inadequate
- *Data science:* Tools to risk-stratify patients to identify those who can most benefit from a specific therapeutic screening and/ or intervention
- *Data visualization:* The process of analyzing large amounts of data and communicating the results in visual context to make them more easily digestible and actionable
- *Data mining:* Tools for discovering patterns in large data sets

**Figure 24-11 •** Expanding Scope of Analytics. (Source: Dale Sanders, Presentation to the Wharton School, Fall 2018.)

**Population Health Analytics**

NOW
- Cost & utilization
- Member analysis
- Registries/gaps in care
- Readmissions
- Transitions of care
- Generic drug utilization
- Provider performance
- Value-based payer reporting
- Contract scorecard

In validation
- HCC/RAF
- Bundle payment–CJR
- Social vulnerability index analysis
- 3rd Party (groupers, TCRRV)

NEXT
- Care management
- Patient targeting
- Provider efficiency
- Employer analytics
- DSRIP program
- State Medicaid program
- Potentially avoidable events
- Bundle payment–commercial
- Network management
- Contract management
- 3rd Party (service categories)
- Open data–expanded use

**Revenue Cycle**

NOW

In Validation
- Accounts receivable
- Cash
- Revenue
- Adjustments
- Census
- Case Mix

In Development
- Denials and variance
- RVU
- Charge and claims level analysis
- Work items
- GL analysis

NEXT
- Access metrics & reports
- HIM metrics & reports
- Predictive analytics
- Benchmarking

**Care Continuum Analytics**

NOW
- Home health–patient & financials

NEXT
- Long-term care
- Behavioral health
- Rehab

**Operational Analytics**

NOW
- Throughput–ED

NEXT
- Command center
- Patient throughput discovery
- Cost and variance
- Pharmacy spend analysis
- Turn around time analysis

**Clinical Analytics**

NOW
- Gaps in care
- AHRQ PQI

NEXT
- Core measures
- Complications
- Infection control
- Clinical variance discovery
- Quality management

**Service Line Analytics**

NEXT
- Service line–general
- Perioperative
- Emergency medicine
- Behavioral health
- Practice management

485

- *Supply chain management:* Demand forecasting, visibility of orders to customers, product location in the channel, and product barcoding.

Analytics and big data have received a lot of attention. There are several "tailwinds" behind this movement and "headwinds" confronting it. The tailwinds include many of the themes addressed in this book: the perception that "healthcare is broken," the perception that healthcare can benefit from disruptive new technologies to fix this broken system, the utility of new technology to improve worker productivity in a labor-intensive sector, the opportunity to reduce medical errors, and the opportunity to improve the quality of physicians' decisions. It is also important to point out 3 "data opportunities" that lend themselves to analytics: the higher *volume of data* generated (eg, by smartphones, wearables, sensors, EMRs, genetic sequencing), the larger *variety of data* being collected (eg, the NIH's "All of Us" program, which is collecting genetic and medical and sociodemographic data on patients), and the faster *velocity of data* resulting from more devices capturing data in real time. The data formats in which this information comes are also multiplying to include hospital discharge and EMR data, claims data, clinical trials data, patient health survey data, patient disease registry data, genomics data, social media data, and sensor data.

The headwinds include the explosion of data and the resulting "signal-to-noise" data problem (ie, separating what are useful signals about the patient's condition from a *lot* of background noise). As noted in Chapter 5, physicians are bombarded with too many measures of quality. The Centers for Medicare and Medicaid Services (CMS) Quality Payment Program (QPP) contains 271 measures; 37% are reportedly invalid, and another 28% have questionable validity. According to one study, of the 1,958 quality metrics in the National Quality Measures Clearinghouse (NQMC), only 7% of those measure clinical outcomes and less than 2% of those are based on patient-reported outcomes[45]; as of 2018, there were over 2,500 quality metrics in the NQMC. We may be measuring the wrong things.

There is also the issue of poor data quality—also known as GIGO (garbage in, garbage out)—that plagues some of the information in the EMR. Other data problems include incomplete data, inadequate formatting of data required for machine learning, the loss of the physician's personal contact with the patient, the lack of physician enthusiasm for the EMR, and fears over breaches of privacy.

Some of the characteristics of data needed for good clinical decision making are listed in Figure 24-12. The data need to be robust and span multiple domains (Figure 24-13).[46] Some of the knotty issues that will need to be managed include data capture (due to poor EMR operability and poor integration with clinician workflows), data quality and accuracy, data structure and readability, data storage and backup (especially for smaller firms), data sharing and interoperability, and data ownership and privacy.

## Artificial Intelligence and Machine Learning

Analytics focuses on figuring out what is happening and why, and uses statistical models and algorithms to derive insights to support decision making; predictive analytics focuses on projecting what will happen. Analytics is an important precursor to AI—the ability of machines to perform tasks that normally require human intelligence using visual perception, speech recognition, decision making, and language translation. Analytics is also an important precursor to *machine learning* (ML)—enabling computers to self-learn from data using advanced algorithms, to understand patterns in large data sets, to make predictions as they encounter new data using pattern recognition, and to adapt independently. *Natural language processing* (NLP) enables computers to understand, interpret, and manipulate human language using contextual patterns.

IBM Watson employed several of these approaches. Launched in 2006 as a research project, IBM expected Watson to become a multi-billion-dollar business that would collate information from the physician's office (including patient notes, test results, and patient questionnaires), combine it with genetic sequencing data on patient tumors, and then help providers to improve their diagnosis and treatment of cancer. This included a well-publicized partnership with MD Anderson Cancer Center to better match cancer patients with clinical trials; MD Anderson spent $62 million on the collaboration project (before cancelling it).

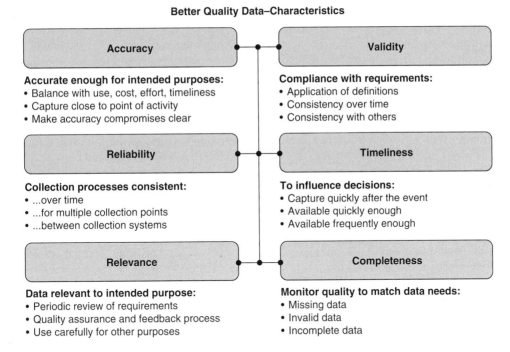

**Figure 24-12 •** Characteristics of Data for Good Decision Making. (Source: Dale Sanders, Presentation to the Wharton School, Fall 2018.)

IBM's bold attempt to revolutionize healthcare began in 2011, when Watson defeated 2 human champions on a TV gameshow (*Jeopardy!*) using its skills in NLP.[47] IBM gradually turned Watson loose on healthcare. In 2014, IBM invested $1 billion in Watson, formed a separate health division in 2015, and spent another $4 billion in 2016 to acquire 4 health data companies. In an attempt to find the business case for medical AI, IBM pursued several projects aimed at decision support by applying AI to massive data sets and using its computing

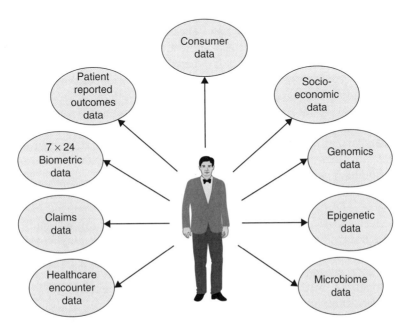

**Figure 24-13 •** The Data Ecosystem of Human Health. (Source: Dale Sanders, Presentation to the Wharton School, Fall 2018.)

power to examine hundreds of variables in patient records (eg, demographics, tumor characteristics, treatments, and outcomes) and discover patterns undetectable to humans. Watson's NLP struggled to make sense of medical text and its inherent ambiguities, however, and failed to pick up on subtle clues that doctors would notice.

It is important to recognize several different functions of AI in clinical care: *detection* of the patient's current health status, *prognostication* of the likelihood of some future state, and *prediction* of the patient's response to an intervention.[48] AI algorithms need to be matched with the problem to be addressed and the function to be performed. That is, AI needs to be better integrated into the clinician's workflow and delivery of care; simply developing lots of algorithms may not be helpful and thus may not be used by clinicians.

Two additional observations about AI and ML are worth noting. First, with regard to AI, the volume of data may be more important than the sophistication (and complexity) of AI models and algorithms. That is, what is needed are *more data points on a given patient* and across all patients within a physician's panel, which help to improve statistical power and reliability. As one researcher has explained, AI is good at distinguishing a zebra from a horse since it can store lots of images of the 2 animals, but AI is not good at understanding rare diseases where there is less information in the database. Second, the AI algorithms and ML code are but a small piece of the ML ecosystem and are perhaps commoditized. A number of other tools and infrastructure are required for AI and ML beyond just "code," including data collection, feature extraction, data verification, analysis tools, process management tools, and serving infrastructure. Part of this infrastructure includes the clinicians, their drawing of inferences from limited data, and developing causal interpretations. At present, AI cannot perform such tasks.[49]

With regard to incomplete data, it may be that "big data" are not really big enough. Some observers suggest that, at best, EMRs contain only 8% of the data needed for population health and personalized medicine. Consider the following observation: Only 10% of the factors that affect health status and health outcomes fall inside traditional healthcare delivery.

On average, patients have only 3 healthcare encounters per year, leaving researchers with missing data for the other 362 days of the year. Healthy patients thus represent the ideal AI training set, but there are no data on them.[50]

Market observers point to some additional, more fundamental problems with AI and ML. One includes the "hype" that fuels these technology efforts, just as they propelled the PHR movement. A little background on hype (defined as the effort to promote or publicize a product intensively, often exaggerating its importance or benefits) will help. In 1992, Howard Fosdick, a computer scientist, published an analysis of technology adoption that rested on two different curves (see top panel of Figure 24-14).[51] The first curve depicts the gradual increase in the usability and usefulness of a new technology to practitioners; the increase is tied to engineering improvements and technological maturation. The second curve depicts the growing public attention, visibility, and expectations surrounding this technology—all of which precedes and outstrips its utility; the growth is tied to a collective movement among technology observers attracted by the "new shiny object" and a social contagion process that fuels expectations. Fosdick referred to the early publicity in the second curve as "the hype phase," where public claims—often advanced by stakeholders (eg, trade press, industry analysts, technology vendors) with vested interests—are totally (and perhaps deliberately) divorced from the experience of actual users.

In 1996, analysts at The Gartner Group combined Fosdick's 2 graphs into 1 and labeled it the "Hype Cycle" (see bottom panel of Figure 24-14). The hype cycle purportedly characterizes the typical progression of technological innovation and its adoption over time. Gartner's model rests on a 5-stage process that includes (1) an initial wave of enthusiasm regarding the triggering of a new technology, (2) a peak in these inflated expectations, akin to overexuberance, followed by (3) disappointing results, expectations not met, and technology start-ups that crash and burn ("valley of despair"), followed by (4) more moderate expectations as surviving start-ups extract benefits from the technology, and (5) a period in which a handful of companies and technologies may finally succeed, leading to more realistic valuations.

**Technology Adoption Curves**

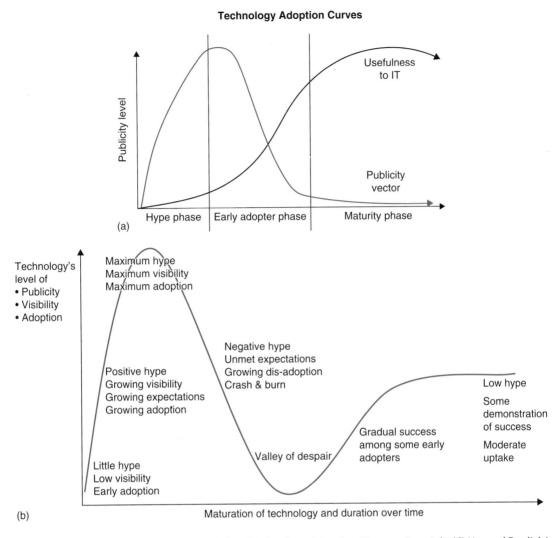

**Figure 24-14 •** (a) Two Different Curves Behind Technology Adoption. (Source: Copyright (C) Howard Fosdick.) (b) The Hype Cycle in Technology Adoption.

Researchers have subsequently noted that the hype cycle is really an amalgamation of Fosdick's different models, does not enjoy a strong theoretical foundation, and lacks empirical validation.[52] This should not be surprising: Fosdick himself acknowledged that he had not quantitatively verified his curves. In other words, the hype cycle may itself be nothing more than hype. Nevertheless, the hype cycle is widely cited and used in industry, which likely believes it to be true. More disturbingly, it can be used as an excuse for technological failure, an explanation for substandard technological performance (eg, "it's just a seasonable dip in the curve"), and the justification for hopeful progress ahead. One should therefore be wary of the publicity surrounding these new healthcare technologies. Perhaps the best conclusion to be drawn from the information craze sweeping healthcare is that we likely overestimate its impact in the short term and underestimate its impact in the long term.

Another problem concerns the neuropsychology of data. Simply stated, a purely data-driven approach to changing people's behavior—doctors and patients—is unlikely to succeed. One cannot force data on people and expect them to change; data and analytics are not enough. What is needed (ie, "ground zero") is the ability to deliver data to the point of decision making when both parties (doctors and patients) are willing to use it. As Daniel Pink wrote about physicians, "What data and decision support do you want and need to feel more informed, more autonomous, and more connected to your sense of purpose?"[53] Evidence suggests that clinicians are 15 times more likely to act on a best practice when presented with the opportunity at the point of care.[54] Of course, physicians may also need published evidence on the effectiveness of AI and ML—evidence that so far is in short supply.[55] Patients must be included in the picture as well. It probably doesn't help that hospitals and clinics employ AI-powered decision support tools—many of them lacking an evidence base for their efficacy—without notifying the patient.[56]

## Telehealth and Telemedicine

Telemedicine and telehealth are often confused. They are both concerned with delivering "from a distance" (original meaning of telemedicine). Although telemedicine has been commonly used in the past, telehealth has become the more universal term for the current broad array of applications in the field. That reflects the rise of consumer-directed healthcare, the shift to value-based care, the rising importance of population health, and the emphasis on wellness and care management. Some applications of home-based telehealth are depicted in Figure 24-15.

In 2014, the Department of Health and Human Services distinguished the 2 terms as follows: "Telehealth is different from telemedicine because it refers to a broader scope of remote healthcare services than telemedicine. While telemedicine refers specifically to remote clinical services, telehealth can refer to remote non-clinical services, such as provider training, administrative meetings, and continuing medical education, in addition to clinical services." The World Health Organization defined telehealth as "the delivery of healthcare services, where distance is a critical factor, by all healthcare professionals using information and communication technologies for the exchange of valid information for diagnosis, treatment and prevention of disease and injuries, research and evaluation, and for the continuing education of healthcare providers, all in the interests of advancing the health of individuals and their communities."

Telemedicine can be decomposed into 4 distinct categories: *mobile health* (mHealth: the practice of medicine and public health supported by mobile devices such as mobile phones, tablets, personal digital assistants, and wireless infrastructure); *remote patient monitoring* (ie, digital technologies that collect medical and other health data from patients in one location and electronically transmit that information securely to healthcare providers in other locations who can track the patient's health status); *store-and-forward care* (ie, asynchronous telemedicine: electronic transmission of patient data from one provider to another for evaluation or consultation); and *live video* (synchronous telemedicine: real-time patient encounters with the provider). It can include the following activities and modalities:

- Fitness/lifestyle tracking
- Chronic disease monitoring
- Semi-urgent care
- Clinician-to-clinician consultation
- Visit substitution
- Remote interpretation
- Tele-mentoring
- Critical care
- Virtual care teams
- Virtual emergency department
- Virtual urgent care
- Virtual patient rounds
- Remote monitoring of patients in the intensive care unit (tele-ICU)
- Live, 2-way management of stroke patients (tele-stroke)
- Live, 2-way management of patients with Parkinson disease (tele-Parkinson)
- Postoperative patient visits in the patient's home

Telemedicine has several tailwinds at its back. These include provider shortages that make access to care more important, the move to VBP such as bundled payment and accountable care organizations (ACOs), increased interest from both the Medicare and Medicaid programs, growing Medicare coverage (eg, under the Bipartisan Budget Act of 2018), and growing interest among private insurers in using telemedicine to substitute for urgent care and emergency department use. While there has been a heavy increase in telemedicine visits, they still accounted for a miniscule portion of Medicare beneficiaries (0.3%) and spending under the physician fee schedule (0.4%) in 2016. Another possible tailwind is the announced $18.5 billion merger in August 2020 of Teladoc (telemedicine

Home Teleheath

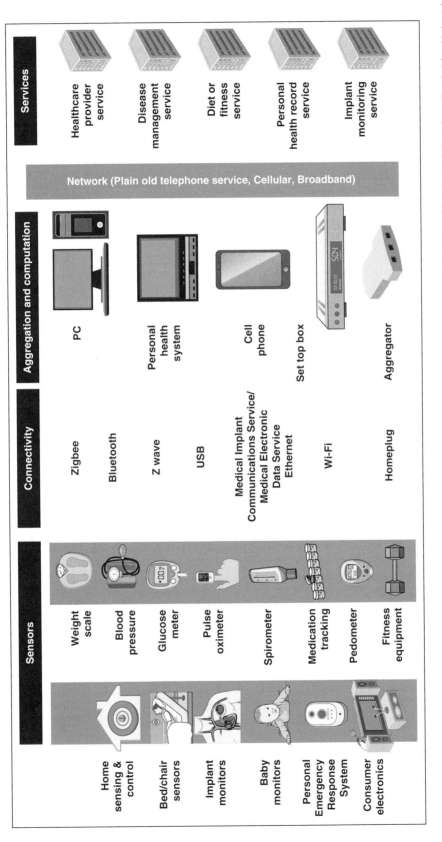

**Figure 24-15 •** Home Telehealth. (Source: Figure 7.6, in Lawton R. Burns [Ed.], *The Business of Healthcare Innovation*, 3rd ed. Cambridge, United Kingdom: Cambridge University Press; 2020.)

platform) with Livongo Health (chronic disease management coaching platform)—a deal that could offer employers more virtual care options for their workers.

The COVID-19 crisis has served as perhaps the biggest tailwind to telemedicine. In late March of 2020, Congress passed the Coronavirus Aid, Relief, and Economic Security (CARES) Act, which supported telehealth to expand access to virtual care. Specific provisions included the following:

- $29 million a year through 2025 to the Health and Resource Service Administration's Telehealth Resource Center to improve funding of telehealth initiatives
- $25 million for rural utilities to prepare for telemedicine services and broadband service
- A temporary lifting of restrictions on federally qualified health centers (FQHCs) and rural health clinics (RHCs) that permit them to see patients at home using telehealth
- A temporary lifting of face-to-face visit requirements for home dialysis patients
- A way to reestablish hospice care eligibility via telehealth
- $200 million for use by the Federal Communications Commission to launch a new telehealth program aimed to improve broadband connectivity for connected health services
- $1.032 billion to the Department for Health and Human Services for Indian Health Services, including telehealth and information technology upgrades
- $180 million to the Public Health and Social Services Emergency Fund to support telehealth and rural health activities

As the virus spread, CMS allowed Medicare providers to bill for telemedicine visits at the same rate as in-person visits; many commercial insurers followed suit. A sharp spike in virtual visits ensued in March and April, but then began to slowly decline in May and June.[57] From 14% of doctor visits in April, virtual care's share fell to only 8% by June. In August of 2020, President Trump signed an executive order directing the administration to permanently extend Medicare's broader coverage for virtual doctor visits via phone or video after the emergency is over.

The rise and fall of telemedicine visits in the spring of 2020 suggests that virtual care programs face a number of operational challenges. The challenges pose barriers to (1) the organizations that wish to pursue a telemedicine strategy, (2) clinicians who need to participate in these programs, and (3) patients who want to use these programs. These challenges include the cost of establishing the program (including both technology and staff training), limited reimbursement for patient encounters, the need for a revenue stream to compensate providers for going virtual, the need to demonstrate to providers that virtual care is financially sustainable, questions over Medicaid coverage and reimbursement for virtual care, legal liability, state variations in informed consent requirements, maintaining patient confidentiality, the need to maintain full compliance with licensure standards and other regulations, the need to achieve consumer buy-in, the need for an evidence base to support its appeal as a high-quality alternative to in-person care, consumer understanding of e-health, and consumers' computer literacy (eg, getting the elderly comfortable with the technology to embark on a video office visit). For example, physicians who wish to practice telemedicine may need a full medical license in both the state in which they live and the state in which the patient lives. Similarly, telemedicine programs that link multiple hospitals may require each physician involved to be credentialed at each hospital in the program.

Overall, according to the Medicare Payment Advisory Commission, telemedicine's impact on the iron triangle has been mixed, demonstrating increased access to care but not with a demonstrable improvement in quality or reduction in cost (Figure 24-16).[58] Huge uncertainties remain going forward, including consumers' willingness to stick with virtual care once stay-at-home orders are relaxed and fears of contagion diminish. It is also unclear whether virtual care in the absence of physical exams, in-office testing, and personal doctor-patient trust can really substitute for office visits and improve value. Perhaps its real value rests on supplementing office care for the chronically ill and reducing unnecessary emergency department visits. However, the discerning reader will recall that such promises have been advanced before in support of retail clinics and pharmacies as healthcare hubs.

## Critical Thinking Exercise: Jefferson Health and Telemedicine

Jefferson Health is a major healthcare system in the Philadelphia market, anchored by Thomas Jefferson University Hospital and its affiliated medical school. In 2015, Jefferson Health initiated a substantial investment in its telemedicine program, "JeffConnect." According to its website:

> JeffConnect serves patients, physicians, employers and our community with easy to access, high-quality care delivered by our talented medical staff and telehealth professionals. Successful telemedicine programs understand that the key to their success lies in the human factor engagement and operational workflows in concert with the right technology to meet their goals and objectives. Telemedicine programs provide patients and physicians with convenient access to each other through video visits that save time and money while providing a higher quality healthcare experience to patients interacting with your healthcare system.

According to system executives, Jefferson believes that "patients want care when and where they want it" and value immediate access (eg, walk in without an appointment) more than they value price. Jefferson's overarching goal is to "deliver comprehensive, high quality, coordinated care to patients when and where they need it or want it." Opportunities to tap include (1) low-risk encounters such as virtual inpatient rounds and on-demand outpatient care, and (2) more transformative models such as virtual emergency department visits, urgent care, and critical care network. In a presentation to the Wharton School, Jefferson executives portrayed their approach using the diagram below.[59]

What makes the Jefferson Health initiative so interesting is its sharp contrast with the strategic approach taken by its local competitor, the University of Pennsylvania Health System (UPHS). UPHS has also developed telemedicine and telehealth capabilities but has focused much of its clinical investments in tertiary and (especially) quaternary patient services, such as transplants and oncological care. Jefferson Health and UPHS are the two major health systems in the Philadelphia metro market. No one really knows which approach is better suited to the future environment. Jefferson is betting on virtual and primary care, although it has also acquired a lot of hospitals in the market (suggesting a brick-and-mortar strategy); UPHS is betting on high-tech inpatient care (and has just built a new flagship hospital). What do you think?

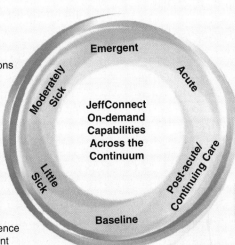

**Virtual ED**
↓Preventable ED use
↑Comprehensive access
↓Risk of care delays; admissions

**Urgent Care (Virtual and In-Person)**
↓Preventable ED use
↑Timeliness, access
↑Risk of becoming emergent

**On-Site Clinics**
↑Employee and dependent health
↑Presenteeism, productivity

**E-Visits**
↑Cost-effectiveness, convenience
↑Complance; self-management

**Critical Care and Specialty Consultation/telemedicine**
↓Avoidable/redundant testing
↓Length of stay
↓Total encounters

**Virtual Rounds**
↑Coordination, communication
↑Patient/family engagement

**Post-Discharge E-Management**
↓Readmissions
↑Compliance and engagement

**Remote Monitoring**
↓Readmissions
↑Compliance and engagement

Source: Dr. Judd Hollander, An Enterprise Wide Approach to Telemedicine. Presentation to the Wharton School (November 2018).

| TeleMedicine Service | Cost | Access | Quality |
|---|---|---|---|
| Telestroke | Small Increase | Expanded | Improved |
| Physical Disability | Small Increase | Expanded | Improved |
| Mental Health | Large Increase | Expanded | Some but Outcomes Unclear |
| DTC (Primary Care) | Very Large Increase | Expanded | Unclear |
| Nursing Home | Decrease | Unclear | Unclear |
| Remote Patient Monitoring | Very Large Increase | Expanded | Improved |

**Figure 24-16** • Impact of Telemedicine on the Iron Triangle. DTC, Direct to Consumer.

## BIG TECH: DANCING WITH ELEPHANTS

Disruption does exist. Consider the following:

- The world's largest taxi company … owns no taxis
- The world's largest voice/video communications companies … own no "telco"
- The most popular media company … owns no content
- The largest lodging company … owns no property
- The world's most valuable retailer … owns no inventory
- The world's largest software vendors … don't write the apps[60]

However, disruption does not usually originate inside healthcare. Perhaps the most potentially disruptive event in healthcare over the past 2 decades has been the entrance of "the big tech elephants"—Amazon, Apple, Google, and Facebook (among others)—with whom providers and other industry incumbents must now dance. Following are some thumbnail descriptions of these elephants' efforts. Although there is no definition of "big tech," it might include large technology firms that are publicly traded (eg, with market caps ranging from $12 billion to $1 trillion) and are category leaders (eg, with a clear competitive advantage in their core competence). Figure 24-17 offers one view of the big tech landscape and their operations in healthcare.[61]

### Amazon

Amazon's core competences include its customer obsession, logistics and distribution, and support platforms such as Amazon Fulfillment (shipping platform) and Amazon Web Services (cloud computing). The company currently operates in 3 sectors of the healthcare space: providers (eg, Amazon Care, Health Navigator, Omron), payers (eg, Haven), and producers (eg, PillPack, PharmacyOS, Basic Care, Grail). These are briefly described in the following list:

- Amazon Care is a virtual primary care clinic available to Amazon employees and family on a pilot basis. Amazon Care includes virtual care (Chat/Video), in-person visits (Mobile Care), and prescription delivery (Care Courier). Its focus is on urgent issues/preventative health consults. Amazon has recently teamed up with a primary care provider, Crossover Health, to pilot test physical clinics ("Neighborhood Health Centers") near its fulfillment centers and operations facilities in Texas to provide care to employees and families.
- Health Navigator provides online symptom checking and triage tools to companies seeking to route patients to the right place.

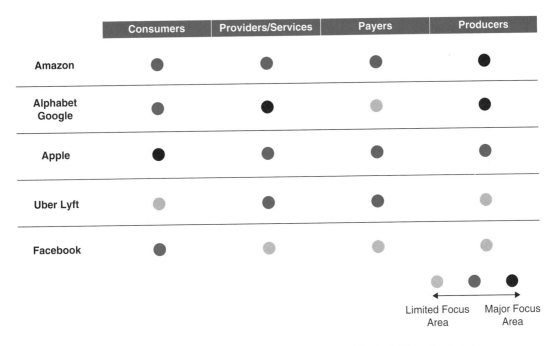

**Figure 24-17 •** Big Tech's Current Focus in Healthcare. (Source: Lazard Analysis, Team Analysis.)

- Omron sells blood pressure monitors.
- Haven is a joint venture between Amazon, Berkshire Hathaway, and JP Morgan to revamp their health insurance coverage to employees.
- PillPack consolidates a patient's multiple medications, simplifies dosing and administration, and provides detailed summaries, with delivery to door, automatic refills, and on-demand customer service. The service is free, requiring customers to pay only for the medications.
- PharmacyOS organizes patient and pharmaceutical data and makes it easy for both pharmacists and customers to manage multiple daily medications. The platform and workflow are designed around a customer's entire set of medications, instead of just designed to efficiently process individual prescriptions.
- Basic Care is Amazon's line of over-the-counter generic medicines (Advil, Mucinex) and Perrigo's GoodSense generic products (Perrigo is a private-label manufacturer).
- Grail is a start-up seeking to use deep sequencing technology to detect cancer in the blood at a treatable stage, which will require a lot of data processing and data storage. The latter could be a large business opportunity for Amazon Web Services. Amazon Web Services is competing with Google Genomics in the DNA data storage space—a business that analysts expect to be worth billions of dollars.

Amazon may leverage its mail-order pharmacy (PillPack) with the grocery store chain (Whole Foods) to offer retail clinics and pharmacies (see Chapter 13). Amazon can also possibly play in both the medical product and drug distribution businesses given its current role of supplier of low-risk products to hospitals and physicians, its interests in business-to-business (B2B) solutions, and its goal to have an interoperable tracking system for all of its businesses by 2023. Other possible businesses include claims management, considering it is selling software to digitize patient medical records and clinical notes, using ML to extract key data from EMRs, and ongoing experiments with Alexa's use in hospitals. The Alexa voice assistant is now a Health Insurance Portability and Accountability Act–compliant voice tool for use in home and hospitals. Another business opportunity is diagnostics and genomics by providing computer power and data storage, given its participation in Grail's $900 million Series B financing.

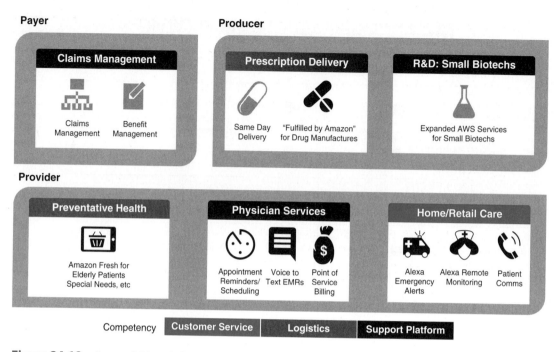

**Figure 24-18** • Amazon's Many Roles in the Healthcare Value Chain. (Source: CB Insights, "Amazon in Healthcare: The E-Commerce Giant's Strategy for a $3 Trillion Market.")

Finally, in an effort to compete with Google's Fitbit (see later discussion), Amazon has recently entered the health tracking space with Halo, a wrist-wearable device that can monitor sleep, body temperature, physical activity, body fat, and voice patterns. Amazon might also further penetrate the wellness and home health space by leveraging Alexa to monitor adherence as well as use cameras to monitor patients' vital signs. Amazon's future in healthcare may diversify to occupy multiple spaces (Figure 24-18).

## Apple

Apple's core competences include its integrated system (devices, applications, IOS software), consumer trust in the company's handling of private information, and its secure payment and transaction systems. Apple has differentiated its hardware using its software. Apple has also built a customer base that is 1.5 to 2.0 times larger than many of the largest health insurers (like Anthem and United Healthcare). Its key competitive advantage includes its considerable brand and customer experience, its potential to aggregate the leverage of its entire user base, its ability to package hardware and software, and thus its potential to create, structure, and interpret data.

In 2014, Apple launched the Health app, which now comes preinstalled on every iPhone.

The app includes features such as activity tracking, sleep monitoring, and mindfulness support. Apple has also created 3 "kits" that help developers build health-related apps for the iPhone and Apple Watch: HealthKit (developers feed information to and from the app and provide a framework for connecting new apps), ResearchKit (developers can create apps for medical research or clinical trials), and CareKit (aimed at connecting patients with providers). With regard to research, Apple can leverage its iPhone and Apple Watch user base to recruit participants for clinical studies. The Apple Heart Study recruited 400,000 participants via their iPhones; this can be contrasted with the typical need to recruit 50 medical centers to enroll 10,000 patients in a medical study.

Apple Watches today have the ability to monitor migraines, blood pressure, and adherence in psychiatric care and to even act as a virtual therapist for arm recovery in stroke patients. Apple has filed patents suggesting that future versions of its devices might let users measure their blood pressure, body fat, and heart rate simply by pressing their finger on the screen. The company has been in talks with Medicare Advantage plans about providing subsidized Apple Watches to the plans' patients in hopes of early detection of atrial fibrillation. Current partnerships include contracts with Aetna and UnitedHealthcare to provide discounted watches to health plan beneficiaries who walk at least 10,000 steps a day.

Apple has entered the EMR and PHR spaces and is seeking to leverage its iPhone platform for lots of healthcare applications. The PHR is the central pillar of Apple's healthcare strategy. In 2015, Apple launched ResearchKit as a tool to let medical researchers conduct studies using the iPhone. In 2018, Apple announced that it was bringing EMR data into the phone's health record. Apple rolled out a feature in its Health app that allows users to download, store, and share parts of their medical records; in turn, participating providers can send lab test results, medication regimens, and other data directly to a patient's iPhone. The company has several dozen partnerships with providers (eg, Cedars-Sinai, Geisinger Health System, Dignity Health, and Johns Hopkins Medicine) and EMR vendors (eg, athenahealth, Cerner, and Epic). Apple is building out an ecosystem around healthcare patient data, but it could move into medical service offerings (Figure 24-19).

## Google/Verily

Google's core competences include (1) search and data; (2) user experience, including AI and ML; and (c) capital, both human and financial. The company's healthcare investments span HCIT, wearables, provider-facing AI tools, and life sciences research and development (R&D). Businesses include Google Health, Google

Cloud, Google Hardware, Verily, Calico, and Google Ventures. These businesses are briefly described here:

- Google Health began as the company's PHR but has since migrated into the AI space, subsuming the company's Deep Mind division in 2018.
- Google Cloud is the company's cloud computing services product. Google recently invested in Amwell, a large telehealth provider, which will use Google Cloud as its preferred telehealth platform (eg, for video capabilities).
- Google Hardware is the company's effort to enter the hardware business (smartphones and fitness trackers like Fitbit that can monitor stress levels, changes in body temperature, and heart rhythms).
- Verily Life Sciences is a research organization dedicated to the study of the life sciences.
- Calico was founded in 2013 as an R&D science firm to study longevity, wellbeing, and health.
- Google Ventures is the VC arm of Google's parent company, Alphabet, and invests in a broad range of industries. These include One Medical (see Chapter 10), Oscar (see Chapter 17), and Grail.

Google's life sciences venture (Verily) has entered the population health data space, along with diabetes patient management and AI to

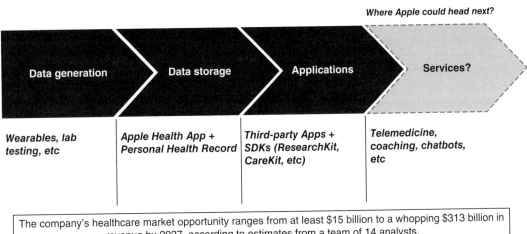

Figure 24-19 • Apple Ecosystem Built Around Healthcare Patient Data.

improve diagnosis of lung cancer. Verily applies Google's core competences to genomics and health data. The goal of Verily's Project Baseline (begun in 2017) is to map human health and create a stronger, more diverse clinical evidence base by engaging the 90%+ of the population that don't participate in clinical trials through new data gathering methods such as EMRs, sensors, and wearables. Verily also seeks to form a clinical research ecosystem with industry research partners and clinical trials that range from cardiovascular disease to oncology to mental health. Google has also applied its core competences to imaging and diagnostics workflow automation. Projects here include AI for Detection of Diabetic Eye Disease (eg, computer vision system for reading retinal images for diabetic retinopathy) and AI for Cancer Detection on Pathology Slides. In 2018, under the leadership of David Feinberg, the company refocused its Google Health effort to apply AI to the following areas: EHR upgrades, wearables, home health monitoring, and genomics research.

Verily has entered into several interesting partnerships with a variety of providers (eg, Duke University, Stanford Health) in a longitudinal, observational study to collect and analyze broad phenotypic health data from approximately 10,000 participants. This is part of a broad effort to develop a baseline of good health and a rich data platform to (1) better understand the transition from health to disease and (2) identify additional risk factors for disease. It has also entered partnerships with drug companies (eg, Sanofi) to offer a virtual diabetes solution to diabetic patients and with suppliers (Dexcom) to develop miniaturized continuous glucose monitors with miniaturized sensor electronics on an adhesive patch to make continuous monitoring less disruptive. Verily has partnered with Nikon to leverage the software and ML models created by Google Research to develop technology for the earlier detection of diabetic retinopathy and diabetic macular edema. They are seeking to combine the technology with Nikon's leadership in optical engineering and Optos's ultra-wide-field technology and strong commercial presence among eye care specialists.

Google has had some missteps, however. As noted earlier, its "direct-to-consumer" PHR product was a failure due to a lack of adoptions. Its Deep Mind project's deal with the United Kingdom's National Health Service violated data protection laws and was cancelled. Similar partnerships to gather patient data via 2 health systems in the United States (University of California–San Francisco, University of Chicago) also stirred up controversy when it was discovered that patients were not informed. Google faces several headwinds going forward, including poor public perception in handling patient data, an overall lack of trust in Google's use of health data, the need for new business models to supplant the company's traditional reliance (86% of revenue) on selling advertisements that use consumer data, and undeveloped competency in consumer hardware (the Fitbit space).

## Facebook

Facebook's core competences include connectivity ("bringing the world closer together"), gathering and analyzing user data, and user engagement. Like some of Apple's projects, Facebook has encountered several stumbles in trying to enter the healthcare space. Principal among these was the Cambridge Analytica scandal. The company also shuttered Moves (its fitness activity and tracker app) in 2018, just 4 years after acquiring it, and was outbid by Google for Fitbit. The Chan Zuckerburg Initiative's mission is to "find new ways to leverage technology, community-driven solutions, and collaboration to accelerate progress in Science, Education, and within our Justice and Opportunity work."

Facebook's latest healthcare initiative, the Preventive Health Tool, is relatively simple, reflecting a need to regain user trust and credibility in this space. The tool's purpose is to "connect people to health resources and checkup recommendations from leading health organizations." Features include leveraging users' age and gender information to make recommendations (initially focused on heart disease, cancer, and the flu). Users can schedule reminders to act upon these recommendations and search for affordable delivery options (eg, FQHCs).

The company is also going to great lengths to reassure the public over their privacy concerns. According to Facebook's Preventive Health Privacy Statement:

> Health is particularly personal, so we took privacy and safety into account from the beginning. For example, Preventive Health allows you to set reminders for your future checkups

and mark them as done, but it doesn't provide us, or the health organizations we're working with, access to your actual test results. Personal information about your activity in Preventive Health is not shared with third parties, such as the health organizations or insurance companies, so it can't be used for purposes like insurance eligibility. We don't show ads based on the information you provide in Preventive Health – that includes things like setting a reminder for a test, marking it as done or searching for a health care location. As always, other actions that you take on Facebook could inform the ads you see, for example, liking the Facebook page of a health organization or visiting an external website linked to Preventive Health.

## Microsoft

Microsoft has entered telehealth, medical imaging, cloud storage, and remote patient monitoring and is applying AI to all of these. In 2019, Microsoft entered a 7-year partnership with Walgreens Boots Alliance (WBA) to make a multiyear R&D investment to build healthcare solutions and explore the potential to establish joint innovation centers in key markets. For 2019, WBA will pilot up to 12 store-in-store "digital health corners" aimed at the merchandising and sale of select healthcare-related hardware and devices.

## Uber and Lyft

Uber and Lyft's core competences include on-demand logistics, a 2-sided platform connecting riders and drivers, and consumer focus. Ride-sharing dominates Lyft's business more than it does Uber's, where "eats" also earns substantial revenues. Uber is seeking to complement its food delivery business with prescription delivery by partnering with NimbleRx to offer next-day service. The major healthcare opportunity that both may try to exploit is addressing the social determinants of health. Transportation barriers significantly affect an individual's access to needed medical care, resulting in increased health expenditures and poorer health outcomes. Data suggest that the number of missed or delayed appointments may be as high as 3.6 million, at a cost of $150 billion. In August 2020, Lyft announced some encouraging results from several states showing that use of Lyft may be associated with fewer visits to emergency departments and shorter wait times for nonemergency transport.[62]

According to CMS, "Medicaid non-emergency medical transportation (NEMT) is an important benefit for beneficiaries who need to get to and from medical services but have no means of transportation. The Code of Federal Regulations requires States to ensure eligible, qualified Medicaid beneficiaries have NEMT to take them to and from providers." Each year, states book millions of rides for Medicaid patients. The government has reportedly spent at least $1.3 billion on NEMT each year, mostly attributed to Medicaid beneficiaries. A 2017 report on the landscape by the Center for Healthcare Strategies states, "Key challenges, including lack of responsiveness to schedule changes, difficulty in providing on-demand transportation, insufficient data collection and oversight, and complaints regarding customer service, have driven efforts across the country to improve NEMT options." The biggest headwind facing these companies is their lack of current profitability, which could make it difficult for them to invest appropriate resources to ensure these businesses work.

## Other Applications

There are a myriad of other applications that "big tech" is exploring. These applications span the provider, payer, and producer (eg, pharma, biotech) sectors. They are too numerous to describe here in detail but are dealt with extensively elsewhere.[63] For pharma, AI applications span molecular profiling and biomarker identification, validation of drug candidates, generation of novel drug candidates, preclinical testing, clinical testing, drug repurposing, and CRO activity. These may encompass the following:

- Molecular profiling and biomarker identification: aggregate and synthesize large biological data sets, use of the "omics" to improve sequencing to better understand diseases, screen new drug candidates, and discover new combination drugs.
- Validation of drug candidates: use neural networks to assess drug safety and efficacy, accelerate preclinical decision

making by generating accurate leads, and prototype and edit drug candidates according to newly discovered molecular properties.

- Generation of novel drug candidates: iterate small molecules to find the most suitable candidate, curate and mine gene variants, and gene mapping for specific diseases.
- Preclinical testing: automate selection and manipulation and analysis of cells, centralize the configuration of experiments, and optimize the reproducibility of experiment protocols and results.
- Clinical testing: predict patient responses to therapies to improve patient inclusion and exclusion criteria and leverage NLP to analyze existing clinical trial protocols that have been successful and unsuccessful to identify areas for improvement.
- Drug repurposing: reposition known drugs and shelved drug candidates, extend drug intellectual property protection by expanding their indications, and identify synergistic combinations of repositioned drugs.
- CRO: use predictive analytics to improve site selection and patient recruitment (eg, identify high-potential sites based on profiles to expedite recruitment and diversify the patient population), use ML to help patients find the right clinical trial, and improve investigator productivity by digitizing standard clinical assessments and automating data capture and data sharing.

## SUMMARY

Although biotechnology is "hot," HCIT is "cool." The sector has not only garnered considerable attention from Wall Street and VC funds as a major investment opportunity, but it has also attracted the market entry of several "FANG" (Facebook, Amazon, Netflix, and Google/Alphabet) companies into the HCIT space. Big tech firms have received a lot of the "ink." There are also a myriad of small companies that have received a lot of the investment money and offer great promise. A great primer on the activity here is summarized in a report prepared last year by Lazard and presented at the Wharton School.[64] See if you can lay your hands on it. Regardless, the lessons of the EMR suggest you still need to "curb your enthusiasm"; the promise may take a while to be realized.

---

### QUESTIONS TO PONDER

1. HCIT seems to hold out so much promise for the entire healthcare ecosystem. Why hasn't this promise been realized?
2. At first glance, EMRs seem to be such a useful tool for physicians in caring for their patients. And, yet, many physicians dislike their EMRs. What explains this? Is it just hostility to new technology and a reluctance to change?
3. What is the promise of new HCIT innovations such as wearables? Analytics? AI?
4. Telemedicine received an enormous boost during the COVID-19 pandemic that started in the spring of 2020. What does telemedicine need in order to become a more central, mainstream feature in healthcare delivery?

---

### REFERENCES

1. For details on the meaningful use program, see: https://www.cms.gov/Regulations-and-Guidance/Legislation/EHRIncentivePrograms/downloads/MU_Stage1_ReqOverview.pdf. See also: https://www.cms.gov/apps/stage-2-meaningful-use-attestation-calculator/.
2. The data presented here are courtesy of Stephanie Demko, Joy Zhang, and Jason Hoffman. *Healthcare Technology* (New York, NY: SVB-Leerink, April 2020).
3. Rebecca Pifer. "Digital Health Funding Shatters Records with $6.3B in 1st Half of 2020," *HealthcareDive* (July 14, 2020).
4. R. Scott Evans. "Electronic Health Records: Then, Now, and in the Future," *Yearbook of Medical Informatics* (Suppl 1) (2016): S48-S61. This section of the chapter relies heavily on this article.
5. Institute of Medicine. *The Computer-Based Patient Record: An Essential Technology for Health Care*. Revised Edition. Richard S. Dick, Elaine B. Steen, Don E. Detmer (Eds.) (Washington, DC: National Academy Press, 1997).
6. Tom Sullivan. "Why EHR Data Interoperability Is Such a Mess in 3 Charts," *Healthcare IT News*

(May 16, 2018). Available online: https://www.healthcareitnews.com/news/why-ehr-data-interoperability-such-mess-3-charts. Accessed on May 2, 2020.

7. Ilana Graetz, Mary Reed, Stephen Shortell, et al. "The Association Between EHRs and Care Coordination Varies by Team Cohesion," *Health Serv Res.* 49 (1) (Part II) (2014): 438-452. Ilana Graetz, Mary Reed, Stephen Shortell, et al. "The Next Step Towards Making Use Meaningful: Electronic Information Exchange and Care Coordination Across Clinicians and Delivery Sites," *Med Care.* 52 (12) (2014): 1037-1041.

8. Diane Rittenhouse, Stephen Shortell, Robin Gillies, et al. "Improving Chronic Illness Care: Findings From a National Study of Care Management Processes in Large Physician Practices," *Med Care Res Rev.* 67 (3) (2010): 301-320.

9. Cheryl Damberg, Stephen Shortell, Kristina Raube, et al. "Relationship Between Quality Improvement Processes and Clinical Performance," *Am J Managed Care.* 16 (8) (2010): 601-606.

10. Stephen Shortell, Robin Gillies, Juned Siddique, et al. "Improving Chronic Illness Care: A Longitudinal Cohort Analysis of Large Physician Organizations," *Med Care.* 47 (9) (2009): 932-939.

11. Ann O'Malley, Ann Tynan, Genna Cohen, et al. *Coordination of Care by Primary Care Practices: Strategies, Lessons and Implications.* Research Brief No. 12 (Washington, DC: Center for Studying Health System Change, 2009). Arthur Kellerman and Spencer Jones. "What It Will Take to Achieve the As-Yet-Unfulfilled Promises of Health Information Technology," *Health Affairs* 32 (1) (2013): 63-68.

12. Chun-Ju Hsiao, Jennifer King, Esther Hing et al. "The Role of Health Information Technology in Care Coordination in the United States," *Med Care.* 53 (2) (2015): 184-190.

13. Ilana Graetz, Mary Reed, Stephen Shortell, et al. "The Association Between EHRs and Care Coordination Varies by Team Cohesion," *Health Serv Res.* 49 (1) (Part II) (2014): 438-452. Ilana Graetz, Mary Reed, Stephen Shortell, et al. "The Next Step Towards Making Use Meaningful: Electronic Information Exchange and Care Coordination Across Clinicians and Delivery Sites," *Med Care.* 52 (12) (2014): 1037-1041.

14. Suzanne Morton, Sarah Shih, Chloe Winther, et al. "Health IT-Enabled Care Coordination: A National Survey of Patient-Centered Medical Home Clinicians," *Ann Fam Med.* 13 (3) (2015): 250-256. Randall Brown. "Lessons for ACOs and Medical Homes on Care Coordination for High-Need Beneficiaries," Presentation to Academy-Health Annual Research Meeting (Baltimore, MD: June 2013). Congressional Budget Office. *Lessons From Medicare's Demonstration Projects on Disease Management, Care Coordination, and*

*Value-Based Payment* (Washington, DC: CBO, January 2012). Marlon Mundt, Valerie Gilchrist, Michael Fleming et al. "Effects of Primary Care Team Social Networks on Quality of Care and Costs for Patients With Cardiovascular Disease," *Annals of Family Medicine* 13 (2) (2015): 139-148.

15. Michael Furukawa, Jennifer King, Vaishali Patel, et al. "Despite Substantial Progress in EHR Adoption, Health Information Exchange and Patient Engagement Remain Low in Office Settings," *Health Aff.* 33 (9) (2014): 1672-1679.

16. Suzanne Morton, Sarah Shih, Chloe Winther, et al. "Health IT-Enabled Care Coordination: A National Survey of Patient-Centered Medical Home Clinicians," *Ann Fam Med.* 13 (3) (2015): 250-256.

17. Suzanne Morton, Sarah Shih, Chloe Winther, et al. "Health IT-Enabled Care Coordination: A National Survey of Patient-Centered Medical Home Clinicians," *Ann Fam Med.* 13 (3) (2015): 250-256."

18. The American Recovery and Reinvestment Act (ARRA, 2009) authorized the Centers for Medicare and Medicaid Services (CMS) to extend financial incentives to physicians who adopt information technology (IT) systems and demonstrate "meaningful use" of them in their clinical practices. Meaningful use had 3 stages: (1) electronic capture of patient health record data, which could then be used in reporting and tracking clinical conditions; (2) use clinical data to guide and support care processes and coordination; and (3) improve performance and health system outcomes. ARRA required 25 functionalities under the meaningful use regulations; only some of these have been studied.

19. Trent Spaulding, Michael Furukawa, T. S. Raghu, et al. "Event Sequence Modeling of IT Adoption in Healthcare," *Decis Support Syst.* 55 (2) (2013): 428-437. Jeffrey McCullough, Michelle Casey, Ira Moscovice, et al. "The Effect of Health Information Technology on Quality in US Hospitals," *Health Aff.* 29 (4) (2010): 647-654.

20. Basil Chaudhry, Jerome Wang, Shinyi Wu, et al. "Systematic Review: Impact of Health Information Technology on Quality, Efficiency, and Costs of Medical Care," *Ann Intern Med.* 144 (2006): E12-E22. Eta Berner. *Clinical Decision Support Systems: State of the Art* (Washington, DC: Agency for Healthcare Research and Quality, 2009). President's Council of Advisors on Science and Technology. *Report to the President—Realizing the Full Potential of Health Information Technology to Improve Healthcare for Americans: The Path Forward* (Washington, DC: PCAST, 2010). Lorenzo Moreno, Deborah Peikes, and Amy Krilla. *Necessary but Not Sufficient: The HITECH Act and Health Information Technology's Potential to Build Medical Homes*

(Washington, DC: Agency for Healthcare Quality and Research, 2010). Melinda Beeuwkes Buntin, Matthew F. Burke, Michael C. Hoaglin, and David Blumenthal. "The Benefits of Health Information Technology: A Review of the Recent Literature Shows Predominantly Positive Results," *Health Aff.* 30 (3) (2011): 464-471. Lawton R. Burns and Mark V. Pauly. "Accountable Care Organizations May Have Difficulty Avoiding the Failures of Integrated Delivery Networks of the 1990s," *Health Aff.* 31 (11) (2012): 2407-2416. Neil Fleming, Edmund Becker, Steven Culler, et al. "The Impact of Electronic Health Records on Workflow and Financial Measures in Primary Care Practices," *Health Serv Res.* 49 (1) (Part II) (2014): 405-420. Julia Adler-Milstein, Jordan Everson, and Daniel Shoou-Yih. "EHR Adoption and Hospital Performance: Time-Related Effects," *Health Serv Res.* 50 (6) (2015): 1751-1771. Hemant Bhargava and Abhay Mishra. "Electronic Medical Records and Physician Productivity: Evidence From Panel Data Analysis," *Manag Sci.* 60 (10) (2014): 2543-2562.

21. Mathematica Policy Research. *Hospital Acquisition of Physician Practices: Higher Value or Higher Costs?* (Washington, DC: Center on Health Care Effectiveness Policy Forum, November 2015).

22. Stephen Shortell, Robin Gillies, Juned Siddique, et al. "Improving Chronic Illness Care: A Longitudinal Cohort Analysis of Large Physician Organizations," *Med Care.* 47 (9) (2009): 932-939.

23. Spencer Jones, Robert Rudin, Tanja Perry, et al. "Health Information Technology: An Updated Systematic Review with a Focus on Meaningful Use," *Ann Intern Med.* 160 (2014): 48-54.

24. Leila Agha. "The Effects of Health Information Technology on the Costs and Quality of Medical Care," *J Health Econ.* 34 (2014): 19-30.

25. David Classen, A. Jay Holmgren, Zoe Co, et al. "National Trends in the Safety Performance of Electronic Health Record Systems From 2009 to 2018," *JAMA Network Open* (May 29, 2020).

26. Lisa Kern, Yolanda Barrón, Rina Dhopeshwarkar, et al. "Electronic Health Records and Ambulatory Quality of Care," *J Gen Intern Med.* 28 (4) (2013): 496-503. Max J. Romano and Randall S. Stafford. "Electronic Health Records and Clinical Decision Support Systems," *Arch Intern Med.* 171 (10) (2011): 897-903.

27. Zilma Reis, Thais Maia, Milena Marcolini, et al. "Is There Evidence of Cost Benefits of Electronic Medical Records, Standards, or Interoperability in Hospital Information Systems? Overview of Systematic Reviews," *JMIR Med Inform.* 5 (3) (2017 Jul-Sep): e26.

28. CDSS might increase quality by improving physician decision making, reducing medication errors, and facilitating the prevention and use of evidence-based recommended therapy. CDSS effects are stronger for increasing preventive care than reducing costs. Evidence on the benefits of diagnostic assistance offered by electronic systems is mixed, partly because physicians often ignore the systems' advice. Theoretically, decision support systems can reduce adverse drug events and thereby reduce costs, but evidence of the effects on costs, testing, and clinicians' time is again mixed. Likewise, CPOE can reduce costs and improve quality by reducing medication error rates, but evidence of this often comes from advanced integrated delivery networks with customized systems. Literature reviews report mixed success of the technology in averting adverse drug events, increasing adherence to guidelines, and prescribing efficiency.

29. Aziz Jamal, Kirsten McKenzie, and Michele Clark. "The Impact of Health Information Technology on the Quality of Medical and Health Care: A Systematic Review," *Health Inform Manag J.* 38 (3) (2009): 26-37.

30. Eta Berner. *Clinical Decision Support Systems: State of the Art* (Washington, DC: Agency for Healthcare Research and Quality, 2009).

31. Alexander Low, Andrew B. Phillips, Jessica S. Ancker, et al. "Financial Effects of Health Information Technology: A Systematic Review," *Am J Managed Care.* 19 (11) (2013): 369-376.

32. Julia Adler-Milstein, Jordan Everson, and Daniel Shoou-Yih. "EHR Adoption and Hospital Performance: Time-Related Effects," *Health Serv Res.* 50 (6) (2015): 1751-1771.

33. Neil Fleming, Edmund Becker, Steven Culler, et al. "The Impact of Electronic Health Records on Workflow and Financial Measures in Primary Care Practices," *Health Serv Res.* 49 (1) (Part II) (2014): 405-420. Hemant Bhargava and Abhay Mishra. "Electronic Medical Records and Physician Productivity: Evidence from Panel Data Analysis," *Manag Sci.* 60 (10) (2014): 2543-2562.

34. Spencer Jones, Robert Rudin, Tanja Perry, et al. "Health Information Technology: An Updated Systematic Review with a Focus on Meaningful Use," *Ann Intern Med.* 160 (2014): 48-54.

35. Leila Agha. "The Effects of Health Information Technology on the Costs and Quality of Medical Care," *J Health Econ.* 34 (2014): 19-30.

36. This section draws on the following sources. Adam Powell and John Glaser. "The Healthcare Information Technology Sector," in Lawton R. Burns (Ed.), *The Business of Healthcare Innovation*, 3rd ed. (Cambridge, United Kingdom: Cambridge University Press, 2020): Chapter 7. Clemens Kruse, Caitlin Kristof, Beau Jones, et al. "Barriers to Electronic Health Record Adoption: A Systematic Literature Review," *J Med Syst.* 40 (12) (2016): 252.

37. Ton Spil and Rich Klein. "Personal Health Records Success: Why Google Vault Failed and

What Does That Mean for Microsoft Health Vault?" 2014 47th Hawaii International Conference on System Science. Available online: https://ieeexplore.ieee.org/document/6758953. Accessed on August 30, 2020.

38. Marianne McGee. "5 Reasons Why Google Health Failed," *InformationWeek* (June 29, 2011). Available online: https://www.informationweek.com/healthcare/electronic-health-records/5-reasons-why-google-health-failed/d/d-id/1098623. Accessed on April 30, 2020.

39. Mike Critelli. "The Unfulfilled Promise of Electronic Health Records and Patient Health Management," *OpenMike*. Available online: https://www.mikecritelli.com/blog/unfulfilled-promise-of-electronic-health-records-patient-health.html. Accessed on July 31, 2020.

40. Fred Schulte and Erika Frye. "Death by 1,000 Clicks: Where Electronic Health Records Went Wrong," *Fortune* (March 18, 2019).

41. Gartner. *Forecast Analysis: Wearable Electronic Devices, Worldwide* (October 24, 2019).

42. Rock Health. *Digital Health Consumer Adoption Survey.*

43. Saee Hamine, Emily Gerth-Guyette, Dunia Faulx, et al. "Impact of mHealth Chronic Disease Management on Treatment Adherence and Patient Outcomes: A Systematic Review," *J Med Internet Res.* 17 (2) (2015): e52.

44. Some content here is courtesy of Dale Sanders. Presentation to the Wharton School (November 2018).

45. Michael E. Porter, Stefan Larrson, and Thomas H. Lee. "Standardizing Patient Outcomes Measurement," *N Engl J Med.* 374 (February 11, 2016): 504-506.

46. Figures 24-12 and 24-13 are courtesy of Dale Sanders.

47. Eliza Strickland. "How IBM Watson Overpromised and Underdelivered on AI Health Care," *IEEE Spectrum* (April 2, 2019).

48. Christopher Lindsell, William Stead, and Kevin Johnson. "Action-Informed Artificial Intelligence: Matching the Algorithm to the Problem," *JAMA.* 323 (2020): 2141-2142.

49. Angel Desai. "Artificial Intelligence: Promise, Pitfalls, and Perspective," *JAMA.* 323 (2020): 2448-2449.

50. Dale Sanders. Presentation to the Wharton School (November 2018).

51. Howard Fosdick. "The Sociology of Technology Adaptation," *Enterprise Systems Journal* (September 1992).

52. Martin Steinert and Larry Leifer. "Scrutinizing Gartner's Hype Cycle Approach," *PICMET*

*2010 Proceedings* (Phuket, Thailand: July 18-22): 254-266. Ozgur Dedehayir and Martin Steinart. "The Hype Cycle Model: A Review and Future Directions," *Technological Forecasting and Social Change* 108 (2016): 28-41.

53. Daniel H. Pink. *Drive* (New York, NY: Riverhead Books, 2009).

54. Kensaku Kawamoto, Caitlin A. Houlihan, E. Andrew Balas, and David F. Lobach. "Improving Clinical Practice Using Clinical Decision Support Systems: A Systematic Review of Trials to Identify Features Critical to Success," *BMJ.* 330 (74794) (April 2, 2005): 765. Available online: https://www.ncbi.nlm.nih.gov/pmc/articles/PMC555881/. Accessed on August 12, 2020. Tiffani J. Bright, Anthony Wong, Ravi Dhurjati, et al. "Effect of Clinical Decision-Support Systems: A Systematic Review," *Ann Intern Med.* 157 (2012): 29-43. Available online: http://annals.org/aim/article/1206700/effect-clinical-decision-support-systems-systematic-review. Accessed on August 12, 2020.

55. Myura Nagendran, Yang Chen, Christopher Lovejoy, et al. "Artificial Intelligence Versus Clinicians: Systematic Review of Design, Reporting Standards, and Claims of Deep Learning Studies," *Br Med J.* 368 (2020): m689.

56. Rebecca Robbins and Erin Brodwin. "An Invisible Hand: Patients Aren't Being Told About the AI Systems Advising Their Care," *Stat* (July 15, 2020).

57. Ateev Mehrotra, David Linetsky, and Hilary Hatch. "This Is Supposed to Be Telemedicine's Time to Shine. Why Are Doctors Abandoning It?" *Stat* (June 25, 2020).

58. Medicare Payment Advisory Commission. "Telehealth Services and the Medicare Program," in *Report to the Congress: Medicare Payment Policy* (Washington, DC: MedPAC, March 2018): Chapter 16.

59. Judd Hollander. *An Enterprise Wide Approach to Telemedicine.* Presentation to the Wharton School (November 2018).

60. Answers: Uber, Skype, Facebook, AirBNB, Alibaba, and Apple/Google. Courtesy of Dale Sanders.

61. This section and figures are based on: Monica Adibe, Ross Brown, Radhika Gupta, et al. "Big Tech Enters Healthcare," Presentation to the Wharton School (November 2019).

62. Erin Brodwin, Rebecca Robbins, and Casey Ross. "How Teladoc Won and Lyft's Medicaid Transportation Business," *Stat* (August 19, 2020).

63. David Gluckman. Presentation to the Wharton School (November 2019).

64. Lazard. *Perspectives on the Future of BioPharma* (New York, NY: Lazard, May 2019).

# SECTION V

## The Public Sector of the Ecosystem

# The Federal Bureaucracy, the US Congress, and Healthcare Policy

25

## INTRODUCTION

Prior chapters have discussed the role of the federal government in payment programs, such as Medicare and Medicaid (see Chapters 18 and 19). The following chapter describes the government's role in promoting public health, including the Centers for Disease Control and Prevention (CDC), which have played a major role in the COVID-19 crisis. This chapter describes the responsibilities for healthcare that are widely distributed and exercised throughout the congressional and executive branches of the US government. It also sketches some of the major policy initiatives these branches have undertaken over the past few decades.

## THE FEDERAL GOVERNMENT's DIVERSE ROLES

The federal government's role in healthcare was never systematically designed; rather, it evolved and developed incrementally over time. In general, the serial involvement of the federal government has spanned (1) the direct delivery of care, (2) welfare payments and public assistance, (3) support for the capital and manpower infrastructure to deliver this healthcare, (4) financing biomedical innovation and payment for that healthcare, and finally (5) regulating the system to control the cost and improve the quality of the healthcare it had spawned.

Federal involvement began with sponsorship of Public Health Services hospitals for merchant seamen at the turn of the 20th century (see Chapter 26). The scale and variety of federal activity has grown since the 1930s, starting with the Social Security Act of 1935. Some of the stimuli for federal involvement have included the Depression of the 1930s, World War II and technological discoveries (1940s and 1950s), and dealing with price inflation (1970s).

This growing involvement has been described in 2, polar opposite ways. One view is that the federal government executed a "takeover" of the healthcare system and inserted itself into everything. The other view is that the federal government has been engaged in a long-term collaboration, partnership, and symbiotic relationship with the healthcare industry, which owes its current size and shape to federal efforts. According to this latter view, every core element of the healthcare ecosystem was fashioned in one way or another by the government, which guided the industry over the course of the 20th century.[1]

Regardless of which view you endorse, why did the federal role develop this way? Problems arose incrementally, and policies then developed incrementally to deal with them. To implement these policies, the federal bureaucracy expanded incrementally. The result is a dynamic, changing structure that is widely spread across the federal government and its divisions. The dispersion of health activities reflects the variety of stimuli that gave rise to federal program development, the diversity in constituencies served, the variety of issues addressed, and the diversity in emphasis by specific agencies.

The federal government plays at least 3 major roles: financing (payer of healthcare), delivery (provider of healthcare), and regulation (oversight of healthcare). With regard to **financing**, the federal government underwrites the provision of *services* through the extension of insurance benefits (eg, Medicare and Medicaid, State Children's Health Insurance Program [SCHIP], Department of Defense, Civilian Health and Medical Program of the Uniformed Services) and coverage for new technology; *education* and *manpower* development (medical school construction, Bureau of Health Professions, health education and assistance loans); *capital* (Hill-Burton Act to finance rural hospitals, Medicare reimbursement of capital investment); *training* (Medicare funding of graduate medical education); and *research* (National Institutes of Health [NIH], Agency for Health Research and Quality).[2]

With regard to **delivery**, the federal government provides healthcare via the Veterans Administration (VA) and its national network of hospitals, clinics, and nursing homes; the Health Resources and Services Administration (HRSA), which operates Public Health Service hospitals, community health centers, and community mental health centers; the NIH, which operates a 500+ bed hospital; the Indian Health Service (IHS), which operates hospitals and health centers; the Department of Defense (DOD), which operates hospitals for branches of the military (eg, Army, Navy); and the Bureau of Medical Services (BMS), which operates Coast Guard and prison hospitals.

Many of these activities fall under the aegis of the Department of Health and Human Services (DHHS). The DHHS aims "to enhance and protect the health and well-being of all Americans" by "providing for effective health and human services and fostering advances in medicine, public health, and social services." The DHHS houses several agencies and operating divisions, 8 of which touch on public health (see Chapter 26).[3] Other divisions and agencies touch on human services. For example, the Centers for Medicare and Medicaid Services (CMS) administers the Medicare, Medicaid, and SCHIP programs. The Administration for Community Living (ACL) provides grants to support home-based and community-based services for older adults and the disabled.

With regard to **regulation**, the federal government operates through the Food and Drug Administration (FDA), the Department of Justice (DOJ), the Federal Trade Commission (FTC), and the Office of the Inspector General (OIG), among others.[4] Through these bodies, the government exercises oversight of the private sector marketplace. Such oversight is

frequently intended to address the iron triangle (increase access, control costs, or improve quality) rather than tackle the triple aim.

## CONSEQUENCES OF FEDERAL INVOLVEMENT

One cannot overestimate the impact of the federal government on the US healthcare ecosystem, despite the latter's largely voluntary and nonprofit character. Healthcare policy can originate from lots of places, such as the executive branch or the legislative branch. The healthcare policy-making process is torturous, and the policy implementation process is detailed and bureaucratic. "Incrementalism" is the name of the game—both for policy making and for policy implementation. Indeed, long ago, political scientist Charles Lindblom labeled the policy process as "disjointed incrementalism," where lots of disparate efforts get patched together in an iterative, semi-coherent fashion to advance some agenda.[5] To fully appreciate the government's role, one needs to get to know the "players" in Congress (eg, key committees and their leaders), the players in the executive branch (eg, key agencies and departments and their leaders), and the rules for enacted legislation embodied in the *Federal Register* and *Code of Federal Regulations*. One also needs to keep in mind that the federal government is but 1 of 3 levels of government; the responsibilities of the other 2 levels are portrayed in Figure 25-1.

## THE US CONGRESS's ROLES[6]

The US Congress fulfills a key role in healthcare policy making by setting the broad parameters and priorities of healthcare programs, determining their funding levels, and overseeing their implementation. Congress, the legislative branch of government, has 2 chambers: the Senate and the House of Representatives. Their efforts are supported by congressional staffers as well as such offices as the Congressional Budget Office (CBO), the Government Accountability Office (GAO), and the Congressional Research Service (CRS).

Just as there is fragmentation in the delivery and financing of healthcare, there is also fragmentation in congressional jurisdiction over healthcare. Between 1980 and 1991, the distribution of congressional committee hearings on

| State Government | Local Government |
|---|---|
| Medicaid funding | Public health departments |
| Mental healthcare | Local public hospitals |
| Medical education (schools, programs) | Safety net providers |
| Licensing of health professionals and provider facilities | Behavioral health (bulk of budget) |
| Regulation of insurers | Substance abuse programs |
| Public health departments | Partnerships with other agencies: child welfare, family court, schools, prisons |

**Figure 25-1** • Multiple Governments.

health-related issues was divided among more committees than hearings in any other policy domain.

As testimony, the Senate and House contain multiple committees and subcommittees that deal with healthcare. There are 16 "standing" (ie, permanent) committees in the Senate (www.senate.gov), 20 standing committees in the House (www.house.gov), and 4 joint (Senate and House) committees.[7] Each branch of Congress also has special committees (4 in the Senate, 3 in the House) and select committees (eg, Intelligence and Climate Crisis).[8] Moreover, most committees have several subcommittees. These committees can be classified by what they do: (1) Taxing Committees, which raise revenues, (2) Authorization Committees, which develop and oversee programs, and (3) Appropriations Committees, which set program spending levels. Both the Senate and the House have appropriations committees with several subcommittees. There is a division of labor and oversight among these subcommittees, with separate responsibility for specific agencies (eg, DHHS, FDA, and VA).

Several key committees in the **US Senate** deal with healthcare. The *Committee on Finance* has jurisdiction over taxation and other revenue measures, including programs under the Social Security Act (including Medicare, Medicaid, and SCHIP). This committee has 6 subcommittees, including the Subcommittee on Health Care.

The Senate *Committee on Health, Education, Labor, and Pensions* has jurisdiction over aging, biomedical research, and development of public health. It has a Subcommittee on Primary Health and Retirement Security with jurisdiction over several issues, including the Health Resources and Services Act, substance abuse and mental health, healthcare disparities, and the Pension Benefit Guaranty Corporation through the Employee Retirement Income Security Act (ERISA).

The Senate *Appropriations Committee* has a Subcommittee on Labor, Health and Human Services, Education, and Related Agencies with jurisdiction over appropriations to DHHS. It also has a Subcommittee on Agriculture, Rural Development, Food and Drug Administration, and Related Agencies that has jurisdiction over appropriations to the FDA.

Finally, the Senate *Committee on Commerce, Science, and Transportation* has jurisdiction over interstate commerce, consumer affairs, and regulation of consumer products. It contains the Subcommittee on Consumer Protection, Product Safety, Insurance, and Data Security, which authorizes and oversees efforts of several federal consumer protection agencies.

Several key committees in the **House of Representatives** also deal with healthcare. The House *Committee on Ways and Means* has jurisdiction over revenue measures, the nation's bonded debt, trade and tariff legislation, and national Social Security programs (Medicare, Medicaid). Its key Subcommittee on Health has legislative and oversight jurisdiction over many activities, including legislative jurisdiction over drug policy. The House *Committee on Energy and Commerce* oversees consumer protection, food and drug safety, public health research, and environmental quality. It also oversees several Cabinet departments including DHHS. Its Subcommittee on Health has broad jurisdiction over the health sector, including the Patient Protection and Affordable Care Act (PPACA), Medicare, Medicaid, SCHIP, biomedical research, hospital construction, mental health, health information technology, the regulation of drugs, DHHS, NIH, and CDC.

The House *Committee on Appropriations* has 3 subcommittees. The Subcommittee on Labor, Health and Human Services, Education, and Related Agencies has jurisdiction over appropriations to DHHS; the Subcommittee on Agriculture, Rural Development, Food and Drug Administration, and Related Agencies has jurisdiction over FDA appropriations; and the Subcommittee on the Interior, Environment, and Related Agencies has jurisdiction over appropriations for the Agency for Toxic Substances and Disease Registry, the Indian Health Service, and the superfund activities of the National Institute of Environmental Health Sciences. The House *Committee on Education and the Workforce* contains the Subcommittee on Health, Employment, Labor, and Pensions, which has jurisdiction over employment-related health and retirement security, including health benefits.

The 2 chambers of Congress also have purview over global healthcare issues. These issues are overseen by different committees in the 2 branches (eg, House Committee on Foreign Affairs, Senate Committee on Foreign Relations).

Congressional committees have 2 broad functions: legislation and oversight. *Legislation* before Congress may consist of either a resolution or a bill, which serve different functions. Resolutions often recognize an issue or express a position on an issue but are generally nonbinding and do not become law. By contrast, bills may become law if they pass both chambers of Congress and are subsequently sent to the president, who then decides whether to sign or veto them. Bills typically function to *authorize* funding, programs, and activities or to *appropriate* funding for such programs and activities. An authorization bill may lay out congressional priorities for healthcare programs, including approaches, strategies, targeted populations, and targeted goals. It may also define the period during which such activities may be operated and provide guidance on the amount of funding.

While authorization bills specify congressional intent with regard to funding, the actual funding comes through appropriations bills. An appropriations bill provides funding for specific programs and activities. Support for healthcare programs can be *discretionary* or *mandatory*;

funding for the former is typically determined (appropriated) on an annual basis by Congress. Congress is not required to appropriate the level of funding that is authorized for a *discretionary* program.

While these 2 kinds of bills are designed to be interrelated as part of a 2-step process, Congress has increasingly used them for similar purposes (although appropriations bills remain the only legislative vehicle for providing funding). As a result, Congress can include provisions in both types of bills that provide guidance or requirements for how funds are spent and/or how programs are implemented. These provisions may include spending directives as well as other legislative requirements and restrictions.

With regard to *oversight*, Congressional committees conduct several activities: (1) hearings that draw public and congressional attention to recent developments and issues as well as inform the legislative process; (2) reviews of legislatively mandated reports to Congress; (3) approvals of changes to program funding allocations through the review of congressional notifications from government agencies; (4) reviews of the rules, regulations, and policies promulgated by departments and agencies to implement laws, policies, and congressional recommendations; and (5) issuance of congressional reports on issues under their jurisdiction that they are investigating.

Congressional oversight also extends to agencies in the executive branch. Regulatory agencies derive their authority from the legislative branch. Congress enacts broad policy and then delegates the specification of the details (including implementation) to the appropriate regulatory agency. Regulatory agencies must act within the bounds of any specific legislation. As a result, congressional committees play important roles in healthcare regulation in terms of authorizing the issuance of such regulations and then exercising oversight to ensure the regulatory process is consistent with legislative intent.

## OVERVIEW OF THE LEGISLATIVE PROCESS

The legislative process starts with a draft legislative proposal. This can originate in either chamber of Congress or in the executive branch. The Health Security Act (popularly known as the Clinton Health Plan) originated in the executive branch in a series of meetings and task forces assembled by Hilary Clinton and Ira Magaziner. The package they delivered to Congress was not warmly received because Congress was not included in the process.[9]

Congressional "sponsors" introduce the proposal as a "bill," which is numbered according to the sequence of its introduction in that chamber, with a letter in front of the number denoting Senate (S) or House (H). The bill is "referred" to the appropriate committee(s) with jurisdiction in that area for further study and consideration; there can be simultaneous or sequential consideration by multiple committees. For example, the Health Security Act was assigned to 2 Senate and 10 House committees. The committee may assign hearings to one of its subcommittees. Many general healthcare bills get referred to the Senate Committee on Health, Education, Labor, and Pensions and the House Committee on Energy and Commerce. Bills involving taxes and revenues are typically referred to the Senate Committee on Finance and the House Ways and Means Committee.

Committee membership is divided between the 2 parties; proportionate membership is determined by the party with the majority in that chamber of Congress. Appointment of the chairs of the committees and subcommittees is also controlled by the majority party; those chairs determine the order and pace by which legislative proposals are considered before them. Committees employ professional staffs ("staffers") to assist them.

Following hearings, committee members "mark up" the bill under consideration and vote on it in committee. If approved, the committee "reports out" the bill to the full chamber of the Senate or the House for a vote. The bill includes a "committee report," written by staffers, that describes the purpose and scope of the bill, the reasons why the committee recommends it, and all changes required to existing law. The bill is considered in the full chamber and may be further amended via a debate process (if there is broad support to do so). If passed in one chamber, the bill is sent to the other chamber, where it is again considered in the appropriate committee or subcommittee, with another round of hearings and votes. If passed in both chambers, differences between the 2 versions of the bill are reconciled in a conference committee, voted on again by both chambers, and then sent to the president's desk for signature. The president can sign the bill, veto the bill, or do nothing ("pocket veto") at the end of a congressional session.

This is not the only source of health policy making. Some policies are increasingly contained within massive pieces of legislation known as "Omnibus Budget Reconciliation Acts" (OBRA) and "Consolidated Omnibus Budget Reconciliation Acts" (COBRA). OBRA and COBRA legislation are generally passed on an annual basis to reconcile expenditures to the projected budget. However, to aid passage, these acts are generally loaded down with numerous other legislative initiatives. Often significant healthcare legislation is included. These are not small pieces of legislation. In fact, OBRA 1989 consisted of some 1,140 pages, and OBRA 1990 consisted of some 1,758 pages.[10] These have been extensively used in the past (eg, the Balanced Budget Act) to adjust the Medicare and Medicaid programs. Some pieces of legislation are not specific "policies" but rather compilations of lots of bills floating through both chambers of Congress that get packaged together and passed with minimal deliberation (see breakout section below on the Bipartisan Budget Act of 2018). Finally, some health policy is formulated within the federal budgetary process, due to its budgetary implications.

## IMPLEMENTATION OF HEALTHCARE POLICY

Although Congress enacts policy via legislation, several departments and agencies in the executive branch (eg, DHHS, CMS, FDA) implement Congress's intent behind public laws. This is a huge managerial undertaking, since these departments and agencies have to "add meat to the bones" via 2 activities (Figure 25-2). *First*, they flesh out legislative intent via a process of "rulemaking" (ie, operationalize the intent embodied in the legislation via a set of proposed and final rules). The process begins when the agency publishes a "Notice of Proposed Rulemaking" in the *Federal Register*. Stakeholders then have a certain time period to submit comments; after reviewing these comments, the agency may choose to revise the regulation. It then publishes the final regulation in the *Federal Register*, along with its responses to the comments. The final regulation is then incorporated into the *Code of Federal Regulations*. In an increasingly popular, alternative approach

## The Bipartisan Budget Act of 2018

The Bipartisan Budget Act (BBA 2018) was enacted as Public Law 115-123 on February 9, 2018. The passage of this large legislative package addressed 2 major issues before Congress: (1) the need for an extension of temporary appropriations set to expire on February 8, 2018, that would fund the federal government through March 23, 2018, and (2) a bipartisan desire to end a brief government shutdown.[11] The BBA also highlighted the government's willingness to spend money on critical healthcare services, even at the risk of increasing federal debt. BBA raised the spending caps imposed by the Budget Control Act of 2011 (BCA) for 2 years, paving the way for a longer-term spending agreement. To pay for BBA 2018's policy and funding changes, it included another 2-year extension of the Medicare sequester.

The road leading to BBA's passage began inauspiciously as House Resolution 1892, originally introduced on April 4, 2017, in the House Judiciary Committee as the "Honoring Hometown Heroes Act." The bill was marked up on May 3, 2017, and reported by the Committee on May 15, 2017. On May 18, 2017, it was passed on and agreed to in the House by a vote of 411-1. On May 22, 2017, it was referred to the Senate Judiciary Committee and then discharged from the committee on November 28, 2017, by unanimous consent. After that, things got more interesting: the bill became part of the BBA. As described by the Congressional Research Service,[12]

An early version of this [BBA funding] package was added by the House to H.R. 1892 (an unrelated measure), in the form of an amendment to an amendment that had been previously adopted by the Senate during its consideration of H.R. 1892. The House adopted its amendment on February 6, 2018, by a vote of 245-182. The Senate subsequently took up the House proposal and adopted a further amendment to it on February 9, by a vote of 71-28. The House agreed to the Senate actions that same day by a vote of 240-186. The final version of H.R. 1892, enacted as the Bipartisan Budget Act of 2018 (P.L. 115-123),

contained FY2018 temporary continuing appropriations, FY2018 supplemental appropriations, an increase to the debt limit, increases to the statutory spending limits for FY2018 and FY2019, tax provisions, and numerous provisions extending or making changes to mandatory spending programs, among other topics.

There were a *lot* of legislative proposals floating around both branches of Congress that made it into BBA 2018 when it was passed. As compiled by Republicans in the House's Ways and Means Committee, these proposals included the Medicare Part B Improvement Act of 2017 (H.R. 3178), which made a series of targeted improvements to Medicare Part B programs. The legislation included several bipartisan ideas from members of the committee, including policies reflected in the following bills:

- H.R. 3163, which creates a transition payment for home infusion therapies for Medicare beneficiaries to ensure there is no gap in care
- H.R. 3171, which protects access to orthotics and prosthetics for Medicare beneficiaries who need them
- H.R. 3166, which improves the accreditation process for dialysis facilities so Medicare beneficiaries with chronic kidney disease living in rural communities can more easily access the treatments they need
- H.R. 3164, which expands the use of telehealth technologies for Medicare beneficiaries receiving dialysis in their homes
- H.R. 3173, which puts into law existing regulations to modernize Medicare's physician self-referral laws, known as "Stark laws"

These proposals also contained the following portions of the CHRONIC Care Act (S. 870):

- H.R. 3168, which extends and strengthens Medicare Special Needs Plans (SNPs) to increase efficiency and plan quality
- H.R. 3044, which expands supplemental benefits to meet the needs of chronically ill Medicare Advantage enrollees under the Medicare program

- H.R. 3727, which includes telehealth services as a basic benefit for Medicare Advantage enrollees and increases access for beneficiaries by allowing plans to incorporate telehealth services into their bids
- H.R. 3992, which postpones the implementation of the Home Health Groupings model (HHGM) until 2020
- H.R. 2663, which requires CMS to consider the entire patient's record when deciding if a patient is eligible for home healthcare services
- H.R. 1955, which extends the Medicare Dependent Hospital Program and the Low-Volume Adjustment Program
- H.R. 1995, which expands the Medicare Advantage value-based insurance design to all 50 states to meet the needs of chronically ill Medicare Advantage enrollees
- H.R. 3271, which bolsters protections for Medicare beneficiaries who purchase blood glucose testing supplies from the National Mail Order Competitive Bidding Program
- H.R. 3263, which grants a 2-year extension for the Independence at Home Medical Practice Demonstration Program (IAH) through fiscal year 2019
- H.R. 807, which permanently repeals the cap on therapy services in Medicare and instead codifies a more stringent medical review threshold

- H.R. 4520, which prevents Medicare's enforcement of unreasonable and inflexible direct supervision rules for outpatient therapy services at critical access hospitals (CAHs) and other small, rural hospitals for 2017; an annual extension bill has been passed into law since 2014
- H.R. 4136, which increases the amount of available services and raises participation for providers in intensive cardiac rehabilitation programs in Medicare
- H.R. 3447, which allows standalone Medicare Part D plans to have access to Medicare Fee-for-Service A and B claims data.

These proposals were cobbled together by Senators Mitch McConnell and Chuck Schumer as part of an extensive negotiation among congressional leaders and the White House—a process resembling "disjointed incrementalism." As Politico noted, quoting Chuck Schumer, "The budget deal doesn't have everything Democrats want. It doesn't have everything the Republicans want. But it has a great deal of what the American people want. . . . After months of legislative logjams, this budget deal is a genuine breakthrough."[13] Indeed, healthcare analysts said that passage of the legislation validates "the power of major advocacy organizations to push through incremental legislative change in an otherwise gridlocked political environment."[14]

called "negotiated regulation," the regulatory agency meets with the affected industry to develop an approach that is acceptable to each side to avoid contentious and time-consuming litigation.

Second, they operate the public laws, run the programs, and enforce the regulations. There can be feedback effects among these 2 activities. The Congress maintains oversight of policy implementation by the executive branch via (1) the appropriations committees and annual funding decisions, (2) direct contact between committee staffers and bureaucrats in the executive branch, and (3) congressional oversight bodies, such as the CBO and GAO. These efforts are complemented by administrative law judges within the implementing agencies that hear appeals of those adversely affected by implemented policy.

More generally, the US judiciary (the third branch of government after the executive and legislative) may be called upon to adjudicate or interpret ambiguous laws in light of the US Constitution.

## REGULATION

### Essence of Regulation

The thrust of regulation can be interpreted in different ways. One view is that it provides impartial external oversight to protect the public interest and achieve the goals in the iron triangle. A different view is that it allows the "visible hand" of centralized decision makers, using regulatory controls, to determine the

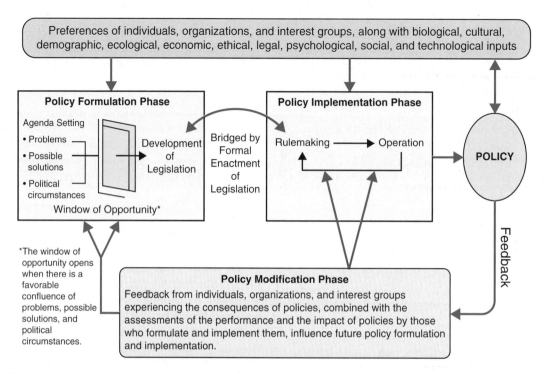

**Figure 25-2** • A Model of the Public Policymaking Process in the United States. (Source: Beaufort Longest. Health Policymaking in the United States.)

allocation of resources—in contrast with competitive approaches that rely on the "invisible hand" of the market to aggregate the choices of decentralized decision makers, using markets of supply and demand, to determine resource allocation.

According to Stuart Altman, former administrator of the Health Care Financing Administration (HCFA; the forerunner of CMS), the United States operates halfway between regulatory and market approaches. The US healthcare system is, at once, one of the most intensively regulated sectors in the United States and one of the most market-oriented systems in the world. The rationale for regulation rests largely on "market failure" (ie, well-functioning markets do not exist; a topic discussed in Chapter 1).

The "theory" of regulation can be summarized in several arguments (*note*: these are not statements of fact). First, healthcare is a social good and a right (due to "externalities"; ie, when one person's actions affect another person's well-being and the relevant costs and benefits are not reflected in market prices), as well as a topic of public interest (due to high costs that are borne by the population). Second, healthcare is subject to unrestrained provider

discretion in organizing and pricing of care, which needs to be restrained. Third, providers have incentives to augment their incomes by inducing demand for their services, which increases utilization and costs. Fourth, supply of services and technologies may create demand for those services and technologies, which also needs to be restrained.[15] Fifth, the nonprofit hospital operates according to different incentives that lead to (wasteful and duplicative) investments in prestige, quality, and quantity. Sixth, economic risk is disproportionately absorbed by the government and insurers. Seventh, there is a lack of consumer information.

This last point is perhaps the most compelling. However, according to economist Mark Pauly, the case for government regulation requires that (1) consumers do not know, (2) the government knows better, and then (3) the government does the right thing (and only the right thing). There are at least 3 reasons why these conditions may not hold. First, the common regulatory requirement to certify individuals and organizations as conforming with regulations imposes administrative costs on certifiers and certifiees. Second, the existence of rules and regulations often calls forth its counterpart: "rent-seeking behavior" engendered by the rules (ie, seek one's own wealth without generating societal benefits), usually via the legal system. Third, regulations that do an imperfect job of defining behavior are confusing and may lead to degradations of behavior down to the minimum standard defined by law.

As partial evidence for the first reason, the American Hospital Association issued a report on the costs of regulation.[16] According to their analysis, every hour of patient care requires 60 minutes of paperwork for emergency department care, 36 minutes of paperwork for surgery and inpatient care, 30 minutes of paperwork for skilled nursing care, and 48 minutes of paperwork for home healthcare. Moreover, providers bear additional costs in conforming with lengthy patient assessment and quality measurement tools. Providers also face ripple effects across their departments with each new rule/regulation, which then get multiplied with the multitude of new/revised rules and the multitude of agencies regulating providers.

As additional evidence, it is important to note that many of the regulatory initiatives undertaken during the 1970s either failed or were seriously curtailed.

## Shift in Thrust of Regulation Over Time

The country's regulatory approach has shifted its focus from quality to access and then to cost. During the period from 1900 to 1960, the emphasis was on improving quality. This was pursued via efforts to ensure the safety of food and drugs, upgrade and standardize medical education, enact state licensing laws, close substandard medical schools, fund biomedical research, and fund hospital construction in rural areas.

During the period from 1960 to 1972, the emphasis shifted to improving access to care. This included the expansion of insurance coverage to the elderly and the poor, increasing medical manpower (number of physicians and medical schools), improving the geographic and specialty distribution of that manpower (eg, the National Health Service Corps), and improving new sites of care (community health centers, community mental health centers). It also included the Comprehensive Health Planning and Services Act (1966) that funded state public health functions and encouraged states to coordinate programs to achieve comprehensive geographic coverage.

The rise in healthcare expenditures that followed from the 1960s' insurance expansions led to a shift in regulatory focus to cost. The initial regulatory approaches during the 1972 to 1980 period were to control capital expansion through "health system agencies" (HSAs) and the use of "certificate of need" (CON), enacted as part of Public Law 93-641 in 1974 (an amendment to the 1966 Planning Act). CON was designed to reduce expensive duplication of services and facilities as follows: A healthcare facility could not be constructed, renovated, or expanded without obtaining a CON if the cost exceeded a threshold amount ($600,000). Numerous research studies concluded that CON was a weak cost containment measure; indeed, Congress allowed the federal health planning mandate to lapse in 1986. Since then, several states have repealed their CON statutes, shifting from a regulatory to a market competition strategy. Nevertheless, by 2016, 37 states still had some form of CON.

Other, contemporaneous efforts focused on reducing costs and use of technology via (1) "professional standards review organizations" (PSROs), which were physician panels designed to review hospital admissions and lengths of stay for Medicare and Medicaid patients; (2) "utilization review" techniques (1972) to scrutinize the appropriateness of care (before admission, during admission, and after discharge); (3) the Health Maintenance Organization (HMO) Act of 1973; (4) wage and price controls; and (5) "hospital rate setting" and "rate review" programs. Most of these efforts failed.

During the subsequent period from 1980 to 1994, the federal government pursued a more diverse set of regulatory approaches (including a mix of market remedies, budget remedies, and legal remedies) to tackle all 3 angles of the iron triangle. With regard to *cost*, several efforts relied on the market and competition. These included efforts to reduce utilization via the Inpatient Prospective Payment System (IPPS; 1983), increase incentives for efficiency by the repeal of CON laws, and increase reliance on antitrust laws and enforcement (covered later). Other strategies included the use of private sector HMOs to cover beneficiaries of public insurance programs like Medicare and Medicaid (as part of OBRA, 1981). With regard to *quality*, regulators sought improvements by publishing the National Practitioner Data Bank, by publishing hospital mortality data and nursing home inspection data, and by legislation such as the

Emergency Medical Treatment and Labor Act (EMTALA, 1986), which stopped private hospitals from "dumping" (transferring) uninsured patients to public hospitals without first evaluating them and then stabilizing their condition. Finally, with regard to access, the Clinton Health Plan sought (unsuccessfully) to set up accountable health plans and health insurance purchasing cooperatives.

During the next period from 1994 to 2010, the focus was almost exclusively on reducing healthcare costs, but this time with some attention to quality of care. The Balanced Budget Act (1997) whacked federal spending on hospitals, skilled nursing facilities, and other providers. It also enacted the sustainable growth rate (SGR) to try to contain physician spending covered under Part B of Medicare. In 2005, the failure of the SGR approach led the government to shift to (1) pay-for-performance (P4P) initiatives that tied reimbursement and rewards to meeting quality metrics and (2) value-based purchasing (VBP).

## Major Regulatory Initiatives

Three major regulatory initiatives include (1) fraud and abuse, (2) the Health Insurance Portability and Accountability Act (HIPAA), and (3) antitrust. These are discussed in the following sections.

### Fraud and Abuse

The government began its pursuit of fraud and abuse in its payment programs with the creation of the OIG in 1976. The following year, the Medicare and Medicaid Anti-Fraud and Abuse Amendments passed in Congress, followed by the establishment of State Medicare/Medicaid Fraud Control Units. Under President Reagan, the OIG was headed by Richard Kusserow, a former Federal Bureau of Investigation (FBI) agent who took the active stance of "junkyard dog." His high-profile prosecutorial activities led to an expansion of OIG's stature and legislative authority in the 1980s.

Fraud and abuse received a lot of attention during the late 1980s and the 1990s for several reasons. The era focused on addressing the rising cost of care; fraud and abuse were viewed as key drivers of those rising costs. Moreover, this was also the era of provider consolidation, and such larger firms became more prominent targets as possible perpetrators of fraud and abuse. Finally, fraud and abuse also potentially impacted quality of care via the ordering of unnecessary referrals, tests, and procedures. The DOJ declared fraud and abuse as both the crime and the crisis of the 1990s.[17] Under the Medicare program, 3 main areas of fraud and abuse were identified: submission of false claims, inducements or kickbacks, and self-referrals.

### False Claims

The False Claims Act was passed by Congress in 1863 to prevent suppliers to the Union Army from defrauding the government. More than 120 years later, 1986 amendments to the act clarified that it applied to Medicare and Medicaid. OIG investigators focused on fraudulent provider "billing" cases, often initiated by private whistleblowers on the inside (who could obtain a percentage of any recovered funds). The cases were investigated by the FBI or the OIG (the enforcement arm of DHHS); convictions carried triple damages of the amount of false claim as well as a penalty up to $10,000 per false claim. The government could also suspend or delay payment of later claims. Such actions also carried an enormous public relations and reputational damage (as well as economic damages) to the provider, who tended to settle quickly with the government.

A report issued by the OIG claimed that Medicare overpaid providers by $20 billion in 1997. Fraud and abuse efforts constituted an attempt by the federal government to recoup these monies and use them to bolster the ailing Hospital Insurance Trust Fund (which supported Part A of Medicare). Here is a summary of FBI and OIG efforts during this period:

- Healthcare fraud investigations by the FBI increased from 657 in fiscal year (FY) 1992 to 2,200 by FY 1996.
- Criminal prosecutions increased from 83 cases and 116 defendants in FY 1992 to 246 cases and 450 defendants by FY 1996.
- Convictions (guilty pleas and guilty verdicts) rose from 90 defendants in FY 1992 to 307 defendants in FY 1996.
- The number of civil fraud investigations rose from 270 in FY 1992 to 2,488 in FY 1996.

A notable investigation during this period involved the largest hospital chain in the country, Columbia/HCA. In March 1997, federal agents raided Columbia/HCA's hospital in El Paso with search warrants; 4 months later, federal agents raided Columbia hospitals in 6 states. The chain was charged with civil fraud violations, including (among others) upcoding of diagnoses, improper payments to physicians, Medicare cost reporting violations (ie, keeping 2 sets of books), overcharging Medicare for its home health businesses, and illegal billing for laboratory services (among others). Three years later, in May 2000, Columbia/HCA reached a tentative agreement with the Justice Department to pay $745 million to settle civil fraud allegations dealing with the upcoding and home health issues; total fines ended up being $840 million. As fallout from this investigation, Columbia/HCA shrank in size from 341 hospitals to 200 hospitals. The investigation served as a "shot across the bow" for all hospitals and was quickly followed by an investigation of another for-profit hospital chain (Tenet) for overcharging Medicare for diagnosis-related group (DRG) outlier payments. In 2006, Tenet agreed to pay $900 million in fines.

## Inducements and Kickbacks

Congress passed the Anti-Kickback Statute (AKS) in 1972 to deter healthcare decisions that would result in unnecessary (and potentially harmful) care. AKS is embodied in Section 1128B(b) of the Social Security Act, which provides criminal penalties for those who knowingly or willfully offer/pay/solicit/receive remuneration in order to induce business reimbursable under the federal or state healthcare programs. "Business" included referring an individual for a service or item (or purchasing/leasing/ordering any good/service/item/facility) reimbursable by the government. Types of "remuneration" included kickbacks, bribes, and rebates. AKS carried a $25,000 fine and 5 years in prison (maximum) and constituted grounds for exclusion from the relevant federal program. There were exceptions to AKS, however, known as regulatory "safe harbors."

In 1987, Congress put some meat on these bones in Section 14 of P.L. 100-93, the Medicare and Medicaid Patient and Program Protection Act (MMPPPA). Section 14 became more widely known as "the Stark laws," named for

Congressman Fortney "Pete" Stark, Chairman of the House Ways and Means Subcommittee on Health, who sponsored the legislation. The Stark laws were designed to protect consumers from inappropriate referrals or purchases of services. The laws imposed restrictions on the ability of physicians to refer patients to facilities (eg, clinical laboratories) in which they had an ownership interest. Such restrictions were based on academic research that showed higher utilization of such facilities in the presence of an ownership interest. This broad statute required the development and promulgation of regulations (safe harbors) to specify payment and business practices that, although potentially capable of inducing referrals and business, would not be treated as criminal offenses (not considered kickbacks).

The Stark laws were enacted in 2 stages. "Stark I," passed in 1989 and enacted in 1992, outlawed referral of Medicare patients to clinical labs tied financially to the referring physician, as well as billing for lab services furnished under a prohibited referral. Stark I also specified safe harbors in 13 areas.[18] These regulations were published in the *Federal Register* on July 29, 1991. "Stark II" expanded the ban on self-referrals to Medicaid patients and to referrals for a variety of other medical services: home health, inpatient and outpatient hospital services, physical therapy, occupational therapy, radiology services, radiation therapy, durable medical equipment, parenteral and enteral nutrients, prosthetics/orthotics and prosthetic devices, and outpatient prescription drugs. Stark II consumed 100 pages in the *Federal Register* published at the end of 2000. In addition, during 1993 to 1994, 8 new safe harbors were proposed and then finalized (in 1999).[19]

## The Health Insurance Portability and Accountability Act (1996)

The HIPAA reinforced some of the government's fraud and abuse efforts. It authorized the HCFA Medicare Integrity Program and created a dedicated fund for fraud and abuse activities drawn from Medicare Part A Trust Funds. These funds were distributed among the OIG, HCFA, Office of General Counsel, the FBI, and others. Such funding ($137 million in 1999) supplemented direct appropriations of DHHS and DOJ for healthcare fraud enforcement. Collections in 1999 for cases brought forward totaled $490 million. HIPAA established new criminal offenses for healthcare fraud, expanded the AKS to cover all federal healthcare programs, and gave the attorney general subpoena authority in criminal healthcare fraud investigations.

Fraud and abuse are not what HIPAA is known for, however. HIPAA prohibited group health plans from discriminating against employees or their dependents based on health risks in determining eligibility or premiums. HIPAA also improved access to the individual health insurance market by helping individuals gain individual insurance coverage if they lost or left their jobs (and thus their group coverage) without preexisting condition exclusions.

HIPAA's protections extended even further beyond regulation of insurance coverage. It sought to safeguard the privacy and security of protected health information (PHI; ie, anything that could identify an individual patient). The use of medical records, billing information, and other personally identifiable health data now had to follow stringent guidelines. Absent specific authorization from patients, PHI could only be shared for certain purposes, such as provider payment, treatment, and healthcare operations. Institutions were required to have security measures in place to protect the data from unnecessary dissemination to parties that were not involved in a patient's care and to ensure that contracted entities protected the information as well. Employees had to be trained to follow appropriate procedures to safeguard PHI. HIPAA also required providers to grant patients access to their own medical records.

Finally, HIPAA contained an "Administrative Simplification Section" designed to reduce the costs and administrative burdens borne by healthcare providers and insurers. This section made possible the standardized, electronic transmission of many administrative and financial transactions that were paper based. This encompassed coding standards for reporting diagnoses and procedures; unique identifiers for providers, health plans, and employers; the requirement that providers and clearinghouses transmit their transactions in electronic form in conformity with these rules; and thus, an effort to standardize the estimated 400 different formats for electronic healthcare claims used in the United States.

## Antitrust

The government shifted to antitrust actions to reduce barriers to professional competition. Until 1975, courts considered physicians largely exempt from antitrust laws (eg, Sherman Act, Clayton Act), leaving doctors free to charge their own prices and impose restrictions on business practices. This situation changed when the US Supreme Court ruled in *Goldfarb v. Virginia State Bar* (1975) that the "learned professions" (like medicine and law) are not exempt from antitrust and could not engage in restraint of trade. This reduced any reluctance to challenge elite professions and their supposed ability to self-regulate their own behavior. Competitors who felt they unfairly lost in market competition could now go to court for redress of grievances. Their efforts were bolstered by a growing belief that market competition could be protected and used to foster iron triangle outcomes.

The government enjoyed some early success. During 1984 to 1994, the FTC and DOJ brought several cases challenging horizontal provider mergers, winning most of them. Many others were settled by consent decree or were abandoned by providers after government inquiries spotlighted potential antitrust claims. Thereafter, the government experienced several failures. Starting in 1995, the government (both federal and state agencies) lost 7 cases litigated in court and began to limit the number of horizontal merger cases they filed. These failures encouraged greater horizontal consolidation in the hospital sector. By contrast, the government was more successful litigating vertical physician-hospital mergers and alliances. The government also turned its attention to the pharmaceutical sector. The FTC successfully challenged (1) Mylan for overcharging on generic drugs and (2) Hoechst for paying generic drug makers to delay bringing products to market.

To address the dip in their success, the FTC and DOJ sought to sharpen their understanding of provider consolidations and the guidelines for providers who undertook consolidation. In 1993, the FTC and DOJ jointly issued their Statements of Antitrust Enforcement Policy in Health Care; these were revised in 1994 and 1996. In 2002, the FTC conducted a workshop on competition and antitrust that focused on hospitals, insurers, and generic drug makers.

Starting in 2004, the FTC and DOJ experienced a reversal of fortunes and went on a winning streak in opposing horizontal provider mergers. One major reason was the agencies' ability to convince the courts that geographic markets for hospital services are local—no bigger than metropolitan areas and often far smaller—rather than the larger geographic regions used in earlier, failed litigations. The impact was broadly felt, from mergers that were successfully blocked, to others that were abandoned. The 2019 investigation of Sutter Health in Northern California is a recent example of successful government enforcement.

## OTHER FEDERAL INITIATIVES

### Tax Exemption Law

The US healthcare ecosystem includes a large number of organizations that are exempt from paying taxes (income, property, and sales). Many of these tax-exempt organizations include nonprofit hospitals and nonprofit providers. Organizations qualify for federal income tax exemption under Section 501(c)(3) of the Internal Revenue Code, which applies to corporations organized and operated exclusively for religious, charitable, scientific, or educational purposes. Most 501(c)(3)-exempt healthcare organizations have qualified on the basis of having a charitable purpose. Organizations that qualify for a federal tax exemption are also able to issue tax-exempt bonds to finance capital improvements.

The Internal Revenue Service (IRS) decides an organization's qualification for exemption based on 2 tests: one organizational and one operational. Regarding the former, the IRS examines the organization's articles of incorporation to gauge its pursuit of an exempt purpose (eg, charitable, scientific). Regarding the latter, the IRS examines whether the organization is operated to achieve an exempt purpose based on a community benefit standard. The community benefit standard consists of several factors: providing charity care to the extent of the hospital's financial ability, operating a 24-hour emergency room, accepting payment from the Medicare and Medicaid programs on a nondiscriminatory basis, extending medical privileges to all qualified physicians in the area, and maintaining a

governing board drawn largely from representatives of the community. The IRS also prohibits any distribution of the nonprofit's earnings to individuals as dividends (private benefit and inurement); rather, any earnings must be used to further the organization's exempt purpose. The IRS also forbids exempt organizations from political activity.

In recent years, hospitals have faced new requirements to maintain their federal tax exemption. In 2009, tax-exempt hospitals were required to report annually to the IRS how much they spent for each of 7 defined community benefits (eg, charity care, unreimbursed costs for Medicaid enrollees, community health improvement). The following year, the PPACA added 4 new requirements, including the need to conduct a community health needs assessment (CHNA) every 3 years and develop an implementation plan to address community needs as identified in the CHNA. The other 3 requirements relate to hospitals' own financial assistance policies and bill collection practices.[20]

Hospitals have also faced challenges to their tax exemption from state and local governments. In August 2011, the Illinois Department of Revenue denied the property tax-exempt status of 3 nonprofit hospitals because they did not provide a sufficient amount of charity care for the poor and indigent populations to warrant exemption. In 2013, Pittsburgh's mayor sued the University of Pittsburgh Medical Center to challenge its exempt status; the suit was ultimately dropped. In 2015, a New Jersey judge ruled that Morristown Medical Center had to pay property taxes because it was not fulfilling its obligations for receiving an exemption.

### Health Care Quality Improvement Act

The Health Care Quality Improvement Act (HCQIA, 1986) was intended to strengthen the process of "peer review" and surveillance of substandard physicians. HCQIA addressed these issues by encouraging physicians to identify and discipline fellow physicians who were incompetent or who engaged in unprofessional behavior by providing them limited immunity. It also established the National Practitioner Data Bank (NPDB) as a repository of information on physicians' professional competence and conduct, medical liability awards and settlements, and peer review sanctions. Hospitals, state licensing bodies, and entities making malpractice payments must report information on these actions to the NPDB, which hospitals must consult when considering offering new physicians staff privileges and must consult every 2 years for all members with staff privileges.

## Transparency

The relatively higher cost of care in the United States, compared to the rest of the world, is largely caused by higher input prices charged by providers and suppliers. Determination of these prices has been shrouded in secrecy by both parties, as well as by health insurers who negotiate the provider fees; the situation is complicated by a fragmented payer market in the private sector. As a result, there has been a continuing, widespread push by government to make the prices of healthcare services more transparent to consumers. The main goal is to promote consumer shopping; secondary goals include promoting provider competition and reducing pricing variation for identical medical services in the same geographic market.

The Commonwealth of Massachusetts adopted a pricing transparency approach in its 2012 cost containment legislation. More recently, on June 24, 2019, the Trump administration issued a new executive order to compel hospitals (not physicians or imaging centers) to provide information on the prices they charge or receive from all insurers (not just Medicare) for a set of services.

There is some evidence that employees who use information platforms such as Castlight Health (referred to as "searchers") incur lower total costs for 3 common medical services: imaging tests, laboratory tests, and office visits. Similar results have been observed for efforts to promote price transparency of medical imaging by benefit managers and public government websites.

The problem is that few consumers (<10%) actually use the websites and their price data. Studies show that consumers rely not on websites but on their physicians (and their physicians' referrals) in selecting providers. Distance and convenience of appointments matter, too. Due to issues of trust, consumers also rely on friends, relatives, and colleagues rather than employers or insurers. Finally, even when armed with pricing information, consumers frequently fail to think about how to translate it into action or do not think it matters.

Evidence published by the GAO reveals that public and private initiatives vary in the price information (eg, completeness) they make available to consumers, thereby limiting comparable and accurate estimates of total cost. A Vermont law requiring pharmaceutical firms to justify price hikes only required such information on the list prices for 10 drugs and failed to slow down drug price increases. One study showed that half of price transparency tools offered to consumers by health plans did not include quality information, thus preventing consumers from making rough determinations of the "value" (quality divided by cost) of what they purchased. Moreover, patients who either have little or no deductible or who have exceeded their deductible may face no incentive to shop for healthcare based on price. This conclusion is reinforced by recent data that suggest only a small percentage (7%) of consumer out-of-pocket spending is for "shoppable services." The problem of low consumer use of transparent data is exacerbated by low consumer awareness and engagement in their own health.[21]

## Value-Based Payment[22]

Part of the initial push for VBP began with P4P models. P4P operated by giving providers a small payment bonus if they hit specified quality targets. The P4P strategy served as an escape hatch from the SGR problem in physician payment enacted as part of the 1997 Balanced Budget Act. Congressional reluctance to make an intended 4.8% SGR cut in physician payment in the early 2000s (dictated by the Balanced Budget Act) led CMS administrators to advocate for a political solution, which became known as the "doc fix." The solution postponed the annual SGR cut and ushered in P4P, even though there was little research evidence that paying providers to meet specific performance indicators improved quality of care.

P4P programs could be targeted at both physicians and hospitals. For physicians, an initial effort was the 2006 Physician Voluntary Reporting Program (PVRP). PVRP began by promoting reporting requirements: It rewarded physicians with a 1-time lump sum if they sufficiently reported on at least 3 quality measures. The program subsequently morphed into a P4P program called the Physician Quality Reporting Initiative (PQRI), and again evolved under PPACA into the Physician Quality Reporting

System (PQRS). PQRS included penalties (starting in 2015) for failing to report data and broadened to performance-based penalties and bonuses in what was called the Value-Base Payment Modifier (Value Modifier). The Value Modifier program mandated payment adjustments based on risk-adjusted quality and cost metrics to Medicare physician payments.

These programs continued to operate until 2018, when they were replaced by the Merit-based Incentive Payment System (MIPS) created in the Medicare Access and CHIP Reauthorization Act (MACRA, 2015), which combined several federal quality programs (see later discussion). MIPS is a fee-for-service–based VBP program beginning in 2019 with payment linked to a composite score on quality, resource use, clinical improvement, and the use of electronic medical records. For providers, substantial amounts of Medicare payments will be in play, with positive or negative adjustments up to 4% in 2019 and increasing over time to up to 9% in 2022.

An early P4P program targeted at hospitals was the Medicare Premier Hospital Quality Incentive Demonstration (Premier HQID), a 6-year P4P demonstration funded by CMS from 2003 to 2009. Premier HQID hospitals could receive a 1% to 2% bonus or, starting in 2006, penalty adjustments, based on performance on 33 measures. This demonstration was one of the most widely studied P4P programs. Evidence on its ability to improve quality or reduce costs was tepid, at best.[23]

The PPACA ushered in a larger P4P initiative called the Medicare Hospital VBP Program (HVBP). HVBP built upon the existing Hospital Inpatient Quality Reporting Program (IQR) pay-for-reporting program for hospitals that started in 2003. The IQR program paid hospitals that successfully reported specific quality measures a higher annual update to their payment rates and reduced payments to hospitals that did not do so. Starting in 2012, HVBP used IQR's infrastructure to introduce Medicare payment adjustments for acute inpatient services. The program created an incentive payment fund by reducing inpatient Medicare payments by a percentage that increased over time, then distributed that fund to hospitals by applying a value-based adjustment factor determined by the hospital's "Total Performance Score." The latter initially consisted of 2 domains of clinical processes of care and a survey of patient experience. As the program evolved, it added measures in additional domains including outcomes (mortality), safety, and efficiency. Performance (and thus incentive payment) was based both on attaining a certain level and on improvement compared to the hospital's baseline and benchmark.

Beyond HVBP, CMS launched 2 other P4P programs: the Hospital Readmissions Reduction Program (HRRP) and the Hospital-Acquired Condition (HAC) reduction. Like HVBP, they were designed to move hospitals away from fee-for-service to value-based payment by withholding some Medicare reimbursements to penalize providers based on their performance on certain quality metrics. HRRP and HAC programs were thus strictly penalty programs. HRRP issued a penalty of up to 3% for hospitals with excessive avoidable readmissions, whereas HAC issued a 1% penalty for hospitals whose performance was in the bottom quartile for hospital-acquired infections. A summary of HVBP, HRRP, and HAC is provided in Figure 25-3. Research suggested that a hospital's performance under VBP was not correlated with its performance under other alternative payment programs, like accountable care organizations.

## Single-Specialty Hospitals

The Stark laws, which were intended to prevent physician self-referrals, contained an exception for physician referrals to hospitals in which they had an ownership stake. By virtue of ownership in the entire facility rather than a particular service, a physician-owner would not directly benefit from a specific patient referral. Physicians acquired ownership stakes in particular hospitals, usually those offering a single, profitable service such as cardiac surgery or orthopedic surgery, which just happened to be the specialty of the physicians.

The "whole hospital exemption," along with the profitability of the services involved, contributed to the growth of specialty heart and orthopedic hospitals. Chains of such hospitals, such as MedCath, emerged during the 1990s and garnered a lot of interest. Investors saw them as a growth vehicle. Researchers labeled them as "focused factories" that, by virtue of focus, could deliver higher-quality, lower-cost care. These hospitals also caught the eye, and incurred the ill will, of their competitors (general medical-surgical hospitals) who provided

**Summary of Medicare Value-Based Purchasing Programs**

| Program | | 2013 | 2014 | 2015 | 2016 | 2017 |
|---|---|---|---|---|---|---|
| | **Payment Year:** | | | | | |
| | **Potential Penalty:** | 1% withheld | 1.25% withheld | 1.50% withheld | 1.75% withheld | 2.0% withheld |
| Hospital Value-Based Purchasing Program | Metrics: | • Clinical process of care (70%)<br>• Patient experience of care (30%) | • Clinical process of care (45%)<br>• Clinical outcomes (25%)<br>• Patient experience of care (30%) | • Clinical process of care (20%)<br>• Clinical outcomes (30%)<br>• Patient experience of care (30%)<br>• Efficiency (20%) | • Clinical process of care (10%)<br>• Clinical outcomes (40%)<br>• Patient experience of care (25%)<br>• Efficiency (20%) | • Clinical process of care (5%)<br>• Clinical outcomes (25%)<br>• Patient experience of care (25%)<br>• Efficiency (25%)<br>• Safety (20%) |
| | Performance Period: | • Clinical process of care (7/1/11-3/31/12)<br>• Patient experience of care (7/1/11-3/31/12) | • Clinical process of care (4/1/12-12/31/12)<br>• Clinical outcomes (7/1/11-6/30/12)<br>• Patient experience of care (4/1/12-12/31/12) | • Clinical process of care (1/1/13-12/31/13)<br>• Clinical outcomes (10/1/12-12/31/13)<br>• Patient experience of care (1/1/13-12/31/13)<br>• Efficiency (5/1/13-12/31/13) | • Clinical process of care (1/1/14-12/31/14)<br>• Clinical outcomes (10/1/12-12/31/14)<br>• Patient experience of care (1/1/14-12/31/14)<br>• Efficiency (1/1/14-12/31/14) | • Clinical process of care (1/1/15-12/31/15)<br>• Clinical outcomes (10/1/13-6/30/15)<br>• Patient experience of care (1/1/15-12/31/15)<br>• Efficiency (1/1/15-12/31/15)<br>• Safety (10/1/13-12/31/15) |
| | **Potential Penalty:** | 1% reduction | 2% reduction | 3% reduction | 3% reduction | 3% reduction |
| Hospital Readmission Reduction Program | Metrics: | • Acute MI<br>• Heart failure<br>• Pneumonia | • Acute MI<br>• Heart failure<br>• Pneumonia | • Acute MI<br>• Heart failure<br>• Pneumonia<br>• Total hip/knee replacement<br>• COPD | • Acute MI<br>• Heart failure<br>• Pneumonia<br>• Total hip/knee replacement<br>• COPD | • Acute MI<br>• Heart failure<br>• Pneumonia<br>• Total hip/knee replacement<br>• COPD<br>• CABG surgery |
| | Performance Period: | 7/1/08-6/30/11 | 7/1/09-6/30/12 | 7/1/10-6/30/13 | 7/1/11-6/30/14 | 7/1/12-6/30/15 |
| | **Potential Penalty:** | | Preliminary analysis | 1% reduction to lowest-performing quartile | 1% reduction to lowest-performing quartile | 1% reduction to lowest-performing quartile |
| Hospital-Acquired Conditions Reduction Program | Metrics: | | • PSI-90 composite (AHRQ)<br>• CAUTI & CLASBI (CDC NHSN) | • Domain 1: PSI-90 composite (AHRQ) (35%)<br>• Domain 2: CAUTI & CLASBI (CDC NHSN) (65%) | • Domain 1: PSI-90 composite (AHRQ) (25%)<br>• Domain 2: CAUTI, CLASBI, SSI colon surgeries & abdominal hysterectomies (CDC NHSN) (75%) | • Domain 1: PSI-90 composite (AHRQ)<br>• Domain 2: CAUTI, CLASBI, SSI colon surgeries & abdominal hysterectomies (CDC NHSN), MRSA, CDI |
| | Performance Period: | | 7/1/12-6/30/13 | • Domain 1: 7/1/11-6/30/13<br>• Domain 2: 1/1/12-2/31/13 | • Domain 1: 7/1/12-6/30/14<br>• Domain 2: 1/1/13-12/31/14 | • Domain 1: 7/1/13-6/30/15<br>• Domain 2: 1/1/14-12/31/15 |

**Figure 25-3** • Medicare Value-Based Purchasing. AHRQ indicates Agency for Healthcare Research and Quality; CABG, coronary artery bypass graft; CAUTI, catheter-associated urinary tract infection; CDC NHSN, Centers for Disease Control and Prevention National Healthcare Safety Network; CDI, Clostridium difficile infection; CLABSI, central line associated bloodstream infection; COPD, chronic obstructive pulmonary disease; MI, myocardial infarction; MRSA, methicillin-resistant staphylococus aureus; PSI, patient safety indicator; SSI, surgical site infection. (Source: David Muhlestein.)

less profitable services (eg, psychiatric care) that needed to be subsidized by the more profitable cardiac and orthopedic patient services.

The accumulating evidence base suggested these single-specialty hospitals were no more efficient and no higher in quality than general medical-surgical hospitals. Some evidence suggested they "cherry picked" the healthiest patients, which made it easier for them to generate net margins. Such results resulted in

(1) a temporary moratorium on their construction imposed by the Medicare Modernization Act (2003), followed by (2) a permanent moratorium imposed by the PPACA (2010). Physician-owned hospitals established before the PPACA were grandfathered into receiving government reimbursement but were permitted to expand only under limited circumstances.

Nevertheless, there have been recent calls to lift the PPACA moratorium (or at least consider doing so) and allow such hospitals to return and instill more competition into the hospital market.[24] According to proponents, the focused model is well suited to the new environment that emphasizes "patient experience," "value," and cost transparency. The specialty hospital model is also consistent with the emphasis on "focus" (specialization) and "experience" (volume), both of which contribute to quality and efficiency in patient care.[25] Research evidence indicates that the presence of such hospitals is not associated with higher per-capita Medicare spending.[26] Other research, however, suggests that the presence of specialty hospitals leads to patient cherry-picking, jeopardizes the profit margins of competitor hospitals (especially for-profit facilities), and spurs more hospital consolidation.[27]

---

### Critical Thinking Exercise: Medcath and Single-Specialty Heart Hospitals

A Harvard Business School (HBS) case outlined the history of the Medcath Corporation, one of the early pioneers in developing chains of single-specialty hospitals.[28] Medcath began life (1988-1996) as a provider of mobile and stationary cardiac catheterization labs to service rural hospitals and then added a division of physician practice management in 1995. In 1996, Medcath opened the first of several "heart hospitals" (ie, hospitals that did primarily open-heart surgical procedures, such as coronary artery bypass with graft [CABG]). The first hospital was in McAllen, Texas, a town that gained notoriety in an article by Atul Gawande in *The New Yorker*[29]; by 1998, Medcath had opened 4 such facilities.

Medcath's business model was quite innovative. First, the hospitals adopted Michael Porter's classic strategy of "focus" on a single set of patients and procedures, which might promote efficiencies in staffing and equipment, as well as in standardization of operations. Second, they offered a "differentiated" product by designing the hospital around universal patient rooms, centrally located inpatient services, distributed nursing stations, efficient work flow, and extra capacity for critical cardiac procedures—all of which purportedly lent Medcath competitive advantage over its rivals. Third, heart surgeons were invited to have an ownership interest in the facilities that they operated in; they were also "engaged" in the governance and managerial decision making of the hospitals. Fourth, the hospitals focused on a specific condition, cardiovascular disease, that was growing in prevalence and afflicted the growing population of elderly covered by the Medicare program. Fifth, the HBS casewriters, 2 of whom are highly respected and prominent healthcare management researchers, advanced several additional benefits offered, including a novel service strategy, a unique model of physician engagement, and the physician's ability to directly impact the quality of care as well as improve outcomes and efficiency. What's not to like about this model of hospital operation?

And, yet, Medcath went out of business by 2012. Its demise raises a boatload of questions. Was its demise due to the moratorium imposed by the PPACA? Were there other weaknesses in Medcath's business model that hampered its growth? Did Medcath really spur competition with general acute care medical-surgical hospitals like those profiled earlier in Chapter 11? Is offering a product organized around a single specialty a novel idea in healthcare delivery? Is the "focused factory" what consumers really want? Are such providers usually more efficient and higher in quality than those who provide a broader range of services? After considering these questions, what do you think about current calls to resuscitate the single-specialty hospital model and allow it back into the marketplace?

## SUMMARY

The complexity of the federal government's role in healthcare financing, delivery, and regulation is matched by the complexity of the bureaucratic apparatus used by the federal government to perform all of these functions. This chapter basically serves as a "lesson in civics" (ie, what you need to know about your government and how it spends your money on healthcare). The government's role in healthcare is pervasive and increasing over time, in tandem with the growing cost of healthcare and public interest in access and quality. There are entire books written on the content of this chapter that are well worth your reading.

## QUESTIONS TO PONDER

1. Why do some people view the growing role of the federal government in healthcare as a "government takeover"? Has such a view been expressed in prior decades?
2. Of the 3 roles played by the federal government (financing, delivery, regulation), which one seems most important? Why do you think so?
3. What does passage of the Bipartisan Budget Act (2018) teach you about the policy development process in Washington, DC? Is this process transparent?
4. How successful has healthcare regulation been in addressing the "iron triangle," particularly the angles of cost and quality? Does regulation serve other purposes?
5. Does the moratorium on developing new single-specialty hospitals still make sense?

## REFERENCES

1. Robert Field. *Mother of Invention* (New York, NY: Oxford University Press, 2014): 24, 41.
2. The various institutes included under NIH are the National Cancer Institute (NCI), National Eye Institute (NEI), National Heart, Lung, and Blood Institute (NHLBI), National Human Genome Research Institute (NHGRI), National Institute on Aging (NIA), National Institute on Alcohol Abuse and Alcoholism (NIAAA), National Institute of Allergy and Infectious Diseases (NIAID), National Institute of Arthritis and Musculoskeletal and Skin Diseases (NIAMS), National Institute of Child Health and Human Development (NICHD), National Institute of Deafness and Other Communication Disorders (NIDCD), National Institute of Dental and Craniofacial Research (NIDCR), National Institute of Diabetes and Digestive and Kidney Diseases (NIDDK), National Institute on Drug Abuse (NIDA), National Institute of Environmental Health Sciences (NIEHS), National Institute of General Medical Sciences (NIGMS), National Institute of Mental Health (NIMH), National Institute of Neurological Disorders and Stroke (NINDS), and National Institute of Nursing Research (NINR).
3. DHHS also has 6 staff divisions: Assistant Secretary for Health (ASH)/Surgeon General, Assistant Secretary for Administration and Management, Assistant Secretary for Budget, Technology and Finance, Assistant Secretary for Legislation, Assistant Secretary for Planning and Evaluation, and Assistant Secretary for Public Affairs.
4. For a more thorough treatment of healthcare regulation, see Robert Field. *Health Care Regulation in America: Complexity, Confrontation, and Compromise* (New York, NY: Oxford University Press, 2007).
5. Charles Lindblom. "The Science of Muddling Through," *Public Admin Rev.* 19 (2) (Spring 1959): 79-88.
6. This section draws upon several sources. See: Kellie Moss and Jennifer Kates. *The U.S. Congress and Global Health: A Primer.* Kaiser Family Foundation (February 20, 2019). Available online: https://www.kff.org/global-health-policy/report/the-u-s-congress-and-global-health-a-primer/. Accessed on May 15, 2020. Ada Cornell. *Health Policy: Resources for Congressional Staff* (June 12, 2018). Available online: https://fas.org/sgp/crs/misc/R43889.pdf. Accessed on May 15, 2020.
7. The 4 joint committees are: Taxation, Printing, the Library, and the Joint Economic Committee.
8. Select or special committees are generally established by a separate resolution of the chamber, sometimes to conduct investigations and studies and, on other occasions, also to consider measures. Often, select committees examine emerging issues that do not fit clearly within existing standing committee jurisdictions or cut across jurisdictional boundaries. A select committee may be permanent or temporary. Select committees may have certain restrictions on member tenure or may include certain specified representatives

(eg, party leaders or certain standing committee chairs) as ex officio members. Instead of the term select, the Senate sometimes uses special committee (eg, the Special Committee on Aging).

9. Jacob Hacker. *The Road to Nowhere* (Princeton, NJ: Princeton University Press, 1999).

10. Michael Geldart. "OBRA/COBRA and Other Dangerous Reptiles," *Home Health Care Manag Pract.* 10 (6) (1998): 11-18.

11. John Bresnahan, Jennifer Scholtes, and Heather Caygle. "Shutdown Ends After Trump Signs Budget Deal," *Politico* (February 18, 2018). Available online: https://www.politico.com/story/2018/02/08/congress-massive-budget-deal-2018-398189. Accessed on August 13, 2020.

12. Paulette C. Morgan. "Bipartisan Budget Act of 2018 (P.L. 115-123): Brief Summary of Division E—The Advancing Chronic Care, Extenders, and Social Services (ACCESS) Act" (Washington, DC: Congressional Research Service, March 9, 2019). Available online: https://fas.org/sgp/crs/misc/R45126.pdf. Accessed on August 13, 2020.

13. Burgess Everett and John Bresnahan. "Congressional Leaders Reach Budget Deal," *Politico* (February 7, 2018). Available online: https://www.politico.com/story/2018/02/07/government-shutdown-senate-budget-deal-395984. Accessed on August 13, 2020.

14. "3 Reasons the Bipartisan Budget Act of 2018 Might Signal Bad News to Come for Providers," *Advisory Board* (March 18, 2018). Available online: https://www.advisory.com/research/revenue-cycle-advancement-center/at-the-margins/2018/03/bipartisan-budget-act. Accessed on August 13, 2020.

15. Max Shain and Milton Roemer. "Hospital Costs Relate to the Supply of Beds," *Modern Hosp.* 92 (1959): 71-73.

16. American Hospital Association. *Patients or Paperwork? The Regulatory Burden Facing America's Hospitals* (Chicago, IL: AHA, 2015).

17. US Department of Justice. *U.S. Department of Justice Health Care Fraud Report Fiscal Years 1995 and 1996.* Available online: https://www.justice.gov/archives/opa/us-department-justice-heatlh-care-fraud-report-fiscal-years-1995-1996. Accessed on August 13, 2020.

18. The safe harbors included investments in large publicly held companies, investments in small joint ventures, space rental, equipment rental, personal services and management contracts, sales of retiring physician practices to other physicians, referral services, warranties, discounts, employee compensation, group purchasing organizations, waivers of Medicare part A inpatient cost-sharing amounts, and managed care practices (reduced cost sharing, reduced premiums, increased coverage, price reductions offered by providers).

19. These included investments in ambulatory surgery centers, joint ventures in underserved areas, practitioner recruitment in underserved areas, sales of physician practices to hospitals in underserved areas, subsidies for obstetrical malpractice insurance in underserved areas, investments in group practices, specialty referral arrangements between providers, and cooperative hospital services organizations.

20. Specifically, hospitals must establish a written financial assistance policy and a written policy governing emergency medical care. Also, in the case of emergency or medically necessary care, hospitals are prohibited from charging patients eligible for financial assistance more than amounts generally billed to insured patients. One additional requirement is that hospitals must make reasonable efforts to determine whether patients are eligible for financial assistance before initiating extraordinary collection efforts for unpaid bills.

21. For a deeper analysis of price transparency, see: Mark V. Pauly and Lawton R. Burns. "When Is Medical Care Price Transparency a Good Thing (And When Isn't It)?" forthcoming in *Advances in Health Care Management-Transforming Health Care: A Focus on Consumerism and Profitability* (Bingley, United Kingdom: Emerald Press, 2020, Volume 19: 75-97).

22. This section draws on several sources. For example, see: Tingyin Chee, Andrew Ryan, Jason Wasfy, et al. "Current State of Value-Based Purchasing Programs," *Circulation.* 133 (22) (2016): 2197-2205. Lawton Burns and Mark Pauly. "Transformation of the Health Care Industry: Curb Your Enthusiasm?" *Milbank Q.* 96 (1) (2018): 57-109.

23. Ash Jha, Karen Joynt, John Orav, et al. "The Long-Term Effect of Premier Pay for Performance on Patient Outcomes," *N Engl J Med.* 366 (2012): 1606-1615. Gregory Kruse, Daniel Polsky, Elizabeth Stuart, et al. "The Impact of Hospital Pay-for-Performance on Hospital and Medicare Costs," *Health Serv Res.* 47 (6) (2012): 2118-2136.

24. Gail Wilensky and Brian Miller. "Time to Consider a New Look at Physician-Owned Hospitals to Increase Competition in Health Care?" *JAMA.* 323 (19) (2020): 1884-1885.

25. E. David Zepeda, Gilbert Nyaga, and Gary Young. "On the Relations Between Focus, Experience, and Hospital Performance," *Health Care Manag Rev.* (April 2020). doi: 10.1097/HMR.0000000000000283.

26. John Schneider, Pengxiang Li, and Robert Ohsfeldt. "The Effects of Endogenous Market Entry of Physician-Owned Hospitals on

Medicare Expenditures: An Instrumental Variables Approach," *Contemp Econ Policy.* 29 (2) (2010): 151-162.

27. Sujoy Chakravarty. "Much Ado About Nothing? The Financial Impact of Physician-Owned Specialty Hospitals," *Int J Health Econ Manag.* 16 (2016): 103-131.

28. Regina Herzlinger, Kevin Schulman, and Fallon Upke. *Medcath Corporation (C).* HBS Case # 9-315-018 (Revised February 11, 2015). (Boston, MA: Harvard Business School).

29. Atul Gawande. "The Cost Conundrum: What a Texas Hospital Can Teach Us About Health Care," *The New Yorker* (May 25, 2009).

# The Public Health System

26

## INTRODUCTION

Chapter 3 defined "health" as a state of complete physical, mental, spiritual, and social well-being and not merely the absence of disease or infirmity. This chapter focuses on "public health." While there is no standard definition, public health has been described as "what we as a society do collectively to assure the conditions in which people can be healthy."[1]

So, what is it that public health does to assure the conditions for people to have health? According to the Centers for Disease Control and Prevention (CDC), public health does the following:

- Prevents epidemics and the spread of disease
- Protects against environmental hazards
- Prevents injuries
- Promotes and encourages healthy behaviors
- Responds to disasters and assists communities in recovery
- Assures the quality and accessibility of health services

Another way to describe public health is to contrast it with allopathic medicine. Allopathic physicians save lives one at a time; public health saves peoples' lives a million at a time.

## PROBLEMS ADDRESSED BY PUBLIC HEALTH

Public health is directly concerned with several of the major causes of death in the United States. These include cancer, accidents, and intentional self-harm, as well as health promotion activities that can address several other causes (heart disease, diabetes). Below are the death rates per 100,000 population for the top 10 causes of death in 2018[2]:

- Heart disease                                 163.6
- Cancer                                        149.1
- Accidents (unintentional injuries)             48.0
- Chronic lower respiratory diseases             39.7
- Stroke (cerebrovascular diseases)              37.1
- Alzheimer disease                              30.5
- Diabetes                                       21.4
- Influenza and pneumonia                        14.9
- Kidney disease                                 12.9
- Intentional self-harm (suicide)                14.2

It is important to point out that the recent spread of COVID-19 catapulted the virus to the number 3 cause of death in the United States by August 2020, just 8 months after the first case was diagnosed. It is unclear at this point how long it will remain in "the top 10" going forward.

Many people are unaware of public health's contribution to health status. Consider the great public health achievements during the 20th century:

- Vaccinations
- Safer workplace
- Safer and healthier food

- Motor vehicle safety
- Control of infectious diseases
- Decline in deaths from coronary heart disease and stroke
- Fluoridation of drinking water
- Family planning
- Recognition of tobacco use as a health hazard
- Healthier mothers and babies

Also consider some of the recent threats to public health during the current millennium (apologies for not listing everything that has happened):

- COVID-19 (2020)
- Border-crossing deaths of migrants (2017-)
- Orlando night club shooting (2016)
- Opioid crisis (2015)
- Drinking water in Flint, Michigan (2014)
- Hurricane Sandy (2012)
- *Salmonella* in peanut butter (2011)
- H1N1 epidemic (2009)
- Hurricane Katrina (2005)
- Anthrax attacks through the mail (2001)
- 9/11 attack (2001)

These events required responses from more than one geographical area and more than one government agency. In general, a well-functioning system of public health entails strong partnerships where partners recognize they are part of the public health system, effective channels of communication among government levels and partners, collaboration and cooperation, system-wide health objectives that are shared, robust resource levels that are shared, strong leadership by governmental public health agencies, and feedback loops between governmental levels and public health partners.

Despite these accomplishments and the important role that public health has played (and continues to play), the US public health system is challenged on several fronts. First, there is little understanding about public health and the public health system. When most people think of public health, they think of state and local health departments, which have traditionally been responsible for public health services. Such topics are not always covered in textbooks on the US healthcare system. Moreover, the public health system suffers from a complex division of labor between federal, state, and local government. Like Medicaid (see Chapter 19),

public health is largely a state responsibility that is (1) dependent on federal funding and (2) implemented with great variation across the states. All of this makes the system opaque, uneven, and resistant to any uniform solutions or generalizations.

Second, funding for public health has been fragmented, limited, and variable over time, despite its importance in promoting the public's health status. Like the late comedian Rodney Dangerfield, public health "gets no respect." The vast majority (95%+) of US healthcare spending goes toward medical care and biomedical research. However, there is strong evidence that behavioral and environmental factors are responsible for 70% of avoidable mortality, and medical care is just one of several determinants of health.[3] It then follows that the nation's heavy investment in the delivery of medical care is a limited future strategy for promoting health (see Figure 3-8). Social and environmental factors create unnecessary health risks for individuals (see Chapter 4).

Third, the Institute of Medicine has released 3 reports over time (1988, 2003, and 2013) on public health.[4] The reports are upbeat and point to progress in several areas; they also display a persistent attention to the importance of public health. Nevertheless, they are unfortunately consistent in terms of their major conclusion: The public health system in the United States "is in disarray."

This chapter seeks to elevate the visibility and challenge of public health. It first outlines some notable problems and some successes in public health that highlight the importance of this sector. It then describes the historical development of public health in the United States, the core purpose and functions of public health overall, and the roles of federal, state, and local government in the provision of public health.

## PROGRESS AND CONTINUED PROBLEMS[5]

### Injuries

A principal public health problem is injury. It affects primarily the young and touches 1 of every 3 Americans each year. Roughly 167,000 Americans died from preventable injuries in 2018, an increase of 93% over the 86,000 deaths in 1992; another 46 million sustained

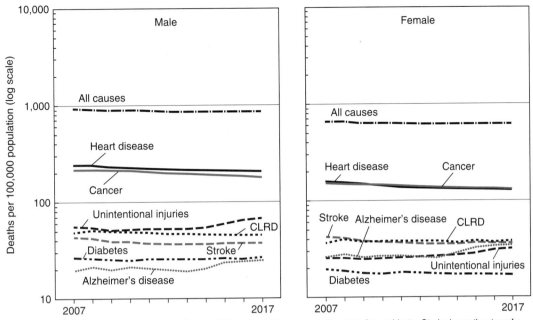

NOTES: CLRD is chronic lower respiratory disease. Unintentional injuries is another term for accidents. Stroke is another term for cerebrovascular disease.

**Figure 26-1** • Age-Adjusted Death Rates for Selected Causes of Death for all Ages by Gender: United States 2007 to 2017. (Source: NCHS, National Vital Statistics System [NVSS], Mortality. Excel and PowerPoint: https://www.cdc.gov/nchs/hus/contents2018.htm#Figure_003.)

nonfatal injuries. The majority of these occurred in the home. Injury is the leading cause of death for children and young adults. Accidents and unintentional injuries are one of the causes of death that is growing in incidence (Figure 26-1). The 3 leading causes of preventable injury-related death are poisoning, motor vehicle accidents, and falls; they account for 83% of all preventable deaths (37%, 24%, and 22%, respectively). Motor vehicle accidents are the leading cause of severe injury and death, responsible for over 33,000 deaths and roughly 3 million injuries annually. Seatbelts can reduce mortality from such injuries by 45%.

## Teen Pregnancy

There is some good news to report here. The teen birth rate (births per 1,000 girls aged 15-19) declined 72% between 1991 and 2018. There were 179,000 teen births in the United States in 2018. Births to teenagers represented about 5% of all births in the nation in 2017, down from 13% in the early 1980s. Nevertheless, rates of teen pregnancy and delivery in the United States are significantly higher than those of comparable countries; 75% of teen pregnancies are unplanned. Moreover, there are wide racial disparities: The teen birth rate is roughly twice as high among Latina teens (27 births per 1,000) and African American teens (26 births per 1,000) compared with non-Hispanic white teens (12 births per 1,000).

Teen pregnancies have several negative, downstream consequences for health. These include higher rates of miscarriages, complications, stillbirths, and infant and maternal deaths (compared to pregnant adults). Low-income teenagers are more likely than adults to have premature births, increasing the likelihood of poor pregnancy outcomes. Surviving children of teenage mothers are more likely to suffer injuries and more likely to be hospitalized by age 5 than children of adult mothers. Adolescent pregnancies and births also cause significant health problems for the teenage mothers. Finally, teenage pregnancy is linked to school dropout rates, low future incomes, and poorer health in the future.

## Tobacco

The smoking rate among adults has declined over time from 42% 50 years ago to just under

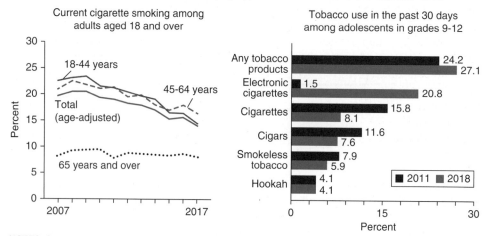

**Figure 26-2** • Prevalence of Smoking. (Source: NCHS, National Health Interiview Survey and CDC, National Youth Tobacco Survey.)

14% by 2017 (Figure 26-2). What caused this favorable trend? The public's literacy about the health effects of tobacco use greatly increased with the 1964 Surgeon General's report.[6] That report concluded that smoking causes lung and laryngeal cancer and is a major cause of cardiovascular disease. The report paved the way for subsequent policies and antismoking campaigns that reduced smoking levels, albeit gradually over time. Such efforts were bolstered by hikes in the prices of cigarettes, which put them out of the financial reach of teens, as well as by passage of smoke-free laws and access to smoking cessation programs.

Since the 1964 report's publication, science has linked the use of tobacco to cancer, heart disease and stroke, lung disease, and reproductive and other effects (eg, type 2 diabetes). Tobacco use is the largest preventable cause of death and disease in the United States. Roughly 480,000 people die annually from tobacco-related illnesses, while 16+ million people suffer from at least one disease caused by smoking. Smoking-related illness costs more than $300 billion each year, including $168 billion for direct medical care for adults and more than $156 billion in lost productivity. At present, 34 million people in the United States still smoke; 20+ million Americans have died because of smoking.

The tobacco issue is morphing, however, due to the emergence of new products such as e-cigarettes or "vapes." Researchers are trying

to identify the health effects of these products at the same time as their popularity increases among young people. While they contain fewer toxic chemicals and are less harmful than regular cigarettes, they are not harmless. They can contain harmful and potentially harmful substances, including nicotine, heavy metals (lead), volatile organic compounds, and cancer-causing agents. According to the CDC, the nicotine they contain is highly addictive, can harm adolescent brain development (which continues into the early to mid-20s), and is a health danger to pregnant women and their developing babies. They can also cause injuries such as fire and explosions.

Use of such products may be on the rise in certain age groups. According to the CDC, 11.7% of high schoolers in 2016 said they had used an e-cigarette, up from 1.5% in 2011. Between 2014 and 2018, the prevalence of reported current and daily use of e-cigarettes increased among young US adults but declined or remained stable in older age groups. The 46.2% increase (5.2% to 7.6%) in current e-cigarette use from 2017 to 2018 among young adults paralleled concurrent 48.5% and 77.8% increases among middle and high school students, respectively.[7] Interviews reveal that youths use the most popular brand of e-cigarettes because "Juul is cool." Social influences such as fitting into peer groups or experimentation play a major role in using such products.[8]

## Behavioral Health

One other tobacco-related issue is the fact that individuals with behavioral (mental) health problems smoke at far higher rates than their peers and have done so for decades. Recent research documents one possible explanation: Smoking is a "coping response" to deal with distress. High rates of smoking among adolescents may be a response to 2 events that trigger acute mental distress: violent crime victimization and death of a non–family member the respondent felt close to.[9]

It is important to note that patients with behavioral health issues (eg, anxiety, depression, substance use disorder) play a major role in rising healthcare costs. A recent analysis found that the 27% of the commercially insured population who had a behavioral health condition accounted for 57% of total annual healthcare costs (paid by both the insurer and the patient).[10] Patients with such conditions had total annual costs of $12,272 versus an average of only $5,932 per person among the commercially insured. Nevertheless, spending on treating their behavioral health conditions accounted for a paltry 4.4% of costs. Half of those with such conditions received treatment costing less than $68; the average spend on such conditions was $965 per patient. Most of the higher spending on patients with behavioral health conditions was devoted to their physical health needs. Researchers surmise that the behavioral conditions exacerbate the medical conditions. Other compounding issues include lower reimbursements paid to providers of such services, the tendency of the latter to remain out-of-network in insurance plans (which raises the cost to patients), and the low detection of such conditions by primary care physicians.

Behavioral health issues seem to be particularly acute in certain segments of the US population. For example, young adults aged 18 to 25 are among the most at risk of major mental health problems but are among the least likely to seek treatment. In 2018, nearly 9% of this cohort reported having a major episode of depression that was so severe it hindered their daily lives, but only half received treatment. This age group is also at risk for serious thoughts about suicide. Researchers suggest this group is hit by a "double whammy": the stresses of reaching adulthood and the loss of a usual source of care when leaving home for college.

## Substance Abuse

According to the World Health Organization (WHO), "substance abuse" refers to the harmful or hazardous use of psychoactive substances, including alcohol and illicit drugs. According to the National Survey on Drug Use and Health, 19.7 million adults (aged 12+ years) battled a substance abuse disorder in 2017. Nearly three-quarters (74%) of these adults also struggled with alcohol use. About 38% of adults in 2017 battled an illicit drug use disorder, and 1 out of every 8 adults struggled with both alcohol and drug use disorders at the same time. In 2018, the United States witnessed 67,367 drug overdose deaths. From 2007 to 2017, the age-adjusted death rate for drug overdose deaths increased 82%, from 11.9 to 21.7 deaths per 100,000 (Figure 26-3).

In 2017, 8.5 million American adults suffered from both a mental health disorder and a substance use disorder or co-occurring disorders. Drug abuse and addiction cost the United States more than $740 billion annually in lost workplace productivity, healthcare expenses, and crime-related costs, as follows:

| Disorder | Health Costs | Overall Costs | Year |
|---|---|---|---|
| Tobacco | $168 billion | $300 billion | 2010 |
| Alcohol | $27 billion | $249 billion | 2010 |
| Illicit drugs | $11 billion | $193 billion | 2007 |

Federal, state, and local governments spend close to $500 billion annually on addiction and substance abuse; for every dollar they spend, only 2 cents are spent on prevention and treatment.

Genetics, including the impact of one's environment on gene expression, account for about 40% to 60% of a person's risk of addiction. Environmental factors that may increase a person's risk of addiction include a chaotic home environment and abuse, parental drug use and attitude toward drugs, peer influences, community attitudes toward drugs, and poor academic achievement. Teenagers and people with mental health disorders are more at risk for drug use and addiction than other populations. More than 90% of people with a substance problem began smoking, drinking or using other drugs before age 18.

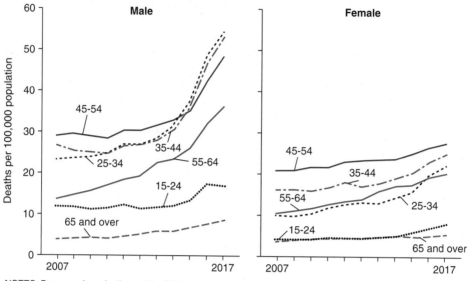

**Drug Overdose Death Rates Among Persons Aged 15 Years and Over, by Sex and Age: United States, 2007-2017**

NOTES: Drug overdose deaths are identified using *International Classification of Diseases, 10th revision* (ICD-10) underlying cause of death codes X40-X44 (unintentional drug poisoning), X60-X64 (suicide by drug poisoning), X85 (homicide by drug poisoning), and Y10-Y14 (drug poisoning of undetermined intent).

**Figure 26-3** • Death Rates from Drug Overdose. (Source: NCHS, National Vital Statistics System [NVSS], Mortality, 2007-2017.)

## Opioids

Prescription and illegal opioids account for more than 60% of overdose deaths in the United States, a toll that has quadrupled over the past 2 decades, according to the CDC. More than 175 people die every day from drug overdoses. More people died from opioid-related causes in 2016 than from car accidents or firearms. According to the CDC, the costs of healthcare, lost productivity, addiction treatment, and criminal justice involvement due to opioid misuse alone are $78.5 billion a year.

From 1999 to 2018, almost 450,000 people died from an overdose involving any opioid, including prescription and illegal opioids. Opioids are currently the main driver of these deaths and were involved in 46,802 (69.5%) of these cases. After a steady increase in the overall national opioid prescribing rate starting in 2006, the total number of prescriptions dispensed peaked in 2012 at more than 255 million, with a prescribing rate of 81.3 prescriptions per 100 persons. The overall national opioid prescribing rate thereafter declined to the lowest rate over the next 13 years at 51.4 prescriptions per 100 persons (168 million total opioid prescriptions). Nevertheless, the prescribing rates continue to

remain very high in certain parts of the country (eg, some counties had prescribing rates 6 times higher than the average).

## Bioterrorism

A biological attack, or "bioterrorism," is the intentional release of viruses, bacteria, or other germs that can sicken or kill people, livestock, or crops. *Bacillus anthracis*, the bacteria that causes anthrax, is one of the most likely agents to be used in a biological attack. The threat of bioterrorism became reality in 2001, exposing weaknesses in the country's public health infrastructure. Just 7 days after the 9/11 attacks, envelopes containing *B anthracis* spores were mailed to several East Coast media outlets and 2 US senators' offices, leading to 22 anthrax cases and 5 deaths.[11]

The 2001 events marked the first time that public health came to be considered central to emergency response and national security. It also showed how public health officials can respond to these types of attacks. In such situations, the CDC (and its partners) can respond by sending samples through the Laboratory Response Network (LRN), testing samples to learn more about the strain of anthrax, deploying field staff to talk to patients and learn more about how they were exposed, shipping out medicine and supplies from the Strategic National Stockpile (SNS) to local points of dispensing, providing guidance to clinicians, health departments, and other partners on how to respond, and communicating life-saving information to the public.

The US Public Health Service (USPHS) and primary healthcare providers must be prepared to address various biological agents, including pathogens that are rarely seen in the United States. The CDC categorizes these agents into 3 categories.[12]

## Firearm Violence

Firearms are heavily implicated in 2 leading causes of death: homicides and suicides. During 2015 to 2016, homicide was the 16th leading cause of death among all persons and the third leading cause among youths (10-19 years); firearm injuries were the underlying cause of death in 74% of all homicides and in 87% of youth homicides. Previously observed decreases in firearm homicide rates were not sustained and were followed by recent rate increases nationally. Firearm homicide rates among persons of all ages and among youths in the large metropolitan areas have both remained higher than corresponding national rates.

During the 2015 to 2016 period, suicide was the 10th leading cause of death nationally among all persons aged 10 years or older and the second leading cause among youths; a firearm injury was the underlying cause of death in 50% of all suicides and in 42% of youth suicides. Previously observed increases in firearm suicide rates among all persons have persisted in recent years; youth firearm suicide rates have also increased at the national level. In contrast to firearm homicide rates, firearm suicide rates among persons of all ages and among youths in the large metropolitan areas overall have both remained lower than corresponding national rates. This is consistent with previous research showing that rates of suicide, considering all causes, have been persistently lower in more urban areas than in less urban areas.

Preventing firearm homicides can be a challenge for cities across the country. Previous research has demonstrated that efforts to modify the physical and social environment by eliminating abandoned buildings and vacant lots, greening activities, street outreach, low-income housing tax credits, and business improvement districts are associated with lower levels of gun assaults, youth homicides, and other violent crimes.

Rates of firearm suicide began increasing with the economic recession of 2007-2008 and have continued to increase, despite the subsequent recovery of the economy. Annual rates of firearm suicide increased 21% from 2006 to 2016 (from 6.5 to 7.8 per 100,000 residents aged ≥10 years). Although urban areas recovered more quickly than did rural areas from the recession, their continued increase in firearm suicide rates suggests that other factors are at play and that a multifaceted prevention strategy may be required. Such interventions (eg, efforts to strengthen household financial security; stabilize housing; teach youths coping and problem-solving skills; identify and support persons at risk; and implement proactive prevention policies in schools, workplaces, and other organizational settings) are associated with reductions in suicide, suicide attempts, and/or co-occurring risks such as substance abuse, depression, and social isolation.

Another factor likely affecting both firearm homicide and suicide is access to firearms by those at risk for harming themselves or others. Previous studies have shown that the interval between deciding to act and attempting suicide can be as brief as 10 minutes or less. Strategies that can protect those at risk, especially juveniles, might include safe storage of firearms or temporary removal from the home. Preventing persons convicted of (or under a restraining order for) domestic violence from possessing a firearm has been associated with reductions in intimate partner-related homicide, including firearm homicide. Efforts to strengthen the background check system to better identify persons convicted of violent crimes or at risk for harming themselves or others might also prevent lethal firearm violence, although such policies warrant further study.

## Pandemics: SARS and COVID-19

In 2002, a respiratory virus called severe acute respiratory syndrome (SARS) appeared first in mainland China and then in Hong Kong. Within months, SARS had spread to more than 2 dozen countries in Europe, North America, South America, and Asia. By the time the contagion was contained, the virus had infected more than 8,000 people worldwide and killed almost 800. At that time, the Chinese government was criticized for responding slowly to the outbreak and concealing the seriousness of the illness. According to a 2004 report, China's initial response to SARS was plagued by a "fatal period of hesitation regarding information sharing and action." It took several months before the Chinese government started sharing information with the WHO. SARS was called the first pandemic of the 21st century.

SARS was eventually contained by means of active case detection ("syndromic surveillance"), prompt isolation of patients, contact tracing, strict enforcement of quarantine of all contacts, and in some areas, top-down enforcement of community quarantine. By interrupting all human-to-human transmission, SARS was effectively eradicated.

History repeated in late 2019 and early 2020. A deadly virus known as Coronavirus Disease 2019 (COVID-19) broke out in Wuhan, China, and then rapidly spread to the rest of Asia, Africa, Europe, and the United States. China was again heavily criticized for concealing the seriousness of the contagion and allowing its population to travel to other countries, which

likely fostered the virus's spread. The CDC took the lead among federal agencies in dealing with the virus in the United States but has had to work in tandem with state and local governments in terms of population measures to slow the spread of the virus, including social distancing, quarantining, use of personal protective equipment (PPE) such as facemasks, working remotely, and shutting down commercial activities. At the time of this writing, it is unclear whether the spread of the virus has been stopped.

Also at the time of this writing, it is unclear whether our public officials and healthcare industry understood what they were facing and whether they could have taken steps to limit the spread of the virus. Your answer to this question may reflect your political persuasion. Entire books will be written on this topic as this volume goes to press. Suffice it to say that there has been a lot of "second-guessing," "backseat driving," and "Monday morning quarterbacking."[13] There have also been several accounts acknowledging the confusion and uncertainty facing both experts and decision makers in fashioning an effective, organized response.[14]

## Critical Thinking Exercise: Managing the COVID-19 Crisis

The COVID-19 crisis has some interesting contrasts and parallels with the 1918 influenza (H1N1) pandemic, although the latter is regarded as much more serious.[15] Unlike COVID-19, there was no consensus regarding where the 1918 virus originated, and unlike COVID-19, the 1918 influenza did not shut down the economy. The 2020 shutdown brought home the message explicated in Chapter 2 of the linkage between "health and wealth."

Like COVID-19, the H1N1 virus spread worldwide in 3 waves during 1918 to 1919; and like COVID-19 (as of this writing), the properties that made it so devastating are not well understood. An estimated 500 million people, or one-third of the world's population, became infected with the H1N1 virus. The number of worldwide deaths was estimated to be at least 50 million, with roughly 675,000 occurring in the United States. With no vaccine to protect against influenza infection and no antibiotics to treat secondary bacterial infections that can be associated with influenza infections,

control efforts worldwide were limited to non-pharmaceutical interventions such as isolation, quarantine, good personal hygiene, use of disinfectants, and limitations of public gatherings, which were applied unevenly. Sound familiar? One major difference between the 1918-1919 virus and COVID-19 is that the United States did not shut down the economy in the former.

Amazingly, these lessons were not quickly disseminated when COVID-19 struck the United States in early Spring 2020. Did people forget the history lessons from a century ago? Did they even know the history and its lessons? Or was the United States confronted by something shrouded in such total mystery and uncertainty that no one in the government (at any level) knew what was going on, let alone what to do in response? If the latter view is correct, what is the best way to manage our way through such a crisis? What is the role of leadership during such times? Is it concerned with strategic planning or more with adaptation to rapidly changing circumstances?

The fragmentation of the governmental public health infrastructure is in part a direct result of the way in which governmental roles and responsibilities have evolved over time. This history also explains why the United States lacks a comprehensive national health policy that could be used to align health sector investment, governmental public health agency structure and function, and incentives for the private sector to work more effectively as part of a broader public health system.

Most public health funding comes from 3 governmental sources: federal, state, and local levels. Such funding is split due to a combination of federalism (division of authority between federal vs state government), home rule, and happenstance. Moreover, public health agencies are allocated specific budgets to accomplish specific tasks, with little discretionary funding.[16] Compounding such fragmentation is the fragmented responsibility for healthcare delivery (illness orientation) and public health (prevention and promotion orientation) between the medical care system and the public health system, respectively.

## Historical Background and Development of Public Health

### The 19th Century

The drivers of improved health status (reduced mortality in particular) have changed over time.[17] During the period from 1750 to 1850, improved nutrition and economic growth (eg, increased agricultural yields, improved caloric intake, reduced susceptibility to bacterial disease) were responsible. During the period from 1870 to 1920, the main driver (and the focus of this chapter) was public health. Since the 1930s, the main driver has been advances in medical technology.

Prior to the 1870s, contagious illness was viewed as the result of poisonous vapors ("miasmas") that were offensive to the smell. Cholera was the most dramatic of the infectious diseases (along with typhoid, diphtheria, yellow fever, tuberculosis, and malaria) that fed on urbanization, poor hygiene, overcrowding, and increased public interactions in the latter half of the

19th century. Medical treatments were generally ineffective. Initial public health functions were conducted on more of a committee oversight basis in coastal cities to quarantine ships that might introduce cholera and yellow fever. These committees constituted precursors to the "local health departments" that exist today. The first department established at the state level did not occur until 1869.

With the invention of the microscope and other technologies, medical science discovered that the causes of many infectious diseases were micro-organisms or pathogens. Such pathogens were too small to be seen by the human eye. This became known as the germ theory of disease. Building on the work of Louis Pasteur (who discovered in 1877 that anthrax is caused by bacteria), Robert Koch identified the tubercule bacillus in 1882 and the cholera bacillus in 1884. Such discoveries marked the ascendance of bacteriology and shifted thinking away from miasmas toward contagions as the cause of epidemics. This began a long-term trend in the reduction of infectious disease (that would run through 1960) that resulted in a dramatic 40% decline in US mortality rates and a 34% increase in life expectancy at birth (from 1900 to 1940).[18]

The growing acceptance of the germ theory of disease allowed public health to play a larger role. *Micro*-level public health activities, such as health behavior campaigns in the late 19th and early 20th centuries, targeted hand and food washing, the boiling of milk and washing of milk bottles, protecting food from insects, ventilation, and breastfeeding. *Macro*-level public health activities, such as large-scale public projects, included clean water technologies, sanitation, refuse management, milk pasteurization, swamp drainage, and meat inspection. This period has been characterized as "the great sanitary awakening" (ie, the identification of filth as both a cause of disease and a vehicle of transmission, as well as the ensuing embrace of cleanliness). Sanitation changed the way society thought about health. Illness came to be seen as an indicator of poor social and environmental conditions, not just poor moral and spiritual conditions.

The germ theory of disease provided a sound scientific basis for public health. Public health measures continued to be focused predominantly on specific contagious diseases, but the means of controlling these diseases changed dramatically. During this period, public agencies that conducted and enforced sanitary measures expanded their purview into laboratory science and epidemiology. Laboratory research identified exact causes and specific strategies for preventing specific diseases. Science also revealed that both the environment and people could be the agents of disease. Public responsibility for health came to include both environmental sanitation and individual health.

Public health agencies began at the local and state levels in the United States in the late 1800s, in the guise of state boards of health, state health departments, and local health departments. To develop and apply the new scientific knowledge, in the 1890s, state and local health departments in the United States began to establish laboratories. The burgeoning social problems of industrial cities convinced legislatures to form more elaborate and professional public health administrations within municipal governments.[19] City boards of health were established to obtain effective agency supervision and control of health threats facing the population.

## The 20th Century

Clean water technologies are likely the most important public health intervention of the 20th century. In 1900, waterborne diseases accounted for nearly one-quarter of reported infectious disease deaths in major cities. In the next few decades, waterborne disease mortality fell dramatically. The introduction of water filtration plants and chlorination systems led to major reductions in mortality, explaining nearly half of the overall reduction in mortality between 1900 and 1936. Clean water was responsible for three-quarters of the decline in infant mortality and nearly two-thirds of the decline in child mortality. The magnitude of these effects is striking. Clean water also appears to have led to the near eradication of typhoid fever, a waterborne scourge of the 19th and early 20th centuries.

Nutritional and public health efforts were both, in turn, supplemented by advances in medical treatment interventions such as vaccinations and antibiotics. While vaccination had been introduced at the end of the 18th century (Edward Jenner), research on vaccines had to wait upon the germ theory of disease. Starting in the late 19th century and extending into the 20th century, there was a wave of vaccines: rabies

(1885), plague (1897), diphtheria (1923), pertussis (1926), tuberculosis (1927), tetanus (1927), yellow fever (1935), polio (1955 and 1962), measles (1964), mumps (1967), rubella (1970), and hepatitis B (1981). Antibiotics, developed in the 1930s and 1940s, were the first of the new wave of medical therapies. Sulfa drugs and penicillin (used to treat bacterial infections) facilitated a decline in infectious disease in the first half of the 20th century. Subsequent declines in mortality rates are largely due to medical interventions (drugs, medical devices) but are also attributable to public health activities such as smoking/tobacco use campaigns and greater use of seatbelts.

## Federal Public Health Efforts in the 20th Century

Federal activities in health were initially limited to public hospitals that cared for merchant seamen as part of the Marine Hospital Service (begun in 1798). The Marine Hospital on Staten Island established a National Hygienic Laboratory to apply the new science of bacteriology to the diagnosis and study of contagious disease. In 1912, the Marine Hospital Service was renamed the USPHS, and its director, the surgeon general, was granted more authority. The USPHS assumed the quarantine function of the Marine Service. Although early USPHS activities were modest, by 1918, they included administering physical and mental examinations of aliens, demonstration projects in rural health, and control and prevention of venereal diseases. Federal activities also grew to include promoting programs for individual health and providing assistance to states for campaigns against specific health problems. This marked the beginning of "categorical funding" to cover specific diseases, populations, or health problems:

- The formation of the Children's Bureau (1912)
- The Sheppard-Towner Act of 1922 established the Federal Board of Maternity and Infant Hygiene, which funded the Children's Bureau and funded states to establish programs in maternal and child health. The act was the impetus for the federal practice of setting guidelines for public health programs and providing funding to states to implement programs meeting the guidelines. Although

federally initiated, the programs were fully state run.

- The Social Security Act (1935) provided federal funds to the states for maternal and child health. One title of the act established a federal grant-in-aid program to the states for establishing and maintaining public health services and for training public health personnel. Another title increased the responsibilities of the Children's Bureau in maternal and child health and capabilities of state maternal and child health programs.
- The National Hygienic Laboratory relocated to the Washington, DC, area in 1930 and was renamed the National Institutes of Health (NIH). In 1937, the institute greatly expanded its research functions to include the study and investigation of all diseases and related conditions, and the National Cancer Institute was established as the first of the research institutes focused on particular diseases or health problems.
- Congress passed a venereal disease control act in 1938, which provided federal funds to states for investigation and control of venereal diseases.
- In 1939, the Federal Security Agency, housing the Public Health Service and national programs in education and welfare, was established. The Public Health Service also continued to expand.
- During World War II, the CDC was established and, shortly thereafter, the National Center for Health Statistics.
- The National Mental Health Act, establishing the National Institute of Mental Health as a part of the NIH, was passed in 1946. This institute was also authorized to finance training programs for mental health professionals and to finance development of community mental health services in local areas, as well as to conduct and support research.
- The Partnership in Health Act of 1966 established a "block grant" approach for a variety of programs, providing federal funding of state and county activities in general health.

As the federal bureaucracy in health grew and programs requiring federal-state partnerships for health programs were developed, the need for expertise and leaders in public health increased at both federal and state levels.

To participate in Medicaid, states had to designate a single state agency to direct the program, setting up a dichotomy between public health services and Medicaid services. Also, most states experienced a sudden growth in programs and program costs with the advent of Medicare and Medicaid. For example, federal funding for the institutionalized mentally ill became available for the first time through Medicaid, allowing expansion of these services and their costs in many states. Some federal programs of the 1960s also inspired growth of health services in local health departments and in private health organizations. Maternal and child health, family planning, immunization, venereal disease control, and tuberculosis control offered financial and technical assistance to local health departments to provide these services. Other federal programs developed at this time allowed funds and technical assistance to be provided directly to private health care providers, bypassing state and local government authorities. One example, the Comprehensive Health Planning Act (1966), allowed federal funding of neighborhood or community health centers, which were governed by boards composed of a consumer majority and related directly to the federal government for policy and program direction and finances.

## THE CORE FUNCTIONS AND ESSENTIAL SERVICES OF PUBLIC HEALTH

Public health has 3 core functions: assessment, policy development, and assurance. These 3 functions subsume 10 "essential" public health services (Figure 26-4).[20] *Assessment* includes monitoring the health status of the population (eg, via community health assessments and disease registries) to identify and solve problems and diagnosis and investigation of health hazards and health problems (eg, investigate infectious and vector-borne disease outbreaks). *Policy development* includes informing, educating, and empowering people about health issues (eg, health education and health promotion); mobilizing community partnerships (eg, with the private sector, civic groups, and faith organizations); and developing policies and

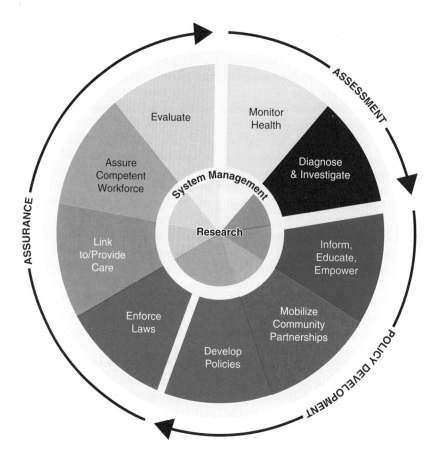

**Figure 26-4** • Essential Public Health Services. (Source: Centers for Disease Control and Prevention. 10 Essential Public Health Services. https://www.cdc.gov/publichealthgateway/publichealthservices/originalessentialhealth services.html.)

plans that support individual and community health efforts (eg, community health improvement planning). *Assurance* includes enforcement of laws and regulations that protect health and safety; linking people to needed personal healthcare services (eg, access to care, primary care); assuring a competent public health workforce; evaluating the effectiveness, accessibility, and quality of personal and population-based health services; and conducting research on innovative solutions to health problems.

regulate interstate commerce and its power to tax and spend for the public welfare, the federal government acts in areas such as environmental protection, occupational health and safety, and food and drug purity. The federal government acts in 6 main areas related to population health: (1) policy making, (2) financing, (3) public health protection, (4) collecting and disseminating information about US health and healthcare delivery systems, (5) capacity building for population health, and (6) direct management of services.

## THE FEDERAL GOVERNMENT's ROLE IN PUBLIC HEALTH

### Source of Federal Authority

For most of US history, the US Supreme Court has granted the federal government broad powers under the Constitution to protect the public's health and safety. Under the power to

### General Responsibilities in Public Health

The federal government has several public health responsibilities. First, it must ensure that all government levels have the capabilities to provide essential public health services (see Figure 26-4). Second, it must act when the country is confronted by health threats that span more than one state. Third, it must act where the solutions to address such threats lie beyond the jurisdiction of a particular state or assist states when they lack the expertise or resources to respond to emergencies such as natural disasters (hurricanes), bioterrorism (Anthrax threat), or emerging diseases (SARS, COVID-19). Fourth, it collaborates with other government levels in formulating public health goals.

The federal government also serves to (1) set public health goals, policies, and standards through its regulatory powers; (2) contribute financial resources to several federal agencies and to the states; and (3) finance research (eg, through the NIH) and education. However, in contrast to state and local public health agencies, the federal government has a limited role in the direct delivery of essential public health services.

## Federal Public Health Structure

The Public Health Service of the Department of Health and Human Services (DHHS) is the main federal authority in health. Its primary efforts are in assessment, research, and policy and program development. Most of its assurance activities are conducted through funding contracts with states, local areas, and providers, who actually carry out the service. Some assurance activities are directly carried out by the federal government.

### Agencies

The executive branch of the US federal government conducts public health activities through the DHHS. DHHS has designated 8 of its 11 agencies as components of the USPHS:

- The *Agency for Healthcare Research and Quality* (AHRQ) funds research on improving the quality and delivery of healthcare.
- The *CDC* is the federal government's lead public health agency. It is the main assessment and epidemiologic unit for the nation, directly serves the population, and provides technical assistance to states and localities.
- The *Agency for Toxic Substances and Disease Registry* (ATSDR) investigates the public health impact of exposure to hazardous substances and focuses on environmentally related diseases.

- The *Food and Drug Administration* (FDA) regulates drugs, medical devices, food, and tobacco products, among other consumer products. It directly tests and assesses safety of food, drugs, and some consumer goods, and sets standards for safe use of these items.
- The *Health Resources and Services Administration* (HRSA) funds programs and systems that provide healthcare services to the uninsured and medically underserved. It is primarily concerned with developing manpower and other resources.
- The *Indian Health Service* (IHS) supports a healthcare delivery system for Native Americans.
- The *NIH* funds basic, clinical, and translational biomedical and behavioral research. It is the primary research arm of the government, conducting internal and supporting external research projects across the nation.
- The *Substance Abuse and Mental Health Services Administration* (SAMHSA) funds mental health and substance abuse prevention and treatment services.

Additionally, several offices relating directly to the Assistant Secretary for Health deal with public health issues, such as the Office of Health Promotion and Disease Prevention and the Office of Planning and Evaluation. These offices are concerned with management; health policy, research, and statistics; planning and evaluation; intergovernmental affairs; health promotion; and other special concerns.

Responsibility for certain health programs is scattered across various White House agencies such as the Office of Science and Technology Policy and the Office of National Drug Control Policy, 14 cabinet-level departments and agencies (eg, Department of Agriculture, Department of Transportation, Environmental Protection Agency, Department of Veterans Affairs [VA], and Department of Defense [DOD]), and more than 10 public corporations and commissions and subcabinet agencies. The US Congress oversees the activities of federal agencies through committees that review the authorization of programs and the appropriation of funds. Multiple committees in both the House of Representatives and the Senate have jurisdiction over DHHS programs and health-related activities in other departments (see Chapter 25). These multiple authorities and congressional jurisdictions are an important reason for the "disarray" noted in previous Institute of Medicine (IOM) reports.

## Funding and Oversight

Federal agency funding of public health is primarily discretionary rather than mandatory spending. Each USPHS agency receives discretionary budget authority through annual appropriations processes. AHRQ, CDC, HRSA, NIH, and SAMHSA are funded through one appropriations act; ATSDR and IHS are funded through a second appropriations act. FDA is funded through a third appropriations act. The DHHS secretary has limited authority to transfer funds from one budget account to another within the department. The secretary may transfer up to 1% of the funds in any given account; the recipient account may not be increased by more than 3%. Congressional appropriators must be notified in advance of any transfer.

Although the bulk of USPHS agency funding is based on discretionary appropriations, agencies also receive a mix of mandatory funding, user fees, and third-party collections. Such funding sources can be a substantial component of the budget of some USPHS agencies. With regard to mandatory funding, the Patient Protection and Affordable Care Act (PPACA) included numerous appropriations to support specified grant programs and activities. PPACA also established and funded 3 trust funds to help support USPHS agency programs and activities: the Community Health Center Fund (CHCF), which supports the federal health centers program and the National Health Service Corps (NHSC); the Prevention and Public Health Fund (PPHF), which supports prevention, wellness, and other public health programs and activities; and the Patient-Centered Outcomes Research Trust Fund (PCORTF), which supports comparative effectiveness research. Several USPHS agencies assess user fees on third parties to help fund their programs and activities.

## Federal Public Health Funding

Unlike medical care and biomedical research, the federal government has never invested heavily in public health infrastructure (eg, clinical laboratories, surveillance systems, or environmental monitoring systems). Over the past 60 years, federal funding of public health activities has waxed and waned, without waxing very much. The figures below list total national health expenditures (NHEs), government public health spending, and the percentage of NHE accounted for by public health spending, by decade.

| Year | NHE ($ billions) | Public Health ($ billions) | % of NHE |
|------|------------------|----------------------------|----------|
| 1960 | $27.2 | $0.4 | 1.47% |
| 1970 | $74.6 | $1.4 | 1.88% |
| 1980 | $255.3 | $6.4 | 2.51% |
| 1990 | $721.4 | $20.0 | 2.77% |
| 2000 | $1,369.2 | $43.0 | 3.14% |
| 2010 | $2,593.2 | $75.7 | 2.92% |
| 2018 | $3,649.4 | $93.5 | 2.56% |

The data indicate that federal spending on public health has remained below 4% historically. Such spending as a percentage of NHE peaked at the turn of the millennium and has steadily declined to roughly 1980s levels.

These figures lend credence to some of the recent criticism of the federal government's response to the COVID-19 crisis, particularly the view that our public health system has been "hollowed out." Decades of underfunding and a current lack of resources may have prevented it from fashioning any effective response to the virus. Some attribute the hollowing out to a gridlocked Congress that opted for continuing resolutions and budget caps rather than making tough decisions about funding needed infrastructure. They also note the public's falling trust and confidence in government, as well as growing antigovernment rhetoric.[21] Others point to the antiquated technology and notification systems inside the CDC, which relies on assembling information supplied by local public health officials (using phone calls, faxes, and spreadsheets attached to e-mails).[22] In addition to the dwindling funding at the federal level noted earlier, state public health department funding dropped 16% per capita since 2010, while local public health department funding dropped 18% per capita.[23] The public health workforce at the local level has shrunk by nearly one-quarter since 2008, the time of the last major economic recession.[24]

## STATE AND LOCAL GOVERNMENTS' ROLE IN PUBLIC HEALTH

### State Authority

States carry out most of their responsibilities through their power to enact and enforce laws to protect and promote the health, safety, and general welfare of the people. In the Tenth Amendment to the US Constitution, states and the people are designated as the repository of all government powers not specifically designated to the federal government. Because the Constitution does not mention the protection and promotion of health, these functions fall to the states. States have thus become the central authorities in the nation's public health system. Each of the 50 states and 4 US territories designates an agency responsible for public health.

### State Organization

State health agencies are organized in 1 of 2 models: (1) as a freestanding, independent agency responsible directly to the governor or the Board of Health, or (2) as a component of a superagency (eg, health and human services program). Several state health departments are also the main environmental agency in their state; several are the mental health agency; and several are also the state Medicaid agency. Physicians and nurses often lead state public health agencies. At the local level, however, general managers with business training rather than formal training in public health or medicine may lead public health agencies.

Organizational units within agencies also vary. Some states have divisions based on regulatory and nonregulatory activities; some have divisions based on different service populations; some have divisions based on different health problems; and some have divisions based on environmental and population services. State health agency operations also differ in their level of centralization at the state level. About one-third are completely centralized, operating whatever local health agency units exist

in the state. The remainder share operation of programs with local health agencies. Some local health agencies operate completely independently of the state health agency, but state agencies are semi-centralized in most states, operating some programs completely, sharing some with locals, and acting as an adviser on some programs.

### State Public Health Funding

Nearly half of state health agency funding comes from the federal government (45% in 2011). The next major source of funding is the state's general funds (23%), which come from state taxes. Additional sources include other state funds (16%), fees and fines (7%), Medicare and Medicaid (4%), and other (5%).

### State Functions

States' public health agencies carry out many of the same general functions, although the scope of activities and specific activities vary tremendously. Activities such as immunization, infectious disease control and reporting, health education, and health statistics are common to most public health agencies. States are also responsible for licensing and regulating the institutional and individual providers that deliver healthcare services. However, states differ in whether the public health agency has responsibility for programs such as mental health and substance abuse, environmental health, and Medicaid. These organizational differences make it more complicated to frame and pursue a coherent national agenda concerning changes and improvements in the governmental public health infrastructure.

Some states conduct a wide array of services, and some only a few. Some concentrate on assessment and policy development activities; some concentrate almost solely on assuring access and delivering personal health services. State resources designated to health also vary. Finally, state public health agencies differ in their relationships with other state agencies involved in health, in their relationships with local health authorities (see later discussion), and in their relationships with the private sector. Some work closely together, some rarely communicate, and some openly compete.

States perform an array of roles in public health. These include screening for diseases and conditions, treatment for diseases, technical assistance and training, provision of state laboratory services, and epidemiology and surveillance. Among their functions, state health agencies may do the following:

- Collect and analyze information
- Conduct inspections
- Plan
- Set policies and standards
- Carry out national and state mandates
- Manage and oversee environmental, educational, and personal health services
- Assure access to healthcare for underserved residents
- Help in resources development
- Respond to health hazards and crises

## State Versus Local Governance

States differ in terms of the relationship between the state agency and the agencies serving localities within the state. The degree of centralization or decentralization of public health below the federal level thus varies considerably. Analysts have detected 4 major relationship models. In "local/decentralized" models, local health departments (LHDs) developed independently from the state agency; they are units led by local governments (county, township), which make most of the fiscal decisions and report directly to local boards of health or health commissioners. In "mixed" models, some LHDs are led by state government, and some are led by local government, with no one arrangement predominating. In "state/centralized" models, all LHDs are units of state government; the state agency has direct control and authority for supervision of local public health activities and makes most fiscal decisions. Finally, in "shared" models, all LHDs are governed by both state and local authorities. In some states, there may be no local public health agencies.

## Local Health Departments

LHDs are the critical actors that directly deliver public health services to the population. The National Association of County and City Health Officials (NACCHO) defines an LHD as "an administrative or service unit of local or state government, concerned with health, and carrying some responsibility for the health of a jurisdiction smaller than the state." Roughly 2,800

agencies or units meet this definition. Nearly two-thirds of LHDs (62%) serve populations of less than 50,000 people; such jurisdictions account for only 10% of the total population. By contrast, only 6% of LHDs serve populations of 500,000 or more people; these LHDs cover 51% of the population. Some states have a public health system structure that includes both regional and local offices of the state health agency.[25] Of the 2,533 LHDs included in the 2016 NACCHO survey, 1,946 are locally governed, 396 are units of the state health agency, and 191 have shared governance. Nearly one-fifth (19%) of LHDs are part of a combined Health and Human Services Agency.

Although LHDs may carry out each of the 3 public health functions outlined earlier, they are substantially more involved in *assurance* activities, particularly the service provision. LHDs are generally responsible for direct delivery of the following public health services:

- Conduct communicable disease control programs
- Provide screening and immunizations
- Collect health statistics
- Provide health education services and chronic disease control programs
- Conduct sanitation, sanitary engineering, and inspection programs
- Run school health programs
- Deliver maternal and child health services, public health nursing services, mental health services, and other home care

Differences in geography and systems of government lead to even greater differences among LHDs than among state agencies. Some LHDs are municipal, some serve a county, and some serve groups of counties, or districts. Some LHDs are directed by full-time physician health officers with public health experience; some are run by part-time administrators with little public health experience. Some local areas have large, sophisticated LHDs that carry out all public health functions with little dependence on the state. Many areas have smaller, more limited LHDs that work in conjunction with, or as a branch of, the state health department. LHDs also vary considerably in their procurement and allocation of resources. Finally, LHDs vary in their relationships with other local agencies and with private providers. Many rely on private providers to augment services; some have little to do with private providers. Figure 26-5 provides

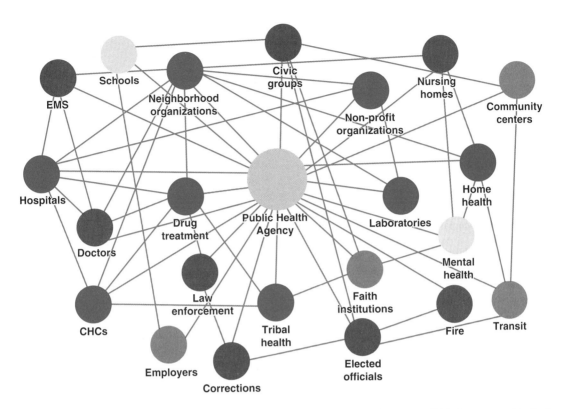

**Figure 26-5** • Local Partnerships in Public Health. CHCs, Community Health Centers; EMS, Emergency Medical Services. (Source: Centers for Disease Control and Preventions. 10 Essential Public Health Services. https://www .cdc.gov/publichealthgateway/publichealthservices/originalessentialhealthservices.html.)

an idea about how broadly these partnerships may need to be constructed. Figure 26-6 highlights the intensity of these linkages with LHDs in 2 ways: the existence of any partnership and the extent of more formalized partnerships with sharing of resources.

## Local Health Agency Funding and Services

LHDs derive their annual revenues from a host of sources. Roughly one-quarter (30%) are local revenues. Another 21% comes from direct state support. The remainder is split between Medicare and Medicaid payments for clinical services (12%), fees and fines (7%), federal pass-throughs (17%), federal direct support (7%), and other. A sizeable portion of LHD funds comes from federal government grants awarded by the CDC. The CDC's funding has barely increased over time, rising from roughly $7 billion in 2010 to $8 billion by 2020.[26]

A recent NACCHO (2016) survey of local public health infrastructure documents the variation in service provision at the local level

(Figure 26-7). The vast majority of LHDs provide immunizations; a majority provide a variety of screening services, with tuberculosis as the most widespread in terms of screening and treatment. Some maternal and child health services are frequently provided (eg, women, infants, and children; home visits), while others are surprisingly not (eg, well-child care, prenatal care). A host of other services are not widely offered, such as school-based clinics, oral health, substance abuse, and behavioral/mental health.

The NACCHO survey data also depict the degree to which LHDs provide population-based programs and services (Figure 26-8). The most prevalent epidemiological programs concern communicable/infectious disease and environmental health. The most prevalent primary prevention programs cover nutrition and tobacco. The other portions of Figure 26-8 indicate the major areas of concern in terms of regulation, inspection, and environmental health.

There are considerable variations in the provision of these programs and services between urban and rural areas. Programs and services that are more prevalent in rural areas (vs urban

### LHD Partnerships and Collaborations in the Past Years

- Percent of LHDs working with partner in any way (exchanging information, regularly scheduling meetings, with written agreements, or sharing personnel/resources)
- Percent of LHDs regularly scheduling meetings, with written agreements, or sharing personnel/resources with partner

**Healthcare partners**

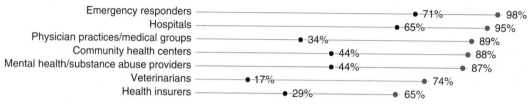

| Partner | % | % |
|---|---|---|
| Emergency responders | 71% | 98% |
| Hospitals | 65% | 95% |
| Physician practices/medical groups | 34% | 89% |
| Community health centers | 44% | 88% |
| Mental health/substance abuse providers | 44% | 87% |
| Veterinarians | 17% | 74% |
| Health insurers | 29% | 65% |

**Community-based partners (eg, education, nongovernment)**

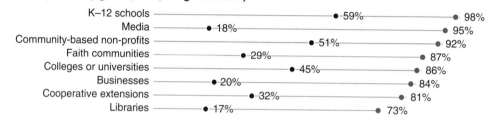

| Partner | % | % |
|---|---|---|
| K–12 schools | 59% | 98% |
| Media | 18% | 95% |
| Community-based non-profits | 51% | 92% |
| Faith communities | 29% | 87% |
| Colleges or universities | 45% | 86% |
| Businesses | 20% | 84% |
| Cooperative extensions | 32% | 81% |
| Libraries | 17% | 73% |

**Government agencies**

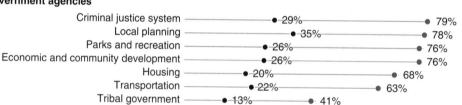

| Partner | % | % |
|---|---|---|
| Criminal justice system | 29% | 79% |
| Local planning | 35% | 78% |
| Parks and recreation | 26% | 76% |
| Economic and community development | 26% | 76% |
| Housing | 20% | 68% |
| Transportation | 22% | 63% |
| Tribal government | 13% | 41% |

**Figure 26-6** • Prevalence of Local Public Health Partnerships. LHD, Local Health Department. (Source: National Association of County and City Health Officials.)

### Clinical Programs and Services Provided Directly in the Past Year

| Program/service | % LHDs | Program/service | % LHDs | Program/service | % LHDs |
|---|---|---|---|---|---|
| **Immunization** | | **Treatment for communicable diseases** | | **Other clinical services** | |
| Adult immunizations | 90% | Tuberculosis | 79% | Laboratory services | 38% |
| Childhood immunizations | 88% | Other STDs | 63% | School-based clinics | 34% |
| **Screening for diseases/conditions** | | HIV/AIDS | 35% | Oral health | 28% |
| Tuberculosis | 84% | **Maternal and child health services** | | Asthma prevention and/or management | 22% |
| Other STDs | 65% | Women, Infants, and Children (WIC) | 66% | Home healthcare | 20% |
| HIV/AIDS | 62% | | | Correctional health | 13% |
| Blood lead | 61% | Home visits | 60% | Substance abuse | 11% |
| High blood pressure | 54% | Family planning | 53% | Comprehensive primary care | 11% |
| Body Mass Index (BMI) | 53% | Early and periodic screening, diagnosis, and treatment | 38% | Behavioral/mental health | 10% |
| Diabetes | 34% | Well child clinic | 29% | Emergency medical services | 4% |
| Cancer | 32% | Prenatal care | 27% | | |
| Cardiovascular disease | 25% | Obstetrical care | 8% | | |

**Figure 26-7** • Local Public Health Clinical Programs. LHD, Local Health Department; STD, Sexually Transmitted Disease. (Source: National Association of County and City Health Officials.)

**Population-Based Programs and Services Provided Directly in the Past Years**

| Program/service | % LHDs | Program/service | % LHDs | Program/service | % LHDs |
|---|---|---|---|---|---|
| **Epidemiology and surveillance** | | **Regulation, inspection, and/or licensing** | | **Other environmental health services** | |
| Communicable/infectious disease | 93% | Food service establishments | 79% | Food safety education | 77% |
| Environmental health | 85% | Schools/daycare | 74% | Nuisance abatement | 76% |
| Maternal and child health | 69% | Recreational water (eg, pools, lakes, beaches) | 68% | Vector control | 53% |
| Syndromic surveillance | 61% | | | Groundwater protection | 44% |
| Chronic disease | 49% | Septic systems | 67% | Surface water protection | 35% |
| Behavioral risk factors | 45% | Smoke-free ordinances | 65% | Indoor air quality | 35% |
| Injury | 32% | Body art (eg, tattoos, piercings) | 60% | Hazmat response | 21% |
| **Population-based primary prevention** | | | | Radiation control | 21% |
| Nutrition | 74% | Private drinking water | 60% | Air pollution | 20% |
| Tobacco | 74% | Children's camps | 59% | Land use planning | 19% |
| Physical activity | 60% | Hotels/motels | 58% | Hazardous waste disposal | 18% |
| Chronic disease programs | 57% | Lead inspection | 53% | Noise pollution | 16% |
| Unintended pregnancy | 51% | Campgrounds & RVs | 46% | **Other population-based services** | |
| Injury | 42% | Tobacco retailers | 38% | Vital records | 62% |
| Substance abuse | 34% | Health-related facilities | 38% | Outreach and enrollment for medical insurance | 44% |
| Violence | 22% | Public drinking water | 37% | School health | 41% |
| Mental illness | 17% | Food processing | 36% | Collection of unused pharmaceuticals | 18% |
| | | Mobile homes | 32% | Animal control | 18% |
| | | Housing (inspections) | 31% | Occupational safety and health | 15% |
| | | Solid waste haulers | 31% | | |
| | | Solid waste disposal sites | 30% | | |
| | | Milk processing | 18% | | |

**Figure 26-8 •** Local Population Health Programs. LHD, Local Health Department. (Source: National Association of County and City Health Officials.)

areas) include childhood immunizations (95% vs 77%), maternal and child health surveillance (76% vs 59%), maternal and child health home health visits (64% vs 51%), women, infants, and children (WIC; 72% vs 53%), blood lead screening (72% vs 49%), body mass index screening (65% vs 43%), and high blood pressure screening (62% vs 51%). Programs and services that are more prevalent in urban areas are lead inspection (63% vs 40%), housing inspection (45% vs 15%), indoor air quality control (44% vs 23%), noise pollution control (31% vs 6%), air pollution control (30% vs 10%), and all forms of regulation.

There is also variation over time in the percentage of LHDs offering each of these programs and services. Areas of increase in their provision between 2008 and 2016 include syndromic surveillance (22% increase), HIV/AIDS treatment (15%), laboratory services (13%), behavioral risk factors surveillance (12%), vital records (12%), regulation of tobacco retailers (11%), and chronic disease surveillance (10%). Areas of decreased provision include high blood pressure screening (14% decrease), well-child clinic (11%), diabetes screening (11%), cardiovascular disease screening (10%), and cancer screening (10%). Approximately one-fifth of

LHDs (19%) report a lower budget for emergency preparedness in the current fiscal year compared to the previous fiscal year, whereas 11% report a higher budget.

## Local Health Agency Contribution

Researchers have quantified the contribution of LHDs over the period from 1998 to 2014. They examined local public health systems in 360 communities serving 100,000+ populations in terms of their (1) scope: availability of 20 recommended population health activities; (2) network density: degree to which multisector organizations contribute to each activity; and (3) network centrality: presence of a central actor (designated public health agency) to coordinate these efforts. They found that 32.7% of communities (representing 47.2% of the population) were served by "comprehensive public health systems" that scored highly on all 3 dimensions; such communities exhibited significantly lower levels of mortality and morbidity than other communities. Figure 26-9 shows the percentage of the 20 recommended public health activities that were delivered, as well as the change in the prevalence of these activities over time (1998 vs 2014).

| 1998-2014 | | | |
|---|---|---|---|
| Public Health Activity | 1998 | 2014 | % Change |
| 1 Community health needs assessment | 71.5% | 86.0% | 20.2% |
| 2 Behavioral risk factor surveillance | 45.8% | 70.2% | 53.2% |
| 3 Adverse health events investigation | 98.6% | 100.0% | 1.4% |
| 4 Public health laboratory testing services | 96.3% | 96.5% | 0.2% |
| 5 Analysis of health status and health determinants | 61.3% | 72.8% | 18.7% |
| 6 Analysis of preventive services utilization | 28.4% | 39.4% | 38.8% |
| 7 Health information provision to elected officials | 80.9% | 84.8% | 4.8% |
| 8 Health information provision to the public | 75.4% | 83.8% | 11.1% |
| 9 Health information provision to the media | 75.2% | 87.5% | 16.3% |
| 10 Prioritization of community health needs | 66.1% | 82.3% | 24.6% |
| 11 Community participation in health improvement planning | 41.5% | 67.7% | 63.0% |
| 12 Development of community health improvement plan | 81.9% | 86.2% | 5.2% |
| 13 Resource allocation to implement community health plan | 26.2% | 43.2% | 64.9% |
| 14 Policy development to implement community health plan | 48.6% | 57.5% | 18.4% |
| 15 Communication network of health-related organizations | 78.8% | 84.8% | 7.6% |
| 16 Strategies to enhance access to needed health services | 75.6% | 50.2% | −33.6% |
| 17 Implementation of legally mandated public health activities | 91.4% | 92.4% | 1.0% |
| 18 Evaluation of public health programs and services | 34.7% | 38.4% | 10.8% |
| 19 Evaluation of local public health agency capacity/performance | 56.3% | 55.0% | −2.4% |
| 20 Implementation of quality improvement processes | 47.3% | 49.6% | 5.0% |

**Figure 26-9** • Percentage of the 20 Recommended Public Health Activities Delivered and the Change in the Prevalence of These Activities Over Time (1998 vs 2014). (Source: National Longitudinal Survey of Public Health Systems. NALSYS Resources and Results. http://systemsforaction.org/projects/national-longitudinal-survey-public-health-systems?&tab=reports.)

## THE PUBLIC HEALTH WORKFORCE

Public health infrastructure at the federal, state, and local levels consists of physical resources (eg, laboratories), information networks, and human resources. Public health is heavily reliant on human resources, although the exact size of those resources is somewhat uncertain. At the turn of the millennium, there were an estimated 450,000 workers in salaried public health positions, with many more in nongovernmental organizations or volunteer positions. Trend data suggest downsizing in public health personnel to roughly 326,602 governmental public health workers by 2012, and down further to 290,988 public health workers in governmental agencies by 2014.[27] For 2014, 51% of these workers were in LHDs, 30% worked in state public health agencies, and the remainder worked in federal settings. The top 3 occupations were administrative or clerical personnel (19%), public health nurses (16%), and environmental health workers (8%). Similar trends in downsizing are found at the LHD level, from 166,000 full-time equivalents (FTEs) in 2008 to 133,000 by 2016. There has also been a decrease in LHD funding per capita, from a mean of $63 to $48.

Public health practitioners have training in a variety of disciplines, including the biological and health sciences, psychology, education, nutrition, ethics, sociology, epidemiology, biostatistics, business, computer science, political science, law, public affairs, and urban planning. Studies have suggested that the public health workforce is improperly prepared to meet the challenges of public health, with an estimated 80% of workers lacking formal public health training. The number and training mix of LHD staff vary by size of the population served (Figure 26-10). Almost three-quarters (73%) of the FTEs work in LHDs serving urban areas; the remaining 27% work in LHDs designated as micropolitan and rural. Small areas typically have 1 to 2 nurses and perhaps an environmental health worker; by contrast, large areas have many nurses and environmental health workers, along with health educators, nutritionists, community health workers,

**Staffing Patterns at LHDs by Size of Population Served (in Median Full-Time Equivalents [FTEs])**

| 10,000–24,999 | 50,000–99,999 | 100,000–249,999 | 500,000–999,999 |
|---|---|---|---|
| **8 Total FTEs** | **27 Total FTEs** | **58 Total FTEs** | **230 Total FTEs** |
| 2 Registered nurses | 6 Registered nurses | 9 Registered nurses | 29.3 Registered nurses |
| 2 Office support staff | 5 Office support staff | 8.5 Office support staff | 30.5 Office support staff |
| 1 Agency leadership | 1 Agency leadership | 3 Agency leadership | 6 Agency leadership |
| 1 Environmental health worker | 3 Environmental health workers | 7 Environmental health workers | 20.5 Environmental health workers |
| | 1 Health educator | 2 Health educators | 6 Health educators |
| | 0.9 Preparedness staff | 1 Preparedness staff | 3 Preparedness staff |
| | 1 Nutritionist | 2 Nutritionists | 6 Nutritionists |
| | 1 Business operations staff | 1.5 Business operations staff | 5.8 Business operations staff |
| | | | 4 Community health workers |
| | | | 2.9 Epidemiologist/statisticians |
| | | | 1 Information systems specialist |
| | | | 1 Public health physician |
| | | | 1 Public information professional |

**Figure 26-10** • Staff Mix in Local Health Departments. LHD, Local Health Department. (Source: National Association of County and City Health Officials.)

epidemiologists, and a public health physician. The composition of LHD employees is depicted in Figure 26-11. LHDs have an average of 50 FTEs. Eighty percent of LHDs employ fewer than 50 FTEs: 37% employ fewer than 10 FTEs, and 42% employ between 10 and 50 FTEs. Ten percent of LHDs employ 100 or more FTEs.

All of the public health inputs described earlier—government levels in the public health system, partnerships with other local organizations, professional workforce, and invested resources—serve to promote the "operational capacity" (or infrastructure) of public health. These inputs and investments exert impacts on community programs and local public health activities. Such impacts are designed to promote better health outcomes, reductions in health disparities, and improved preparedness for emergencies. This "theory of action" of public health is presented in Figure 26-12.

## SOURCES OF TENSION FACING PUBLIC HEALTH

Public health is also faced with 2 sources of tension: politics and organized medicine. There is a tension between public health professionals and

politics. Public health professionals are experts in such fields as epidemiology and biostatistics and draw on such skills to identify and deal with the population's health needs. Their focus is on accurate data and professional judgment to make decisions in the public's welfare. But these decisions are usually made (and publicly made) in periods of crisis on topical issues. By contrast, political decisions are made in the face of competing interest groups, bargaining, and influence rather than statistically derived analysis. Such tension was evident during the summer of 2020 in the relationship between Dr. Anthony Fauci, Director of the CDC, and President Trump's administration. This has likely weakened the voice of public health officials in political decisions. The situation is not helped by the rapid turnover among public health officials, the trend to have top public health officials be political appointees rather than career professionals, and the demise of many state boards of health.

There is also a tension with organized medicine. This tension began with the ascendance of public health in the wake of the bacteriological revolution. Vaccinations are the purview of physicians, not public health agencies, and brought the two into competition. Beyond competition, there is also some public health

**Workforce Composition**

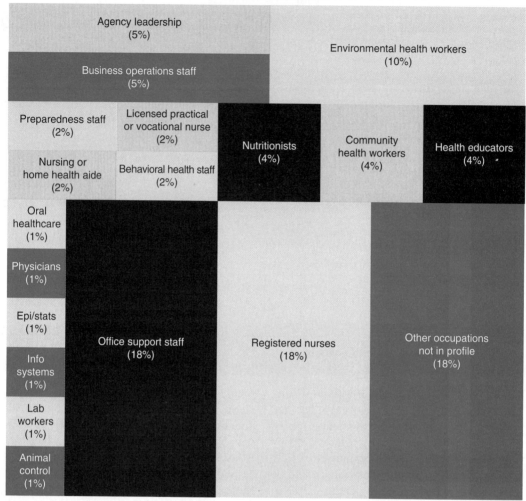

**Figure 26-11** • Workforce Composition of Local Health Departments. (Source: National Association of County and City Health Officials.)

**Framework for Improving the Performance of Public Health**

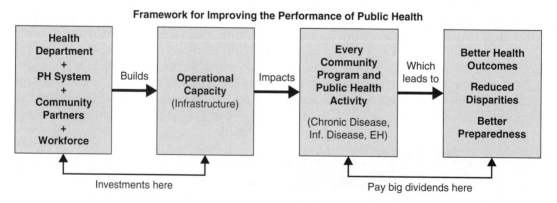

**Figure 26-12** • Theory of Action of Public Health (PH). EH, Environmental Health; Inf., Infectious. (Source: D. Lenaway, Centers for Disease Control and Prevention, Office of Chief of Public Health Practice, 2019.)

distrust of physicians and/or lack of physician understanding of public health's role. This is despite the fact that the 2 parties play complementary roles.

## SUMMARY

There is nothing like a global pandemic to increase the importance of public health. In response to the COVID-19 crisis, the Trump administration held daily press briefings on the handling of the crisis, encouraged the private sector to manufacture ventilators for COVID-19 victims, and increased government stockpiling of PPEs to retard the virus's spread. State governors exerted their public health responsibilities by shutting down commercial activity in their states and mandating the use of PPEs in public.

Public Health, like Rodney Dangerfield later in his career, has finally gotten (at least some) respect. Moreover, it has carried the rest of the healthcare system on its back. The US population made visible demonstrations (banners, signs) of its appreciation for healthcare workers (eg, physicians, nurses, emergency personnel) who treated the many COVID-19 victims. No one said during this time of crisis that "the US healthcare system is broken."

### QUESTIONS TO PONDER

1. Despite its clear importance, public health does not get much respect, let alone much funding. Why is this?
2. In the same vein, the Institute of Medicine (now part of the National Academies) has issued multiple reports on public health over a 25-year period. And, yet, we have seen very little progress in public health. Why is this?
3. Why don't state and local governments invest more funding and resources in the public health functions they are responsible for?
4. What might be done to elevate the stature and recognition of public health in the United States?

## REFERENCES

1. Institute of Medicine. *The Future of Public Health* (Washington, DC: National Academies Press, 1988).
2. Centers for Disease Control and Prevention. *Mortality in the United States, 2018* (Washington, DC: CDC, 2020). NCHS Data Brief No. 355.
3. J. Michael McGinnis and William Foege. "Actual Causes of Death in the United States," *JAMA.* 270 (18) (1993): 2207-2212. J. Michael McGinnis, Pamela Williams-Russo, and James Knickman. "The Case for More Active Policy Attention to Health Promotion," *Health Aff.* 21 (2) (2002): 78-93.
4. Institute of Medicine. *The Future of Public Health* (Washington, DC: National Academies Press, 1988). Institute of Medicine. *The Future of the Public's Health in the 21st Century* (Washington, DC: National Academies Press, 2003). Institute of Medicine. *U.S. Health in International Perspective* (Washington, DC: National Academies Press, 2013).
5. This section draws heavily on the following: Centers for Disease Control and Prevention. *Mortality in the United States, 2018* (Washington, DC: CDC, 2020). NCHS Data Brief No. 355.
6. US Public Health Service. *Smoking and Health: Report of the Advisory Committee to the Surgeon General of the Public Health Service* (Washington, DC: US Department of Health, Education, and Welfare, 1964).
7. Hongying Dai and Adam Levinthal. "Prevalence of e-Cigarette Use Among Adults in the United States, 2014-2018," *JAMA* (September 16, 2019). Available online: https://jamanetwork.com/journals/jama/fullarticle/2751687. Accessed on March 10, 2020.
8. Georgia Wood, Marika Waselewski, Arrice Bryant, et al. "Youth Perceptions of Juul in the United States," *JAMA Pediatr.* 174 (8) (2020): 800-802.
9. Abigail Friedman. "Smoking to Cope: Addictive Behavior as a Response to Mental Distress," *J Health Econ.* 72 (July 2020): article 102323.
10. Shelby Livingston. "Behavioral Health Patients Spur 57% of Commercial Healthcare Spending," *Modern Healthcare* (August 13, 2020). Stoddard Davenport, Travis Gray, and Stephen Melek. *How Do Individuals With Behavioral Health Conditions Contribute to Physical and Total Healthcare Spending?* Milliman Research Report (August 13, 2020).
11. Based on a 7-year investigation, the FBI concluded that the attacker came from the US Army Medical Research Institute of Infectious Diseases.

12. *High-priority agents* include organisms that pose a risk to national security because they (1) can be easily disseminated or transmitted from person to person; (2) result in high mortality rates and have the potential for major public health impact; (3) might cause public panic and social disruption; and (4) require special action for public health preparedness. These agents include anthrax, botulism, plague, smallpox, tularemia, and vital hemorrhagic fevers. The *second highest priority agents* include those that (1) are moderately easy to disseminate; (2) result in moderate morbidity rates and low mortality rates; and (3) require specific enhancements of CDC's diagnostic capacity and enhanced disease surveillance. These agents include ricin toxin, typhus fever, *Salmonella*, encephalitis, and water safety threats, among others. The *third highest priority agents* include emerging pathogens that could be engineered for mass dissemination in the future because of (1) availability; (2) ease of production and dissemination; and (3) potential for high morbidity and mortality rates and major health impact. These include emerging infectious diseases such as Nipah virus and hantavirus.

13. J. David Goodman. "How Delays and Unheeded Warnings Hindered New York's Virus Fight," *The New York Times* (April 8, 2020). Ed Yong. "How the Pandemic Defeated America," *The Atlantic* (September 2020). David Quammen. "Why Weren't We Ready for the Coronavirus?" *The New Yorker* (May 4, 2020).

14. Anthony Fauci, Clifford Lane, and Robert Redfield. "Covid-19—Navigating the Uncharted," *N Engl J Med.* 382 (13) (2020): 1268-1269. Ed Yong. "Why the Coronavirus Is So Confusing," *The Atlantic* (April 29, 2020). Joanne Kenen and Rachel Roubein. "Why America Is Scared and Confused: Even the Experts Are Getting It Wrong," *Politico* (March 31, 2020).

15. Information presented here on the 1918 pandemic is taken from the Centers for Disease Control and Prevention (CDC). See the following: https://www.cdc.gov/flu/pandemic-resources/1918-pandemic-h1n1.html. Accessed on August 18, 2020.

16. Jonathan Leider, Beth Resnick, David Bishai, et al. "How Much Do We Spend? Creating Historical Estimates of Public Health Expenditures in the United States at the Federal, State, and Local Levels," *Ann Rev Public Health.* 39 (2018): 471-487.

17. David Cutler, Angus Deaton, and Adriana Lleras-Muney. "The Determinants of Mortality," *J Econ Perspect.* 20 (3) (2006): 97-120. David Cutler and Grant Miller. "The Role of Public Health Improvements in Health Advances: The 20th Century United States," NBER Working Paper 10511 (Cambridge, MA: National Bureau of Economic Research, May 2004).

18. David Cutler and Grant Miller. "The Role of Public Health Improvements in Health Advances: The 20th Century United States" (February 2004). Available online: https://scholar.harvard.edu/cutler/files/cutler_miller_cities.pdf. Accessed on August 18, 2020.

19. John Duffy. *The Sanitarians: History of American Public Health* (Champaign-Urbana, IL: University of Illinois Press, 1990).

20. Institute of Medicine. *The Future of Public Health* (Washington, DC: The National Academies Press, 1988). See also CDC website: https://www.cdc.gov/publichealthgateway/publichealthservices/essentialhealthservices.html. Accessed on August 18, 2020.

21. Dan Balz. "Crisis Exposes How America Has Hollowed Out Its Government," *The Washington Post* (May 16, 2020).

22. Eric Lipton, Abby Goodnough, Michael Shear, et al. "The C.D.C. Waited 'Its Entire Existence for This Moment.' What Went Wrong?" *The New York Times* (Updated August 14, 2020).

23. Lauren Weber, Laura Ungar, and Michelle Smith. "Hollowed-Out Public Health System Faces More Cuts Amid Virus," *Kaiser Health News* (July 1, 2020).

24. Chelsea Janes. "The Nation's Public Health Agencies are Ailing When They're Needed Most," *The Washington Post* (August 31, 2020).

25. National Association of County and City Health Officials. *2016 Profile of Local Health Departments* (Washington, DC: NACCHO, 2017).

26. Centers for Disease Control and Prevention and the Health Resources and Services Administration. "Discretionary Public Health Spending." Available online: https://www.apha.org/-/media/files/pdf/aphatraining/200124_cdc_hrsa.ashx. Accessed on September 1, 2020.

27. Angela Beck, Matthew Boulton, and Fatima Coronado. "Enumeration of the Governmental Public Health Workforce, 2014," *Am J Prev Med.* 47 (2014): S306-S313.

# Index

Note: Page numbers followed by b indicate boxed material; those followed by f indicate figures; those followed by t indicate tables.